Clinical Reproductive Neuroendocrinology

Clinical Reproductive Neuroendocrinology

Editor: Christine Abbey

AMERICAN
MEDICAL PUBLISHERS
www.americanmedicalpublishers.com

AMERICAN
MEDICAL PUBLISHERS
www.americanmedicalpublishers.com

Cataloging-in-Publication Data

Clinical reproductive neuroendocrinology / edited by Christine Abbey.
p. cm.
Includes bibliographical references and index.
ISBN 979-8-88740-010-5
1. Human reproduction--Endocrine aspects. 2. Neuroendocrinology. 3. Obstetrical endocrinology.
4. Endocrine glands--Diseases--Treatment. I. Abbey, Christine.
RC648 .C55 2023
6164--dc23

American Medical Publishers,
41 Flatbush Avenue,
1st Floor, New York,
NY 11217, USA

ISBN 979-8-88740-010-5 (Hardback)

Contents

Preface

Every book is initially just a concept; it takes months of research and hard work to give it the final shape in which the readers receive it. In its early stages, this book also went through rigorous reviewing. The notable contributions made by experts from across the globe were first molded into patterned chapters and then arranged in a sensibly sequential manner to bring out the best results.

Neuroendocrinology is a branch of biology that studies the interaction between the nervous system and the endocrine system, such as the regulation of hormonal activity in the body by the brain. Progesterone and estrogen are the reproductive hormones in women while testosterone is present in men. These hormones are produced by primary reproductive glands, which include testes in men and ovaries in women. They are regulated through hormone signals generated by the follicle stimulating hormone, luteinizing hormone and pituitary gland. The neuroendocrine system regulates reproduction, metabolism, eating and drinking behavior, energy utilization, osmolarity and blood pressure. The neuroendocrine system regulates all aspects of reproduction, from bonding to sexual behavior. Spermatogenesis, the ovarian cycle, parturition, lactation, and maternal behavior are all controlled by this system. It also controls the body's reaction to stress and infection. This book explores all the important aspects of clinical reproductive neuroendocrinology in the present day scenario. It is a vital tool for all researching and studying this field. The book will serve as a valuable source of reference for graduate and post graduate students.

It has been my immense pleasure to be a part of this project and to contribute my years of learning in such a meaningful form. I would like to take this opportunity to thank all the people who have been associated with the completion of this book at any step.

Editor

1

Androgen modulation of social decision-making mechanisms in the brain: an integrative and embodied perspective

Gonçalo A. Oliveira[1] and Rui F. Oliveira[1,2,3]*

[1] Unidade de Investigação em Eco-Etologia, ISPA – Instituto Universitário, Lisboa, Portugal
[2] Integrative Behavioural Biology Lab, Instituto Gulbenkian de Ciência, Oeiras, Portugal
[3] Champalimaud Neuroscience Program, Champalimaud Center for the Unknown, Lisboa, Portugal

***Correspondence:**
Rui F. Oliveira, ISPA – Instituto Universitário, R. Jardim do Tabaco 34, 1149-041 Lisboa, Portugal
e-mail: ruiol@ispa.pt

Apart from their role in reproduction androgens also respond to social challenges and this response has been seen as a way to regulate the expression of behavior according to the perceived social environment (Challenge hypothesis, Wingfield et al., 1990). This hypothesis implies that social decision-making mechanisms localized in the central nervous system (CNS) are open to the influence of peripheral hormones that ultimately are under the control of the CNS through the hypothalamic-pituitary-gonadal axis. Therefore, two puzzling questions emerge at two different levels of biological analysis: (1) Why does the brain, which perceives the social environment and regulates androgen production in the gonad, need feedback information from the gonad to adjust its social decision-making processes? (2) How does the brain regulate gonadal androgen responses to social challenges and how do these feedback into the brain? In this paper, we will address these two questions using the integrative approach proposed by Niko Tinbergen, who proposed that a full understanding of behavior requires its analysis at both proximate (physiology, ontogeny) and ultimate (ecology, evolution) levels.

Keywords: androgens, testosterone, ultimate causes, proximate causes, embodiment, challenge hypothesis

INTRODUCTION

In his classical paper "On aims and methods of Ethology," Niko Tinbergen (1963) identified proximate causation, survival value, ontogeny and evolution as the four major questions in the study of behavior. Although these four questions can be interpreted as culminating into the proximate-ultimate dichotomy of biological causation proposed by Mayr (1961), Tinbergen's formulation clearly distinguishes cause from function and calls not the separateness of his questions, but rather for their integration when investigating a particular phenotype. Only such an integrative approach would allow a truly comprehensive understanding of the behavior in question. Indeed, on one hand knowledge of the proximate mechanisms underlying a given behavior is crucial to understanding its costs, limits and evolutionary consequences, therefore highlighting the fact that proximate mechanisms contribute to the dynamics of selection. On the other hand, knowledge on the ecological function and evolution of a given behavior will clarify how the proximate mechanisms underlying it evolved. Thus, reciprocal causation analysis of biological phenomena (i.e., considering the interaction between immediate factors and evolutionary explanations) can be a more useful approach than the traditional proximate-ultimate dichotomy (e.g., Laland et al., 2013).

Following Tinbergen's footsteps, here we aim to integrate the study of function with the study of proximate mechanisms of the social modulation of androgens. For this purpose we will start by reviewing the current hypothesis for the social modulation of androgen levels, we will then address its proximate and ultimate mechanisms, and we will finish by integrating both levels of analysis in addressing the ultimate question of why are social decision-making mechanisms in the brain open to modulation by peripheral hormones. The term function will be used here in reference to the current utility of a character, as it makes no assumptions about the processes from which function emerged and emphasizes that current and original function may not match (Bateson and Laland, 2013).

RECIPROCAL MODELS OF ANDROGEN-SOCIAL BEHAVIOR INTERACTIONS

Over the last decades, accumulated evidence has revealed a reciprocal relationship between androgen levels and the social environment. As a result, androgens are no longer seen exclusively as sex steroids involved in reproduction. Early models for the interaction between hormones and behavior (Leshner, 1975, 1979; Mazur, 1976), already presented the core ideas that would be further developed in subsequent formal explanations, namely that androgen levels influence the behavioral response to social stimuli and that changes in androgens can be elicited by the social environment, thus creating a reciprocal interaction between androgens and behavior [i.e., biosocial model, (Mazur, 1985); challenge hypothesis, (Wingfield et al., 1990)].

The reciprocal model of androgens and social behavior has been formalized in two different hypotheses, each presenting different theoretical constraints and generating its own predictions. The biosocial model, initially proposed by Mazur (Mazur, 1985; Mazur and Booth, 1998), establishes a dynamic and mutual reinforcing relationship between androgens and social dominance. According to this model, androgens promote status seeking behaviors, and the achievement of higher status through dominance contests feeds back on the individuals' androgen levels, according to the individual's new position in the social hierarchy. Therefore, the biosocial model predicts that dominant individuals should have higher baseline levels of androgens than subordinates and while it is expected that winning an agonistic interaction results in increased androgen levels, establishing a positive feedback loop between status and androgens, losing such an interaction should result in decreased androgens and an inhibition of the individuals' engagement in further dominance contests (Mazur and Booth, 1998).

While the biosocial model focused essentially on androgens and social dominance, Wingfield and co-workers proposed the "challenge hypothesis" with the goal of providing an explanation for the interspecific seasonal variation of androgen levels, linking fluctuations in androgen levels with its functions in reproductive and aggressive contexts (Wingfield et al., 1990). The "challenge hypothesis" (**Figure 1**) predicts that androgen levels increase from a non-breeding constitutive baseline (level A) to breeding season levels (level B) to allow for the expression of secondary sex characters and reproductive behaviors; short term further increases in androgen levels up to a maximum physiological level (level C) may occur in response to agonistic encounters (e.g., territorial intrusions). Recent revisions of the "challenge hypothesis" have shown that B to C increases do not reflect the effect of social challenges and in fact, across species, no correlation was found between seasonal androgen responsiveness and the androgen response to an experimental territorial challenge (Goymann et al., 2007). These two time scales of the androgen response to the social environment are expected to rely on different mechanisms (e.g., non-genomic and genomic steroid action: Baker, 2003; Balthazart et al., 2006), and thus should be seen as separate phenomena. For example, while the dynamic reciprocal changes of the biosocial model and of the acute response to a territorial intrusion in the "challenge hypothesis," are acute and short-lived and therefore are expected to rely on either non-genomic or on transient changes in gene expression, seasonal changes in androgen responses are gradual and long-lasting, and therefore are expected to rely on genomic and epigenetic mechanisms.

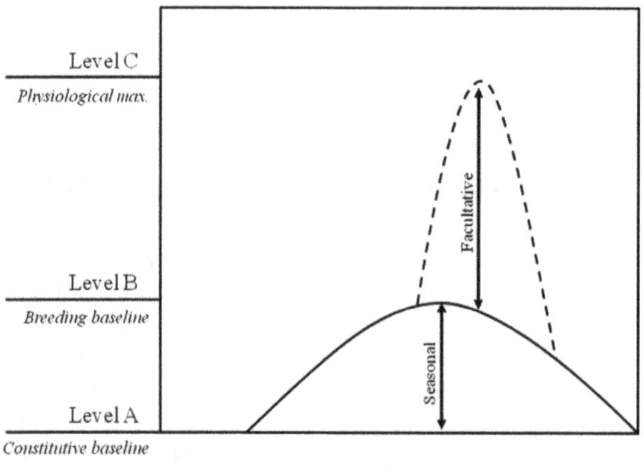

FIGURE 1 | Representation of the androgen changes proposed by the challenge hypothesis: (A) constitutive androgen levels; (B) breeding baseline levels needed for successful reproduction; and (C) maximum physiological levels.

MECHANISMS OF ANDROGEN RESPONSE TO SOCIAL CHALLENGES

Most androgen production results from the activation of the hypothalamic-pituitary-gonadal (HPG) axis in which a sequential pulsatile hormonal cascade targets the Leydig cells in male gonads, to elicit testosterone (T) production and its release into circulation (Gleason et al., 2009). Androgens can also be produced in the brain *de novo* from cholesterol and can be converted into other hormones (Schmidt et al., 2008) and both processes can be modulated by social context (e.g., Pradhan et al., 2010; Cornil et al., 2012). In fact, studies in several taxa (fish, birds, mammals) suggest that the effects of androgens on agonistic behavior is mediated by their rapid aromatization into estrogens in the brain (Soma et al., 2003; Trainor et al., 2006; Charlier et al., 2011; Huffman et al., 2013). Additionally, tissue sensitivity to androgens can also be socially modulated through rapid changes in androgen receptor expression (Burmeister et al., 2007; Fuxjager et al., 2010).

The adjustment of androgen levels according to the social environment requires mechanisms that can translate and integrate multi-modal social information relevant to the organism and modulate neuroendocrine activity responsible for the production of androgens. Cichlid fish have been a very successfully model in this respect. Experiments with cichlid fish have shown how changes in social status can induce rapid changes in HPG axis activity leading to changes in circulating androgens (for comprehensive reviews see Oliveira, 2009; Maruska and Fernald, 2013). When opportunities to ascend in social status arise subordinates can rapidly exhibit the traits of dominant fish (e.g., coloration and aggressive behavior), and sequentially increase the expression of GnRH1 in the preoptic area, pituitary gonadotropins and androgen levels (Maruska et al., 2013). Conversely, dominant males experiencing a decrease in social status present a reduced expression of GnRH1 and pituitary gonadotropins, and a decrease of androgen levels (Maruska et al., 2013). Furthermore, the social information signaling social opportunity seems to be conveyed by changes in the expression of the immediate early gene *egr-1* in high density GnRH1 neuron areas of the anterior preoptic area, indicating that *egr-1* is interfacing social information with the activity of the HPG (Burmeister et al., 2005). Interestingly, experiments where the use of mirror elicited fights allowed for decoupling the effects of expressing aggressive behavior from those of assessing the fight outcome indicate that the androgen response to social status depends on the fish appraisal of the interaction outcome (Oliveira et al., 2005; see also Oliveira and Canário, 2011 for a debate on contradictory results on this topic). Evidence also exists in support of appraisal as a modulator of the androgen response to social contests in birds (e.g., Japanese quail; Hirschenhauser et al., 2008) and in humans (for a recent review see Oliveira and Oliveira, 2014). For example, T changes in female competitors that lost a face to face contest are moderated by the subjective evaluation of the outcome as a threat and the perception of opponent familiarity, with the highest increases of T appearing in situations of perceived high threat with unfamiliar opponents (Oliveira et al., 2013).

THE FUNCTION OF ANDROGEN RESPONSE TO SOCIAL CHALLENGES

The fact that androgen levels change in response to the perceived outcome of an interaction, and not merely by experiencing an agonistic interaction raises the hypothesis that socially driven changes in androgen levels will not directly affect the current interaction, for which the outcome has already been established, but should rather modulate behavioral expression in subsequent social interactions (Oliveira, 2009). Interestingly, Leshner's (1975) proposal for the reciprocal model had already hinted that the hormone response should modify future behavior when the individuals are facing a similar challenge, and both the biosocial model and the challenge hypothesis have also implicitly assumed that the adaptive function of the social modulation of androgen levels is to fine tune the expression of androgen-dependent behavior according to the perceived social environment.

More recently, this view has been formalized as the Winning hypothesis (Oyegbile and Marler, 2005) according to which changes in the probability of winning future interactions driven by the success in previous ones (i.e., winner/loser effect, Hsu et al., 2006), could be mediated by post-contest transient changes in androgen levels. This hypothesis is currently supported by several lines of evidence. In cichlid fish winner effects can be blocked (i.e., reduction of the winning probability of previous winners from ca. 90% back to chance levels) by the exogeneous administration of the anti-androgen cyproterone acetate to the winners of the first interaction between the agonistic encounters (Oliveira et al., 2009). In California mice (*Peromyscus californicus*), in the emergence of the winner effect during successive social interactions is paralleled by increased levels of androgens after cumulative winning experience (Oyegbile and Marler, 2005). Furthermore, unlike the California mice, the white-footed mouse (*Peromyscus leucopus*) does not form a winner effect or respond to a contest with increased T, but a robust winner effect can be induced in this species via a post-contest administration of T (Fuxjager et al., 2011). As it has been previously suggested, it is possible that these effects could result from the aromatization of T in the brain (e.g., Trainor et al., 2006). In humans, although to the best of our knowledge no formal tests have been conducted, it is known that increased androgen levels after a competition predict the willingness to engage in further contests, even after losing the first interaction (Mehta and Josephs, 2006; Carré and McCormick, 2008).

One assumption of the Winning hypothesis is that socially driven changes in androgen levels modulate the expression of variables relevant for success in subsequent social contests. Given the time frame of this response these variables are expected to be of the cognitive (i.e., information-processing) domain. Most of the evidence for the effects of androgens on cognitive variables comes from research using paradigms that involve the administration of exogenous T to animals and humans (for a review see Bos et al., 2012), which have been shown to reduce vigilance (Van Honk et al., 2005), startle reflex (Hermans et al., 2006) and threat detection in human females (Van Honk and Schutter, 2007), and to reduce fear in other animals (Frye and Seliga, 2001; Aikey et al., 2002). Furthermore, in women T also reduces trust (Bos et al., 2010), increases risk-taking accompanied by increased sensitivity to rewards and reduced sensitivity to punishment (Van Honk et al., 2004), and also facilitates resource acquisition and high status via cooperation (Eisenegger et al., 2010). Thus, the available data indeed suggests that increased levels of T induce competitive cognitive traits that are beneficial in competitive settings. However, these results should be interpreted with caution since most manipulations used dosages way above the androgens levels observed in response to social challenges. Another issue to consider is that in some species of birds the levels of high aggression toward the intruder are accompanied by lowering T levels (Goymann, 2009). The ecological and adaptive function of this decrement of androgens is still unknown and currently stands outside the predictions of the challenge hypothesis and the biosocial model.

MODULATION OF SOCIAL DECISION-MAKING MECHANISMS IN THE BRAIN BY PERIPHERAL HORMONES

If one considers that the social environment is sensed by the brain and that the androgen response to it is a top-down process conveyed by the HPG axis, then, under classical models of cognition, the involvement of peripheral androgens in the modulation of a central decision-making process seems redundant, since the decision-making mechanism already has the relevant information on the social environment and could provide a faster and more economic response *per se*. However, if one shifts perspective toward embodiment as an essential component of cognition, then neuroendocrine axes can be seen as an example of brain-body-environmental coupling, in which upstream and downstream information relevant for the expression of appropriate social behavior are integrated, and therefore can function as a pathway for coordinated convergent adaptive responses to social change (e.g., Oliveira, 2009; Adkins-Regan, 2012). This view follows a soft definition of embodiment, since it still assumes the brain as a central processor that is merely permeable to bodily as well as environmental raw inputs. A more stringent definition of embodiment goes further, by proposing a distributed cognitive system that goes beyond the brain to include the body (therefore spreading the computational load) in an interacting goal-oriented, problem-solving system, that can be exploited by the agent replacing the need for complex internal mental representations (Beer, 2009; Wilson and Golonka, 2013).

But just as the brain is embedded in a body, the body is embedded in an environment. This implies a connection between the behavioral agent and the physical or social environment (situatedness) and therefore the characteristics of the environment and the properties arising from this interaction can also be used by the agent to solve adaptive problems (Beer, 2009; Nolfi, 2011). What arises from this situated-embodied-dynamic framework (**Figure 2**) is a multi-level complex system in which adaptive

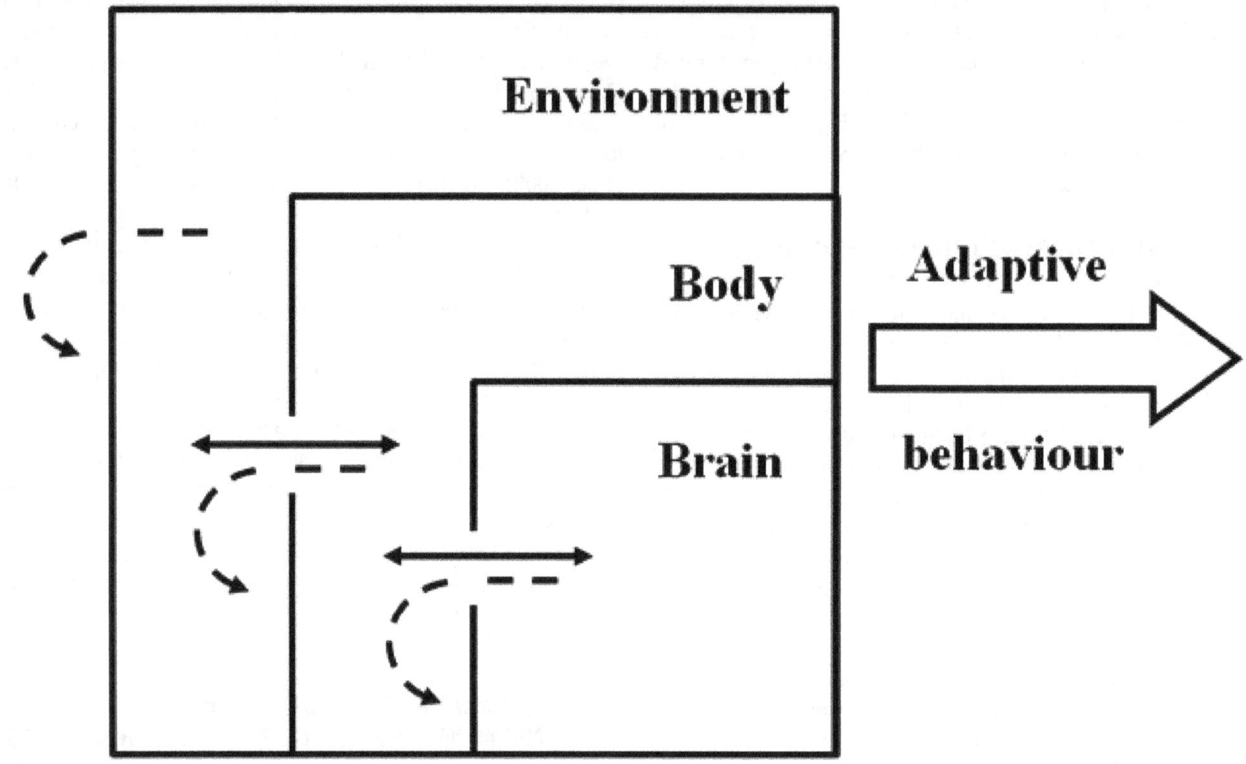

FIGURE 2 | Schematic representation of the situated-dynamic-embodied framework with adaptive behavior resulting from the emergent characteristics of brain-body-environment coupling and not from singular contribution of the components. Full arrows represent dynamic processes between the components. Dashed arrows represent the dynamic processes within the components.

behavior and cognition cannot be inferred from any of the elements in isolation as it emerges from the non-linear, dynamical interactions between and within these three foundational elements (Chiel and Beer, 1997; Nolfi, 2011; Williams and Beer, 2013). Examples of this multi-level coupling can be seen in animals, in which adequate locomotion depends not on simple neural commands, but on a multimodal integration of information that must include body and environment feedback (for a review see Dickinson et al., 2000). Also supporting this idea, the body and the morphological characteristics of artificial agents do not simply feed the control center (e.g., brain) with sensory inputs; instead they allow the agent to create or elicit appropriate inputs by actively self-structuring flows of multimodal and temporally specific environmental information into sensorimotor networks, linking information structure from motor activity and information processing in the brain (Lungarella and Sporns, 2005, 2006).

Therefore in embodied agents, a neuromodulatory system, such as the androgen reciprocal model discussed here, must be able to continually guide plasticity, while stabilizing and maintaining previously acquired adaptive structures, and to adapt the agent to variation in behavior, physiology, and external stimuli (Alexander and Sporns, 2002). This definition is compatible with the current hypothesis for the role of androgens on social decision-making mechanisms that has lost the assumptions of causality to focus more on a systems perspective. Empirical evidence for this process can be found in the examples described above (section IV) referring to the effects of T administration, which within a situated-embodied-dynamical framework, can be seen as an experimental manipulation of the information carried by the peripheral signaling of T that is being translated into systemic changes in the brain-body-environment coupling.

Although the neuromodulatory effects of peripheral androgens are well documented, a challenging puzzle arises when one has to account for the dynamics of evolution and the function that peripheral androgens have in this process. If adaptive behavior emerges from brain-body-environment continuous and dynamical interaction, evolution should not select individual components but variations of systemic couplings responsible for the emergent characteristics that originated behavioral efficacy (Beer, 2009). Androgens may play a role in this process by stabilizing the system via pleiotropic effects on neural-dynamics and on relevant body components that could be rapidly enhanced by transient increases in androgens (Oliveira, 2009). Evidence for non-genomic effects on bodily components can be found in the literature (e.g., review by Rahman and Christian, 2007). For example, acute increases of T enhanced 2-deoxyglucose uptake in cultured myotubules within 1 min (Tsai and Sapolsky, 1996) and increased the intracellular concentration of calcium suggesting the existence of a G protein-linked membrane receptor in skeletal muscle cells (Estrada et al., 2003). Also, rapid effects of T on vasorelaxation at micromolar concentrations has been reported in several species (Jones et al., 2004).

In conclusion, the evidence presented here substantiates the need to integrate the proximate mechanisms of behavior with their ecological and evolutionary function as it was proposed by Tinbergen (1963). The apparent paradox of social challenges eliciting increases in peripheral androgen levels at a greater cost (e.g., Wingfield et al., 2001) when brain androgen synthesis is available to the organism, may be better understood by integrating its' action both on neural circuits and on bodily parameters relevant to behavioral performance, influencing the emergent characteristics of the brain-body-environment coupling itself and thus reducing the fitness variability of the expressed phenotypes. Although further research is required to support these claims, previous work by Johnson and Whalen (1988) proposed that in male mice the signaling of gonadal hormones on brain areas is required to regulate and reduce the inter-individual differences in aggressive behavior observed in gonadectomized animals, that are not present in gonadally-intact or castrated mice treated with T. In our view, these experiments can be seen as an example of how the characteristics of the systemic coupling can be skewed into more variable behavioral outputs when body signaling is disrupted, and restored to a finer context dependent response by restituting the signal to congruent levels. This suggests that body signaling is necessary for effective couplings that generate more adaptive patterns of response and this goal could be achieved by narrowing the degrees of freedom for possible fitness outcomes that could be obtained from the multiple combinations of the components involved in the dynamical system. Although most of the research presented here focused on males, this conceptual framework is expectable to also apply to females, at least for humans where recent studies suggest the similar patterns of androgen responsiveness to social competition in both sexes (Jiménez et al., 2012). However, given the possible sex differences in androgen modulation and signaling integration in central systems across different taxa, further research is needed to fully establish this approach in both sexes.

ACKNOWLEDGMENTS

The writing of this paper was supported by a research grant (EXCL/BIA-ANM/0549/2012) from Fundação para a Ciência e a Tecnologia (FCT, Portugal). Rui F. Oliveira is a member of the FCT Eco-Ethology R&D Unit (PEst-OE/MAR/UI0331/2011). Gonçalo A. Oliveira is supported by a PhD fellowship from FCT (SFRH/BD/68528/2010).

REFERENCES

Adkins-Regan, E. (2012). Hormonal organization and activation: evolutionary implications and questions. *Gen. Comp. Endocrinol.* 176, 279–85. doi: 10.1016/j.ygcen.2011.12.040

Aikey J. L., John Nyby, G., David Anmuth, M., and James, P. J. (2002). Testosterone rapidly reduces anxiety in male house mice (Mus musculus). *Horm. Behav.* 42, 448–460. doi: 10.1006/hbeh.2002.1838

Alexander, W. H., and Sporns, O. (2002). An embodied model of learning, plasticity, and reward. *Adapt. Behav.* 10, 143–159. doi: 10.1177/1059712302010003001

Baker, M. E. (2003). Evolution of adrenal and sex steroid action in vertebrates: a ligand-based mechanism for complexity. *Bioessays* 25, 396–400. doi: 10.1002/bies.10252

Balthazart, J., Baillien, M., and Ball, G. F. (2006). Rapid control of brain aromatase activity by glutamatergic inputs. *Endocrinology* 147, 359–366. doi: 10.1210/en.2005-0845

Bateson, P., and Laland, K. N. (2013). Tinbergen's four questions: an appreciation and an update. *Trends Ecol. Evol.* 28, 712–718. doi: 10.1016/j.tree.2013.09.013

Beer, R. D. (2009). Beyond control: the dynamics of brain-body-environment interaction in motor systems. *Adv. Exp. Med. Biol.* 629, 7–24. doi: 10.1007/978-0-387-77064-2_2

Bos, P. A., Panksepp, J., Bluthé, R. M., and Van Honk, J. (2012). Acute effects of steroid hormones and neuropeptides on human social-emotional behavior: a review of single administration studies. *Front. Neuroendocrinol.* 33:17–35. doi: 10.1016/j.yfrne.2011.01.002

Bos, P. A., Terburg, D., and van Honk, J. (2010). Testosterone decreases trust in socially naive humans. *Proc. Natl. Acad. Sci. U.S.A.* 107, 9991–9995. doi: 10.1073/pnas.0911700107

Burmeister, S. S., Jarvis, E. D., and Fernald, R. D. (2005). Rapid behavioral and genomic responses to social opportunity. *PLoS Biol.* 3:e363. doi: 10.1371/journal.pbio.0030363

Burmeister, S. S., Kailasanath, V., and Fernald, R. D. (2007). Social dominance regulates androgen and estrogen receptor gene expression. *Horm. Behav.* 51, 164–170. doi: 10.1016/j.yhbeh.2006.09.008

Carré, J. M., and McCormick, C. M. (2008). Aggressive behavior and change in salivary testosterone concentrations predict willingness to engage in a competitive task. *Horm. Behav.* 54, 403–409. doi: 10.1016/j.yhbeh.2008.04.008

Charlier, T. D., Newman, A. E., Heimovics, S. A., Po, K. W., Saldanha, C. J., and Soma, K. K. (2011). Rapid effects of aggressive interactions on aromatase activity and oestradiol in discrete brain regions of wild male white-crowned sparrows. *J. Neuroendocrinol.* 23, 742–753. doi: 10.1111/j.1365-2826.2011.02170.x

Chiel, H. J., and Beer, R. D. (1997). The brain has a body: adaptive behavior emerges from interactions of nervous system, body and environment. *Trends Neurosci.*20, 553–557.

Cornil, C. A., Ball, G. F., and Balthazart, J. (2012). Rapid control of male typical behaviors by brain-derived estrogens. *Front. Neuroendocrinol.* 33, 425–446. doi: 10.1016/j.yfrne.2012.08.003

Dickinson, M. H., Farley, C. T., Full, R. J., and Koehl, M. A. R. (2000). How animals move: an integrative view. *Science* 288, 100–106. doi: 10.1126/science.288.5463.100

Eisenegger, C., Naef, M., Snozzi, M., Heinrichs, M., and Fehr, E. (2010). Prejudice and truth about the effect of testosterone on human bargaining behaviour. *Nature* 463, 356–359. doi: 10.1038/nature08711

Estrada, M., Espinosa, A., Müller, M., and Jaimovich, E. (2003). Testosterone stimulates intracellular calcium release and mitogen-activated protein kinases via a g protein-coupled receptor in skeletal muscle cells. *Endocrinology* 144, 3586–3597. doi: 10.1210/en.2002-0164

Frye, C. A., and Seliga, A. M. (2001). Testosterone increases analgesia, anxiolysis, and cognitive performance of male rats. *Cogn. Affect. Behav. Neurosci.*1, 371–381. doi: 10.3758/CABN.1.4.371

Fuxjager, M. J., Forbes-Lorman, R. M., Coss, D. J., Auger, C. J., Auger, A. P., and Marler, C. A. (2010). Winning territorial disputes selectively enhances androgen sensitivity in neural pathways related to motivation and social aggression. *Proc. Natl. Acad. Sci. U.S.A.* 107, 12393–12398. doi: 10.1073/pnas.1001394107

Fuxjager, M. J., Montgomery, J. L., and Marler, C. A. (2011). Species differences in the winner effect disappear in response to post-victory testosterone manipulations. *Proc. Biol. Sci.* 278, 3497–3503. doi: 10.1098/rspb.2011.0301

Gleason, E. D., Fuxjager, M. J., Oyegbile, T. O., and Marler, C. A. (2009). Testosterone release and social context: when it occurs and why. *Front. Neuroendocrinol.* 30:460–469. doi: 10.1016/j.yfrne.2009.04.009

Goymann, W. (2009). Social modulation of androgens in male birds. *Gen. Comp. Endocrinol.* 163, 149–157. doi: 10.1016/j.ygcen.2008.11.027

Goymann, W., Landys, M. M., and Wingfield, J. C. (2007). Distinguishing seasonal androgen responses from male-male androgen responsiveness-revisiting the challenge hypothesis. *Horm. Behav.* 51, 463–476. doi: 10.1016/j.yhbeh.2007.01.007

Hermans, E., Putman, P., Baas, J. M., Koppeschaar, H. P., and van Honk, J. (2006). A single administration of testosterone reduces fear-potentiated startle in humans. *Biol. Psychiatry* 59, 872–874. doi: 10.1016/j.biopsych.2005.11.015

Hirschenhauser, K., Wittek, M., Johnston, P., and Möstl, E. (2008). Social context rather than behavioral output or winning modulates post-conflict testosterone responses in japanese quail (*Coturnix japonica*). *Physiol. Behav.* 95, 457–463. doi: 10.1016/j.physbeh.2008.07.013

Hsu, Y., Earley, R. L., and Wolf, L. L. (2006). Modulation of aggressive behaviour by fighting experience: mechanisms and contest outcomes. *Biol. Rev. Camb. Philos. Soc.* 81, 33–74. doi: 10.1017/S146479310500686X

Huffman, L. S., O'Connell, L. A., and Hofmann, H. A. (2013). Aromatase regulates aggression in the african cichlid fish *Astatotilapia Burtoni*. *Physiol. Behav.* 112–113, 77–83. doi: 10.1016/j.physbeh.2013.02.004

Jiménez, M., Aguilar, R., and Alvero-Cruz, J. R. (2012). Effects of victory and defeat on testosterone and cortisol response to competition: evidence for same response patterns in men and women. *Psychoneuroendocrinology* 37, 1577–1581. doi: 10.1016/j.psyneuen.2012.02.011

Johnson, F., and Whalen, R. E. (1988). Testicular hormones reduce individual differences in the aggressive behavior of male mice: a theory of hormone action. *Neurosci. Biobehav. Rev.* 12, 93–99.

Jones, R. D., Hugh Jones, T., and Channer, K. S. (2004). The influence of testosterone upon vascular reactivity. *Eur. J. Endocrinol.* 151, 29–37. doi: 10.1530/eje.0.1510029

Laland, K. N., Odling-Smee, J., Hoppitt, W., and Uller, T. (2013). More on how and why: cause and effect in biology revisited. *Biol. Philos.* 28, 719–745. doi: 10.1007/s10539-012-9335-1

Leshner, A. I. (1975). A model of hormones and agonistic behavior. *Physiol. Behav.* 15, 225–235.

Leshner, A. I. (1979). Kinds of hormonal effects on behavior: a new view. *Neurosci. Biobehav. Rev.* 3, 69–73.

Lungarella, M., and Sporns, O. (2005). "Information self-structuring: key principle for learning and development," in *Proceedings of the 4th International Conference on Development and Learning, 2005* (Osaka: IEEE) 25–30. doi: 10.1109/DEVLRN.2005.1490938

Lungarella, M., and Sporns, O. (2006). Mapping information flow in sensorimotor networks. *PLoS Comput. Biol.* 2:e144. doi: 10.1371/journal.pcbi.0020144

Maruska, K. P., and Fernald, R. D. (2013). Social regulation of male reproductive plasticity in an african cichlid fish. *Integr. Comp. Biol.* 53, 938–50. doi: 10.1093/icb/ict017

Maruska, K. P., Zhang, A., Neboori, A., and Fernald, R. D. (2013). Social opportunity causes rapid transcriptional changes in the social behaviour network of the brain in an african cichlid fish. *J. Neuroendocrinol.* 25, 145–57. doi: 10.1111/j.1365-2826.2012.02382.x

Mayr, E. (1961). Cause and effect in biology. *Science* 134, 1501–1506.

Mazur, A. (1976). Effects of testosterone on status in primate groups. *Folia Primatol.* 26, 214–226. doi: 10.1159/000155752

Mazur, A. (1985). A biosocial model of status in face-to-face primate groups. *Soc. Forces* 64, 377–402. doi:10.2307/2578647

Mazur, A., and Booth, A. (1998). Testosterone and dominance in men. *Behav. Brain Sci.* 21, 353–363. discussion: 363–397.

Mehta, P. H., and Josephs, R. (2006). Testosterone change after losing predicts the decision to compete again. *Horm. Behav.* 50, 684–692. doi: 10.1016/j.yhbeh.2006.07.001

Nolfi, S. (2011). "Behavior and cognition as a complex adaptive system: insights from robotic experiments," in *Handbook of the Philosophy of Science: Philosophy of Complex Systems*, eds D. M. Gabbary, C. A. Hooker, P. Thagard, and J. Woods (Oxford: North Holland), 443–463. doi:10.1016/B978-0-444-52076-0.50016-X

Oliveira, G. A., and Oliveira, R. F. (2014). Androgen responsiveness to competition in humans: the role of cognitive variables. *Neurosci. Neuroecon.* 3, 19–32. doi: 10.2147/NAN.S55721

Oliveira, G. A., Uceda, S., Oliveira, T., Fernandes, A., Garcia-Marques, T., and Oliveira, R. F. (2013). Threat perception and familiarity moderate the androgen response to competition in women. *Front. Psychol.* 4:389. doi: 10.3389/fpsyg.2013.00389

Oliveira, R. F. (2009). Social behavior in context: hormonal modulation of behavioral plasticity and social competence. *Integr. Comp. Biol.* 49, 423–440. doi: 10.1093/icb/icp055

Oliveira, R. F., and Canário, A. V. M. (2011). Nemo through the looking-glass: a commentary on desjardins & fernald. *Biol. Lett.* 7, 487–488. doi: 10.1098/rsbl.2010.0760

Oliveira, R. F., Carneiro, L. A., and Canário, A. V. M. (2005). Behavioural endocrinology: no hormonal response in tied fights. *Nature* 437, 207–208. doi: 10.1038/437207a

Oliveira, R. F., Silva, A., and Canário, A. V. M. (2009). Why do winners keep winning? Androgen mediation of winner but not loser effects in cichlid fish. *Proc. Biol. Sci.* 276. 2249–2256. doi: 10.1098/rspb.2009.0132

Oyegbile, T. O., and Marler, C. A. (2005). Winning fights elevates testosterone levels in california mice and enhances future ability to win fights. *Horm. Behav.* 48, 259–267. doi: 10.1016/j.yhbeh.2005.04.007

Pradhan, D. S., Newman, A. E. M., Wacker, D. W., Wingfield, J. C., Schlinger, B. A., and Soma, K. K. (2010). Aggressive interactions rapidly increase androgen synthesis in the brain during the non-breeding season. *Horm. Behav.* 57, 381–389. doi: 10.1016/j.yhbeh.2010.01.008

Rahman, F., and Christian, H. C. (2007). Non-Classical actions of testosterone: an update. *Trends Endocrinol. Metab.* 18, 371–378. doi: 10.1016/j.tem.2007.09.004

Schmidt, K. L., Pradhan, D. S., Shah, A. H., Charlier, T. D., Chin, E. H., and Soma, K. K. (2008). Neurosteroids, immunosteroids, and the balkanization of endocrinology. *Gen. Comp. Endocrinol.* 157, 266–274. doi: 10.1016/j.ygcen.2008.03.025

Soma, K. K., Schlinger, B. A., Wingfield, J. C., and Saldanha, C. J. (2003). Brain aromatase, 5 alpha-reductase, and 5 beta-reductase change seasonally in wild male song sparrows: relationship to aggressive and sexual behavior. *J. Neurobiol.* 56, 209–221. doi: 10.1002/neu.10225

Tinbergen, N. (1963). On aims and methods of ethology. *Zeitschrift Für Tierpsychologie* 20, 410–433.

Trainor, B. C., Kyomen, H. H., and Marler, C. A. (2006). Estrogenic encounters: how interactions between aromatase and the environment modulate aggression. *Front. Neuroendocrinol.* 27:170–179. doi: 10.1016/j.yfrne.2005.11.001

Tsai, L. W., and Sapolsky, R. M. (1996). Rapid stimulatory effects of testosterone upon myotubule metabolism and sugar transport, as assessed by silicon microphysiometry. *Aggress. Behav.* 22, 357–364.

Van Honk, J., Peper, J. S., and Schutter, D. J. L. G. (2005). Testosterone reduces unconscious fear but not consciously experienced anxiety: implications for the disorders of fear and anxiety. *Biol. Psychiatry* 58, 218–225. doi: 10.1016/j.biopsych.2005.04.003

Van Honk, J., and Schutter, D. J. L. G. (2007). Testosterone reduces conscious detection of signals serving social correction: implications for antisocial behavior. *Psychol. Sci.* 18, 663–667. doi: 10.1111/j.1467-9280.2007.01955.x

Van Honk, J., Schutter, D. J. L. G., Hermans, E., Putman, P., Tuiten, A., and Koppeschaar, H. (2004). Testosterone shifts the balance between sensitivity for punishment and reward in healthy young women. *Methods* 937–943. doi: 10.1016/j.psyneuen.2003.08.007

Williams, P., and Beer, R. (2013). "Environmental feedback drives multiple behaviors from the same neural circuit," in *Advances in Artificial Life, ECAL 2013* (Taormina), 268–275. doi: 10.7551/978-0-262-31709-2-ch041

Wilson, A. D., and Golonka, S. (2013). Embodied cognition is not what you think it is. *Front. Psychol.* 4:58. doi: 10.3389/fpsyg.2013.00058

Wingfield, J. C., Hegner, R. E., Dufty, A. M. Jr., and Ball, G. F. (1990). The challenge hypothesis: theoretical implications for patterns of testosterone secretion, mating systems, and breeding strategies. *Am. Nat.* 136, 829–846. doi: 10.1086/285134

Wingfield, J. C., Lynn, S., and Soma, K. K. (2001). Avoiding the 'Costs' of testosterone: ecological bases of hormone-behavior interactions. *Brain Behav. Evol.* 57, 239–251. doi: 10.1159/000047243

2

Estradiol-sensitive projection neurons in the female rat preoptic area

Yasuo Sakuma *

Laboratory of Physiology, University of Tokyo Health Sciences, Tokyo, Japan

Correspondence:
Yasuo Sakuma, Laboratory of Physiology, University of Tokyo Health Sciences, 11 Ochiai 4, Tama 206-0033, Tokyo, Japan
e-mail: y-sakuma@u-ths.ac.jp

Electrical stimulation of the preoptic area (POA) interrupts the lordosis reflex, a combined contraction of back muscles, in response to male mounts and the major receptive component of sexual behavior in female rat in estrus, without interfering with the proceptive component of this behavior or solicitation. Axon-sparing POA lesions with an excitotoxin, on the other hand, enhance lordosis and diminish proceptivity. The POA effect on the reflex is mediated by its estrogen-sensitive projection to the ventral tegmental area (VTA) as shown by the behavioral effect of VTA stimulation as well as by the demonstration of an increased threshold for antidromic activation of POA neurons from the VTA in ovariectomized females treated with estradiol benzoate (EB). EB administration increases the antidromic activation threshold in ovariectomized females and neonatally castrated males, but not in neonatally androgenized females; the EB effect is limited to those that show lordosis in the presence of EB. EB causes behavioral disinhibition of lordosis through an inhibition of POA neurons with axons to the VTA, which eventually innervate medullospinal neurons innervating spinal motoneurons of the back muscle. The EB-induced change in the threshold or the axonal excitability may be a result of EB-dependent induction of BK channels. Recordings from freely moving female rats engaging in sexual interactions revealed separate subpopulations of POA neurons for the receptive and proceptive behaviors. Those POA neurons engaging in the control of proceptivity are EB-sensitive and project to the midbrain locomotor region (MLR). EB thus enhances lordosis by reducing excitatory neural impulses from the POA to the VTA. An augmentation of the POA effect to the MLR may culminate in an increased locomotion that embodies behavioral estrus in the female rat.

Keywords: sexual behavior, estradiol, preoptic, ventral tegmental area, central gray, lordosis reflex

OVERVIEW

Protracted electrical stimulation of the ventrolateral part of the ventromedial nucleus of the hypothalamus (VMN) at low frequencies has been found to cause lasting facilitation of the lordosis reflex in female rats in the estrus, a combined contraction of the longissimus and other back muscles caused by touch-pressure stimulation on the flank-perineal skin given by male partners (Pfaff and Sakuma, 1979). The resultant dorsiflexion of the female trunk allows penile penetration. A recent study replicated the effectiveness of low frequency stimulation, albeit by optogenic stimulation in male mice, to elicit sexual behavior or aggression from the ventrolateral VMN at different thresholds (Lin et al., 2011). The effects of electrical stimulation at low frequencies may be compatible with the scalable control of mounting and attack at different optogenic stimulation thresholds at the similar frequency range around 10 Hz (Lee et al., 2014).

SYSTEMIC ESTROGEN IS NEEDED FOR EFFECTIVE VMN STIMULATION

Systemic treatment with submaximal doses of estrogen, in particular estradiol benzoate (EB), was needed for electrical stimulation of the VMN to facilitate lordosis in the ovariectomized female rats. EB-induced increase in the excitability of VMN neurons does not fully explain the requirement of systemic EB to stimulation-bound facilitation of lordosis, because VMN stimulation does not promote lordosis in the absence of systemic EB, even at stronger currents. The VMN contains estrogen receptor (ER) α positive projection neurons to the midbrain, but ERα positive neurons are also present in the preoptic area (POA), medial amygdala, midbrain central gray (CG), and lateral septum, to name but a few (Simerly et al., 1990; Doncarlos et al., 1991). In the periphery, EB-induced enlargement of the cutaneous sensory field pertinent to the induction of lordosis has been shown (Kow and Pfaff, 1973).

The medial amygdala exerts an estrogen-dependent facilitatory effect on lordosis, evidence that is based on lesion of the structure (Rajendren and Moss, 1993) and resection of its efferents in the stria terminalis (Takeo et al., 1995). Significant reduction the lordosis quotient following lesion of the amygdala was, however, detected only in the response to repeated coital stimulation. Fos immunohistochemistry attributed the effect secondary to the diminished activation of gonadotropin-releasing hormone neurons. Thus, the medial amygdala cannot be a principal site for estrogen action on the lordosis reflex. The lateral septum is also an origin of a lordosis-inhibiting efferents (Yamanouchi and Arai,

1990), and EB implants in this structure releases the behavioral inhibition (Satou and Yamanouchi, 1999). Morphologically, however, only a small number of estrogen receptor immunoreactive cells have been visualized in this structure (Yokosuka et al., 1997).

THE POA AS A TARGET OF ESTROGEN ACTION

Whereas, the VMN is known to play a key role in the lordosis reflex and other components of estrogen-dependent female sexual behavior, the POA has more often been associated with male behavior and is not traditionally been considered to be vital in the regulation of female behavior. Several earlier studies have shown, however, that the POA is primarily an inhibitory structure for the lordosis reflex. Stereotaxic implantation of minute amount of crystalline EB either in the VMN or the POA supplements a subthreshold EB given systemically to induce lordosis (Barfield and Chen, 1977). Although larger doses were needed to induce lordosis by implants in the POA than in the VMN, this observation has shown that the POA is a target site of estrogen action to induce lordosis.

Pharmacological disruption of aminergic neurotransmission in the POA has been found to promote lordosis (Ward et al., 1975; Carter et al., 1978). Intracerebral implantation of the antiestrogens in the preoptic and anterior hypothalamic continuum has also been found to antagonize systemic EB, which results in a dramatic inhibition of lordosis (Luttge, 1976). Additionally, lesions in the dorsal POA have been found to produce a significant increase in lordosis (Nance et al., 1977). It is worth noting that the CG receives dense projection from the rostral and dorsal parts of the POA (Morrell et al., 1981; Swanson et al., 1987).

POA STIMULATION AND LORDOSIS

In freely moving EB-treated ovariectomized females, neurons associated with bouts of sexual interactions with a male partner in rate-meter and ethograms have been shown to have a mean firing rate of 10.3 Hz (Kato and Sakuma, 2000). Electrical stimulation of the POA at around 10 Hz suppressed lordosis, with a slow onset and gradual suppression which reached a maximum at 90 min. This effect has also been characterized by slow recovery of lordosis after the termination of POA stimulation (Pfaff and Sakuma, 1979; Takeo et al., 1993). The peculiar time course in the behavioral response to the POA stimulation disappeared by the removal of dorsal connection of the POA by a horizontal knife cut (roof cut), or in particular, the disruption of the stria terminalis, resulting in immediate interruption of lordosis in response to current application (Takeo et al., 1993). Therefore, the POA contains a particular set of neurons that are responsible for the inhibition of lordosis. The elimination of facilitatory neural components for this reflex, which enter the POA via the stria terminalis, is responsible for the prompt and exaggerated stimulation effect in the roof-cut animals (**Figure 1**).

THE POA AND THE PROCEPTIVE BEHAVIOR

Of great significance in the observed effects of POA lesions on lordosis is that the effects depend on test situation. For instance, Whitney (1986) found that, in a no-exit paradigm when the females were constrained in the vicinity of males, lordosis was enhanced. In exit tests, in which the females could evade male partners, no lordosis was seen as a consequence of the lack of sexual contacts. Thus, the authors concluded that the enhanced lordosis in the lesioned females detected by no-exit tests was not due to any potentiation in the females' preference to engage in sexual interactions with males.

In the rat, sexual interactions are initiated and paced by females in estrus through patterns of approach toward and withdrawal from sexually active males (Erskine, 1989). Emotional state of the females, determined by activity of the medial amygdala, one major source of estrogen-sensitive POA afferents, may regulate this approach and withdrawal (Kondo and Sakuma, 2005). Preoptic implants of estradiol suppress open-field and increase wheel-running activities in ovariectomized female rats (Fahrbach et al., 1985). These behavioral changes have been interpreted to reflect increased anxiety and fear learning together with locomotor activation, the effects, as investigated in knockout mice (Ogawa et al., 2003), mediated by ERα-positive, but not ERβ-positive, neurons in the POA. In stressed female rats, however, estradiol has been found to decrease anxious behavior on the open field and to enhance radial-arm maze performance (Bowman et al., 2002). Changes in cognitive and emotional activity have been inferred to reflect a general increase in arousal level (Morgan and Pfaff, 2002), with both responses increasing the likelihood of successful reproduction.

PREOPTIC LOCOMOTOR AREA

Thus, an increased locomotor activity in female rats in estrus embodies enhanced sexual motivation (Quadagno et al., 1972; Swanson and Mogenson, 1981; Mink et al., 1983; Edwards and Einhorn, 1986; Rivas and Mir, 1990; Paredes and Vazquez, 1999), and the POA has been positively identified as a site for estrogen-induced activation of wheel running (Fahrbach et al., 1985) through activation of ERα (Hertrampf et al., 2008). The POA contributes to the rostro-caudal neural axis for the locomotor synergy (Mori et al., 1992) with its projections to the midbrain locomotor region (MLR) (Swanson et al., 1984, 1987). The preoptic locomotor region, from which stepping can be initiated by chemical (Sinnamon, 1987) or electrical (Sinnamon, 1992) stimulation, is situated in the medial portion of the lateral POA (mLPO). The locomotor activity can be consistently reduced by cholinergic activation of the periventricular POA (Brudzynski and Eckersdorf, 1984; Brudzynski and Mogenson, 1986).

In the EB-dependent regulation of locomotor activity, two separate POA projections to the MLR that mediate EB effects have been identified (Takeo and Sakuma, 1995). The female rat POA contains neurons that promote proceptive behavior (Hoshina et al., 1994). Females with lesions of the peripeduncular nucleus, through which fibers with origins in the POA and other subpallidal structures descend to the MLR (Swanson et al., 1984), characteristically failed to show darting and other solicitatory behavior (Pfeifle and Edwards, 1983). An observation that lesions of the accumbens does not modify soliciting activity (Rivas and Mir, 1990) may mean that the POA constitutes an independent entity for solicitatory behavior, because the accumbens activates locomotion through innervation of the POA (Swerdlow et al., 1984). In a male rat engaging in sexual interaction, however, our recent study showed that the shell of the accumbens contains

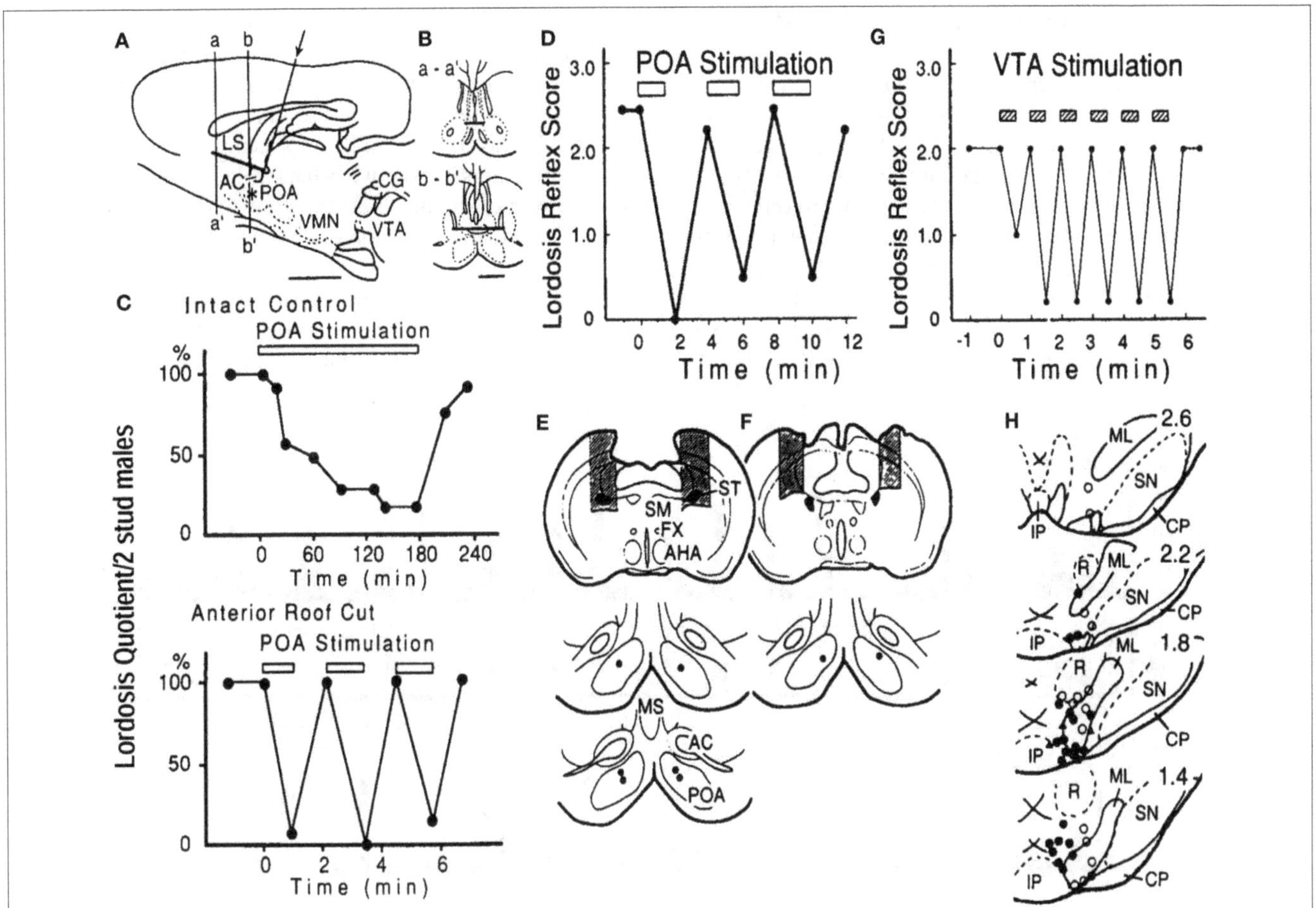

FIGURE 1 | (A) Locations and the extent of the roof cut of the POA in the sagittal **(A)** and frontal **(B)** planes. An L-shaped wire was inserted in the midline (arrow) and rotated 180°. The asterisk shows the stimulation site in the POA. AC, anterior commissure; LS, lateral septum; other abbreviations are in the text. **(C)** Lordosis reflex suppression during bilateral POA stimulation in the intact control (top) and roof-cut (bottom) animals. POA was stimulated at 100 Hz for periods indicated by the bar in each panel. Stimulus intensity was 100 μA per electrode. Note different time scales. **(D)** Interruption of lordosis by POA stimulation in rats with bilateral cuts of the stria terminalis (ST, shaded areas in **E**, top panel). POA stimulation was ineffective when the ST was spared (shaded areas in **F**). Stimulation sites are in lower panels in **(E)** and **(F)** (Takeo et al., 1993). **(G)** Time course of suppression of lordosis by electrical stimulation of the VTA. Pulses of 50 μA, 100 Hz were applied in 30-s trains during the period indicated by shaded bars. **(F)** Locations of stimulation sites in the VTA and adjacent tegmentum plotted on sections 400 um apart. Filled circles, suppression exceeding 50% of prestimulation lordosis reflex score at current intensity below 50 μA; open circles, suppression under 50% or no effect. Abbreviations: CP, cerebral peduncle: IP, interpeduncular nucleus: ML, medial lemniscus: p, pons: R, red nucleus: SN, substantia nigra; III, oculomotor nerve (Sakuma, 1995).

neurons encoding cues or contexts related to sexual behavior, reward-related processing, and the inhibition of sexual behavior after ejaculation (Matsumoto et al., 2012). These results suggest that estrogen inhibits neural impulse flow from the MPO and facilitates that from the lateral POA. The effects of estrogen, when combined, would culminate in increased locomotor activity that is typical of female rats in estrus.

PROJECTION NEURONS IN THE POA

Stereotaxic infusion of ibotenic acid, an excitotoxin which obliterates POA neuronal soma but spares local axons of passage, enhances lordosis by lowering the threshold for EB needed to induce the reflex (Hoshina et al., 1994). At the same time, females with the excitotoxin lesion did not commit themselves to sexual interactions. Far from showing solicitation, these females antagonized and vigorously resisted any males that attempted to mount them in the non-exit test paradigm. Meanwhile, gradual and persistent suppression of the lordosis reflex followed electrical stimulation of the local axons of passage that survived the excitotoxic damage. Apart from the fact that the females with the POA lesion needed less estrogen to obtain comparable prestimulation quotients with the controls, the lesioned and control animals responded similarly to the stimulation.

In the females with ibotenic-acid lesion of the POA, an additional roof cut dorsal to the POA abolished the stimulus-bound suppression of lordosis, and the stimulation effect was thus due to the activation of axons of passage that presumably descend from the septum, cingulate cortex, or other structures. As described above, the septum is an origin of lordosis-inhibiting efferents (Yamanouchi and Arai, 1990). Thus, the POA is a major target for EB in eliciting proceptive behavior; local POA neurons as well as septal efferents appear to inhibit the lordosis, a receptive behavior.

DESCENDING PROJECTION OF THE VENTRAL TEGMENTAL AREA

The midbrain ventral tegmental area (VTA) is one of major projection targets of estrogen concentrating neurons in the POA (Fahrbach et al., 1986). Earlier anterograde tracing studies in the rat (Conrad and Pfaff, 1976) and gerbil (Finn et al., 1993) visualized dense POA projection to the VTA. POA projection may in turn activate both ascending and descending efferents of the VTA (Simon et al., 1979a,b; Matsumoto et al., 2012). Electrical stimulation of the VTA in EB-primed ovariectomized female rats caused immediate and strong interruption of lordosis reflex in response to either male mounts or manual cutaneous stimuli. The intensity and the time course of the disruption bore a resemblance to that induced by POA stimulation in the rat with the roof cut. Likewise, lordosis performance returned promptly to the pre-stimulation level after the termination of stimulation. Interestingly, electrical stimulation specifically blocked lordosis without disturbing proceptive behavior. Pharmacological depletion of dopamine did not affect the stimulation on lordosis.

The VTA disruption of lordosis is a result of an activation of a pathway inhibitory to the reflex arc at the lower brainstem. Indeed, non-dopaminergic descending projections of the VTA have been traced ipsilaterally to the ventral and dorsal tegmental nucleus and the ventral CG (Simon et al., 1979a).

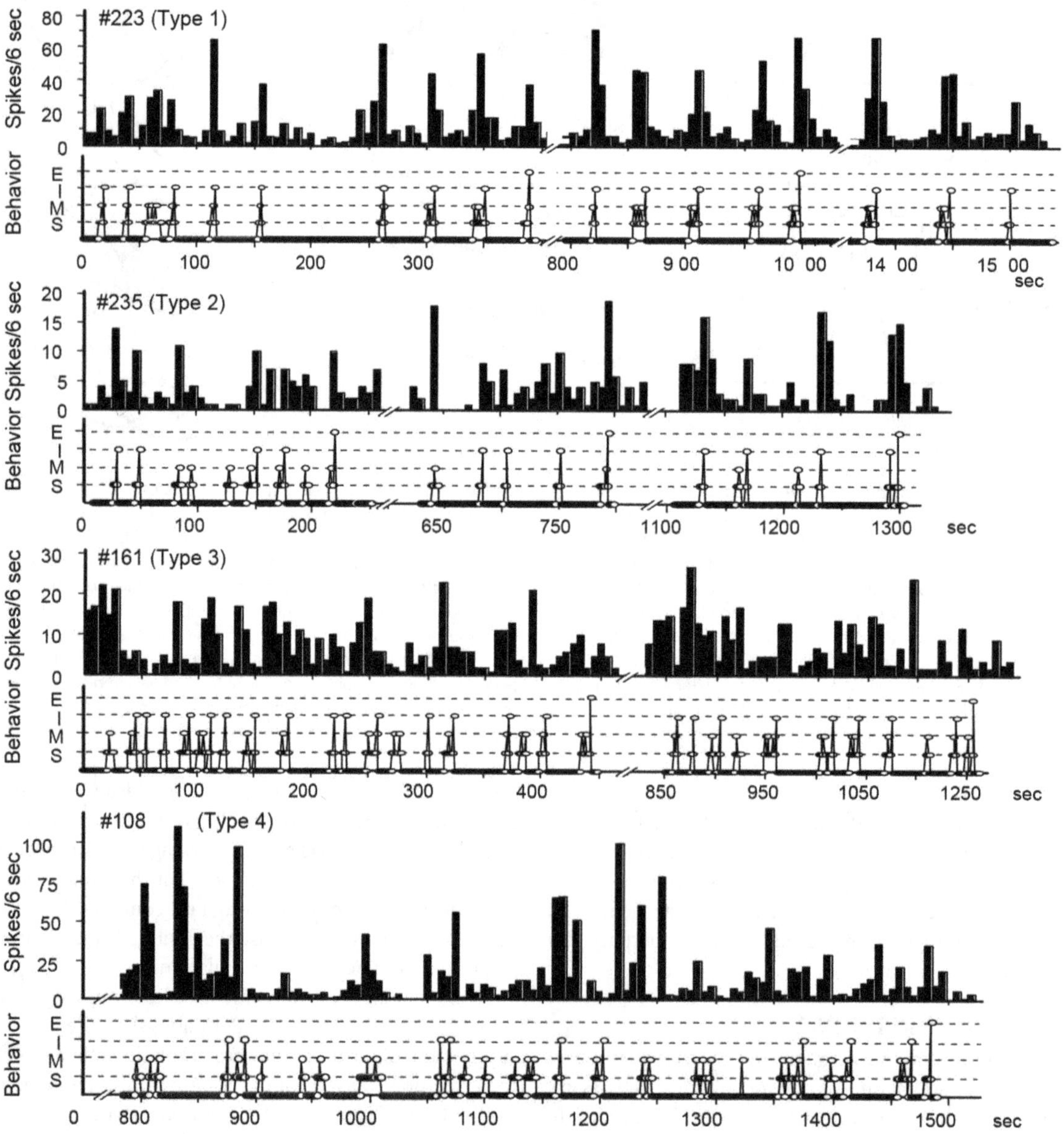

FIGURE 2 | Temporal relationship between neuronal activity and sexual behavior in rate-meter and ethogram charts. The activity of these POA neurons was related to bouts of sexual interactions, which were characterized into four types in peri-event histograms associated with different events in sexual behavior (see text).

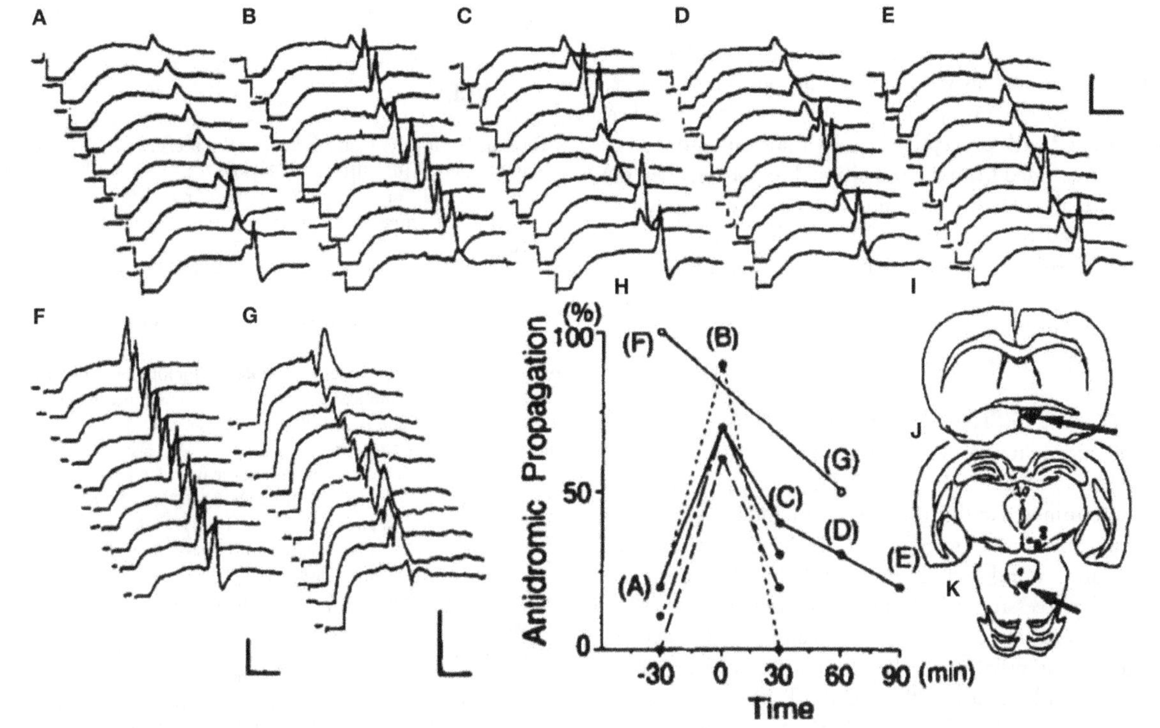

FIGURE 3 | Effects of POA stimulation or lesion on the propagation of CG-induced antidromic potentials into ventral tegmental area neurons. Trains of antidromic stimuli were given at 0.5 Hz, and excerpts of the responses in an ovariectomized, estrogen-treated rat are shown **(A–E)**. The POA was stimulated at 100 Hz for a 30-s period during the period indicated in **(B)**. Acute electrolytic lesion made during the period indicated in **(D)** had no effect on this neuron. **(F)** and **(G)** depict recordings from an ovariectomized, non-treated animal that were made before and after an electrolytic lesion of the POA, respectively. As summarized in **(H)**, all four cells in ovariectomized, EB-treated animals originally showed low rates of antidromic propagation that were temporarily increased by POA stimulation. A POA lesion in an ovariectomized female rat, which originally showed a high rate of antidromic propagation, exerted a contrasting effect to that of POA stimulation, resulting in a decrease in the frequency and a delay in antidromic propagation. The position of tip of each stimulation electrode and the extent of the POA lesion are shown in **(I)**, the location of each recorded neuron in **(J)**, and the antidromic stimulation sites in **(K)**. Calibrations are 5 ms and 1 mV (Sakamoto et al., 1993).

Functional demarcation exists between the dorsal and ventral parts of the CG. Opposite patterns of cardiovascular changes have been found to be elicited from lateral and ventrolateral subregions of the CG (Bandler and Shipley, 1994; Vaughan et al., 1996). Activation of CG sites lateral to the aqueduct produced increased arterial pressure and tachycardia; activation of sites ventrolateral to the aqueduct produced decreased arterial pressure and bradycardia. The lordosis reflex is under a similar antagonistic regulation: the dorsal CG is a target of VMN projection, from which the reflex can be promoted. The ventral CG contains descending VTA axons-of-passage, which inhibits the reflex, and electrical stimulation of this structure elicits antidromic action potentials in VTA neurons (Sakamoto et al., 1993) (**Figure 3**). One of the targets of the VTA projection, the dorsal tegmentum, contains neurons associated with paradoxical sleep (Torterolo et al., 2002). Paradoxical sleep is characterized by somatic muscle atonia (Sakai and Neuzeret, 2011), which would result in the disruption of lordosis.

Consistent with morphological studies, POA neurons have been found to be antidromically driven from the VTA (Hasegawa and Sakuma, 1993). Whereas EB treatment decreased antidromic activation threshold for VMN neurons by CG stimulation (Sakuma, 1984), EB showed an opposite effect on the threshold for activation of POA neurons from the VTA. Besides, in both projections, the authors found that EB was effective in females or neonatally orchidectomized males but not in females given testosterone as pups. EB-induced excitability changes in either VMN or POA axons were observed in the ovariectomized females and neonatally orchidectomized males, but not in androgenized females, in parallel with the capability of EB treatment to induce lordosis.

Changes in antidromic activation thresholds, along with those in refractory periods and axonal conduction velocity, indicate an altered axonal excitability. Our experiment in a model system deploying GT1-7 cells showed that EB at physiological doses, that is 100–300 pM in the medium, enhanced Ni^{2+}-, Cd^{2+}-sensitive BK current after 3 days in culture. BK or KCNM channels have a large conductance, and are voltage-gated. Thus, in this model, the enhanced expression of these channels would decrease excitability (Nishimura et al., 2008).

DIFFERENT SUBSETS OF POA NEURONS

In order to clarify whether separate POA neurons regulate solicitatory and receptive components of female rat sexual behavior, single unit activities were recorded (Kato and Sakuma, 2000) (**Figure 2**). Perievent histograms identified separate groups of neurons that increased their firing rate (1) during the solicitatory period, from the initiation of solicitatory locomotion to the male mounts, (2) when the male mounted, or (3) in response to intromission. There was also another set of neurons that were quiescent prior to and throughout the display of the lordosis. Neurons associated with proceptive behavior and somatosensory responses were recorded from the transitional region between the medial and lateral POAs. Those neurons that behaved exactly as if they inhibited the execution of the lordosis were located medially in the medial POA to other neurons. These results thus showed separate sets of POA neurons each specifically associated with proceptive and receptive components of female rat sexual behavior.

VTA NEURONS ARE EXCITED BY POA EFFERENTS

In urethane-anesthetized, EB-treated ovariectomized rats, antidromic action potentials elicited in VTA neurons by CG stimulation often terminated at the initial segment and rarely invaded the neuronal soma (Sakamoto et al., 1993) (**Figures 3A–K**). The authors also found that POA stimulation increased the probability of successful antidromic invasion up to 90%. Conversely, ovariectomized females showed almost 100% success of antidromic invasion without POA stimulation in the absence of EB; acute electrolytic destruction of the POA decreased the invasion rate down to 50%. Thus, the POA is thought to excite the soma of VTA neurons, and EB decreases the impact of POA effect on the VTA. EB would thus decrease the efficacy of neural transmission from the POA to the CG. The pattern of estrogen-induced changes in the excitability of these descending VTA neurons is that required for the behavioral disinhibition of the lordosis reflex.

PROJECTIONS TO THE MEDULLA

The gigantocellular nucleus of the medullary reticular formation (NGc) and lateral vestibular nucleus (LVN) are the origins of the ipsilateral reticulospinal and vestibulospinal tract, respectively, which innervate spinal motoneurons responsible for the induction of the lordosis. Lesion studies have suggested that the contribution of these tracts is not dependent upon the integrity of the other, and that the magnitude of the lordosis deficit is instead correlated with amount of giant cell loss in NGc and Deiters cell loss in the LVN (Modianos and Pfaff, 1979). Finally, lordosis is facilitated by electrical stimulation of the LVN (Modianos and Pfaff, 1977).

Electrical stimulation of the NGc in urethane-anesthetized female rats induced antidromic activation in neurons in the CG. Antidromically driven cells were in all parts of the CG and adjacent mesencephalic reticular field except within the inner ring of the CG that surrounds the aqueduct.

As with the antidromic potentials induced in the VTA in response to CG stimulation, POA stimulation reduced the rate of successful propagation of NGc-induced antidromic potentials into the soma, whereas VMN stimulation increased the rate. Thus, the pattern of descending effects originating in the EB-sensitive POA and VMN on these CG neurons is required for their control of the lordosis reflex, via the regulation of the activity of medullospinal neuron that govern the contraction of back muscles responsible for the induction of the lordosis reflex.

REFERENCES

Bandler, R., and Shipley, M. T. (1994). Columnar organization in the midbrain periaqueductal gray: modules for emotional expression? *Trends Neurosci.* 17, 379–389. doi: 10.1016/0166-2236(94)90047-7

Barfield, R. J., and Chen, J. J. (1977). Activation of estrous behavior in ovariectomized rats by intracerebral implants of estradiol benzoate. *Endocrinology* 101, 1716–1725. doi: 10.1210/endo-101-6-1716

Bowman, R. E., Ferguson, D., and Luine, V. N. (2002). Effects of chronic restraint stress and estradiol on open field activity, spatial memory, and monoaminergic neurotransmitters in ovariectomized rats. *Neuroscience* 113, 401–410. doi: 10.1016/S0306-4522(02)00156-2

Brudzynski, S. M., and Eckersdorf, B. (1984). Inhibition of locomotor activity during cholinergically-induced emotional-aversive response in the cat. *Behav. Brain Res.* 14, 247–253. doi: 10.1016/0166-4328(84)90192-X

Brudzynski, S. M., and Mogenson, G. J. (1986). Decrease of locomotor activity by injections of carbachol into the anterior hypothalamic/preoptic area of the rat. *Brain Res.* 376, 38–46. doi: 10.1016/0006-8993(86)90897-8

Carter, C. S., Bahr, J. M., and Ramirez, V. D. (1978). Monoamines, estrogen and female sexual behavior in the golden hamster. *Brain Res.* 144, 109–121. doi: 10.1016/0006-8993(78)90438-9

Conrad, L. C., and Pfaff, D. W. (1976). Efferents from medial basal forebrain and hypothalamus in the rat. I. An autoradiographic study of the medial preoptic area. *J. Comp. Neurol.* 169, 185–219. doi: 10.1002/cne.901690205

Doncarlos, L. L., Monroy, E., and Morrell, J. I. (1991). Distribution of estrogen receptor-immunoreactive cells in the forebrain of the female guinea pig. *J. Comp. Neurol.* 305, 591–612. doi: 10.1002/cne.903050406

Edwards, D. A., and Einhorn, L. C. (1986). Preoptic and midbrain control of sexual motivation. *Physiol. Behav.* 37, 329–335. doi: 10.1016/0031-9384(86)90242-8

Erskine, M. S. (1989). Solicitation behavior in the estrous female rat: a review. *Horm. Behav.* 23, 473–502. doi: 10.1016/0018-506X(89)90037-8

Fahrbach, S. E., Meisel, R. L., and Pfaff, D. W. (1985). Preoptic implants of estradiol increase wheel running but not the open field activity of female rats. *Physiol. Behav.* 35, 985–992. doi: 10.1016/0031-9384(85)90270-7

Fahrbach, S. E., Morrell, J. I., and Pfaff, D. W. (1986). Identification of medial preoptic neurons that concentrate estradiol and project to the midbrain in the rat. *J. Comp. Neurol.* 247, 364–382. doi: 10.1002/cne.902470307

Finn, P. D., De Vries, G. J., and Yahr, P. (1993). Efferent projections of the sexually dimorphic area of the gerbil hypothalamus: anterograde identification and retrograde verification in males and females. *J. Comp. Neurol.* 338, 491–520. doi: 10.1002/cne.903380403

Hasegawa, T., and Sakuma, Y. (1993). Developmental effect of testosterone on estrogen sensitivity of the rat preoptic neurons with axons to the ventral tegmental area. *Brain Res.* 611, 1–6. doi: 10.1016/0006-8993(93)91769-O

Hertrampf, T., Seibel, J., Laudenbach, U., Fritzemeier, K. H., and Diel, P. (2008). Analysis of the effects of oestrogen receptor alpha (ERalpha)- and ERbeta-selective ligands given in combination to ovariectomized rats. *Br. J. Pharmacol.* 153, 1432–1437. doi: 10.1038/sj.bjp.0707664

Hoshina, Y., Takeo, T., Nakano, K., Sato, T., and Sakuma, Y. (1994). Axon-sparing lesion of the preoptic area enhances receptivity and diminishes proceptivity among components of female rat sexual behavior. *Behav. Brain Res.* 61, 197–204. doi: 10.1016/0166-4328(94)90160-0

Kato, A., and Sakuma, Y. (2000). Neuronal activity in female rat preoptic area associated with sexually motivated behavior. *Brain Res.* 862, 90–102. doi: 10.1016/S0006-8993(00)02076-X

Kondo, Y., and Sakuma, Y. (2005). The medial amygdala controls the coital access of female rats: a possible involvement of emotional responsiveness. *Jpn. J. Physiol.* 55, 345–353. doi: 10.2170/jjphysiol.RP001105

Kow, L. M., and Pfaff, D. W. (1973). Effects of estrogen treatment on the size of receptive field and response threshold of pudendal nerve in the female rat. *Neuroendocrinology* 13, 299–313. doi: 10.1159/000122214

Lee, H., Kim, D. W., Remedios, R., Anthony, T. E., Chang, A., Madisen, L., et al. (2014). Scalable control of mounting and attack by Esr1+ neurons in the ventromedial hypothalamus. *Nature* 509, 627–632. doi: 10.1038/nature13169

Lin, D., Boyle, M. P., Dollar, P., Lee, H., Lein, E. S., Perona, P., et al. (2011). Functional identification of an aggression locus in the mouse hypothalamus. *Nature* 470, 221–226. doi: 10.1038/nature 09736

Luttge, W. G. (1976). Intracerebral implantation of the anti-estrogen CN-69, 725-27: effects on female sexual behavior in rats. *Pharmacol. Biochem. Behav.* 4, 685–688. doi: 10.1016/0091-3057(76)90220-3

Matsumoto, J., Urakawa, S., Hori, E., de Araujo, M. F., Sakuma, Y., Ono, T., et al. (2012). Neuronal responses in the nucleus accumbens shell during sexual behavior in male rats. *J. Neurosci.* 32, 1672–1686. doi: 10.1523/JNEUROSCI.5140-11.2012

Mink, J. W., Sinnamon, H. M., and Adams, D. B. (1983). Activity of basal forebrain neurons in the rat during motivated behaviors. *Behav. Brain Res.* 8, 85–108. doi: 10.1016/0166-4328(83)90173-0

Modianos, D., and Pfaff, D. (1979). Medullary reticular formation lesions and lordosis reflex in female rats. *Brain Res.* 171, 334–338. doi: 10.1016/0006-8993(79)90338-X

Modianos, D. T., and Pfaff, D. W. (1977). Facilitation of the lordosis reflex in female rats by electrical stimulation of the lateral vestibular nucleus. *Brain Res.* 134, 333–345. doi: 10.1016/0006-8993(77)91077-0

Morgan, M. A., and Pfaff, D. W. (2002). Estrogen's effects on activity, anxiety, and fear in two mouse strains. *Behav. Brain Res.* 132, 85–93. doi: 10.1016/S0166-4328(01)00398-9

Mori, S., Matsuyama, K., Kohyama, J., Kobayashi, Y., and Takakusaki, K. (1992). Neuronal constituents of postural and locomotor control systems and their interactions in cats. *Brain Dev.* 14(Suppl.), S109–S120.

Morrell, J. I., Greenberger, L. M., and Pfaff, D. W. (1981). Hypothalamic, other diencephalic, and telencephalic neurons that project to the dorsal midbrain. *J. Comp. Neurol.* 201, 589–620. doi: 10.1002/cne.902010409

Nance, D. M., Christensen, L. W., Shryne, J. E., and Gorski, R. A. (1977). Modifications in gonadotropin control and reproductive behavior in the female rat by hypothalamic and preoptic lesions. *Brain Res. Bull.* 2, 307–312. doi: 10.1016/0361-9230(77)90087-9

Nishimura, I., Ui-Tei, K., Saigo, K., Ishii, H., Sakuma, Y., and Kato, M. (2008). 17b-estradiol at physiological concentrations augments Ca^{2+}-activated K^+ currents via estrogen receptor b in the gonadotropin-releasing hormone neuronal cell line GT1-7. *Endocrinology* 149, 774–782. doi: 10.1210/en.2007-0759

Ogawa, S., Chan, J., Gustafsson, J. A., Korach, K. S., and Pfaff, D. W. (2003). Estrogen increases locomotor activity in mice through estrogen receptor alpha: specificity for the type of activity. *Endocrinology* 144, 230–239. doi: 10.1210/en.2002-220519

Paredes, R. G., and Vazquez, B. (1999). What do female rats like about sex? Paced mating. *Behav. Brain Res.* 105, 117–127. doi: 10.1016/S0166-4328(99)00087-X

Pfaff, D. W., and Sakuma, Y. (1979). Facilitation of the lordosis reflex of female rats from the ventromedial nucleus of the hypothalamus. *J. Physiol.* 288, 189–202.

Pfeifle, J. K., and Edwards, D. A. (1983). Midbrain lesions eliminate sexual receptivity but spare sexual motivation in female rats. *Physiol. Behav.* 31, 385–589. doi: 10.1016/0031-9384(83)90206-8

Quadagno, D. M., Shryne, J., Anderson, C., and Gorski, R. A. (1972). Influence of gonadal hormones on social, sexual, emergence, and open field behaviour in the rat (*Rattus norvegicus*). *Anim. Behav.* 20, 732–740. doi: 10.1016/S0003-3472(72)80145-3

Rajendren, G., and Moss, R. L. (1993). The role of the medial nucleus of amygdala in the mating-induced enhancement of lordosis in female rats: the interaction with luteinizing hormone-releasing hormone neuronal system. *Brain Res.* 617, 81–86. doi: 10.1016/0006-8993(93)90616-U

Rivas, F. J., and Mir, D. (1990). Effects of nucleus accumbens lesion on female rat sexual receptivity and proceptivity in a partner preference paradigm. *Behav. Brain Res.* 41, 239–249. doi: 10.1016/0166-4328(90)90111-Q

Sakai, K., and Neuzeret, P. C. (2011). Brainstem neurons responsible for postural, masseter or pharyngeal muscle atonia during paradoxical sleep in freely-moving cats. *Arch. Ital. Biol.* 149, 325–347. doi: 10.4449/aib.v149i4.1380

Sakamoto, Y., Suga, S., and Sakuma, Y. (1993). Estrogen-sensitive neurons in the female rat ventral tegmental area: a dual route for the hormone action. *J. Neurophysiol.* 70, 1469–1475.

Sakuma, Y. (1984). Influences of neonatal gonadectomy or androgen exposure on the sexual differentiation of the rat ventromedial hypothalamus. *J. Physiol.* 349, 273–286. doi: 10.1113/jphysiol.1984.sp015156

Sakuma, Y. (1995). Differential control of proceptive and receptive components of female rat sexual behavior by the preoptic area. *Jpn. J. Physiol.* 45, 211–228. doi: 10.2170/jjphysiol.45.211

Satou, M., and Yamanouchi, K. (1999). Effect of direct application of estrogen aimed at lateral septum or dorsal raphe nucleus on lordosis behavior: regional and sexual differences in rats. *Neuroendocrinology* 69, 446–452. doi: 10.1159/000054448

Simerly, R. B., Chang, C., Muramatsu, M., and Swanson, L. W. (1990). Distribution of androgen and estrogen receptor mRNA-containing cells in the rat brain: an *in situ* hybridization study. *J. Comp. Neurol.* 294, 76–95. doi: 10.1002/cne.902940107

Simon, H., Le Moal, M., and Calas, A. (1979a). Efferents and afferents of the ventral tegmental-A10 region studied after local injection of [3H]leucine and horseradish peroxidase. *Brain Res.* 178, 17–40. doi: 10.1016/0006-8993(79)90085-4

Simon, H., Le Moal, M., Stinus, L., and Calas, A. (1979b). Anatomical relationships between the ventral mesencephalic tegmentum–a 10 region and the locus coeruleus as demonstrated by anterograde and retrograde tracing techniques. *J. Neural Transm.* 44, 77–86. doi: 10.1007/BF01252703

Sinnamon, H. M. (1987). Glutamate and picrotoxin injections into the preoptic basal forebrain initiate locomotion in the anesthetized rat. *Brain Res.* 400, 270–277. doi: 10.1016/0006-8993(87)90626-3

Sinnamon, H. M. (1992). Microstimulation mapping of the basal forebrain in the anesthetized rat: the "preoptic locomotor region." *Neuroscience* 50, 197–207. doi: 10.1016/0306-4522(92)90392-F

Swanson, L. W., and Mogenson, G. J. (1981). Neural mechanisms for the functional coupling of autonomic, endocrine and somatomotor responses in adaptive behavior. *Brain Res.* 228, 1–34. doi: 10.1016/0165-0173(81)90010-2

Swanson, L. W., Mogenson, G. J., Gerfen, C. R., and Robinson, P. (1984). Evidence for a projection from the lateral preoptic area and substantia innominata to the 'mesencephalic locomotor region' in the rat. *Brain Res.* 295, 161–178. doi: 10.1016/0006-8993(84)90827-8

Swanson, L. W., Mogenson, G. J., Simerly, R. B., and Wu, M. (1987). Anatomical and electrophysiological evidence for a projection from the medial preoptic area to the 'mesencephalic and subthalamic locomotor regions' in the rat. *Brain Res.* 405, 108–122. doi: 10.1016/0006-8993(87)90995-4

Swerdlow, N. R., Swanson, L. W., and Koob, G. F. (1984). Electrolytic lesions of the substantia innominata and lateral preoptic area attenuate the "supersensitive" locomotor response to apomorphine resulting from denervation of the nucleus accumbens. *Brain Res.* 306, 141–148. doi: 10.1016/0006-8993(84)90362-7

Takeo, T., Chiba, Y., and Sakuma, Y. (1993). Suppression of the lordosis reflex of female rats by efferents of the medial preoptic area. *Physiol. Behav.* 53, 831–838. doi: 10.1016/0031-9384(93)90258-H

Takeo, T., Kudo, M., and Sakuma, Y. (1995). Stria terminalis conveys a facilitatory estrogen effect on female rat lordosis reflex. *Neurosci. Lett.* 184, 79–81. doi: 10.1016/0304-3940(94)11173-G

Takeo, T., and Sakuma, Y. (1995). Diametrically opposite effects of estrogen on the excitability of female rat medial and lateral preoptic neurons with axons to the midbrain locomotor region. *Neurosci. Res.* 22, 73–80. doi: 10.1016/0168-0102(95)00885-W

Torterolo, P., Sampogna, S., Morales, F. R., and Chase, M. H. (2002). Gudden's dorsal tegmental nucleus is activated in carbachol-induced active (REM) sleep and active wakefulness. *Brain Res.* 944, 184–189. doi: 10.1016/S0006-8993(02)02561-1

Vaughan, C. W., Bandler, R., and Christie, M. J. (1996). Differential responses of lateral and ventrolateral rat periaqueductal grey neurones to noradrenaline *in vitro*. *J. Physiol.* 490(Pt 2), 373–381. doi: 10.1113/jphysiol.1996.sp021151

Ward, I. L., Crowley, W. R., and Zemlan, F. P. (1975). Monoaminergic mediation of female sexual behavior. *J. Comp. Physiol. Psychol.* 88, 53–61. doi: 10.1037/h0076202

Whitney, J. F. (1986). Effect of medial preoptic lesions on sexual behavior of female rats is determined by test situation. *Behav. Neurosci.* 100, 230–235. doi: 10.1037/0735-7044.100.2.230

Yamanouchi, K., and Arai, Y. (1990). The septum as origin of a lordosis-inhibiting influence in female rats: effect of neural transection. *Physiol. Behav.* 48, 351–355. doi: 10.1016/0031-9384(90)90326-Y

Yokosuka, M., Okamura, H., and Hayashi, S. (1997). Postnatal development and sex difference in neurons containing estrogen receptor-alpha immunoreactivity in the preoptic brain, the diencephalon, and the amygdala in the rat. *J. Comp. Neurol.* 389, 81–93.

3

Neuroanatomy and sex differences of the lordosis-inhibiting system in the lateral septum

Shinji Tsukahara[1]*, Moeko Kanaya[1] and Korehito Yamanouchi[2]

[1] *Division of Life Science, Graduate School of Science and Engineering, Saitama University, Saitama, Japan*
[2] *Department of Human Behavior and Environment Sciences, Faculty of Human Sciences, Waseda University, Saitama, Japan*

***Correspondence:**
Shinji Tsukahara, Division of Life Science, Graduate School of Science and Engineering, Saitama University, 255 Shimo-Okubo, Sakura-ku, Saitama 338-8570, Japan
e-mail: stsuka@mail.saitama-u.ac.jp

Female sexual behavior in rodents, termed lordosis, is controlled by facilitatory and inhibitory systems in the brain. It has been well demonstrated that a neural pathway from the ventromedial hypothalamic nucleus (VMN) to the midbrain central gray (MCG) is essential for facilitatory regulation of lordosis. The neural pathway from the arcuate nucleus to the VMN, via the medial preoptic nucleus, in female rats mediates transient suppression of lordosis, until female sexual receptivity is induced. In addition to this pathway, other regions are involved in inhibitory regulation of lordosis in female rats. The lordosis-inhibiting systems exist not only in the female brain but also in the male brain. The systems contribute to suppression of heterotypical sexual behavior in male rats, although they have the potential ability to display lordosis. The lateral septum (LS) exerts an inhibitory influence on lordosis in both female and male rats. This review focuses on the neuroanatomy and sex differences of the lordosis-inhibiting system in the LS. The LS functionally and anatomically links to the MCG to exert suppression of lordosis. Neurons of the intermediate part of the LS (LSi) serve as lordosis-inhibiting neurons and project axons to the MCG. The LSi-MCG neural connection is sexually dimorphic, and formation of the male-like LSi-MCG neural connection is affected by aromatized testosterone originating from the testes in the postnatal period. The sexually dimorphic LSi-MCG neural connection may reflect the morphological basis of sex differences in the inhibitory regulation of lordosis in rats.

Keywords: lordosis, lateral septum, midbrain central gray, estradiol, sexual differentiation

INTRODUCTION

Sexual behaviors enable mammals to copulate with the opposite sex and ensure fertilization and consequently reproductive success. One of the most studied sexual behaviors in female mammals is lordosis. Lordosis is a characteristic sexually receptive behavior in female rodents, and this is a postural reflex with dorsiflexion of the vertebral column. The lordosis reflex is observed in sexually receptive female rodents, when their flank perineum region is stimulated by mounting of a vigorous male rodent (**Figures 1A,B**). Sexual receptive activity of female rodents is modulated by ovarian sex steroids and changes with the estrous cycles: estrous females frequently display lordosis, while anestrous females rarely display lordosis.

As well as anestrous female rats, intact male rats rarely exhibit lordosis. Moreover, most male rats (approximately 88%) do not display lordosis, even when castrated and treated with ovarian sex steroids in adulthood (Yamanouchi and Arai, 1976) (**Figure 1C**). Although some estradiol benzoate (EB)- and progesterone-treated castrated male rats (approximately 12%) display lordosis, the lordosis quotient (LQ: number of lordosis/number of mounts × 100) is very low (LQ: approximately 10). However, in laboratory rats, lordosis of male rats can be elicited by lesioning of some brain regions and treatment with a large amount of exogenous estradiol. The lateral septum (LS) is one such region, which when lesioned induces lordosis in male rats (**Figure 1D**). The incidence of lordosis in estradiol-17β (E_2)- or EB-treated castrated male rats can be increased by surgical destruction of the LS (Nance et al., 1975b; Kondo et al., 1990). Thus, the LS suppresses heterotypical sexual behavior in male rats. Furthermore, this finding supports the idea that the male brain has the potential ability to exhibit sexual behavioral patterns of the opposite sex.

The LS of female rats, as well as male rats, plays an inhibitory role in the regulation of lordosis. Lesioning of the LS enhances lordotic activity induced by EB in ovariectomized female rats (Nance et al., 1975a; Gorzalka and Gray, 1981). Direct implantation of E_2 into the LS potentiates lordosis in female rats that have been ovariectomized and treated with EB at a subthreshold dose for increasing sexual receptivity; however, the same hormonal manipulation did not induce lordosis in castrated male rats (Satou and Yamanouchi, 1999). This finding indicates that the function of LS in the inhibition of lordosis differs between sexes with respect to responsiveness to estradiol. Thus, inhibitory regulation of lordosis by the LS contributes to estradiol-dependent control of sexual receptivity in female rats and in the suppression of heterotypical sexual behavior in male rats. Understanding the mechanisms responsible for inhibitory regulation of lordosis by the LS will contribute to our

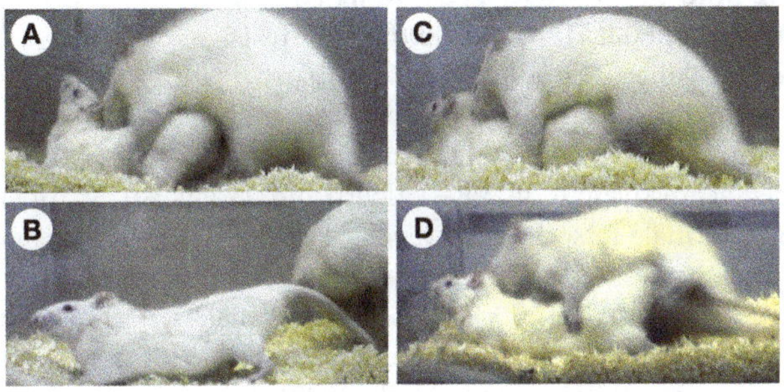

FIGURE 1 | Photographs of rats displaying sexual behaviors. An estradiol-treated ovariectomized female rat displays lordosis in response to the mounting of a vigorous male rat **(A,B)**. An estradiol-treated castrated male rat does not exhibit lordosis **(C)**. However, an estradiol-treated castrated male exhibits lordosis when the lateral septum is surgically destructed **(D)**.

understanding of female reproduction and the sexual differentiation of reproductive behaviors in rodent models.

ESTRADIOL, A KEY MOLECULE FOR MODULATION OF FEMALE SEXUAL RECEPTIVITY

Female rats normally exhibit a 4- or 5-day estrous cycle, and female sexual behaviors are displayed during a limited period from the evening of the day of proestrus to the morning of the day of estrus. Estradiol, the levels of which change throughout the estrous cycle, is a key molecule for modulation of female sexual receptivity. Levels of estradiol are high during proestrus because of increasing production of estradiol in the preovulatory ovarian follicle. This leads to an increase in sexually receptive activity in female rodents and the induction of lordosis. Ovariectomy drastically reduces the sexual receptivity of female rats. Decreased receptivity can be subsequently increased by injection of EB or E_2 (Davidson et al., 1968; Dohanich and Clemens, 1983; Blasberg and Clark, 1997; Tsukahara and Yamanouchi, 2001). One of the important actions of estradiol to induce female sexual receptivity is to activate the facilitatory neural system for lordosis. Neural projections from the ventromedial hypothalamic nucleus (VMN) to the midbrain central gray (MCG) are a critical part of the facilitatory neural system for lordosis (Pfaff et al., 1994, 2008). The VMN expresses estrogen receptors (ERs), transducing estrogen signaling to neural signaling, and then modulating MCG functions to facilitate lordosis (Flanagan-Cato, 2011).

Estradiol evidently acts to increase female sexual receptivity. However, female sexual receptivity is not increased immediately after estradiol affects the brain. In the case of ovariectomized female rats injected with EB followed by progesterone 4 h before testing lordosis, at least 30 h is needed after EB injection to observe the full display of lordosis (Sinchak and Micevych, 2001). Regarding E_2 or EB treatment alone, more than 6 days are needed to induce sexual receptivity in ovariectomized rats (Dohanich and Clemens, 1983; Blasberg and Clark, 1997; Tsukahara and Yamanouchi, 2001). The delayed effects of estradiol are considered to be due to the genomic actions of estradiol to promote protein synthesis, which is requisite to induce female sexual receptivity. Estradiol-induced expression of progesterone receptors requires approximately 16 h following estradiol treatment, and this estradiol-induced expression is required for progesterone to exert its facilitatory effects on lordosis (Parsons et al., 1979, 1980, 1981). Another explanation for the delayed effects of estradiol on female sexual receptivity is that estradiol initially suppresses lordotic activity until female rats show a maximal level of female sexual receptivity. Recently, Micevych and his colleagues proposed a neural system that is activated by rapid actions of estradiol via membrane signaling, resulting in transient suppression of lordosis in female rats (Micevych and Christensen, 2012; Micevych and Sinchak, 2013). Reportedly, estradiol acts rapidly through estradiol membrane signaling to release neuropeptide Y in the arcuate nucleus of the hypothalamus. Subsequently, there is activation of β-endorphin neurons, which express neuropeptide Y-Y1 receptors, which project from the arcuate nucleus to the medial preoptic nucleus. In the medial preoptic nucleus, neurons expressing μ-opioid receptors and projecting to the VMN are stimulated by β-endorphin, resulting in the inhibition of lordosis. Thus, transitory inhibition of lordotic activity by rapid actions of estradiol may be necessary for estrous female rats to exhibit full performance of lordosis.

On diestrous and estrous days, when the levels of estradiol in the blood are low, female rats rarely display lordosis, even if male rats attempt copulation. One reasonable explanation for decreased sexual receptivity during the anestrous phase is that the facilitatory neural system for lordosis is not activated in the absence of certain estradiol levels. In addition, the inhibitory neural system may contribute to the control of sexual receptivity in female rats. Although the detailed mechanisms responsible for inhibition of lordosis are poorly understood, several regions involved in the inhibitory regulation of lordosis have been documented, including the LS, medial preoptic nucleus, and dorsal raphe nucleus (Yamanouchi, 1997). Here, we focus on the lordosis-inhibiting system in the LS, as discussed below.

LORDOSIS-FACILITATING SYSTEM: A COMMON PATHWAY FROM THE VMN TO THE MCG

The VMN is known as an important component of the facilitatory neural system for lordosis. Surgical destruction of the VMN in female rats prevents the display of lordosis (Mathews and Edwards, 1977; Pfaff and Sakuma, 1979a), while electrical stimulation of the VMN facilitates lordosis (Pfaff and Sakuma, 1979b). Injection of EB into the VMN stimulates ovariectomized female rats to display lordosis (Barfield and Chen, 1977). The VMN of the rat brain, especially the ventrolateral part of the VMN (VL-VMN), abundantly expresses estrogen receptor-α (ERα) but not ERβ (Shughrue et al., 1997; Osterlund et al., 1998). The actions of estrogens binding to ERα are essential for the induction of lordosis behavior. This is illustrated by studies showing that lordosis is elicited in ovariectomized female rats by injection of a selective ERα agonist, but not a selective ERβ agonist (Mazzucco et al., 2008). Female mice lacking the ERα gene do not show any lordosis response (Ogawa et al., 1998). In contrast, sexual behaviors of ERβ-knockout female mice are indistinguishable from those of wild-type female mice (Ogawa et al., 1999). Sexually receptive behaviors in female mice are abolished by knock-down of ERα in the VL-VMN (Musatov et al., 2006), suggesting that ERα expressed in this region is necessary to induce lordosis behavior. Thus, the VMN exerts an estrogen-dependent facilitatory influence on the control of lordosis in female rodents.

Some VMN neurons project axons to the MCG, and neural projections from the VMN to MCG are an important part of the neural circuitry underlying lordosis (Daniels et al., 1999). The lordosis response in female rats disappears after lesion of the MCG (Sakuma and Pfaff, 1979b), while it is activated by electrical stimulation of the MCG (Sakuma and Pfaff, 1979a). Electrical stimulation of the VMN facilitates lordosis in female rats, but this effect is nullified by MCG lesions (Sakuma and Pfaff, 1979b). Transection of neural connections between the VMN and MCG results in elimination of the lordosis response in female rats (Hennessey et al., 1990). Neurons of the MCG project axons to the medullary reticular formation of the hindbrain, which controls motoneurons in the lumbar spinal cord, thus innervating axial muscles involved in maintaining the lordosis posture (Pfaff et al., 1994). According to a study demonstrating the central neural circuit innervating the lumber epaxial muscle in female rats, neurons comprising the circuit were concentrated in the ventrolateral column, rather than the dorsal, dorsolateral, or ventral columns of the MCG, and were mainly localized in the VL-VMN rather than other parts of the VMN (Daniels et al., 1999). Thus, neural projections from the VL-VMN to the ventrolateral column of the MCG form a critical neural pathway for facilitatory regulation of lordosis. Interestingly, most VMN neurons projecting to the MCG do not express ERα (Calizo and Flanagan-Cato, 2003). However, the VMN contains many ERα-expressing cells (Shughrue et al., 1997; Osterlund et al., 1998) and ERα expressed in the VMN plays a facilitatory role in lordosis induction (Musatov et al., 2006). After mating, of those VMN neurons expressing Fos, a marker for neuronal activation, approximately 41% neither contain ERα nor project to the MCG, and 35% contain ERα but do not project to the MCG (Calizo and Flanagan-Cato, 2003). Flanagan-Cato proposed that there are at least three different types of VL-VMN neurons participating in the control of lordosis behavior: ERα-containing neurons that may serve as local circuit neurons, MCG-projecting neurons without ERα, and neurons that neither express ERα nor project to the MCG, but are activated during mating (Flanagan-Cato, 2011). Local neural circuitry comprising these neurons in the VL-VMN could underlie lordosis-facilitating functions of the VMN, which detects estrogens and modulates the functions of the MCG. Besides neural projection from the VL-VMN, the MCG also receives neural information from other regions, including the habenular nucleus, medial amygdala, and zona incerta (Beitz, 1995). These brain regions are reported to have facilitatory influences on the regulation of lordosis in female rats (Modianos et al., 1975; Dornan et al., 1991; Rajendren and Moss, 1993). Additionally, the MCG receives sensory information from the flank skin stimulated by male mounting via the lumber spinal cord (Pfaff et al., 1994). Thus, the MCG plays an important role in the integration of neural information from the forebrain, lower brain stem, and spinal cord to regulate lordosis.

LORDOSIS-INHIBITING SYSTEM IN THE LS

INHIBITORY REGULATION OF LORDOSIS BY THE LS

The LS of the forebrain is known to participate in the control of instinctive behaviors related to fear, aggression, and reproduction. LS lesions cause hyperirritability, hyper reactivity, and hyper aggressiveness in rats (Albert and Wong, 1978; Albert, 1980). In male rats, the LS is involved in the facilitation of male sexual behavior and the inhibition of heterotypical sexual behavior. Lesion of the LS effectively suppresses male sexual behavior (Kondo et al., 1990) and facilitates lordosis behavior in male rats (Nance et al., 1975b; Kondo et al., 1990). Injection of a neurotoxin into the LS also induces lordosis in E_2-treated castrated male rats (Tsukahara and Yamanouchi, 2001), indicating that neurons localized in the LS themselves function to inhibit lordosis in male rats. The LS exerts an inhibitory influence on lordosis not only in male rats but also in female rats, because lordosis response is enhanced by lesion of the LS in female rats (Nance et al., 1975a; Gorzalka and Gray, 1981) and in female hamsters (Nance and Myatt, 1987), while electrical stimulation in the LS suppresses lordosis behavior in female hamsters (Zasorin, 1975).

Although the male LS contributes to suppression of heterotypical sexual behavior, LS lesions alone do not result in full display of lordosis in male rats, as seen in female rats. The level of vertebral column dorsiflexion and the LQ in LS-lesioned male rats are lower than those in sexually receptive female rats (**Figures 1A,D, 2B**). Accordingly, inhibitory functions of heterotypical sexual behavior are inherent not only in the LS, but also in other brain regions. The medial preoptic nucleus and the dorsal raphe nucleus have an inhibitory influence on lordosis display in male rats (Van De Poll and Van Dis, 1979; Hennessey et al., 1986; Kakeyama and Yamanouchi, 1992). Lesioning of both the LS and dorsal raphe nucleus induces lordosis display in male rats at a comparable level to that of female rats (Kakeyama and Yamanouchi, 1994). Thus, development of the inhibitory neural systems for lordosis in other regions except the LS is also critical for sexual differentiation of sexual behavioral patterns.

It appears that LS neurons involved in the inhibition of lordosis elongate their axons ventrally, because horizontal deafferentation at the site ventral to the LS elicits the lordosis reflex in rats of both sexes (Yamanouchi and Arai, 1977, 1985, 1990). Neural fibers projecting from the LS join the medial forebrain bundle (MFB) (Veening et al., 1982). Transection of the MFB at the suprachiasmatic level enhances lordosis in female rats (Yamanouchi and Arai, 1989) and induces lordosis in male rats (Yamashita Suzuki and Yamanouchi, 1998). Therefore, it is considered that lordosis-inhibiting neurons of the LS terminate at the brain stem after the neural fibers pass through the MFB. The VMN and MCG are possible projection sites for lordosis-inhibiting neurons of the LS, because both are major components of the facilitatory neural system for lordosis, as mentioned above. However, an anatomical study demonstrated that the VMN does not receive direct input from any part of the LS in rats (Risold and Swanson, 1997b). Furthermore, it indicated that the LS and VMN are functionally independent of each other for regulation of lordosis in female rats (Yamanouchi, 1980; King and Nance, 1985). In this context, lordosis-inhibiting neurons of the LS presumably send their axons to other regions than the VMN. There is anatomical evidence for

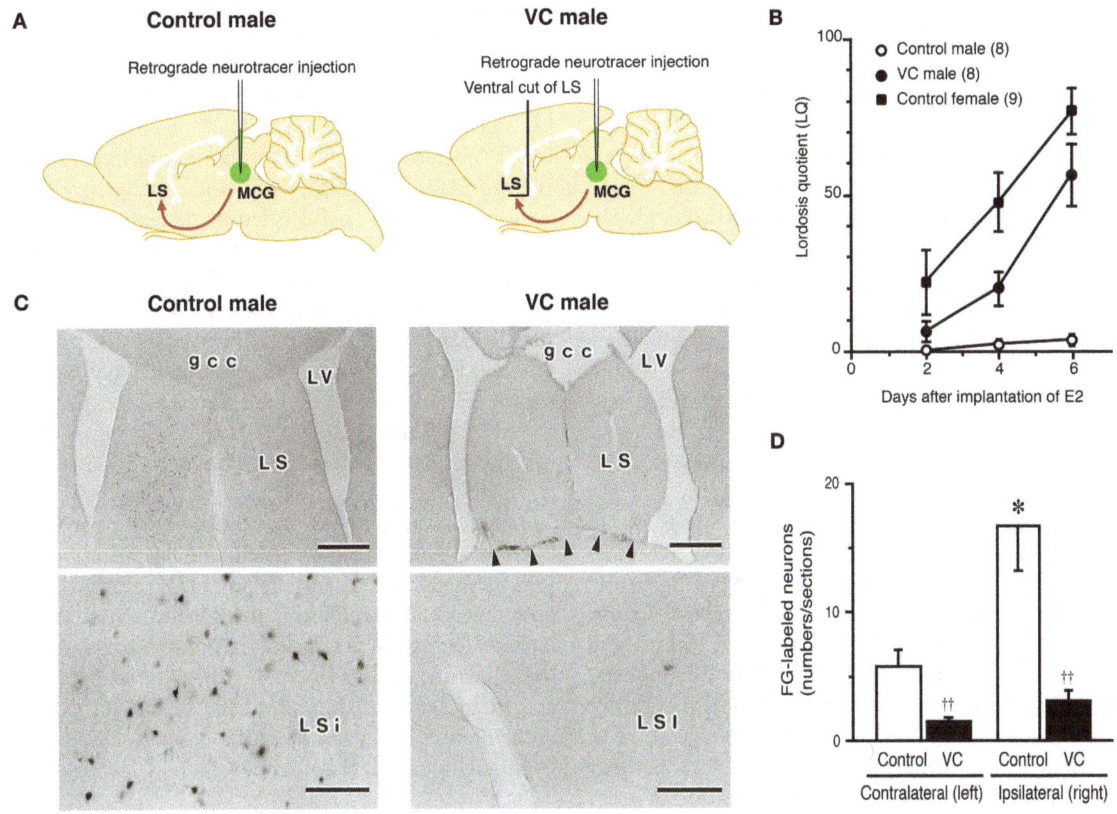

FIGURE 2 | Effects of a ventral cut of the LS (VC) on lordotic activity and neural projection from the LS to MCG in male rats. (A) Estradiol-17β (E_2)-treated castrated male rats with or without VC were tested for lordosis behavior and then injected with Fluoro-Gold (FG), a retrograde neurotracer, into the MCG. FG-labeled neurons in the LS were detected by immunohistochemistry. **(B)** The mean LQ of E_2-treated castrated male rats with VC (VC male) was increased over time (days) after E_2 treatment, like an E_2-treated ovariectomized female (control female), but the mean LQ of E_2-treated castrated male rats without VC (control male) was low. **(C)** Photomicrographs of the LS of control and VC male rats that received FG injection into the MCG on the right side. Many FG-labeled neurons were found in the LSi of control male rats, but not in the LSi of VC male rats. Arrowheads indicate the scar of VC. Scale bars = 500 μm. gcc, genu of the corpus callosum; LS, lateral septum; LSi, intermediate part of the LS; LV, lateral ventricle; MCG, midbrain central gray. **(D)** The number of FG-labeled neurons in the LSi of control male rats was significantly greater than that of VC male rats on the ipsilateral and contralateral side of the FG injection site. The LSi of control male rats contained many more FG-labeled neurons on the ipsilateral side of the FG injection site. $^{††}p < 0.01$ vs. control male rat; $^{*}p < 0.05$ vs. contralateral side (modified from Tsukahara and Yamanouchi, 2001).

direct neural connections from the LS to MCG in guinea pigs (Staiger and Nurnberger, 1991) and rats (Risold and Swanson, 1997b). The lordosis response in female rats is enhanced by a LS lesion, but this effect disappears when the MCG is surgically destroyed in combination with the LS lesion (Kondo et al., 1993). This finding indicates the possibility that the LS functionally links to the MCG to exert an inhibitory influence on the regulation of lordosis.

LS-MCG CONNECTIONS FOR INHIBITION OF LORDOSIS

To clarify whether neural connections between the LS and MCG have a functional role in the inhibition of lordosis, we carried out a neuroanatomical and behavioral study (Tsukahara and Yamanouchi, 2001). We performed behavioral tests for lordosis in E_2-treated castrated male rats, some of which bore neural transections of the ventral outputs from the LS (**Figure 2A**). Mean LQ in castrated male rats that received neural transections of the ventral outputs from the LS gradually increased days after implantation of E_2 (**Figure 2B**), as reported previously (Yamanouchi and Arai, 1975, 1978, 1985). In contrast, most of the E_2-treated castrated male rats without neural transection did not display lordosis, and the mean LQ was low throughout behavioral testing. After behavioral testing, we injected Fluoro-Gold (FG), a retrograde neurotracer, into the MCG to determine the location of FG-labeled neurons in the LS and the effects of the neural transections on retrograde transport of FG from the MCG to LS (**Figure 2A**). In E_2-treated castrated male rats that exhibited lower performance of lordosis, the intermediate part of the LS (LSi), especially the rostral part of the LSi, contained a large number of FG-labeled neurons (**Figures 2C,D**). However, other parts of the LS contained only a few FG-labeled neurons. In E_2-treated castrated male rats that exhibited higher performance of lordosis following neural transections of the ventral outputs from the LS, only a few FG-labeled neurons were found in the LSi. These findings suggest that male rats can display lordosis when the neural projection from the LSi to the MCG is transected.

The LS is classically divided into three parts, the aforementioned LSi, the dorsal LS (LSd), and the ventral LS (LSv) based on the size and density of neurons (Jakab and Leranth, 1995). Of the three parts, the LSi is the largest subdivision and exhibits the most heterogeneous cytoarchitecture, with loosely grouped neurons of different cell sizes. Neurons of the LSi themselves function to suppress the display of lordosis, because E_2-treated castrated male rats can exhibit lordosis when LSi neurons are completely killed by a neurotoxin, but not when chemical lesion of the LSi is incomplete (Tsukahara and Yamanouchi, 2001). The LS contains several types of neurons that produce neuropeptides, opioid peptides, and gamma-aminobutyric acid (GABA) as neurotransmitters (Risold and Swanson, 1997a; Tsukahara and Yamanouchi, 2003). In the rostral part of the LSi, from which many neurons project to the MCG (Risold and Swanson, 1997b; Tsukahara and Yamanouchi, 2001), neurons produce GABA, neurotensin, or enkephalin (Risold and Swanson, 1997a; Tsukahara and Yamanouchi, 2003). Therefore, these substances are candidate neurotransmitters that may transfer neural information for lordosis-inhibiting neurons of the LSi, but this is yet to be determined. The MCG of rats contains $GABA_A$ receptors and $GABA_B$ receptors (Williams and Beitz, 1990b; Barbaresi, 2007). Systemic administration of a $GABA_A$ receptor agonist or a $GABA_B$ receptor agonist inhibits lordosis in rats (Agmo et al., 1989; Luine et al., 1991; Kakeyama and Yamanouchi, 1996). However, local GABAergic neurotransmission via $GABA_A$ receptors in the MCG is involved in facilitatory regulation of lordosis (McCarthy et al., 1991, 1994, 1995). GABAergic neurons are generally divided into local circuit neurons with short axons and projection neurons with longer axons, and most GABAergic neurons function as local circuit neurons (Vincent et al., 1982; Ottersen and Storm-Mathisen, 1984; Ottersen et al., 1995). GABAergic neurons in the MCG may act as local circuit neurons to mediate facilitatory effects on lordosis, although the roles of GABAergic neurons in the LSi in the regulation of lordosis are largely unknown. Enkephalin may serve as a neurotransmitter in the MCG to inhibit lordosis in female rats and the MCG of rats contains enkephalinergic nerve terminals (Williams and Beitz, 1990a; Beitz, 1995). Lordotic activity of EB- and progesterone-treated ovariectomized female rats is decreased by injection of Met-enkephalin into the MCG in combination with an inhibitor of enkephalin degrading enzymes (Bednar et al., 1987). Neurotensinergic nerve terminals and their receptors are found in the MCG of rats (Shipley et al., 1987; Boudin et al., 1996). However, there is no evidence for the involvement of neurotensin in the regulation of lordosis.

Neurons of the LS send axons to a variety of regions in the thalamus, hypothalamus, and midbrain in a subdivision-specific manner, and the septal region that sends the largest number of axons to the MCG is the rostral LSi (Risold and Swanson, 1997b). To determine the lordosis-inhibiting neural tracts from the LS to MCG, we traced the neural projections from the LSi to the MCG in E_2-treated castrated male rats using Phaseolus vulgaris leucoagglutinin (PHAL), an anterograde neurotracer (Tsukahara and Yamanouchi, 2001) (**Figure 3A**). Neural tracts from the LS to MFB (**Figures 3A-1,2**) are essential for lordosis-inhibiting LSi neurons to function, because the lordosis reflex is induced in male rats by transection of the ventral area of the septal region (Yamanouchi and Arai, 1985) and by transection of the MFB (Yamashita Suzuki and Yamanouchi, 1998). Similar surgical manipulations enhance lordotic activity in female rats (Yamanouchi and Arai, 1977, 1989, 1990). Thus, the MFB includes fibers originating from lordosis-inhibiting LSi neurons in both sexes. After passing through the MFB, PHAL-labeled axonal fibers reach the anterior hypothalamic area (**Figure 3A-3**). The VMN did not contain any PHAL-labeled axons, but many PHAL-labeled fibers existed in the region surrounding it (**Figure 3A-4**), supporting previous studies showing that the LS and VMN are functionally independent of each other in the regulation of lordosis (Yamanouchi, 1980; King and Nance, 1985). PHAL-labeled axonal fibers in the posterior hypothalamic area projected along the longitudinal axis from the ventral region (**Figure 3A-5**), and then terminated at the rostral part of the MCG (**Figure 3A-6**). It is likely that lordosis-inhibiting LSi neurons elongate their axons to the MCG by passing through the posterior hypothalamic area, because the expression of lordosis in female rats was increased by transection of neural fibers passing through the medial regions, including the posterior hypothalamic area (Ohnishi et al., 2003). Taking these results together, we propose that lordosis-inhibiting neural tracts from the LSi to MCG include the MFB at the level of the optic chiasma, the ventrolateral hypothalamic regions (including the anterior hypothalamic area, and excluding the VMN), and the medial part of the junction of the diencephalon and mesencephalon (including the posterior hypothalamic area) (**Figure 3B**).

SEXUAL DIFFERENTIATION OF THE LORDOSIS-INHIBITING SYSTEM IN THE LS

Morphological sex difference in the LSi

Nuclei exhibiting morphological differences by sex are generally termed sexually dimorphic nuclei (SDNs) and are found in the central nervous system (Woodson and Gorski, 1999). The LSi is one of the SDNs in the rat brain. The volume of the LSi in prepubertal female rats is larger than that of same-aged male rats, however, there are no sex differences in the volume of the LSd and LSv (Tsukahara et al., 2004). The number of LSi neurons in adult female rats is greater than that in adult male rats, while there are no sex differences in the number of neurons in the LSd and LSv (Segovia et al., 2009). Thus, sexual dimorphism of the LSi is reflected by its larger size and greater number of neurons in female rats than in male rats.

In rodent models, it has been long considered that organizational effect of aromatizable testosterone originating from the testes during the perinatal period is critical for the formation of morphological sex differences in the brain (McEwen et al., 1977; MacLusky et al., 1979; MacLusky and Naftolin, 1981). This is based on the classic concept for understanding the sexual differentiation of the brain by sex steroids, but this view has now been revised. However, testicular testosterone that acts on the brain during the perinatal period is still necessary, but not solely, for the formation of morphological sex differences in the brain. Testosterone synthesis in the testis of rats begins on embryonic day 15.5, rises to a peak around embryonic day 18.5, and then declines after birth (Warren et al., 1973). Temporal change in plasma testosterone levels is similar to that in testosterone synthesis in the testes, and male rats have higher plasma testosterone

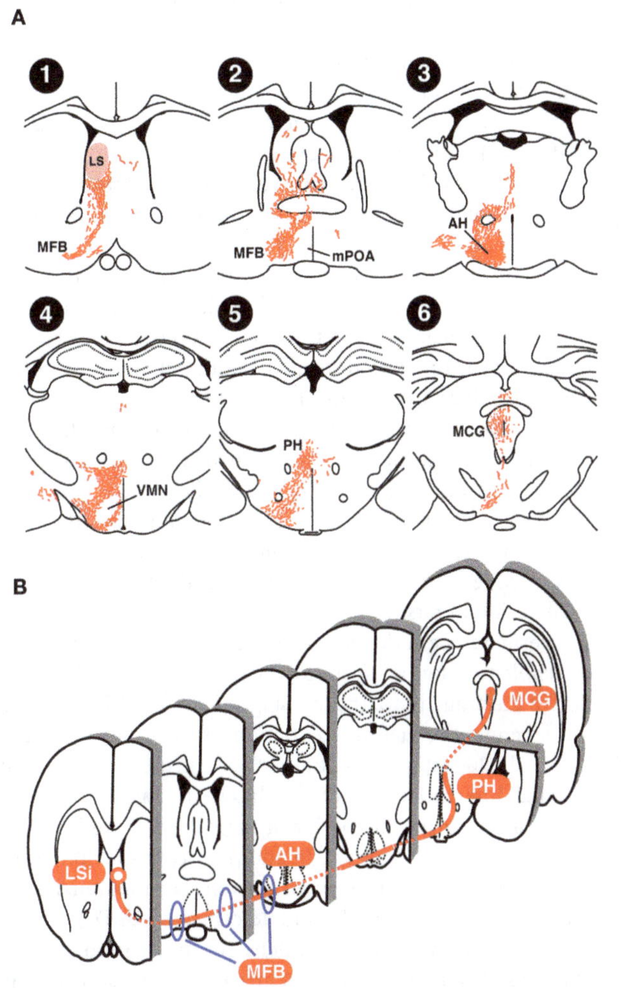

FIGURE 3 | Neural projection of the LS in rats. (A) Distribution of Phasiolus vulgaris leucoagglutinin (PHAL), an anterograde neurotracer, -labeled neural fibers in an estradiol-treated castrated male rat that received PHAL injection into the LS on the right side (modified from Tsukahara and Yamanouchi, 2001). **(B)** Possible lordosis-inhibiting neural tract from the LSi to MCG. AH, anterior hypothalamic area; LS, lateral septum; MCG, midbrain central gray; MFB, medial forebrain bundle; mPOA, medial preoptic area; PH, posterior hypothalamic area; VMN, ventromedial hypothalamic nucleus.

levels from embryonic day 18 to postnatal day 5 (PD5, day of birth = PD1) than do female rats (Weisz and Ward, 1980). This period corresponds to the classically identified critical period, when testosterone effectively masculinizes and defeminizes the brain (MacLusky and Naftolin, 1981). Testosterone in the postnatal period has masculinizing effects on the morphology of the LSi at least in part, because the number of LSi neurons in male rats is increased by castration on the day of birth (Segovia et al., 2009).

In the currently revised view of brain sexual differentiation, the period when the sexually differentiated brain is organized under the influence of sex steroids is not limited to the perinatal period, but is extended to the pubertal/adolescent period (Schulz et al., 2009a; Juraska et al., 2013). Ahmed et al. reported that new cells generated during puberty are added to the anteroventral periventricular nucleus (AVPV), a female-biased SDN, and the sexually dimorphic nucleus of the preoptic area (SDN-POA) and medial amygdala (Me), male-biased SDNs, and that the cell number and volume of the AVPV in female rats and those of the SDN-POA and Me in male rats are greater than those in the opposite sexes (Ahmed et al., 2008), indicating a significant contribution of cell generation during puberty in the formation of morphological sex differences in the brain. They further showed that gonadectomy at PD20 suppresses the increase in the number of new cells and the volume of the female AVPV and of the male SDN-POA and Me, excepting the volume of the male Me, whereas cell number and volume of the opposite sexes do not change with gonadectomy (Ahmed et al., 2008). Sexually dimorphic formation of the principal nucleus of the bed nucleus of the stria terminalis (BNSTp), another male-biased SDN in rodents, is also affected by gonadal hormones during the prepubertal and/or pubertal period. The number of neurons in the male BNSTp is greater than that in the female BNSTp in 20-day-old prepubertal mice, and this sex difference becomes marked in adulthood with increasing neuron number in the male BNSTp and loss of neurons in the female BNSTp (Wittmann and Mclennan, 2013). These findings indicate that ovarian and testicular hormones during puberty act in remodeling the brain after it develops with or without the organizational effect of testicular testosterone during the perinatal period.

In addition to the organizational effects of sex steroids, sex chromosome genes directly influence the sexual differentiation of the brain (McCarthy and Arnold, 2011; Arnold, 2014; Cox et al., 2014). The expression of tyrosine hydroxylase (TH) in dopamine neurons of the murine midbrain differs by sex, and it is higher in male mice. The higher TH expression is due to *Sry*, which is a dominant testis-determining gene of the mammalian Y chromosome (Lovell-Badge and Robertson, 1990), because the TH expression is reduced by suppression of *Sry* expression (Dewing et al., 2006). Moreover, other sex chromosome genes also contribute to sex differences in TH expression, which is revealed by the four core genotypes model (Carruth et al., 2002). The four core genotypes model consists of mice in which the complement of sex chromosomes (XX vs. XY) is made independently of gonadal sex (Arnold and Chen, 2009). It was revealed by studies using the four core genotypes model that vasopressin neural fibers in the LS, which are greater in gonadal males than gonadal females, is also influenced by the complement of sex chromosomes: the amount of vasopressin neural fibers is increased by the existence of the Y chromosome independently of gonadal sex (De Vries et al., 2002; Gatewood et al., 2006).

Regarding the LSi, the decrease in the number of LSi neurons in male rats by neonatal castration is prevented following injection with androstendione every other day during PD1-19 (Segovia et al., 2009). This finding suggests that androgens have an effect during the neonatal to prepubertal periods and are necessary for the formation of the male-typical structures of the LSi. The sex difference in LSi volume of rats is found on PD31, but not on PD16 (Tsukahara et al., 2004), indicating that this sex difference emerges during the prepubertal period between PD16 and PD31. Additionally, control of cell number by apoptotic cell death contributes to creating sex differences in cell number in several SDNs (Forger, 2009; Tsukahara, 2009). We found that the number of apoptotic cells in the male LSi is larger than that of the female LSi on PD16 (Tsukahara et al., 2004). The sex difference in the loss of cells by apoptosis during the late postnatal period is a contributing factor for producing the sex difference in neuron number of the LSi in adulthood.

Sex difference in the lordosis-inhibiting system in the LS

Development of the lordosis-inhibiting neural system is critical for defeminization of sexual behavioral patterns in male rats. In adult female rats, the actions of estradiol in the brain are a prerequisite for increasing sexual receptivity followed by lordosis display. However, estradiol, which induces lordosis in adult female rats, is ineffective in adult male rats, partially because the LS inhibits lordosis independently of estradiol (Satou and Yamanouchi, 1999). The LS of female rats also functions to inhibit lordosis, but this may be exhibited only in the anestrous phase, when the level of estradiol in blood is low. Direct implantation of E_2 into the LS enhances the lordosis response in ovariectomized female rats that are subcutaneously treated with a low dose of EB in combination with progesterone (Satou and Yamanouchi, 1999). However, the treatment with EB and progesterone without E_2-implantation is not sufficient for inducing the maximal level of sexual receptivity in ovariectomized rats (Satou and Yamanouchi, 1999). In contrast, direct implantation of E_2 into the LS does not stimulate lordotic activity in castrated male rats receiving the same hormonal treatment (Satou and Yamanouchi, 1999). The number of Fos-expressing cells in the LS of female rats is increased by vaginocervical stimulation, and this increase in EB- and progesterone-treated ovariectomized rats is significantly smaller than that in vehicle-treated ovariectomized rats (Pfaus et al., 1996). This may support the possibility that the neuronal activity of the female LS, which is related to the inhibition of lordosis, is lowered by estradiol. Thus, it appears that female rats can be relieved of the inhibitory influence over lordosis by the direct actions of estradiol in the LS, while the lordosis-inhibiting function of the male LS cannot be released by estradiol. Moreover, it is reported that implantation of dihydrotestosterone into the LS inhibits lordosis in female rats (Tobet and Baum, 1982).

The mechanisms underlying the difference in the response of the LS to estradiol between the sexes and the resulting sex difference in inhibitory regulation of lordosis are yet to be shown. Long-term treatment with E_2 increases the number of synapses in the LS of adult female rats, whereas this treatment fails to increase the number of synapses in the LS of adult male rats (Miyakawa and Arai, 1987), indicating a possible sexually dimorphic synaptic response to estrogens in the LS. Neural projections from the LSi to MCG, which are involved in the inhibition of lordosis (Tsukahara and Yamanouchi, 2001), are sexually dimorphic. The number of LSi neurons that were labeled by FG, a retrograde neurotracer, injected into the MCG is greater in female rats than male rats (Tsukahara and Yamanouchi, 2002; Tsukahara et al., 2003) (**Figures 4A,B**). The sex difference in the neural connectivity between the LSi and MCG is presumably related to the sex difference in inhibitory regulation of lordosis.

Formation of sexually dimorphic LS-MCG connections

Estradiol, which is locally synthesized in the brain from testosterone by aromatase in the perinatal period, affects the brain by masculinizing and defeminizing sexual behavioral patterns in rodents (McEwen et al., 1977; MacLusky et al., 1979; MacLusky and Naftolin, 1981). Injection of an anti-androgen drug or an aromatase inhibitor into pregnant rats enhances lordotic activity of offspring in both sexes in adulthood (Clemens and Gladue, 1978; Gladue and Clemens, 1978, 1982). Male rats castrated on the day of birth show lordosis behavior when they are treated with ovarian sex steroids in adulthood (Feder and Whalen, 1965). In contrast, treatment with testosterone propionate, an aromatizable androgen, on PD1 decreases lordotic activity in rats of both sexes (Gladue and Clemens, 1982). This effect of testosterone propionate may be mimicked by estradiol, because lordotic activity of female rats and neonatally castrated male rats is reduced by EB injection on PD5 (Whalen and Nadler, 1963; Feder and Whalen, 1965; Brown-Grant, 1975). Thus, defeminization of the neural systems regulating lordosis proceeds under the influence of aromatized testosterone originating from the testes during the perinatal period in rats.

The perinatal period, when aromatizable testicular testosterone is able to act as an agent for masculinization and defeminization of the brain, is not the sole stage but the initial stage of sex steroid-dependent sexual differentiation of the brain in rodents (Schulz et al., 2009a; Juraska et al., 2013). In the classic view of brain sexual differentiation, estradiol has been long considered to affect the brain during the perinatal period to masculinize and defeminize the brain. However, in addition to this action, estradiol was recently shown to play an active role in feminizing the brain during the prepubertal to adolescent period. Female aromatase knockout mice, which are deficient in the production of estradiol from testosterone, showed low levels of lordotic activity even after being treated with E_2 and progesterone at adulthood (Bakker et al., 2002). The decreased lordotic activity in female aromatase knockout mice is recovered by injection of EB between PD16 and PD26, whereas EB injection between PD6 and PD16 has no effect (Brock et al., 2011). On the other hand, treatment with EB during PD6 to PD16 increases female-directed mounting behavior in testosterone-treated ovariectomized mice in adulthood, whereas there is no significant effect of EB treatment during PD16 to PD26 (Brock et al., 2011). In postnatal mice, the synthesis of estradiol in the ovary starts from PD7 (Mannan and O'Shaughnessy, 1991). Thus, the neural substrate involved in the regulation of lordosis is defeminized in males by estradiol originating from testicular testosterone during the perinatal period and conversely feminized in females by estradiol that is synthesized from the ovary during the late postnatal and prepubertal period. In males, testicular testosterone during the prepubertal period seems also to participate in the organization of sexual behavior. Indeed, prepubertal testosterone masculinizes and defeminizes sexual behavioral patterns in male hamsters (Schulz et al., 2004, 2009b).

The number of LSi neurons that were labeled by FG injected into the MCG is greater in ovariectomized female rats than castrated male rats with or without E_2 treatment at adulthood (Tsukahara and Yamanouchi, 2002). This indicates that sexually

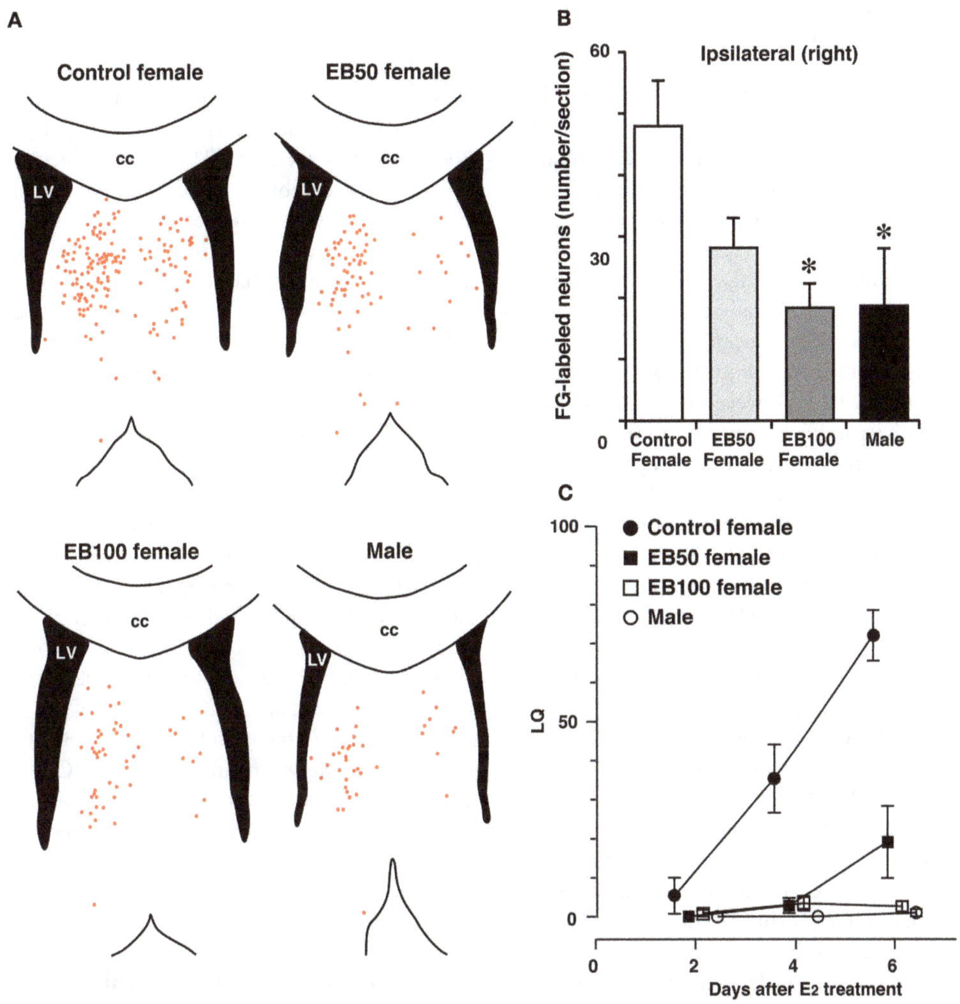

FIGURE 4 | Sex difference in neural projection from the LSi to MCG and effects of postnatal treatment with estradiol benzoate (EB) in the formation of the neural projection. Distribution of Fluoro-Gold (FG)-labeled neurons in the LS **(A)** and the number of FG-labeled neurons in the LSi **(B)** of female and male rats that received FG injection into the MCG. Female rats were subcutaneously injected with 50 or 100 μg of EB or vehicle on postnatal day 5 (day 1 = date of birth), and they were ovariectomized and treated with estradiol in adulthood (EB50, EB100, and control female groups). Male rats were castrated and treated with estradiol in adulthood. Each red dot of the line drawings of **(A)** indicates a FG-labeled neuronal cell body. Postnatal EB treatment dose-dependently decreased the number of FG-labeled neurons in the LSi of female rats, resulting in elimination of sex differences in the number of FG-labeled neurons. cc, corpus callosum; LV, lateral ventricle. *$p < 0.05$ vs. control female. **(C)** The mean LQ of control, EB50, EB100 female rats, and male rats. Postnatal EB treatment dose-dependently decreased lordotic activity of female rats (modified from Tsukahara et al., 2003).

dimorphic neural connectivity between the LSi and MCG is not influenced by estradiol in adulthood. In contrast, estradiol in the postnatal period is a key molecule for the sexually dimorphic formation of LSi-MCG neural connections. The number of LSi neurons projecting to the MCG in female rats is dose-dependently decreased by treatment with EB on PD5 (Tsukahara et al., 2003) (**Figures 4A,B**). Moreover, this hormonal treatment decreases lordotic activity of adult female rats in a dose-dependent fashion (**Figure 4C**). Performance of lordosis in adult female rats can be decreased by neonatal treatment with an ERα agonist, but not an ERβ agonist (Patchev et al., 2004; Kanaya and Yamanouchi, 2012). The LSi of postnatal rats expresses ERα but not ERβ (Perez et al., 2003). Thus, defeminization of sexual behavior partly results from the development of the male LS, which contains less neuron projecting axons to the MCG than the female LS and inhibits lordosis independently of estradiol, under the influence of aromatized testosterone binding with ERα during the postnatal period. In contrast to estradiol originating from testicular testosterone during the postnatal period, estradiol that is secreted from the ovaries before puberty acts to feminize the neural substrate regulating lordosis behavior (Brock et al., 2011). Ovarian estradiol during the prepubertal period may contribute to the development of the female LS, which contains many more neuron projecting axons to the MCG than the male LS, resulting in the release from the inhibitory influence of the LS on lordosis in female rats by the direct action of estradiol at adulthood. The effect of prepubertal estradiol on the formation of sexually dimorphic LSi-MCG neural projection remains to be investigated.

In addition to sex steroids, genetic differences between males having a single X chromosome and a Y chromosome and females having two X chromosomes, which could cause sex-specific gene expression in the brain independently of sex steroids, is a sex-biasing factor in behavioral expression (Cox et al., 2014). Steroidogenic factor 1 (SF-1) is a transcriptional factor required for gonadal development, and therefore SF-1 knockout mice of both sexes are not exposed to endogenous gonadal steroids and have female external phenotypes regardless of genetic sex (Ingraham et al., 1994; Grgurevic et al., 2012). According to one report, lordotic activity was drastically decreased in EB- and progesterone-treated SF-1 knockout mice in comparison to wild-type ovariectomized female mice that bore the same hormonal treatment (Grgurevic et al., 2012). However, there was still a sex difference in lordotic activity in SF-1 knockout mice, and the LQ of SF-1 knockout female mice was significantly higher than that of SF-1 knockout male mice (Grgurevic et al., 2012). This finding suggests that sex chromosome effects partly contribute to the sexual differentiation of sexual behavioral patterns. Genes of the X chromosomes may promote behavioral feminization, or genes of the Y chromosome may induce behavioral defeminization of mice.

The mechanisms responsible for postnatal estradiol-dependent, sexually dimorphic formation of the LSi-MCG neural connections remain to be investigated. There are several potential mechanistic explanations. On PD16, male rats have a significantly greater number of apoptotic cells in the LSi than female rats (Tsukahara et al., 2004). The sex difference in postnatal apoptosis may be partially related to formation of the sexually dimorphic LSi-MCG neural connection. However, not all neurons killed by apoptosis during the postnatal period may be fated to project axons to the MCG, even if they survive and elongate axons. Moreover, sex differences in apoptosis arise on PD16, after PD5 when EB exhibits significant effects on the sexually dimorphic formation of the LSi-MCG neural connection. Epigenetic changes in the developing brain are caused by transitory exposure to estradiol during the perinatal period. The epigenetic changes caused by estradiol exhibit long-lasting effects, inducing permanent sex differences in the morphology and function of the brain (Nugent et al., 2011; Matsuda et al., 2012). Although the time lag between EB actions and sex differences arising in apoptosis may be explained by epigenetic regulation by estradiol, further studies are needed to clarify the involvement of postnatal apoptosis on the estradiol-dependent sexually dimorphic formation of LSi-MCG neural projections. It is also possible that sex differences in LSi-MCG neural projections are due to a sex difference in terminal arborization of LSi neurons at the MCG. The female LSi would contain many more FG-labeled neurons than the male LSi if terminal arborization of LSi neurons projecting to the MCG showed more complexity in female rats. However, there is no evidence for sex differences in the terminal arborization in the MCG. One report shows that daily subcutaneous injections of EB for 20 days increases the number of nerve terminals and synapses in the MCG of ovariectomized rats (Chung et al., 1988). This report suggests that estradiol increases synaptic plasticity in the MCG of female rats. However, sexually dimorphic neural connectivity between the LSi and MCG is not influenced by estradiol in adulthood (Tsukahara and Yamanouchi, 2002).

Several lines of evidence indicate that estradiol modulates axon outgrowth. Axon outgrowth of cultured neurons originating from the fetal hypothalamus is promoted by E_2 (Cambiasso et al., 2000; Carrer et al., 2005). The neural projection from the BNSTp to the AVPV exhibits a sex difference. It is more prominent in male rats and this sex difference is dependent on the effects of testosterone in the AVPV in the postnatal period (Ibanez et al., 2001). This suggests that testosterone, or its metabolite estradiol, induces production of a chemotrophic factor at the target of neural projections. This chemotrophic factor directs the innervation by projection neurons to produce the sexually dimorphic neural projections. It is also known that estradiol has opposite effects on axon outgrowth. The density of mesencephalic serotonergic fibers in the medial preoptic nucleus of male rats is lower than that of female rats, and perinatal treatment with testosterone propionate masculinizes the serotonergic fibers in female rats (Simerly et al., 1985). Neurite growth of cultured serotoninergic neurons, which originate from the mesencephalon of rat embryos and express ERα and ERβ, is inhibited by EB (Lu et al., 2004). Both the LSi and MCG during the postnatal period are presumably the action sites of estradiol, because ERα is expressed in both regions in postnatal rats (Perez et al., 2003). Neurons of the LS elongate axons to the MCG during the period between PD5 and PD15, and most of the axons complete termination at the MCG on PD15 (Kouki and Yamanouchi, 2007). Aromatized testosterone originating from the testes in the perinatal period may affect the LSi and/or MCG to suppress axon outgrowth from the LSi to MCG, resulting in the formation of sexually dimorphic neural connections between the LSi and MCG.

SUMMARY AND FUTURE DIRECTIONS

The LS plays an inhibitory role in the regulation of lordosis in rats of both sexes. For male rats, the LS is important for suppressing heterotypical sexual behavior. For female rats, the LS is important for suppressing sexual behavior in the anestrous phase. The LS functionally and anatomically links to the MCG, but not to the VMN, in the inhibitory regulation of lordosis. Lordosis-inhibiting neurons are located in the LSi, and they project axons to the MCG. The neural connection between the LSi and MCG is sexually dimorphic. There are greater numbers of LSi neurons projecting to the MCG in female rats than in male rats. The inhibitory regulation of lordosis by the LS differs between sexes with respect to responsiveness to estradiol: female rats can be relieved of the inhibitory influence on lordosis by the direct actions of estradiol in the LS, while inhibition of lordosis by the LS cannot be released by estradiol in male rats. Sexually dimorphic neural connections between the LSi and MCG form the morphological basis of the sex difference in the inhibitory regulation of lordosis by the LS. Further studies are needed to examine estrogen signaling in the LSi, and how this modulates activity of lordosis-inhibiting neurons in female rats. Additionally, how LSi neurons project to the MCG and inhibit lordosis independently of estradiol in male rats needs to be investigated. Defeminization of sexual behavioral patterns by estradiol during the postnatal period may partly result from the sexual differentiation of the

LS. Estradiol in the postnatal period serves as a key molecule to form male-like LSi-MCG neural pathways. However, it remains to be determined which mechanisms form these sexually dimorphic LSi-MCG neural projections and how prepubertal estradiol contributes to the formation of female-like LSi-MCG neural connection. Accumulating evidence has provided further insights on the control of sexual behaviors in rodent models. However, the mechanisms responsible for the inhibitory regulation of lordosis are less well understood. Therefore, further studies are needed to better our understanding of female reproduction and sexual differentiation of the brain.

ACKNOWLEDGMENTS

This study was supported by a Grant-in-Aid for Scientific Research from the Ministry of Education, Culture, Sports, Science and Technology of Japan (25670114) to Shinji Tsukahara and Kibankeisei 2010 to Korehito Yamanouchi.

REFERENCES

Agmo, A., Soria, P., and Paredes, R. (1989). GABAergic drugs and lordosis behavior in the female rat. *Horm. Behav.* 23, 368–380. doi: 10.1016/0018-506X(89)90050-0

Ahmed, E. I., Zehr, J. L., Schulz, K. M., Lorenz, B. H., Doncarlos, L. L., and Sisk, C. L. (2008). Pubertal hormones modulate the addition of new cells to sexually dimorphic brain regions. *Nat. Neurosci.* 11, 995–997. doi: 10.1038/nn.2178

Albert, D. J. (1980). Hyperreactivity following temporary chemical lesions in the region ventral to the anterior septum but not in the anterior olfactory nucleus, the lateral olfactory tract, or the olfactory bulb. *Physiol. Behav.* 25, 481–483. doi: 10.1016/0031-9384(80)90292-9

Albert, D. J., and Wong, R. C. (1978). Hyperreactivity, muricide, and intraspecific aggression in the rat produced by infusion of local anesthetic into the lateral septum or surrounding areas. *J. Comp. Physiol. Psychol.* 92, 1062–1073. doi: 10.1037/h0077524

Arnold, A. P. (2014). Conceptual frameworks and mouse models for studying sex differences in physiology and disease: why compensation changes the game. *Exp. Neurol.* 259, 2–9. doi: 10.1016/j.expneurol.2014.01.021

Arnold, A. P., and Chen, X. (2009). What does the "four core genotypes" mouse model tell us about sex differences in the brain and other tissues? *Front. Neuroendocrinol.* 30, 1–9. doi: 10.1016/j.yfrne.2008.11.001

Bakker, J., Honda, S., Harada, N., and Balthazart, J. (2002). The aromatase knockout mouse provides new evidence that estradiol is required during development in the female for the expression of sociosexual behaviors in adulthood. *J. Neurosci.* 22, 9104–9112.

Barbaresi, P. (2007). Cellular and subcellular localization of the GABA(B) receptor 1a/b subunit in the rat periaqueductal gray matter. *J. Comp. Neurol.* 505, 478–492. doi: 10.1002/cne.21509

Barfield, R. J., and Chen, J. J. (1977). Activation of estrous behavior in ovariectomized rats by intracerebral implants of estradiol benzoate. *Endocrinology* 101, 1716–1725. doi: 10.1210/endo-101-6-1716

Bednar, I., Forsberg, G., and Sodersten, P. (1987). Inhibition of sexual behavior in female rats by intracerebral injections of Met-enkephalin in combination with an inhibitor of enkephalin degrading enzymes. *Neurosci. Lett.* 79, 341–345. doi: 10.1016/0304-3940(87)90456-3

Beitz, A. J. (1995). "Periaqueductal gray," in *The Rat Nervous System, 2nd Edn.*, ed G. Paxinos (San Diego, CA: Academic Press), 173–182.

Blasberg, M. E., and Clark, A. S. (1997). Anabolic-androgenic steroid effects on sexual receptivity in ovariectomized rats. *Horm. Behav.* 32, 201–208. doi: 10.1006/hbeh.1997.1422

Boudin, H., Pelaprat, D., Rostene, W., and Beaudet, A. (1996). Cellular distribution of neurotensin receptors in rat brain: immunohistochemical study using an antipeptide antibody against the cloned high affinity receptor. *J. Comp. Neurol.* 373, 76–89.

Brock, O., Baum, M. J., and Bakker, J. (2011). The development of female sexual behavior requires prepubertal estradiol. *J. Neurosci.* 31, 5574–5578. doi: 10.1523/JNEUROSCI.0209-11.2011

Brown-Grant, K. (1975). A re-examination of the lordosis response in female rats given high doses of testosterone propionate or estradiol benzoate in the neonatal period. *Horm. Behav.* 6, 351–378. doi: 10.1016/0018-506X(75)90004-5

Calizo, L. H., and Flanagan-Cato, L. M. (2003). Hormonal-neural integration in the female rat ventromedial hypothalamus: triple labeling for estrogen receptor-alpha, retrograde tract tracing from the periaqueductal gray, and mating-induced Fos expression. *Endocrinology* 144, 5430–5440. doi: 10.1210/en.2003-0331

Cambiasso, M. J., Colombo, J. A., and Carrer, H. F. (2000). Differential effect of oestradiol and astroglia-conditioned media on the growth of hypothalamic neurons from male and female rat brains. *Eur. J. Neurosci.* 12, 2291–2298. doi: 10.1046/j.1460-9568.2000.00120.x

Carrer, H. F., Cambiasso, M. J., and Gorosito, S. (2005). Effects of estrogen on neuronal growth and differentiation. *J. Steroid Biochem. Mol. Biol.* 93, 319–323. doi: 10.1016/j.jsbmb.2004.12.007

Carruth, L. L., Reisert, I., and Arnold, A. P. (2002). Sex chromosome genes directly affect brain sexual differentiation. *Nat. Neurosci.* 5, 933–934. doi: 10.1038/nn922

Chung, S. K., Pfaff, D. W., and Cohen, R. S. (1988). Estrogen-induced alterations in synaptic morphology in the midbrain central gray. *Exp. Brain Res.* 69, 522–530. doi: 10.1007/BF00247306

Clemens, L. G., and Gladue, B. A. (1978). Feminine sexual behavior in rats enhanced by prenatal inhibition of androgen aromatization. *Horm. Behav.* 11, 190–201. doi: 10.1016/0018-506X(78)90048-X

Cox, K. H., Bonthuis, P. J., and Rissman, E. F. (2014). Mouse model systems to study sex chromosome genes and behavior: relevance to humans. *Front. Neuroendocrinol.* doi: 10.1016/j.yfrne.2013.12.004. [Epub ahead of print].

Daniels, D., Miselis, R. R., and Flanagan-Cato, L. M. (1999). Central neuronal circuit innervating the lordosis-producing muscles defined by transneuronal transport of pseudorabies virus. *J. Neurosci.* 19, 2823–2833.

Davidson, J. M., Rodgers, C. H., Smith, E. R., and Bloch, G. J. (1968). Stimulation of female sex behavior in adrenalectomized rats with estrogen alone. *Endocrinology* 82, 193–195. doi: 10.1210/endo-82-1-193

De Vries, G. J., Rissman, E. F., Simerly, R. B., Yang, L. Y., Scordalakes, E. M., Auger, C. J., et al. (2002). A model system for study of sex chromosome effects on sexually dimorphic neural and behavioral traits. *J. Neurosci.* 22, 9005–9014.

Dewing, P., Chiang, C. W., Sinchak, K., Sim, H., Fernagut, P. O., Kelly, S., et al. (2006). Direct regulation of adult brain function by the male-specific factor SRY. *Curr. Biol.* 16, 415–420. doi: 10.1016/j.cub.2006.01.017

Dohanich, G. P., and Clemens, L. G. (1983). Inhibition of estrogen-activated sexual behavior by androgens. *Horm. Behav.* 17, 366–373. doi: 10.1016/0018-506X(83)90046-6

Dornan, W. A., Peterson, M., Matuszewich, L., and Malen, P. (1991). Ibotenic acid-induced lesions of the medial zona incerta decrease lordosis behavior in the female rat. *Behav. Neurosci.* 105, 210–214. doi: 10.1037/0735-7044.105.1.210

Feder, H. H., and Whalen, R. E. (1965). Feminine behavior in neonatally castrated and estrogen-treated male rats. *Science* 147, 306–307. doi: 10.1126/science.147.3655.306

Flanagan-Cato, L. M. (2011). Sex differences in the neural circuit that mediates female sexual receptivity. *Front. Neuroendocrinol.* 32, 124–136. doi: 10.1016/j.yfrne.2011.02.008

Forger, N. G. (2009). Control of cell number in the sexually dimorphic brain and spinal cord. *J. Neuroendocrinol.* 21, 393–399. doi: 10.1111/j.1365-2826.2009.01825.x

Gatewood, J. D., Wills, A., Shetty, S., Xu, J., Arnold, A. P., Burgoyne, P. S., et al. (2006). Sex chromosome complement and gonadal sex influence aggressive and parental behaviors in mice. *J. Neurosci.* 26, 2335–2342. doi: 10.1523/JNEUROSCI.3743-05.2006

Gladue, B. A., and Clemens, L. G. (1978). Androgenic influences on feminine sexual behavior in male and female rats: defeminization blocked by prenatal antiandrogen treatment. *Endocrinology* 103, 1702–1709. doi: 10.1210/endo-103-5-1702

Gladue, B. A., and Clemens, L. G. (1982). Development of feminine sexual behavior in the rat: androgenic and temporal influences. *Physiol. Behav.* 29, 263–267. doi: 10.1016/0031-9384(82)90013-0

Gorzalka, B. B., and Gray, D. S. (1981). Receptivity, rejection and reactivity in female rats following kainic acid and electrolytic septal lesions. *Physiol. Behav.* 26, 39–44. doi: 10.1016/0031-9384(81)90076-7

Grgurevic, N., Budefeld, T., Spanic, T., Tobet, S. A., and Majdic, G. (2012). Evidence that sex chromosome genes affect sexual differentiation of female sexual behavior. *Horm. Behav.* 61, 719–724. doi: 10.1016/j.yhbeh.2012.03.008

Hennessey, A. C., Camak, L., Gordon, F., and Edwards, D. A. (1990). Connections between the pontine central gray and the ventromedial hypothalamus are essential for lordosis in female rats. *Behav. Neurosci.* 104, 477–488. doi: 10.1037/0735-7044.104.3.477

Hennessey, A. C., Wallen, K., and Edwards, D. A. (1986). Preoptic lesions increase the display of lordosis by male rats. *Brain Res.* 370, 21–28. doi: 10.1016/0006-8993(86)91100-5

Ibanez, M. A., Gu, G., and Simerly, R. B. (2001). Target-dependent sexual differentiation of a limbic-hypothalamic neural pathway. *J. Neurosci.* 21, 5652–5659.

Ingraham, H. A., Lala, D. S., Ikeda, Y., Luo, X., Shen, W. H., Nachtigal, M. W., et al. (1994). The nuclear receptor steroidogenic factor 1 acts at multiple levels of the reproductive axis. *Genes Dev.* 8, 2302–2312. doi: 10.1101/gad.8.19.2302

Jakab, R. L., and Leranth, C. (1995). "Septum," in *The Rat Nervous System, 2nd Edn.*, ed G. Paxinos (San Diego, CA: Academic Press), 405–442.

Juraska, J. M., Sisk, C. L., and Doncarlos, L. L. (2013). Sexual differentiation of the adolescent rodent brain: hormonal influences and developmental mechanisms. *Horm. Behav.* 64, 203–210. doi: 10.1016/j.yhbeh.2013.05.010

Kakeyama, M., and Yamanouchi, K. (1992). Lordosis in male rats: the facilitatory effect of mesencephalic dorsal raphe nucleus lesion. *Physiol. Behav.* 51, 181–184. doi: 10.1016/0031-9384(92)90221-M

Kakeyama, M., and Yamanouchi, K. (1994). Two types of lordosis-inhibiting systems in male rats: dorsal raphe nucleus lesions and septal cuts. *Physiol. Behav.* 56, 189–192. doi: 10.1016/0031-9384(94)90278-X

Kakeyama, M., and Yamanouchi, K. (1996). Inhibitory effect of baclofen on lordosis in female and male rats with dorsal raphe nucleus lesion or septal cut. *Neuroendocrinology* 63, 290–296. doi: 10.1159/000126968

Kanaya, M., and Yamanouchi, K. (2012). Defeminization of brain functions by a single injection of estrogen receptor alpha or beta agonist in neonatal female rats. *Neuroendocrinology* 95, 297–304. doi: 10.1159/000332128

King, T. R., and Nance, D. M. (1985). The effects of unilateral frontolateral hypothalamic knife cuts and asymmetrical unilateral septal lesions on lordosis behavior of rats. *Physiol. Behav.* 35, 955–959. doi: 10.1016/0031-9384(85)90265-3

Kondo, Y., Koizumi, T., Arai, Y., Kakeyama, M., and Yamanouchi, K. (1993). Functional relationships between mesencephalic central gray and septum in regulating lordosis in female rats: effect of dual lesions. *Brain Res. Bull.* 32, 635–638. doi: 10.1016/0361-9230(93)90166-9

Kondo, Y., Shinoda, A., Yamanouchi, K., and Arai, Y. (1990). Role of septum and preoptic area in regulating masculine and feminine sexual behavior in male rats. *Horm. Behav.* 24, 421–434. doi: 10.1016/0018-506X(90)90019-T

Kouki, T., and Yamanouchi, K. (2007). Postnatal development of septal projections to the midbrain central gray in female rats: tract-tracing analysis with DiI. *Neurosci. Lett.* 411, 37–41. doi: 10.1016/j.neulet.2006.09.085

Lovell-Badge, R., and Robertson, E. (1990). XY female mice resulting from a heritable mutation in the primary testis-determining gene, Tdy. *Development* 109, 635–646.

Lu, H., Nishi, M., Matsuda, K., and Kawata, M. (2004). Estrogen reduces the neurite growth of serotonergic cells expressing estrogen receptors. *Neurosci. Res.* 50, 23–28. doi: 10.1016/j.neures.2004.06.010

Luine, V., Cowell, J., and Frankfurt, M. (1991). GABAergic-serotonergic interactions in regulating lordosis. *Brain Res.* 556, 171–174. doi: 10.1016/0006-8993(91)90564-C

MacLusky, N. J., Lieberburg, I., and Mcewen, B. S. (1979). The development of estrogen receptor systems in the rat brain: perinatal development. *Brain Res.* 178, 129–142. doi: 10.1016/0006-8993(79)90093-3

MacLusky, N. J., and Naftolin, F. (1981). Sexual differentiation of the central nervous system. *Science* 211, 1294–1302. doi: 10.1126/science.6163211

Mannan, M. A., and O'Shaughnessy, P. J. (1991). Steroidogenesis during postnatal development in the mouse ovary. *J. Endocrinol.* 130, 101–106. doi: 10.1677/joe.0.1300101

Mathews, D., and Edwards, D. A. (1977). Involvement of the ventromedial and anterior hypothalamic nuclei in the hormonal induction of receptivity in the female rat. *Physiol. Behav.* 19, 319–326. doi: 10.1016/0031-9384(77)90345-6

Matsuda, K. I., Mori, H., and Kawata, M. (2012). Epigenetic mechanisms are involved in sexual differentiation of the brain. *Rev. Endocr. Metab. Disord.* 13, 163–171. doi: 10.1007/s11154-012-9202-z

Mazzucco, C. A., Walker, H. A., Pawluski, J. L., Lieblich, S. E., and Galea, L. A. (2008). ERalpha, but not ERbeta, mediates the expression of sexual behavior in the female rat. *Behav. Brain Res.* 191, 111–117. doi: 10.1016/j.bbr.2008.03.016

McCarthy, M. M., and Arnold, A. P. (2011). Reframing sexual differentiation of the brain. *Nat. Neurosci.* 14, 677–683. doi: 10.1038/nn.2834

McCarthy, M. M., Felzenberg, E., Robbins, A., Pfaff, D. W., and Schwartz-Giblin, S. (1995). Infusions of diazepam and allopregnanolone into the midbrain central gray facilitate open-field behavior and sexual receptivity in female rats. *Horm. Behav.* 29, 279–295. doi: 10.1006/hbeh.1995.1020

Mccarthy, M. M., Masters, D. B., Rimvall, K., Schwartz-Giblin, S., and Pfaff, D. W. (1994). Intracerebral administration of antisense oligodeoxynucleotides to GAD65 and GAD67 mRNAs modulate reproductive behavior in the female rat. *Brain Res.* 636, 209–220. doi: 10.1016/0006-8993(94)91019-7

McCarthy, M. M., Pfaff, D. W., and Schwartz-Giblin, S. (1991). Midbrain central gray GABAA receptor activation enhances, and blockade reduces, sexual behavior in the female rat. *Exp. Brain Res.* 86, 108–116. doi: 10.1007/BF00231045

McEwen, B. S., Lieberburg, I., Chaptal, C., and Krey, L. C. (1977). Aromatization: important for sexual differentiation of the neonatal rat brain. *Horm. Behav.* 9, 249–263. doi: 10.1016/0018-506X(77)90060-5

Micevych, P., and Christensen, A. (2012). Membrane-initiated estradiol actions mediate structural plasticity and reproduction. *Front. Neuroendocrinol.* 33, 331–341. doi: 10.1016/j.yfrne.2012.07.003

Micevych, P., and Sinchak, K. (2013). Temporal and concentration dependent estradiol effects on neural pathways mediating sexual receptivity. *J. Neuroendocrinol.* 25, 1012–1023. doi: 10.1111/jne.12103

Miyakawa, M., and Arai, Y. (1987). Synaptic plasticity to estrogen in the lateral septum of the adult male and female rats. *Brain Res.* 436, 184–188. doi: 10.1016/0006-8993(87)91574-5

Modianos, D. T., Hitt, J. C., and Popolow, H. B. (1975). Habenular lesions and feminine sexual behavior of ovariectomized rats: diminished responsiveness to the synergistic effects of estrogen and progesterone. *J. Comp. Physiol. Psychol.* 89, 231–237. doi: 10.1037/h0076805

Musatov, S., Chen, W., Pfaff, D. W., Kaplitt, M. G., and Ogawa, S. (2006). RNAi-mediated silencing of estrogen receptor {alpha} in the ventromedial nucleus of hypothalamus abolishes female sexual behaviors. *Proc. Natl. Acad. Sci. U.S.A.* 103, 10456–10460. doi: 10.1073/pnas.0603045103

Nance, D. M., and Myatt, G. A. (1987). Female sexual behavior in the golden hamster following kainic acid lesions in the lateral septal area. *Brain Res. Bull.* 19, 751–754. doi: 10.1016/0361-9230(87)90064-5

Nance, D. M., Shryne, J., and Gorski, R. A. (1975a). Effects of septal lesions on behavioral sensitivity of female rats to gonadal hormones. *Horm. Behav.* 6, 59–64. doi: 10.1016/0018-506X(75)90023-9

Nance, D. M., Shryne, J., and Gorski, R. A. (1975b). Facilitation of female sexual behavior in male rats by septal lesions: an interaction with estrogen. *Horm. Behav.* 6, 289–299. doi: 10.1016/0018-506X(75)90015-X

Nugent, B. M., Schwarz, J. M., and Mccarthy, M. M. (2011). Hormonally mediated epigenetic changes to steroid receptors in the developing brain: implications for sexual differentiation. *Horm. Behav.* 59, 338–344. doi: 10.1016/j.yhbeh.2010.08.009

Ogawa, S., Chan, J., Chester, A. E., Gustafsson, J. A., Korach, K. S., and Pfaff, D. W. (1999). Survival of reproductive behaviors in estrogen receptor beta gene-deficient (betaERKO) male and female mice. *Proc. Natl. Acad. Sci. U.S.A.* 96, 12887–12892. doi: 10.1073/pnas.96.22.12887

Ogawa, S., Eng, V., Taylor, J., Lubahn, D. B., Korach, K. S., and Pfaff, D. W. (1998). Roles of estrogen receptor-alpha gene expression in reproduction-related behaviors in female mice. *Endocrinology* 139, 5070–5081.

Ohnishi, H., Kondo, Y., and Sakuma, Y. (2003). Oestrogen-induced vigorous mounting in female rats carrying hypothalamic knife cuts. *J. Neuroendocrinol.* 15, 602–606. doi: 10.1046/j.1365-2826.2003.01040.x

Osterlund, M., Kuiper, G. G., Gustafsson, J. A., and Hurd, Y. L. (1998). Differential distribution and regulation of estrogen receptor-alpha and -beta mRNA within the female rat brain. *Mol. Brain Res.* 54, 175–180. doi: 10.1016/S0169-328X(97)00351-3

Ottersen, O. P., Hjelle, O. P., Osen, K. K., and Laake, J. H. (1995). "Amino acid transmitters," in *The Rat Nervous System, 2nd Edn.*, ed G. Paxinos (San Diego, CA: Academic Press), 1017–1037.

Ottersen, O. P., and Storm-Mathisen, J. (1984). Glutamate- and GABA-containing neurons in the mouse and rat brain, as demonstrated with a new immunocytochemical technique. *J. Comp. Neurol.* 229, 374–392. doi: 10.1002/cne.902290308

Parsons, B., MacJusky, N. J., Krey, L., Pfaff, D. W., and Mcewen, B. S. (1980). The temporal relationship between estrogen-inducible progestin receptors in the female rat brain and the time course of estrogen activation of mating behavior. *Endocrinology* 107, 774–779. doi: 10.1210/endo-107-3-774

Parsons, B., MacLusky, N. J., Krieger, M. S., Mcewen, B. S., and Pfaff, D. W. (1979). The effects of long-term estrogen exposure on the induction of sexual behavior and measurements of brain estrogen and progestin receptors in the female rat. *Horm. Behav.* 13, 301–313. doi: 10.1016/0018-506X(79)90047-3

Parsons, B., Rainbow, T. C., Pfaff, D. W., and Mcewen, B. S. (1981). Oestradiol, sexual receptivity and cytosol progestin receptors in rat hypothalamus. *Nature* 292, 58–59. doi: 10.1038/292058a0

Patchev, A. V., Gotz, F., and Rohde, W. (2004). Differential role of estrogen receptor isoforms in sex-specific brain organization. *FASEB J.* 18, 1568–1570. doi: 10.1096/fj.04-1959fje

Perez, S. E., Chen, E. Y., and Mufson, E. J. (2003). Distribution of estrogen receptor alpha and beta immunoreactive profiles in the postnatal rat brain. *Dev. Brain Res.* 145, 117–139. doi: 10.1016/S0165-3806(03)00223-2

Pfaff, D. W., Kow, L. M., Loose, M. D., and Flanagan-Cato, L. M. (2008). Reverse engineering the lordosis behavior circuit. *Horm. Behav.* 54, 347–354. doi: 10.1016/j.yhbeh.2008.03.012

Pfaff, D. W., and Sakuma, Y. (1979a). Deficit in the lordosis reflex of female rats caused by lesions in the ventromedial nucleus of the hypothalamus. *J. Physiol.* 288, 203–210.

Pfaff, D. W., and Sakuma, Y. (1979b). Facilitation of the lordosis reflex of female rats from the ventromedial nucleus of the hypothalamus. *J. Physiol.* 288, 189–202.

Pfaff, D. W., Schwartz-Giblin, S., Mccarthy, M. M., and Kow, L.-M. (1994). "Cellular and molecular mechanisms of female reproductive behaviors," in *The Physiology of Reproduction*, eds E. Knobil and J. D. Neil (New York, NY: Raven Press), 107–220.

Pfaus, J. G., Marcangione, C., Smith, W. J., Manitt, C., and Abillamaa, H. (1996). Differential induction of Fos in the female rat brain following different amounts of vaginocervical stimulation: modulation by steroid hormones. *Brain Res.* 741, 314–330. doi: 10.1016/S0006-8993(96)00985-7

Rajendren, G., and Moss, R. L. (1993). The role of the medial nucleus of amygdala in the mating-induced enhancement of lordosis in female rats: the interaction with luteinizing hormone-releasing hormone neuronal system. *Brain Res.* 617, 81–86. doi: 10.1016/0006-8993(93)90616-U

Risold, P. Y., and Swanson, L. W. (1997a). Chemoarchitecture of the rat lateral septal nucleus. *Brain Res. Rev.* 24, 91–113. doi: 10.1016/S0165-0173(97)00008-8

Risold, P. Y., and Swanson, L. W. (1997b). Connections of the rat lateral septal complex. *Brain Res. Rev.* 24, 115–195. doi: 10.1016/S0165-0173(97)00009-X

Sakuma, Y., and Pfaff, D. W. (1979a). Facilitation of female reproductive behavior from mesensephalic central gray in the rat. *Am. J. Physiol.* 237, R278–R284.

Sakuma, Y., and Pfaff, D. W. (1979b). Mesencephalic mechanisms for integration of female reproductive behavior in the rat. *Am. J. Physiol.* 237, R285–R290.

Satou, M., and Yamanouchi, K. (1999). Effect of direct application of estrogen aimed at lateral septum or dorsal raphe nucleus on lordosis behavior: regional and sexual differences in rats. *Neuroendocrinology* 69, 446–452. doi: 10.1159/000054448

Schulz, K. M., Molenda-Figueira, H. A., and Sisk, C. L. (2009a). Back to the future: The organizational-activational hypothesis adapted to puberty and adolescence. *Horm. Behav.* 55, 597–604. doi: 10.1016/j.yhbeh.2009.03.010

Schulz, K. M., Richardson, H. N., Zehr, J. L., Osetek, A. J., Menard, T. A., and Sisk, C. L. (2004). Gonadal hormones masculinize and defeminize reproductive behaviors during puberty in the male Syrian hamster. *Horm. Behav.* 45, 242–249. doi: 10.1016/j.yhbeh.2003.12.007

Schulz, K. M., Zehr, J. L., Salas-Ramirez, K. Y., and Sisk, C. L. (2009b). Testosterone programs adult social behavior before and during, but not after, adolescence. *Endocrinology* 150, 3690–3698. doi: 10.1210/en.2008-1708

Segovia, S., Garcia-Falgueras, A., Perez-Laso, C., Pinos, H., Carrillo, B., Collado, P., et al. (2009). The effects of partial and complete masculinization on the sexual differentiation of nuclei that control lordotic behavior in the male rat. *Behav. Brain Res.* 196, 261–267. doi: 10.1016/j.bbr.2008.09.017

Shipley, M. T., Mclean, J. H., and Behbehani, M. M. (1987). Heterogeneous distribution of neurotensin-like immunoreactive neurons and fibers in the midbrain periaqueductal gray of the rat. *J. Neurosci.* 7, 2025–2034.

Shughrue, P. J., Lane, M. V., and Merchenthaler, I. (1997). Comparative distribution of estrogen receptor-alpha and -beta mRNA in the rat central nervous system. *J. Comp. Neurol.* 388, 507–525.

Simerly, R. B., Swanson, L. W., and Gorski, R. A. (1985). Reversal of the sexually dimorphic distribution of serotonin-immunoreactive fibers in the medial preoptic nucleus by treatment with perinatal androgen. *Brain Res.* 340, 91–98. doi: 10.1016/0006-8993(85)90777-2

Sinchak, K., and Micevych, P. E. (2001). Progesterone blockade of estrogen activation of mu-opioid receptors regulates reproductive behavior. *J. Neurosci.* 21, 5723–5729.

Staiger, J. F., and Nurnberger, F. (1991). The efferent connections of the lateral septal nucleus in the guinea pig: projections to the diencephalon and brainstem. *Cell Tissue Res.* 264, 391–413. doi: 10.1007/BF00319031

Tobet, S. A., and Baum, M. J. (1982). Implantation of dihydrotestosterone propionate into the lateral septum inhibits sexual receptivity in estrogen-primed, ovariectomized rats. *Neuroendocrinology* 34, 333–338. doi: 10.1159/000123323

Tsukahara, S. (2009). Sex differences and the roles of sex steroids in apoptosis of sexually dimorphic nuclei of the preoptic area in postnatal rats. *J. Neuroendocrinol.* 21, 370–376. doi: 10.1111/j.1365-2826.2009.01855.x

Tsukahara, S., Ezawa, N., and Yamanouchi, K. (2003). Neonatal estrogen decreases neural density of teh septum-midbrain central gray conncetion underlying the lordosis-inhibiting system in rats. *Neuroendocrinology* 78, 226–233. doi: 10.1159/000073706

Tsukahara, S., Inami, K., Maekawa, F., Kakeyama, M., Yokoyama, T., Yuji, M., et al. (2004). Postnatal apoptosis, development, and sex difference in the lateral septum of rats. *J. Comp. Neurol.* 475, 177–187. doi: 10.1002/cne.20184

Tsukahara, S., and Yamanouchi, K. (2001). Neurohistological and behavioral evidence for lordosis-inhibiting tract from lateral septum to periaqueductal gray in male rats. *J. Comp. Neurol.* 431, 293–310. doi: 10.1002/1096-9861(20010312)431:33.0.CO;2-M

Tsukahara, S., and Yamanouchi, K. (2002). Sex difference in septal neurons projecting axons to midbrain central gray in rats: a combined double retrograde tracing and ER-immunohistochemical study. *Endocrinology* 143, 285–294. doi: 10.1210/endo.143.1.8588

Tsukahara, S., and Yamanouchi, K. (2003). Distribution of glutamic acid decarboxylase, neurotensin, enkephalin, neuropeptide Y, and cholecystokinin neurons in the septo-preoptic region of male rats. *J. Reprod. Dev.* 49, 67–77. doi: 10.1262/jrd.49.67

Van De Poll, N. E., and Van Dis, H. (1979). The effect of medial preoptic–anterior hypothalamic lesions on bisexual behavior of the male rat. *Brain Res. Bull.* 4, 505–511. doi: 10.1016/0361-9230(79)90035-2

Veening, J. G., Swanson, L. W., Cowan, W. M., Nieuwenhuys, R., and Geeraedts, L. M. (1982). The medial forebrain bundle of the rat. II. An autoradiographic study of the topography of the major descending and ascending components. *J. Comp. Neurol.* 206, 82–108. doi: 10.1002/cne.902060107

Vincent, S. R., Hokfelt, T., and Wu, J. Y. (1982). GABA neuron systems in hypothalamus and the pituitary gland. Immunohistochemical demonstration using antibodies against glutamate decarboxylase. *Neuroendocrinology* 34, 117–125. doi: 10.1159/000123288

Warren, D. W., Haltmeyer, G. C., and Eik-Nes, K. B. (1973). Testosterone in the fetal rat testis. *Biol. Reprod.* 8, 560–565.

Weisz, J., and Ward, I. L. (1980). Plasma testosterone and progesterone titers of pregnant rats, their male and female fetuses, and neonatal offspring. *Endocrinology* 106, 306–316. doi: 10.1210/endo-106-1-306

Whalen, R. E., and Nadler, R. D. (1963). Suppression of the development of female mating behavior by estrogen administered in infancy. *Science* 141, 273–274. doi: 10.1126/science.141.3577.273

Williams, F. G., and Beitz, A. J. (1990a). Ultrastructural morphometric analysis of enkephalin-immunoreactive terminals in the ventrocaudal periaqueductal gray: analysis of their relationship to periaqueductal gray-raphe magnus projection neurons. *Neuroscience* 38, 381–394. doi: 10.1016/0306-4522(90)90036-4

Williams, F. G., and Beitz, A. J. (1990b). Ultrastructural morphometric analysis of GABA-immunoreactive terminals in the ventrocaudal periaqueductal grey: analysis of the relationship of GABA terminals and the GABAA receptor to periaqueductal grey-raphe magnus projection neurons. *J. Neurocytol.* 19, 686–696. doi: 10.1007/BF01188037

Wittmann, W., and Mclennan, I. S. (2013). The bed nucleus of the stria terminalis has developmental and adult forms in mice, with the male bias in the developmental form being dependent on testicular AMH. *Horm. Behav.* 64, 605–610. doi: 10.1016/j.yhbeh.2013.08.017

Woodson, J. C., and Gorski, R. A. (1999). "Structural sex differences in the mammalian brain: reconsidering the male/female dichotomy," in *Sexual*

Differentiation of the Brain, ed A. Matsumoto (Boca Raton, FL: CRC Press LLC), 229–255.

Yamanouchi, K. (1980). Inhibitory and facilitatory neural mechanisms involved in the regulation of lordosis behavior in female rats: effects of dual cuts in the preoptic area and hypothalamus. *Physiol. Behav.* 25, 721–725. doi: 10.1016/0031-9384(80)90375-3

Yamanouchi, K. (1997). "Brain mechanisms inhibiting the expression of heterotypical sexual behavior in rats," in *Neural Control of Reproduction*, eds K.-I. Maeda, H. Tsukamura, and A. Yokoyama (Basel: Karger), 219–235.

Yamanouchi, K., and Arai, Y. (1975). Female lordosis pattern in the male rat induced by estrogen and progesterone: effect of interruption of the dorsal inputs to the preoptic area and hypothalamus. *Endocrinol. Jpn.* 22, 243–246. doi: 10.1507/endocrj1954.22.243

Yamanouchi, K., and Arai, Y. (1976). Heterotypical sexual behavior in male rats: individual difference in lordosis respones. *Endocrinol. Jpn.* 23, 179–182. doi: 10.1507/endocrj1954.23.179

Yamanouchi, K., and Arai, Y. (1977). Possible inhibitory role of the dorsal inputs to the preoptic area and hypothalamus in regulating female sexual behavior in the female rat. *Brain Res.* 127, 296–301. doi: 10.1016/0006-8993(77)90544-3

Yamanouchi, K., and Arai, Y. (1978). Lordosis behaviour in male rats: effects of deafferentation in the preoptic area and hypothalamus. *J. Endocrinol.* 76, 381–382. doi: 10.1677/joe.0.0760381

Yamanouchi, K., and Arai, Y. (1985). Presence of a neural mechanism for the expression of female sexual behaviors in the male rat brain. *Neuroendocrinology* 40, 393–397. doi: 10.1159/000124104

Yamanouchi, K., and Arai, Y. (1989). Lordosis-inhibiting pathway in the lateral hypothalamus: medial forebrain bundle (MFB) transection. *Zool. Sci.* 6, 141–145.

Yamanouchi, K., and Arai, Y. (1990). The septum as origin of a lordosis-inhibiting influence in female rats: effect of neural transection. *Physiol. Behav.* 48, 351–355. doi: 10.1016/0031-9384(90)90326-Y

Yamashita Suzuki, K., and Yamanouchi, K. (1998). Inhibitory pathway for female sexual behavior in male rat brain: effect of medial forebrain bundle (MFB) cuts. *J. Reprod. Dev.* 44, 393–398. doi: 10.1262/jrd.44.393

Zasorin, N. L. (1975). Suppression of lordosis in the hormone-primed female hamster by electrical stimulation of the septal area. *Physiol. Behav.* 14, 595–599. doi: 10.1016/0031-9384(75)90187-0

4

Visual attention for social information and salivary oxytocin levels in preschool children with autism spectrum disorders: an eye-tracking study

Takashi X. Fujisawa[1,2]**, Shiho Tanaka**[1]**, Daisuke N. Saito**[1,2,3]**, Hirotaka Kosaka**[1,2,4] **and Akemi Tomoda**[1,2]*****

[1] Research Center for Child Mental Development, University of Fukui, Fukui, Japan
[2] Department of Child Development, United Graduate School of Child Development, Osaka University, Kanazawa University, Hamamatsu University School of Medicine, Chiba University, University of Fukui, Fukui, Japan
[3] Biomedical Imaging Research Center, University of Fukui, Fukui, Japan
[4] Department of Neuropsychiatry, Faculty of Medical Sciences, University of Fukui, Fukui, Japan

***Correspondence:**
Akemi Tomoda, Research Center for Child Mental Development, University of Fukui, 23-3 Matsuoka-Shimoaizuki, Eiheiji-cho (Yoshida-gun), Fukui 910-1193, Japan
e-mail: atomoda@u-fukui.ac.jp

This study was designed to ascertain the relationship between visual attention for social information and oxytocin (OT) levels in Japanese preschool children with autism spectrum disorder (ASD). We hypothesized that poor visual attention for social information and low OT levels are crucially important risk factors associated with ASD. We measured the pattern of gaze fixation for social information using an eye-tracking system, and salivary OT levels by the Enzyme-Linked Immunosorbent Assay (ELISA). There was a positive association between salivary OT levels and fixation duration for an indicated object area in a finger-pointing movie in typically developing (TD) children. However, no association was found between these variables in children with ASD. Moreover, age decreased an individual's attention to people moving and pointed-at objects, but increased attention for mouth-in-the-face recognition, geometric patterns, and biological motions. Thus, OT levels likely vary during visual attention for social information between TD children and those with ASD. Further, aging in preschool children has considerable effect on visual attention for social information.

Keywords: oxytocin (OT), autism spectrum disorder (ASD), visual attention, preschool children, eye-tracking

INTRODUCTION

Oxytocin (OT), a neuropeptide secreted from the posterior pituitary, has physiological functions in labor and lactation, and there is increasing evidence that OT plays an important role in modulating social behavior in diverse species (Donaldson and Young, 2008; Insel, 2010). In humans, much research has suggested that OT facilitates the ability to infer the mental state of others from the eye region (i.e., Domes et al., 2007b; Guastella et al., 2008, 2010), and can even selectively enhance the memory encoding of faces (Rimmele et al., 2009). OT also modulates trust and generosity in interpersonal relationships (Kosfeld et al., 2005; Zak et al., 2005, 2007; Baumgartner et al., 2008; Kéri et al., 2009). In fact, OT affects the activation of brain areas responsible for emotion, mentalization, and cognitive control, including the amygdala and prefrontal cortex (Kirsch et al., 2005; Domes et al., 2007a; Baumgartner et al., 2008). In addition, oxytocin receptors (OXTR) are expressed in brain areas, such as medial prefrontal cortex (MPFC), dorsal anterior cingulate cortex (dACC), amygdala and dorsal striatum (Landgraf and Neumann, 2004; Skuse and Gallagher, 2009), that are involved in social behavior, including reproductive and maternal behaviors, affiliation and attachment, and reactivity to social stress in nonhuman mammals (Carter, 1998; Ferguson et al., 2000; Young and Wang, 2004). Further, OXTR gene polymorphisms were associated with prosocial behavior in a dictator game and in social value orientations tasks (Israel et al., 2009).

Autism spectrum disorder (ASD) is a common neurodevelopmental disorder affecting around 3.8/1000 boys and 0.8/1000 girls (Taylor et al., 2013). Revised diagnostic criteria for ASDs recently published in the latest Diagnostic and Statistical Manual of Mental Disorders (DSM-5), include two core areas: communication and social deficits, and fixed or repetitive behaviors (American Psychiatric Association, 2013). A core symptom of ASD is indeed the presence of early and persistent deficits in social interaction and social communication. Individuals with ASD experience difficulties in establishing and maintaining eye contact and in processing facial information and intentions (American Psychiatric Association, 2013). Individuals with ASD have particular difficulty in interpreting nonverbal social information such as facial expressions, vocal expressions (Doi et al., 2013), pointing gestures (Paparella et al., 2011), and body gestures (Centelles et al., 2012) that lead to severe social impairment (Hill and Frith, 2003). Recently, many studies have revealed relations between OT and social functioning (e.g., Munesue et al., 2010; Higashida et al., 2012), and have devoted particular attention to OT as a candidate treatment for social impairments in patients with ASD. In fact, plasma OT levels in patients with ASDs are reportedly low (Modahl et al., 1998). Moreover, nasal administration of OT improve social impairments in patients with ASDs

(Andari et al., 2010; Guastella et al., 2010; Kosaka et al., 2012; Watanabe et al., 2014).

Several studies have revealed that patients with ASD have impaired visual attention for social information when compared to individuals that have undergone typical development (e.g., Klin et al., 2002b, 2009; Nakano et al., 2010; Pierce et al., 2011; Jones and Klin, 2013; Sasson and Touchstone, 2014). In that context, eye-tracking technology can provide great benefits for investigating visual attention regarding social information in ASD. This approach enables researchers to measure, with high precision and accuracy, what a participant is looking at and for how long. Moreover, it offers an optimal balance between ecological validity and methodological constraints (Guillon et al., 2014). Eye tracking is therefore a unique method to detect and characterize subtle variations in the spontaneous viewing patterns of individuals with ASD (Klin et al., 2002a, 2003). Moreover, eye-tracking technology is applicable for all populations, from infants to adults, irrespective of their level of non-verbal and verbal ability (Guillon et al., 2014). Therefore, the different aspects of visual attention for social information can be investigated similarly across various participant statuses, such as age, sex, and clinical condition.

The aim of this study was to investigate the relationship between visual attention for social information and salivary OT levels in preschool children with ASD compared to children with typical development. In terms of peripheral OT, studies have reported correlations between plasma and salivary OT concentrations in humans (Carter et al., 2007; Feldman et al., 2011). Although several studies have examined the relationship between social dysfunction and peripheral OT levels, or between social dysfunction and the pattern of visual attention using eye-tracking, the association between the two in preschool children with ASD and typical development remains unclear. Moreover, developmental patterns change with age, and sex differences could exist; thus, it is surprising that these aspects of ASD have not been investigated. Here, we measured the pattern of visual attention for social information and salivary OT levels using eye-tracking and Enzyme-Linked Immunosorbent Assay (ELISA), respectively, to investigate the relationship among these factors. We hypothesized that poor visual attention for social information and low salivary OT levels are crucially important risk factors associated with ASD.

MATERIALS AND METHODS

ETHICS STATEMENT

The Ethics Committee of the University of Fukui approved the study protocol (Assurance # FU24-123), and the parents of all participants gave written informed consent. The experimental protocol was conducted in accordance with the Declaration of Helsinki.

PARTICIPANTS

In this study, 19 preschool children with ASD (16 boys and 3 girls, mean age, 57.9 months; *SD*, 13.6 months) participated along with 60 typically developing (TD) preschoolers (28 boys and 32 girls, mean age, 48.1 months; *SD*, 22.7 months) (**Table 1**). Subjects in the ASD group were predominantly male (84%), whereas TD controls were skewed slightly female (53%). Six children (4 with ASD, 2 TD) were excluded from our final analyses because of non-compliance during testing, which was attributable to fewer than 50% of valid trials in the eye-tracking task or to insufficient saliva samples.

Table 1 | Characteristics of subjects used in the dataset for statistical analysis.

Characteristic	TD	ASD	*p*-value
Subjects numbers (male/female)	60 (28/32)	19 (16/3)	<0.05 (χ^2-test)
Age (month)	48.1 (22.7)	57.9 (13.6)	*n.s.* (*t*-test)
DQ (Kyoto scale)	–	77.7 (19.5)	–
PARS score (peak)	–	20.9 (8.50)	–
PARS score (current)	–	18.6 (8.68)	–
SDQ score	–	17.7 (4.36)	–

TD, Typical Development; ASD, Autism spectrum disorder; DQ, Developmental Quotient; PARS, Pervasive Developmental Disorders Autism Society Japan Rating Scale; SDQ, Strength and Difficulties Questionnaire.

The patients were referred to our laboratory during 2013–2014 for examination of visual attention and OT measurement in saliva. All patients were referred from the Department of Child and Adolescent Psychological Medicine, University of Fukui Hospital. All participants' race/ethnicity was Japanese. Diagnoses were made by one senior pediatric neurologist through interviews and reviews of clinical records, according to the DSM-5 (American Psychiatric Association, 2013). We assessed their developmental status using the developmental quotient (DQ) (Kyoto Scale of Psychological Development), PARS (Pervasive Developmental Disorders Autism Society Japan Rating Scale), and SDQ (Strength and Difficulties Questionnaire). The validity and reliability of the Japanese version of these scales were confirmed (Ikuzawa et al., 2002; Tsujii et al., 2006; Matsuishi et al., 2008; Iizuka et al., 2010). The detailed characteristics of the participants included in the final analysis are summarized in **Table 1**.

To obtain data from normal age-matched typically developed controls, healthy preschool children were recruited as subjects from the community. Kindergarten students were targeted, and none had any physical problem or had encountered any abnormal developmental milestone.

MEASURES OF OT LEVELS IN SALIVA

Saliva samples were collected using Salivettes® (Sarstedt, Rommelsdorft, Germany). Parents were asked to put a roll of cotton in their child's mouth and instructed their child to chew for 1 min until it was saturated with saliva. Two cotton samples were collected by repeating the chewing process twice. Saliva samples were frozen and stored at −80°C in the laboratory. Before the assay was run, saliva samples were lyophilized overnight and kept at −20°C to concentrate them 2–4 times. The dry samples were reconstructed in the assay buffer immediately before analysis using an OT enzyme immunoassay commercial kit (Assay Designs Inc., Ann Arbor, MI). These protocols were consistent with an earlier study for adults (Carter et al., 2007; White-Traut et al., 2009; Feldman et al., 2011; Gordon et al., 2013), as well as one that had been performed on children at the age of 3 years old (Feldman et al., 2013). Each sample was performed in duplicate and concentrations were calculated using the SpectraMax® (Molecular Device, Sunnyvale, California) micro plate reader, according to relevant standard curves. Average intra- and inter-assay coefficients of variation (CV) were 5.7 and 11.7%, respectively.

MEASURES OF THE GAZE PATTERN

We measured each child's gaze pattern using Gazefinder® (JVC Kenwood; Hamamatsu, Japan) for response to social information by visual stimuli. The Gazefinder® used infrared light sources and cameras that were integrated into a 19-inch-thin film transistor monitor (1280 × 1024 pixels). Using corneal reflection techniques, the Gazefinder® records the X and Y coordinates of each child's eye position at a frequency of 50 Hz (i.e., 3000 data collections/min). Stimuli presented by the Gazefinder® consisted of short movies including four categories of social information, which were (A) human faces, (B) people and geometric patterns, (C) bodily motion of a human, and (D) objects with or without finger pointing. These stimuli were set to two areas as areas-of-interest (AOI), which included the eyes and mouth areas in the human face category (31 s), people and geometric image areas in the people and geometric patterns category (32 s), upright and inverted image areas in the motion category (20 s), and lastly, an object with or without pointing (20 s) (**Figure 1**).

PROCEDURE

Testing was executed in a research laboratory located in the Research Center for Child Mental Development at University of Fukui. Children were seated (on a parent's lap when younger than 18 months) 40 cm in front of the eye-tracking monitor. To obtain calibration information, children were first shown images of an animated animal that appeared in one of five locations on the screen. If the calibration quality was poor for any of these points, then the calibration process was repeated. Before the task, children were told that pictures of faces, people, and objects were to be shown on the computer screen and that they should look at them without looking away for as long as possible. Stimulus movies were displayed in a definitive order. Before each trial, an attention-getting animation with a voice saying "Hey! Look!" was presented in the center of the screen to reorient their attention for stimuli.

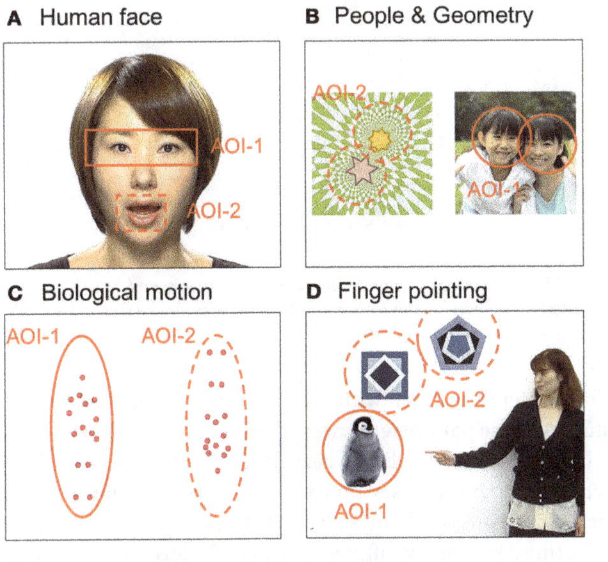

FIGURE 1 | Snapshots of four short movies with each type of social information as stimuli presented by the Gazefinder®: (A) human faces, (B) people and geometric patterns, (C) bodily motions of a human, and (D) objects with or without finger pointing. These stimuli were set as two areas-of-interest (AOI-1 and AOI-2).

STATISTICAL PROCEDURE

We computed the percentage of fixation durations on two AOIs as well as for other areas on the screen, and analyzed them as dependent variables of social attention relevant to the autistic phenotype. Analysis of visual attention for social information between the groups was then conducted using a separate repeated measures analysis of variance (ANOVA) for each primary variable, with a cue type (face, people, motion, and pointing) as the within-subjects variable and group (ASD, TD) as the between group variable. The significance level was set to $p < 0.05$. Statistical analyses were conducted using software (IBM SPSS 20.0 for Windows, Statistical Package for the Social Sciences; IBM).

RESULTS

TYPICAL DEVELOPMENT OF VISUAL ATTENTION FOR SOCIAL INFORMATION AND SALIVARY OT LEVELS

Mean values of salivary OT levels and the mean percentage of fixation durations for each category of social information in TD children are presented in **Table 2**, together with standard errors. Mean values of these variables by sex are also shown. For salivary OT levels and the percentage of fixation durations, we tested the effect of sex difference separately for each variable. First, for the salivary OT levels, no significant difference was observed [$t_{(56)} = 0.35$, *n.s.*], indicating that no sex difference of OT levels existed in either group. Next, for the face stimuli, a significant difference was observed in the % of fixation on the mouth [$t_{(56)} = 1.84$, $p < 0.10$], indicating that female TD children were more attentive to the mouth area in faces than male children, although no sex-related difference of attention for the eye area was found between groups [$t_{(56)} = 0.93$, *n.s.*]. For the people and geometry stimuli, a significant difference was observed in the % of fixation on people stimuli [$t_{(56)} = 3.42$, $p < 0.001$], indicating that female TD children were more attentive to people moving than male children; however, no sex-related difference in attention for geometry patterns was found between groups [$t_{(56)} = 1.52$, *n.s.*]. For bodily motion stimuli, a significant difference was observed in the fixation % on stimuli of upright positions [$t_{(56)} = 3.10$, $p < 0.01$], indicating that female TD children were more attentive to biological motion than were male children, although no sex-related difference in attention for inverted presentation of bodily motion was found between groups [$t_{(56)} = 0.38$, *n.s.*]. Finally, for finger-pointing stimuli, a significant difference was observed in the % of fixation on pointed objects [$t_{(56)} = 2.38$, $p < 0.05$], indicating

Table 2 | Mean values and correlation coefficients of salivary OT levels and gaze fixation parameters in TD children.

		Total ($n = 58$)		Male ($n = 27$)		Female ($n = 31$)		*t*	Correlation		Partial correlation
		Mean	***SD***	**Mean**	***SD***	**Mean**	***SD***		**Age**	**OT level**	**OT level**
Oxytocin levels (pg/ml)		44.5	24.89	45.7	29.78	43.4	20.15	0.35	−0.164	–	–
Face	%Eyes	39.8	13.78	40.1	14.78	39.6	13.09	0.13	−0.090	−0.011	−0.028
	%Mouth	34.4	13.73	**30.9**	13.48	**37.5**	13.42	**1.84**#	**0.401****	−0.106	−0.028
	%Out of AOI	13.4	6.86	14.3	7.89	12.7	5.83	0.93	−0.087	−0.063	−0.087
People and geometry	%People	45.0	15.21	**38.3**	14.95	**50.8**	13.03	**3.42*****	**−0.466****	0.007	−0.059
	%Geometry	29.1	16.54	32.6	19.34	26.0	13.22	1.52	**0.576****	−0.012	0.093
	%Out of AOI	18.0	6.27	18.1	6.02	18.0	6.59	0.06	−0.061	−0.020	−0.032
Biological motion	%Upright	51.6	14.98	**45.6**	14.48	**56.9**	13.50	**3.10****	**0.315***	0.016	0.109
	%Inverted	34.5	13.07	35.2	12.93	33.9	13.38	0.38	0.042	−0.081	−0.078
	%Out of AOI	8.0	7.65	9.6	10.01	6.6	4.46	1.44	−0.154	−0.009	−0.049
Finger pointing	%Pointed	43.0	12.19	**39.1**	12.71	**46.5**	10.80	**2.38***	**−0.352****	**0.281***	**0.273***
	%Non-pointed	10.7	6.77	10.0	6.83	11.2	6.78	0.66	**0.441****	−0.145	−0.075
	%Out of AOI	38.6	10.27	38.2	9.93	38.9	10.70	0.26	0.220	−0.040	−0.001

# $p < 0.10$; *$p < 0.05$; **$p < 0.01$; ***$p < 0.001$.

that female TD children were more attentive to pointed-at objects than male children; however, no sex difference of attention for non-pointed-at objects was found between groups [$t_{(56)} = 0.66$, *n.s.*].

Next, we investigated aging effects for salivary OT levels and fixation durations for each social measure in order to address whether the pattern of attention for social information is dependent on age. We also wanted to address this since the relationship between OT levels and aging in infant and preschool children remains unclear. The correlation coefficients between age, salivary OT levels, and each variable of fixation duration are also presented in **Table 2**. First, no significant correlation was found between age and OT levels. Next, for fixation durations, a significant positive correlation was observed for mouth area of the facial stimuli, geometric pattern stimuli, and upright body position. Significant negative correlations were found for stimuli showing people moving and pointed-at objects in finger-pointing stimuli. These results suggest that aging reduces attention for human movement and for pointed-at objects, but that aging increases a TD child's attention for mouths, geometric patterns, and biological motion. Finally, a significant correlation of salivary OT levels was found only with the fixation % of pointed-at objects in finger-pointing stimuli. To exclude the effects of sex and age, we calculated partial correlation coefficients between salivary OT levels and the % of pointed-at objects, controlled by sex and age. Results showed significant partial correlation coefficients between the variables, indicating that children with high OT levels were more attentive to the pointed-at object than children with low OT levels (**Figure 2**).

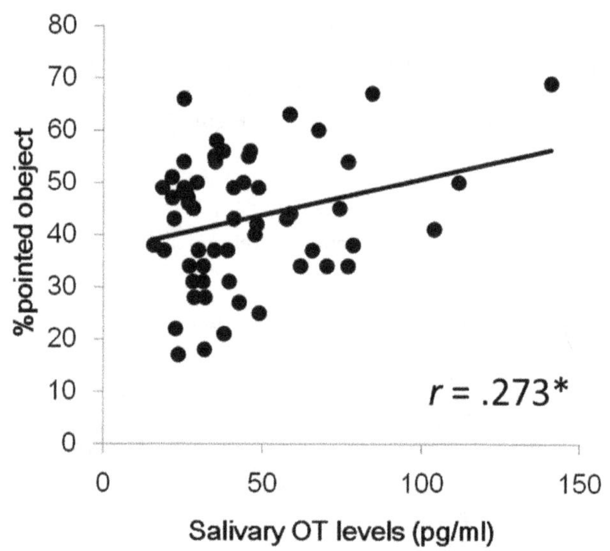

FIGURE 2 | Relationship between salivary OT levels and % of pointed-at objects in the finger pointing movies. *$p < 0.05$.

DEVELOPMENT OF VISUAL ATTENTION FOR SOCIAL SIGNALS AND OT LEVELS WITH ASD

Together with standard errors, mean values of salivary OT and proportions of gaze fixations for each category of social information in children with ASD are presented in **Table 3**. Mean values of these parameters grouped by sex are also shown.

For salivary OT levels and gaze fixation, we first tested whether there was an effect of sex on each parameter. No significant difference was observed for salivary OT levels [$t_{(56)} = 0.35$, *n.s.*], indicating a lack of sex difference among OT levels in both groups.

Regarding the relationship between age, salivary OT levels, and respective gaze fixation parameters, the correlation coefficients for these variables are presented in **Table 3**. First, no significant correlation was found between age and OT levels, as it was for TD children. For variables of gaze fixation, a significant negative

Table 3 | Mean values and the correlations of salivary oxytocin (OT) levels and each gaze fixation parameter in children with autism spectrum disorder (ASD).

		Total ($n = 15$)		Male ($n = 12$)		Female ($n = 3$)		t	Correlation		Partial correlation
		Mean	*SD*	Mean	*SD*	Mean	*SD*		Age	OT level	OT level
Oxytocin levels (pg/ml)		39.33	23.52	40.3	25.02	35.7	20.11	0.29	−0.171	–	–
Face	%Eyes	36.73	10.12	36.5	9.19	37.7	15.82	0.17	−0.274	**0.461**[#]	0.439
	%Mouth	30	12.61	28.2	11.90	37.3	15.28	1.14	−0.123	−0.215	−0.217
	%Out of AOI	16.33	7.86	17.6	8.04	11.3	5.51	1.26	0.292	−0.013	0.004
People and geometry	%People	36.2	17.76	**31.4**	15.89	**55.3**	11.50	**2.42***	**−0.529***	0.268	0.332
	%Geometry	35.4	16.96	**40.0**	15.73	**17.0**	4.36	**2.44***	0.414	−0.271	−0.342
	%Out of AOI	20.07	7.71	19.6	8.11	22.0	6.93	0.47	0.324	0.115	0.216
Biological motion	%Upright	55.53	20.16	**50.9**	18.74	**74.0**	16.52	**1.94**[#]	−0.269	0.251	0.304
	%Inverted	27.4	15.4	28.8	15.71	21.7	15.50	0.71	0.028	−0.043	−0.064
	%Out of AOI	11	10.11	12.9	10.47	3.3	1.53	1.54	0.452	−0.386	−0.421
Finger pointing	%Pointed	41.93	13.36	50.9	18.74	74.0	16.52	1.30	0.060	0.065	0.131
	%Non-pointed	11.6	8.54	28.8	15.71	21.7	15.50	0.73	0.229	0.312	0.354
	%Out of AOI	42.53	9.96	12.9	10.47	3.3	1.53	0.35	−0.280	−0.314	−0.412

[#] $p < 0.10$; * $p < 0.05$.

correlation was found only for the fixation % of people moving. This result suggests that aging in children with ASD also decreases attention for people moving as it does in TD children. Finally, for salivary OT levels, a marginally significant correlation was found with the % of fixation on eyes in the facial stimuli, indicating that children with ASD and high OT levels were more attentive to the eye area in terms of facial recognition than children with low OT levels.

COMPARISON OF VISUAL ATTENTION FOR SOCIAL SIGNALS AND OT LEVELS IN TD CHILDREN AND THOSE WITH ASD

To examine the interaction among sex and developmental status for OT levels and the fixation duration for social information, the ratio of the percentage of fixation duration for each category was calculated as the dependent variable: Face, eyes-to-mouth; People and Geometry, people-to-geometry; Biological motion, upright-to-inverted; Finger pointing, pointed-to-non-pointed. Subsequently a Two-Way (2 × 2) ANOVA was conducted with sex (male, female) and development status (patients, controls) as between-subjects factors.

First, for salivary OT levels, there was no main effect of sex ($p = 0.693$) or developmental status ($p = 0.449$), and no sex × developmental status interaction ($p < 0.897$) (**Figure 3A**).

Next, regarding fixation variables, analysis of the eyes-to-mouth ratio in the face stimuli showed no main effect of either sex ($p = 0.223$) or developmental status ($p = 0.979$), and no sex × developmental status interaction ($p = 0.790$) (**Figure 3B**). Analysis of the people-to-geometry ratio showed a main effect of sex [$F_{(1,69)} = 9.73$, $p < 0.01$], but no main effect of developmental status ($p = 0.815$) or sex × group interaction ($p = 0.118$), indicating that female children were more attentive to people moving than male children, irrespective of developmental status (**Figure 3C**). Analysis of upright-to-inverted biological motion showed no main effect of sex ($p = 0.066$), developmental status [$F_{(1, 69)} = 3.96$, $p < 0.05$], or sex × group interaction ($p = 0.455$), indicating that children with ASD were more attentive to biological motion than TDs irrespective of the sex group (**Figure 3D**). Analysis of pointed-to-non-pointed ratio showed no main effect of sex ($p = 0.323$), development status ($p = 0.907$), or sex × developmental status interaction ($p = 0.385$) (**Figure 3E**).

DISCUSSION

This study examined the relationship between gaze fixation for social information and OT levels in preschool children with ASD or typical development. The results revealed a positive association between salivary OT levels and % pointed-at object area in TD children, although no association was found between these variables in children with ASDs. Thus, TD children with high OT levels pay more attention to a pointed-at object than do those with low OT levels. Most gaze fixation variables were dependent on age, with results revealing a positive association of the % of fixation on mouths, geometric patterns, and biological motion. In contrast, a negative association was found between age and the % of fixation on people and pointed-at objects in TD children. Although there was a negative association between age and the fixation duration on people in children with ASD, those tendencies were clearer in TD than in ASD. These results suggest that attention for people moving and pointed-at objects decreases with aging in preschool children, although attention for the mouth, geometric patterns, and biological motion increased with age.

Many previous studies have suggested that OT has a positive effect on attention for social information (Domes et al., 2007a,b; Donaldson and Young, 2008; Guastella et al., 2008; Insel, 2010). Earlier studies also suggested that impairments in social

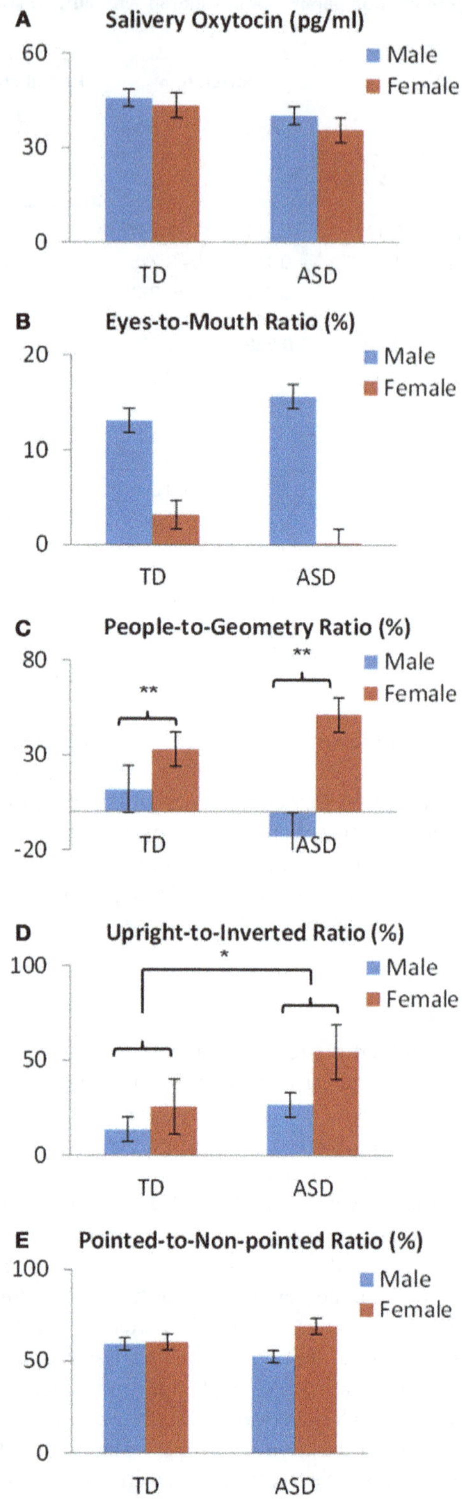

FIGURE 3 | OT levels and fixation variables by sex and developmental status in preschoolers show (A) no difference in salivary OT levels or (B) in eyes-to mouth ratios. (C) A significant difference of sex was found in people-to-geometry ratios. **(D)** A significant difference of developmental status was found in the upright-to-inverted ratios in bodily motion stimuli. **(E)** No difference was found in the pointed-to-non-pointed ratios of finger pointing stimuli. *$p < 0.05$, **$p < 0.01$.

functioning of patients with ASDs were related to dysfunction of the OT mechanism (Andari et al., 2010; Guastella et al., 2010; Kosaka et al., 2012). Moreover, several studies have revealed that patients with ASD have poorer or different visual attention for social information than the amount of visual attention expected to result from typical development (Klin et al., 2002a, 2003). In that context, eye-tracking technology presents numerous advantages for investigating visual social attention in ASD (Guillon et al., 2014). This report is the first study to clarify the association between the pattern of visual attention for social information and OT levels in preschool children with ASD and TD.

We also found a positive association between salivary OT levels and % pointed object areas in the pointing gesture movie for TD children. The ability to follow pointing gestures by others is a significant component in establishing joint attention (Paparella et al., 2011), and various studies have reported a deficit in joint attention as one of the salient signs of ASDs (Warreyn et al., 2007; Redcay et al., 2013). Although there is no direct evidence that OT has a positive effect on joint attention, the idea that social motivation deficits play a central role in ASD has recently gained increasing interest (Chevallier et al., 2012), and it has also been suggested that OT may have a positive effect on enhancing social motivation including joint attention (Stavropoulos and Carver, 2013). In addition, although previous studies have suggested that the mPFC and posterior superior temporal sulcus (pSTS) mediate joint attention (Redcay et al., 2013), recent brain imaging studies have shown that mPFC and pSTS were more activated for social literacy when OT was administered (Gordon et al., 2013). Moreover, several findings have suggested that OXTRs are abundant in the mPFC compared with other brain regions (Skuse and Gallagher, 2009). These findings suggest a positive OT effect for joint attention. Hence, an increase in OT levels may induce enhanced gaze duration at a pointed object.

In the current study, the pattern of visual attention for social information was affected not only by OT levels, but also by age or sex, the development of which represents interactions between these variables. However, results of previous studies have suggested that children with ASD have less attention for social information than TD children; especially for social information variables related to the eyes (Jones and Klin, 2013), people relative to a geometric pattern (Pierce et al., 2011), and biological motion (Klin et al., 2002a,b). In terms of aging effects, our results revealed a positive association with people moving, eye area on the face, and pointed-at objects, and a negative association with geometric patterns in TD preschoolers. These results suggest reduced attention for social information with aging, although this has not received much attention at this point. Furthermore, although this tendency was also observed in children with ASD, the results were not clear because of the insufficient number of samples.

This study confirmed the findings of earlier studies in that female children had more attention for people, whereas male children had more attention for geometric patterns (Pierce et al., 2011). Sex differences reportedly exist for infants' preferences for several properties of the human face and body (Bower, 1989). However, although the present study found that children with ASD were more attentive to biological motion than TD children were, irrespective of sex group, this finding is inconsistent with those of earlier studies (Klin et al., 2002a,b). We were unable to clarify the underlying mechanism, but a possible explanation is the difference of age groups examined in current and previous research. Our participants were preschoolers, whereas most subjects of previous research were infants. As described above, the visual attention for social information can change depending on age. Therefore, aging might be the cause of the discrepancy that we observed. This study also presents some limitations that, if resolved, would improve assessment for ASD. For one, we should analyze the difference between ASD and TD groups using DQ and gender differences as confounding factors. This will be important analyses to conduct since these factors could produce differences in terms of performance and visual attention. Moreover, a larger sample size will be beneficial, therefore, it is necessary to conduct this study again with more participants.

In conclusion, these results demonstrate that OT levels have a positive association with visual attention for finger pointing in TD preschoolers, although no association was found between these variables in children with ASDs. These results suggest that OT is involved in visual attention for social information. Moreover, with the exception of biological motion, age showed a negative relationship with visual attention for social information. However, this study did not directly investigate the neural mechanism underlying this effect. Thus, combining this experimental paradigm with neurophysiological indicators of brain activity (such as imaging techniques) should prove fruitful in further elucidating mechanisms underlying visual attention for social information.

FUNDING

This work was supported by a Grant-in-Aid for Scientific Research (B), Young Scientists (B) and Challenging Exploratory Research from the Ministry of Education, Culture, Sports, Science and Technology (MEXT) of Japan (KAKENHI: grant numbers 24300149 and 25560386 to Akemi Tomoda, grant number 25750405 to Takashi X. Fujisawa). Part of this report is the result of "Integrated Research on Neuropsychiatric Disorders" conducted under the Strategic Research Program for Brain Sciences by MEXT of Japan. This work also was partially supported by a research grant from the "Center of Community (COC)" program from the MEXT of Japan to Takashi X. Fujisawa, Daisuke N. Saito, and Akemi Tomoda. Funding organizations had no role in the design or conduct of the study, such as the collection, management, analysis, or interpretation of the data, or the preparation, review, or approval of the manuscript.

ACKNOWLEDGMENTS

We thank Chisato Ohta, Tohru Fujioka, Rikako Teshigawara, Sakae Mizushima, and Hitomi Suzuki for their excellent technical assistance in evaluating the participants.

REFERENCES

American Psychiatric Association (APA). (2013). *Diagnostic and Statistical Manual of Mental Disorders: DSM-V, 5th Edn.* Washington, DC: American Psychiatric Association.

Andari, E., Duhamel, J. R., Zalla, T., Herbrecht, E., Leboyer, M., and Sirigu, A. (2010). Promoting social behavior with oxytocin in high-functioning autism spectrum disorders. *Proc. Natl. Acad. Sci. U.S.A.* 107, 4389–4394. doi: 10.1073/pnas.0910249107

Baumgartner, T., Heinrichs, M., Vonlanthen, A., Fischbacher, U., and Fehr, E. (2008). Oxytocin shapes the neural circuitry of trust and trust adaptation in humans. *Neuron* 58, 639–650. doi: 10.1016/j.neuron.2008.04.009

Bower, T. G. R. (1989). *The Rational Infant: Learning in Infancy.* New York, NY: W. H. Freeman & Co Ltd.

Carter, C. S. (1998). Neuroendocrine perspectives on social attachment and love. *Psychoneuroendocrinology* 23, 779–818. doi: 10.1016/S0306-4530(98)00055-9

Carter, C. S., Pournajafi-Nazarloo, H., Kramer, K. M., Ziegler, T. E., White-Traut, R., Bello, D., et al. (2007). Behavioral associations and potential as a salivary biomarker. *Ann. N.Y. Acad. Sci.* 1098, 312–322. doi: 10.1196/annals.1384.006

Centelles, L., Assaiante, C., Etchegoyhen, K., Bouvard, M., and Schmitz, C. (2012). Understanding social interaction in children with autism spectrum disorders: does whole-body motion mean anything to them? *Encephale* 38, 232–240. doi: 10.1016/j.encep.2011.08.005

Chevallier, C., Kohls, G., Troiani, V., Brodkin, E. S., and Schultz, R. T. (2012). The social motivation theory of autism. *Trends Cogn. Sci.* 16, 231–239. doi: 10.1016/j.tics.2012.02.007

Doi, H., Fujisawa, T. X., Kanai, C., Ohta, H., Yokoi, H., Iwanami, A., et al. (2013). Recognition of facial expressions and prosodic cues with graded emotional intensities in adults with Asperger syndrome. *J. Autism Dev. Disord.* 43, 2099–2113. doi: 10.1007/s10803-013-1760-8

Domes, G., Heinrichs, M., Gläscher, J., Büchel, C., Braus, D. F., and Herpertz, S. C. (2007a). Oxytocin attenuates amygdala responses to emotional faces regardless of valence. *Biol. Psychiatry* 62, 1187–1190. doi: 10.1016/j.biopsych.2007.03.025

Domes, G., Heinrichs, M., Michel, A., Berger, C., and Herpertz, S. C. (2007b). Oxytocin improves "mind-reading" in humans. *Biol. Psychiatry* 61, 731–733. doi: 10.1016/j.biopsych.2006.07.015

Donaldson, Z. R., and Young, L. J. (2008). Oxytocin, vasopressin, and the neurogenetics of sociality. *Science* 322, 900–904. doi: 10.1126/science.1158668

Feldman, R., Gordon, I., Influs, M., Gutbir, T., and Ebstein, R. P. (2013). Parental oxytocin and early caregiving jointly shape children's oxytocin response and social reciprocity. *Neuropsychopharmacology* 38, 1154–1162. doi: 10.1038/npp.2013.22

Feldman, R., Gordon, I., and Zagoory-Sharon, O. (2011). Maternal and paternal plasma, salivary, and urinary oxytocin and parent-infant synchrony: considering stress and affiliation components of human bonding. *Dev. Sci.* 14, 752–761. doi: 10.1111/j.1467-7687.2010.01021.x

Ferguson, J. N., Young, L. J., Hearn, E. F., Matzuk, M. M., Insel, T. R., and Winslow, J. T. (2000). Social amnesia in mice lacking the oxytocin gene. *Nat. Genet.* 25, 284–288. doi: 10.1038/77040

Gordon, I., Vander Wyk, B. C., Bennett, R. H., Cordeaux, C., and Lucas, M. V., Eilbott, J. A. et al. (2013). Oxytocin enhances brain function in children with autism. *Proc. Natl. Acad. Sci. U.S.A.* 110, 20953–20958. doi: 10.1073/pnas.1312857110

Guastella, A. J., Einfeld, S. L., Gray, K. M., Rinehart, N. J., Tonge, B. J., Lambert, T. J., et al. (2010). Intranasal oxytocin improves emotion recognition for youth with autism spectrum disorders. *Biol. Psychiatry* 67, 692–694. doi: 10.1016/j.biopsych.2009.09.020

Guastella, A. J., Mitchell, P. B., and Dadds, M. R. (2008). Oxytocin increases gaze to the eye region of human faces. *Biol. Psychiatry* 63, 3–5. doi: 10.1016/j.biopsych.2007.06.026

Guillon, Q., Hadjikhani, N., Baduel, S., and Rogé, B. (2014). Visual social attention in autism spectrum disorder: insights from eye tracking studies. *Neurosci. Biobehav. Rev.* 42, 279–297. doi: 10.1016/j.neubiorev.2014.03.013

Higashida, H., Yokoyama, S., Huang, J. J., Liu, L., Ma, W. J., Akther, S., et al. (2012). Social memory, amnesia, and autism: brain oxytocin secretion is regulated by NAD+ metabolites and single nucleotide polymorphisms of CD38. *Neurochem. Int.* 61, 828–838. doi: 10.1016/j.neuint.2012.01.030

Hill, E. L., and Frith, U. (2003). Understanding autism: insights from mind and brain. *Philos. Trans. R. Soc. Lond. B Biol. Sci.* 358, 281–289. doi: 10.1098/rstb.2002.1209

Iizuka, C., Yamashita, Y., Nagamitsu, S., Yamashita, T., Araki, Y., Ohya, T., et al. (2010). Comparison of the strengths and difficulties questionnaire (SDQ) scores between children with high-functioning autism spectrum disorder (HFASD) and attention-deficit/hyperactivity disorder (AD/HD). *Brain Dev.* 32, 609–612. doi: 10.1016/j.braindev.2009.09.009

Ikuzawa, M., Matsushita, H., and Nakazawa, A. (eds.). (2002). *Guides for the Use of the Kyoto Scale of Psychological Development 2001 (Japanese).* Kyoto: Kyoto International Social Welfare Exchange Center.

Insel, T. R. (2010). The challenge of translation in social neuroscience: a review of oxytocin, vasopressin, and affiliative behavior. *Neuron* 65, 768–779. doi: 10.1016/j.neuron.2010.03.005

Israel, S., Lerer, E., Shalev, I., Uzefovsky, F., Riebold, M., Laiba, E., et al. (2009). The oxytocin receptor (OXTR) contributes to prosocial fund allocations in the dictator game and the social value orientations task. *PLoS ONE* 4:e5535. doi: 10.1371/journal.pone.0005535

Jones, W., and Klin, A. (2013). Attention to eyes is present but in decline in 2-6-month-old infants later diagnosed with autism. *Nature* 504, 427–431. doi: 10.1038/nature12715

Kéri, S., Kiss, I., and Kelemen, O. (2009). Sharing secrets: oxytocin and trust in schizophrenia. *Soc. Neurosci.* 4, 287–293. doi: 10.1080/17470910802319710

Kirsch, P., Esslinger, C., Chen, Q., Mier, D., Lis, S., Siddhanti, S., et al. (2005). Oxytocin modulates neural circuitry for social cognition and fear in humans. *J. Neurosci.* 25, 11489–11493. doi: 10.1523/JNEUROSCI.3984-05.2005

Klin, A., Jones, W., Schultz, R., and Volkmar, F. (2003). The enactive mind, or from action to cognition: lessons from autism. *Philos. Trans. R. Soc. Lond. B Biol. Sci.* 358, 345–360. doi: 10.1098/rstb.2002.1202

Klin, A., Jones, W., Schultz, R., Volkmar, F., and Cohen,. D. (2002a). Defining and quantifying the social phenotype in autism. *Am. J. Psychiatry* 159, 895–908. doi: 10.1176/appi.ajp.159.6.895

Klin, A., Jones, W., Schultz, R., Volkmar, F. R., and Cohen, D. J. (2002b). Visual fixation patterns during viewing of naturalistic social situations as predictors of social competence in individuals with autism, *Arch. Gen. Psychiatry* 59, 809–816. doi: 10.1001/archpsyc.59.9.809

Klin, A., Lin, D. J., Gorrindo, P., Ramsay, G., and Jones, W. (2009). Two-year-olds with autism orient to non-social contingencies rather than biological motion. *Nature* 459, 257–261. doi: 10.1038/nature07868

Kosaka, H., Munesue, T., Ishitobi, M., Asano, M., Omori, M., Sato, M., et al. (2012). Long-term oxytocin administration improves social behaviors in a girl with autistic disorder. *BMC Psychiatry* 12:110. doi: 10.1186/1471-244X-12-110

Kosfeld, M., Heinrichs, M., Zak, P. J., Fischbacher, U., and Fehr, E. (2005). Oxytocin increases trust in humans. *Nature* 435, 673–676. doi: 10.1038/nature03701

Landgraf, R., and Neumann, I. D. (2004). Vasopressin and oxytocin release within the brain: a dynamic concept of multiple and variable modes of neuropeptide communication. *Front. Neuroendocrinol.* 25, 150–176. doi: 10.1016/j.yfrne.2004.05.001

Matsuishi, T., Nagano, M., Araki, Y., Tanaka, Y., Iwasaki, M., Yamashita, Y., et al. (2008). Scale properties of the strengths and difficulties questionnaire (SDQ): a study of infant and school children in community samples. *Brain Dev.* 30, 410–415. doi: 10.1016/j.braindev.2007.12.003

Modahl, C., Green, L., Fein, D., Morris, M., Waterhouse, L., Feinstein, C., et al. (1998). Plasma oxytocin levels in autistic children. *Biol. Psychiatry* 43, 270–277. doi: 10.1016/S0006-3223(97)00439-3

Munesue, T., Yokoyama, S., Nakamura, K., Anitha, A., Yamada, K., Hayashi, K., et al. (2010). Two genetic variants of CD38 in subjects with autism spectrum disorder and controls. *Neurosci. Res.* 67, 181–191. doi: 10.1016/j.neures.2010.03.004

Nakano, T., Tanaka, K., Endo, Y., Yamane, Y., Yamamoto, T., Nakano, Y., et al. (2010). Atypical gaze patterns in children and adults with autism spectrum disorders dissociated from developmental changes in gaze behaviour. *Proc. Biol. Sci.* 277, 2935–2943. doi: 10.1098/rspb.2010.0587

Paparella, T., Goods, K. S., Freeman, S., and Kasari, C. (2011). The emergence of nonverbal joint attention and requesting skills in young children with autism. *J. Commun. Disord.* 44, 569–583. doi: 10.1016/j.jcomdis.2011.08.002

Pierce, K., Conant, D., Hazin, R., Stoner, R., and Desmond, J. (2011). Preference for geometric patterns early in life as a risk factor for autism. *Arch. Gen. Psychiatry* 68, 101–109. doi: 10.1001/archgenpsychiatry.2010.113

Redcay, E., Dodell-Feder, D., Mavros, P. L., Kleiner, M., Pearrow, M. J., Triantafyllou, C., et al. (2013). Atypical brain activation patterns during a face-to-face joint attention game in adults with autism spectrum disorder. *Hum. Brain Mapp.* 34, 2511–2523. doi: 10.1002/hbm.22086

Rimmele, U., Hediger, K., Heinrichs, M., and Klaver, P. (2009). Oxytocin makes a face in memory familiar. *J. Neurosci.* 29, 38–42. doi: 10.1523/JNEUROSCI.4260-08.2009

Sasson, N. J., and Touchstone, E. W. (2014). Visual attention to competing social and object images by preschool children with autism spectrum disorder. *J. Autism Dev. Disord.* 44, 584–592. doi: 10.1007/s10803-013-1910-z

Skuse, D. H., and Gallagher, L. (2009). Dopaminergic-neuropeptide interactions in the social brain. *Trends Cogn. Sci.* 13, 27–35. doi: 10.1016/j.tics.2008.09.007

Stavropoulos, K. K., and Carver, L. J. (2013). Research review: social motivation and oxytocin in autism–implications for joint attention development and intervention. *J. Child Psychol. Psychiatry* 54, 603–618. doi: 10.1111/jcpp.12061

Taylor, B., Jck, H., and MacLaughlin, D. (2013). Prevalence and incidence rates of autism in the UK: time trend from 2004–2010 in children aged 8 years. *BMJ Open* 3:e003219. doi: 10.1136/bmjopen-2013-003219

Tsujii, M., Yukihiro, T., Adachi, J., Ichikawa, H., Inoue, M., Uchiyama, T., et al. (2006). Reliability and validity of the infant part of the PARS (PDD-autism society japan rating scale) (Japanese). *Rinshou Seishin Igaku* 35, 1119–1126.

Warreyn, P., Roeyers, H., Van Wetswinkel, U., and De Groote, I. (2007). Temporal coordination of joint attention behavior in preschoolers with autism spectrum disorder. *J. Autism Dev. Disord.* 37, 501–512. doi: 10.1007/s10803-006-0184-0

Watanabe, T., Abe, O., Kuwabara, H., Yahata, N., Takano, Y., Iwashiro, N., et al. (2014). Mitigation of sociocommunicational deficits of autism through oxytocin-induced recovery of medial prefrontal activity: a randomized trial. *JAMA Psychiatry* 71, 166–175. doi: 10.1001/jamapsychiatry

White-Traut, R., Watanabe, K., Pournajafi-Nazarloo, H., Schwertz, D., Bell, A., and Carter, C. S. (2009). Detection of salivary oxytocin levels in lactating women. *Dev. Psychobiol.* 51, 367–373. doi: 10.1002/dev.20376

Young, L. J., and Wang, Z. (2004). The neurobiology of pair bonding. *Nat. Neurosci.* 7, 1048–1054. doi: 10.1038/nn1327

Zak, P. J., Kurzban, R., and Matzner, W. T. (2005). Oxytocin is associated with human trustworthiness. *Horm. Behav.* 48, 522–527. doi: 10.1016/j.yhbeh.2005.07.009

Zak, P. J., Stanton, A. A., and Ahmadi, S. (2007). Oxytocin increases generosity in humans. *PLoS ONE* 2:e1128. doi: 10.1371/journal.pone.0001128

5

Epigenetic changes in the estrogen receptor α gene promoter: implications in sociosexual behaviors

Ken Ichi Matsuda *

Department of Anatomy and Neurobiology, Graduate School of Medical Science, Kyoto Prefectural University of Medicine, Kyoto, Japan

****Correspondence:***
Ken Ichi Matsuda, Department of Anatomy and Neurobiology, Graduate School of Medical Science, Kyoto Prefectural University of Medicine, 465 Kawaramachi Hirokoji, Kamigyoku, Kyoto, 602-8566 Japan
e-mail: matsuken@koto.kpu-m.ac.jp

Estrogen action through estrogen receptor α (ERα) is involved in the control of sexual and social behaviors in adult mammals. Alteration of ERα gene activity mediated by epigenetic mechanisms, such as histone modifications and DNA methylation, in particular brain areas appears to be crucial for determining the extents of these behaviors between the sexes and among individuals within the same sex. This review provides a summary of the epigenetic changes in the ERα gene promoter that correlate with sociosexual behaviors.

Keywords: estrogen receptor α, epigenetics, histone acetylation, histone deacetylation, DNA methylation, sexual differentiation, sexual behavior, sociosexual behavior

ERα AND ITS GENE PROMOTER

Estrogen receptor α (ERα) is a member of the nuclear receptor superfamily of ligand-dependent transcription factors that regulate expression of target genes (Evans, 1988; Kawata, 1995; Parker, 1995; Matsuda et al., 2002; McCarthy, 2008). ERα has a typical nuclear receptor structure with at least three functional domains: the ligand-binding domain located in the C-terminal half of the protein, the DNA-binding domain located centrally, and a variable transactivation domain located in the N-terminal region. Upon activation by a ligand, estradiol, ERα forms a homodimer within the nucleus and the dimer complex binds to specific regulatory DNA sequences, which are referred to as estrogen responsive elements (EREs), in promoter or enhancer regions of target genes. After binding to an ERE, the ERα dimer recruits transcription co-factors, which leads to gene activation and transcription. Following transcription, mRNA is translated into proteins that are the ultimate outcome of the hormone responses. Alternatively, accumulating evidence suggests that rapid non-genomic actions of ERα initiated at the plasma membrane through induction of protein phosphorylation-mediated signal transduction pathways are also crucial in estrogenic responses (Vasudevan and Pfaff, 2008; Sakamoto et al., 2012). These characteristics of ERα are common to the other estrogen receptor subtype, ERβ (Koehler et al., 2005).

Expression of the ERα gene is controlled by multiple promoters located upstream of the first coding exon (Kos et al., 2001; Wilson et al., 2008). In rats, at least four different promoters (C, 0S, 0N, and 0B) that can initiate transcription have been identified and shown to be utilized in an organ- and tissue-specific manner. The ERα gene transcript from the 0B promoter (also designated as the 1B promoter; Freyschuss and Grandien, 1996; Champagne et al., 2006), which corresponds to the C promoter in humans and mice, is expressed in brain areas involved in sociosexual behaviors, such as the bed nucleus of the stria terminalis (BNST) (Emery and Sachs, 1976) (Numan, 1996; Numan and Woodside, 2010), the medial preoptic area (MPOA) (Larsson and Heimer, 1964), and hypothalamic and amygdaloid nuclei (Kawata, 1995; McCarthy, 2008), as well as in the anterior pituitary, ovary and uterus (Kato et al., 1998).

ERα IN SOCIOSEXUAL BEHAVIORS

Gene targeting in mice has shown that ERα contributes to various brain functions, including regulation of sociosexual behaviors in both sexes (Rissman et al., 1997; Tetel and Pfaff, 2010).

FEMALE SEXUAL BEHAVIOR

ERα knockout (ERαKO) female mice, in which the ERα gene is disrupted in both alleles throughout the body, completely lack lordosis behavior, a typical female sexual behavior (Ogawa et al., 1996). ERαKO females are also deficient in sexual interactions that precede the lordosis response (Ogawa et al., 1998a). The estradiol level in gonadally intact ERαKO females is elevated compared to that in wild type females, and thus expression of ERα in the brain is critical for induction of female sexual behavior. However, these studies in ERαKO mice did not clarify whether the deficits were caused by a lack of ERα activation during development or in adulthood.

Spatiotemporal knockdown of ERα mRNA (ERαKD) mediated by infection with adeno-associated virus (AAV) expressing small hairpin (sh) RNA against ERα mRNA has been conducted in adult female mice. When gene silencing was restricted to the bilateral ventromedial nucleus of hypothalamus (VMH), where

ERα is strongly expressed, the mice exhibited no sexual behavior (Musatov et al., 2006), indicating that ERα function in the VMH in adulthood is a key regulator of female sexual behavior. Female mice in which expression of ERα was silenced in the MPOA also exhibited significant reduction in receptive and rejective female sexual behaviors (Ribeiro et al., 2012).

MALE SEXUAL BEHAVIOR

In males, estrogen is produced from testosterone by the enzymatic activity of aromatase in the brain and is known to regulate sexual behavior. Male ERαKO mice show significant impairment in some components of sexual behavior compared with wild type mice. ERαKO mice exhibit a normal motivation to mount females, but reduced levels of intromission and no ejaculation (Ogawa et al., 1997; Wersinger et al., 1997; Ogawa et al., 1998b; Scordalakes and Rissman, 2003).

Brain regions responsible for ERα-mediated regulation of male sexual behavior have been examined using ERαKD by AAV infection. Male sexual behavior was greatly reduced when ERα expression was silenced in the MPOA (Sano et al., 2013). In MPOA ERαKD mice, mount motivation and intromission were reduced, suggesting that ERα expressed in the MPOA in adulthood is involved in the control of male sexual motivation and behavior. Silencing ERα expression in the VMH also caused a reduction in male sexual behavior, particularly in the number of intromissions (Sano et al., 2013). This result indicates that ERα function in the VMH is also important for the expression of male sexual behavior.

FEMALE SOCIAL BEHAVIOR

ERαKO females show increased aggression toward other females (Ogawa et al., 1996). Gonadally intact ERαKO females vigorously attack gonadectomized and steroid-primed female intruder mice. Gonadectomized and steroid-primed ERαKO females placed in the home cage of males that showed sexual behavior to wild type females showed extreme rejection of male mounts, whereas gonadally intact ERαKO females were vigorously attacked by the males (Ogawa et al., 1996, 1998a). Similarly, ERα gene silencing in the VMH caused steroid-primed females to reject males (Spiteri et al., 2010a,b). In contrast, ERαKD in the MPOA decreased aggression toward male intruders, as well as social investigation behaviors consisting of genital sniffing, touching the back and chasing (Spiteri et al., 2012).

ERα signaling also contributes to the induction of maternal behavior toward newborn pups. ERαKO females exhibited greatly reduced pup retrieval behavior compared with wild type controls (Ogawa et al., 1996). Silencing of ERα mRNA in the MPOA almost completely abolished maternal behaviors, including nursing and licking the pups, and significantly increased latency to pup retrieval (Ribeiro et al., 2012).

MALE SOCIAL BEHAVIOR

Estradiol contributes to male aggressive behaviors at least partially via ERα. Male-typical offensive attacks are rarely observed in gonadally intact or gonadectomized and androgen-replaced ERαKO males (Ogawa et al., 1997, 1998b). ERαKD in the VMH reduces aggressive behavior, but this effect is not seen for ERαKD in the MPOA (Sano et al., 2013).

EPIGENETIC CHANGES IN THE ERα GENE PROMOTER

Studies using ERα gene targeting techniques suggest that alteration of sensitivity to estrogen by changing the expression level of ERα in specific brain regions is a crucial feature in the control of sociosexual behaviors.

SEX DIFFERENCE

The sex of the brain is mostly determined by the effects of androgen and its metabolite, estradiol. In rodents, androgen is transiently secreted from the testes during a critical perinatal period, the so-called androgen surge, and organizes the developing brain into a masculinized phenotype (Arnold and Gorski, 1984; Kawata, 1995; Matsuda et al., 2008; McCarthy, 2008). Androgen does not affect the brain directly; instead masculinization is largely mediated by estradiol converted from testosterone by aromatase in the brain. The presence or absence of brief exposure to estradiol during the perinatal period creates permanent sex differences in the brain including lasting sex differences in the expression of several genes. ERα expression in the preoptic area (POA) is higher in females than in males from postnatal day 2 through adulthood (DonCarlos and Handa, 1994; DonCarlos, 1996; Yokosuka et al., 1997). Thus, how the early effects of estrogen on the developing brain are permanently maintained is a fundamental issue in the study of sexual differentiation of the brain. Epigenetic mechanisms are emerging as important mediators for the maintenance of the hormonal effects (Keverne and Curley, 2008; McCarthy and Crews, 2008; Matsuda et al., 2012).

DNA methylation is a well characterized epigenetic change that contributes widely to transcriptional regulation (Nakao, 2001; Felsenfeld and Groudine, 2003). In the genome, the 5 position of the cytosine pyrimidine ring in the 5′-CpG-3′ dinucleotide is frequently modified with a methyl group. In general, the extent of CpG methylation in a promoter region is inversely correlated with the transcription level of the gene: higher methylation causes suppressed gene expression. The DNA methylation status of the CpG-rich region in the 1st intron of the ERα gene across the life span has been examined in the POA and the mediobasal hypothalamus (MBH), which includes the VMH (Schwarz et al., 2010). On postnatal day 1, during the critical period of sexual differentiation, two of seven CpG sites (one of these sites differs between the POA and MBH) have a significantly lower methylation rate in males than in females in both the POA and MBH (**Figure 1**). This difference is a result of estradiol exposure because treatment of females with estradiol 24 h before sample collection induces a methylation pattern identical to that in males. These site specific modifications of DNA methylation may be involved in the maintenance of ERα expression in males to facilitate the effect of estradiol during the androgen surge.

The histone acetylation status in the ERα gene promoter also shows a sex difference during the critical perinatal period. Histone acetylation is a well-characterized epigenetic modification that is important in transcriptional regulation (Kouzarides, 2007; Graff and Tsai, 2013). Histone acetylation neutralizes the positive charge of the histone tail and reduces its attraction to the negatively charged DNA, thereby loosening the nucleosome and allowing access of transcriptional factors, thus enhancing gene transcription. Acetylation levels of histone H4 at the ERα

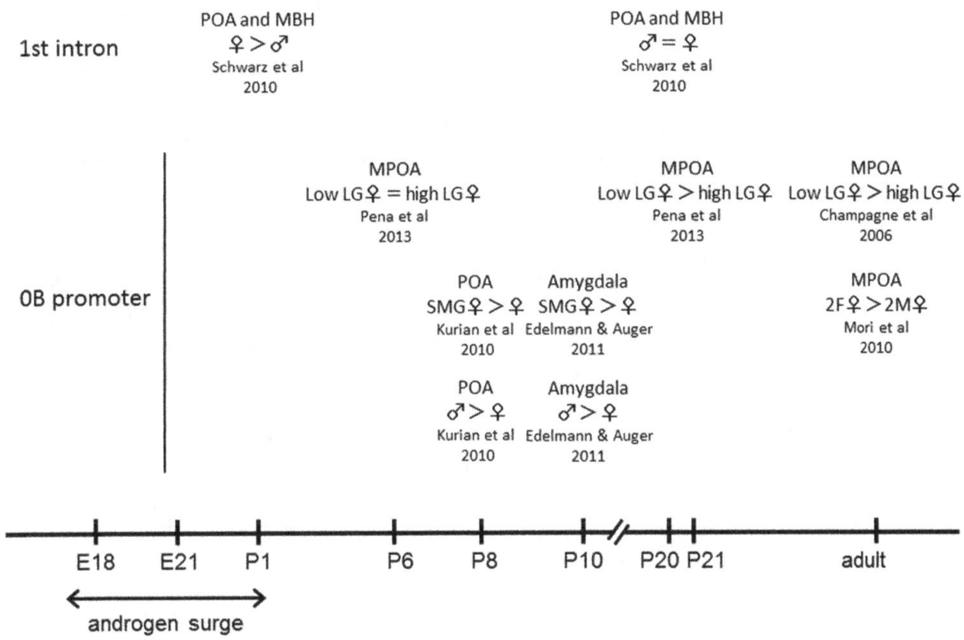

FIGURE 1 | Summary of DNA methylation status in the ERα gene in association with sociosexual behaviors. E, embryonic day; P, postnatal day.

0B promoter in the MPOA are higher in males than females on embryonic day 21 (Matsuda et al., 2011), suggesting prevention of downregulation of ERα expression in males.

The extent of methylation of CpG sites in the 1st intron of the ERα gene increases through development in both male and female MPOA and the sex difference detected on postnatal day 1 is abolished by postnatal day 20 (Schwarz et al., 2010) (**Figure 1**). In addition, an analysis of DNA methylation of the ERα 0B promoter in the POA on postnatal day 8 showed that the average methylation across 17 CpG sites was significantly higher in males compared with females (Kurian et al., 2010) (**Figure 1**). Two of the 17 CpG sites had significantly greater methylation in males and methylation at 6 other CpG sites was detected only in males. Estradiol treatment of females in the neonatal period increased methylation of the ERα promoter to a similar level to that in males. These findings suggest that sex differences in ERα gene expression may result from sex differences in DNA methylation patterns. A similar difference of methylation pattern at a specific CpG site in the ERα promoter has been seen in the amygdala (Edelmann and Auger, 2011), a brain area important for social and emotional processing, on postnatal day 10 (**Figure 1**).

The histone acetylation status is inversely correlated with DNA methylation (Matsuda et al., 2011). Histone H4 acetylation differences in the ERα 0B promoter on embryonic day 21 were rearranged by postnatal day 3, at which time acetylation levels in males declined in correspondence with the developmental decrease in testosterone. The acetylation status of histones is controlled by the balance of enzymatic activity of histone acetyltransferases and histone deacetylases (HDACs), which remove the acetyl group from an acetylated histone. Thus, HDAC activity during the early postnatal period may be involved in the regulation of sexually dimorphic ERα expression in the MPOA (**Figure 2**). HDAC2 and -4, which are expressed in the developing brain and are related to steroid hormone signaling (Leong et al., 2005; Bicaku et al., 2008; Graff and Tsai, 2013), have been identified as candidate molecules regulating this process (Matsuda et al., 2011). The amount of HDAC2 and -4 binding to the ERα promoter on postnatal day 1 is higher in males than in females in the MPOA, while mRNA levels for HDAC2 and −4 do not differ between the sexes. The importance of HDAC activity in masculinization of the brain in the early postnatal period has been shown by both behavioral and morphological analyses. Inhibition of HDACs *in vivo* by intracerebroventricular infusion of a HDAC inhibitor (trichostatin A) or an antisense oligodeoxynucleotide directed against mRNA for HDAC2 and −4 in newborn male rats results in significant reduction of male sexual behavior in adulthood (Matsuda et al., 2011). Administration of another HDAC inhibitor (valproic acid) to male mice on postnatal days 1 and 2 eliminates the development of the sex difference in the volume of

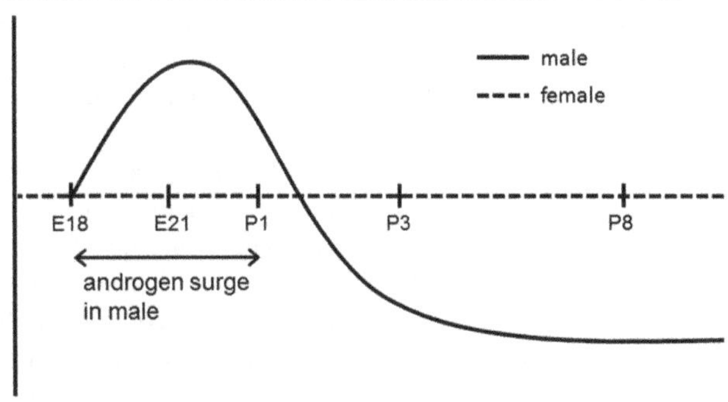

FIGURE 2 | Developmental changes in histone acetylation status in the ERα 0B promoter in the preoptic area in male and female rat.
E, embryonic day; P, postnatal day.

the principal nucleus of the BNST (Murray et al., 2009), which is normally larger in males than females.

These findings provide insights into the molecular mechanisms underlying the developmental consequences of sexually dimorphic ERα expression mediated by epigenetic modifications in the MPOA. During the prenatal androgen surge and subsequent activation of ERα, the acetylation status of histones in the ERα promoter region is increased in males to maintain ERα expression. After the androgen surge, inactivation of ERα due to the decline in ligand levels leads to recruitment of HDAC2 and -4 to promoters and the acetylation status of the promoter is reduced (**Figure 2**). Following the change in histone acetylation, methylation of DNA in the ERα promoter region is increased to a greater extent in males (**Figure 3**). This results in continuous lower expression of ERα compared with females, which is appropriate for execution of masculinized brain functions. These processes are not evident in females due to the absence of an androgen surge, and the consequent higher sensitivity to estrogen with higher expression of ERα may induce feminized brain functions.

INDIVIDUAL DIFFERENCES

As described above, perinatal estradiol exposure contributes to lasting sex differences in ERα expression. However, early social experience can also alter ERα expression and associated behaviors. Variations in maternal care in rats distinguished by levels of whole-body licking and grooming (LG) by the dam exert a lasting influence on some neuroendocrine and behavioral characteristics of offspring in adulthood (Francis et al., 1999; Liu et al., 2000; Champagne et al., 2001; Cameron et al., 2005, 2008a,b; Prior et al., 2013). Offspring of dams that display high levels of LG (high LG) exhibit more modest hypothalamic-pituitary-adrenal responses to stress, enhanced cognitive ability, a higher level of maternal behavior, and altered sexual behavior in comparison to offspring of dams with low levels of LG (low LG). The effect of an individual difference in maternal behavior is transmitted across generations (Champagne and Meaney, 2007). Adult female offspring of high LG mothers display increased pup LG, compared

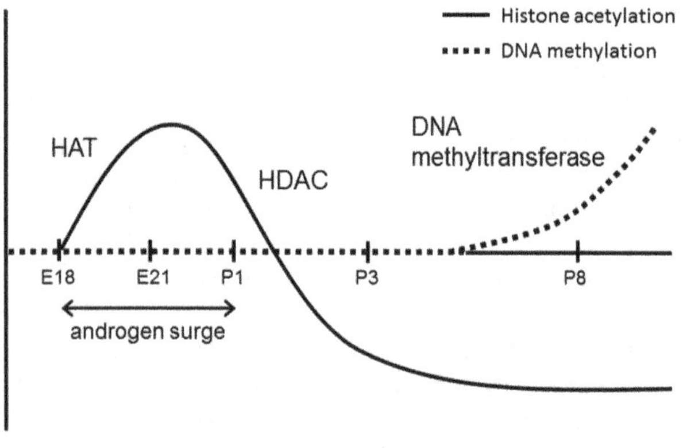

FIGURE 3 | Developmental changes in epigenetic status in the ERα 0B promoter in the preoptic area in male rat. E, embryonic day; P, postnatal day.

with adult female offspring of low LG mothers. Cross-fostering, in which pups born to high-LG mothers are fostered at birth to low-LG mothers and vice versa, has shown a direct relationship between maternal care actually received and individual characteristics, suggesting that an epigenetic mechanism underlies the transgenerational inheritance of the individual behavioral differences. Variation of neonatal maternal care has been associated with ERα expression (Champagne et al., 2003) and DNA methylation of the ERα promoter in the MPOA (Champagne et al., 2006). Females that received high LG exhibited elevated ERα expression in adulthood compared with females that received low LG. DNA methylation patterns across the ERα 0B promoter differed significantly, with 7 of 14 CpG sites exhibiting significantly greater methylation in offspring of low LG dams compared to those from high LG dams (**Figure 1**). These findings suggest that environmental differences during development are programmed in the brain as a different pattern of epigenetic marks, and that this leads to differences in neuroendocrine and behavioral characteristics after maturity.

Examination of the developmental emergence of LG-mediated epigenetic variation (Pena et al., 2013) indicated a significant difference in DNA methylation rate at the ERα 0b promoter between high LG and low LG individuals on postnatal day 21, but not on postnatal day 6 (**Figure 1**), concomitant with the appearance of different ERα mRNA expression. Another epigenetic change, histone methylation, which is catalyzed by histone methyltransferases (HMT), does not change the overall charge of the histone tail, but increases basicity and hydrophobicity, which enhances histone affinity for DNA (Zhang and Reinberg, 2001; Martin and Zhang, 2005). Therefore, histone methylation is generally correlated with transcriptional repression, although methylation of some residues can result in transcriptional activation. Histone H3 trimethylation at lysine 9 (H3K9me3) and lysine 4 (H3K4me3) are epigenetic marks for repressed and active gene transcription, respectively. Comparison of the histone methylation status at the ERα 0B promoter in the MPOA between high LG and low LG females showed reduced H3K9me3 and increased H3K4me3 in high LG offspring on postnatal day 21, but not on postnatal day 6. These findings suggest that the influence of the amount of maternal care on epigenetic effects is apparent between postnatal days 6 and 21.

There is a difference between the sexes in the amount of maternal care. Mother rats preferentially lick and groom their male offspring more than their female offspring (Moore, 1992). This phenomenon implies that somatosensory stimuli associated with maternal grooming, as well as hormone exposure, influence brain masculinization. Simulated maternal grooming (SMG) by stimulation of the anogenital region of female pups with a paintbrush from postnatal days 5 to 7 increases ERα 0B promoter CpG methylation to a similar level to that in males on postnatal day 8 (Kurian et al., 2010) (**Figure 1**). ERα expression in the POA on postnatal day 10 was significantly reduced in female pups that received SMG compared to control female pups. These results suggest that maternal grooming may contribute to brain sex organization through programming differences in ERα expression through the epigenetic machinery. A similar effect of SMG on the methylation pattern at a specific CpG site in the ERα promoter has been detected in the amygdala on postnatal day 10 (Edelmann and Auger, 2011) (**Figure 1**). However, there is a difference in the direction of the effect of maternal care between the two studies: ERα expression was enhanced in high LG females, but reduced in SMG-stimulated females. This may indicate that SMG does not exhibit actual maternal grooming effect, but sensory stimulation during neonatal period has lasting effect on the expression of ERα gene in the POA by altering DNA methylation status of its promoter.

In addition to the postnatal social, physiological and environmental stimuli, differences in the embryonic hormonal milieu can also have a lasting influence on the development of sociosexual behavior in the offspring brain, resulting in individual variation of behavioral characteristics in adulthood within the same sex. In polytocous animals, the sex-specific positioning of fetuses can result in a natural variation of the hormonal environment during intrauterine development due to diffusion of androgen from neighboring male siblings. During the late gestational period, both the blood and brain concentrations of testosterone are higher in female fetuses that grow between two male siblings (2M females) compared with growth between two female siblings (2F females) (vom Saal and Bronson, 1980; Pei et al., 2006). Corresponding to this different level of androgen exposure, 2M females show greater aggressiveness and less sexual receptivity than 2F females in adulthood (vom Saal, 1984, 1989). It can be hypothesized that there may be intrauterine position-related differential ERα expression in the VMH, and ERα expression levels have been found to differ between 2M and 2F female offspring (Mori et al., 2010), with ERα expression in the VMH being higher in 2M females than 2F females. CpG sites across the ERα 0b promoter region in the VMH were more densely methylated in 2F females than in 2M females (**Figure 1**), showing a negative correlation between ERα expression levels in the VMH and DNA methylation frequency in the ERα promoter. These findings indicate that programming effects induced by the intrauterine position may be mediated by epigenetic modification.

CONCLUSION

ERα expressed in specific brain areas controls various sociosexual behaviors in both sexes. The ERα level is correlated with differences in the magnitude of expression of these behaviors between the sexes and among individuals. Epigenetic programming appears to play central roles in the lasting regulation of ERα expression in response to the hormonal, social, and physiological environment during development. It will be of interest to determine the mechanisms that link these environmental cues to patterns of epigenetic modification in the ERα promoter.

REFERENCES

Arnold, A. P., and Gorski, R. A. (1984). Gonadal steroid induction of structural sex differences in the central nervous system. *Annu. Rev. Neurosci.* 7, 413–442. doi: 10.1146/annurev.ne.07.030184.002213

Bicaku, E., Marchion, D. C., Schmitt, M. L., and Munster, P. N. (2008). Selective inhibition of histone deacetylase 2 silences progesterone receptor-mediated signaling. *Cancer Res.* 68, 1513–1519. doi: 10.1158/0008-5472.CAN-07-2822

Cameron, N., Del Corpo, A., Diorio, J., McAllister, K., Sharma, S., and Meaney, M. J. (2008a). Maternal programming of sexual behavior and hypothalamic-pituitary-gonadal function in the female rat. *PLoS ONE* 3:e2210. doi: 10.1371/journal.pone.0002210

Cameron, N. M., Champagne, F. A., Parent, C., Fish, E. W., Ozaki-Kuroda, K., and Meaney, M. J. (2005). The programming of individual differences in defensive responses and reproductive strategies in the rat through variations in maternal care. *Neurosci. Biobehav. Rev.* 29, 843–865. doi: 10.1016/j.neubiorev.2005.03.022

Cameron, N. M., Fish, E. W., and Meaney, M. J. (2008b). Maternal influences on the sexual behavior and reproductive success of the female rat. *Horm. Behav.* 54, 178–184. doi: 10.1016/j.yhbeh.2008.02.013

Champagne, F. A., Diorio, J., Sharma, S., and Meaney, M. J. (2001). Naturally occurring variations in maternal behavior in the rat are associated with differences in estrogen-inducible central oxytocin receptors. *Proc. Natl. Acad. Sci. U.S.A.* 98, 12736–12741. doi: 10.1073/pnas.221224598

Champagne, F. A., and Meaney, M. J. (2007). Transgenerational effects of social environment on variations in maternal care and behavioral response to novelty. *Behav. Neurosci.* 121, 1353–1363. doi: 10.1037/0735-7044.121.6.1353

Champagne, F. A., Weaver, I. C., Diorio, J., Dymov, S., Szyf, M., and Meaney, M. J. (2006). Maternal care associated with methylation of the estrogen receptor-alpha1b promoter and estrogen receptor-alpha expression in the medial preoptic area of female offspring. *Endocrinology* 147, 2909–2915. doi: 10.1210/en.2005-1119

Champagne, F. A., Weaver, I. C., Diorio, J., Sharma, S., and Meaney, M. J. (2003). Natural variations in maternal care are associated with estrogen receptor alpha expression and estrogen sensitivity in the medial preoptic area. *Endocrinology* 144, 4720–4724. doi: 10.1210/en.2003-0564

DonCarlos, L. L. (1996). Developmental profile and regulation of estrogen receptor (ER) mRNA expression in the preoptic area of prenatal rats. *Brain Res. Dev. Brain Res.* 94, 224–233. doi: 10.1016/S0165-3806(96)80014-9

DonCarlos, L. L., and Handa, R. J. (1994). Developmental profile of estrogen receptor mRNA in the preoptic area of male and female neonatal rats. *Brain Res. Dev. Brain Res.* 79, 283–289. doi: 10.1016/0165-3806(94)90133-3

Edelmann, M. N., and Auger, A. P. (2011). Epigenetic impact of simulated maternal grooming on estrogen receptor alpha within the developing amygdala. *Brain Behav. Immun.* 25, 1299–1304. doi: 10.1016/j.bbi.2011.02.009

Emery, D. E., and Sachs, B. D. (1976). Copulatory behavior in male rats with lesions in the bed nucleus of the stria terminalis. *Physiol. Behav.* 17, 803–806. doi: 10.1016/0031-9384(76)90044-5

Evans, R. M. (1988). The steroid and thyloid hormone receptor superfamily. *Science* 240, 889–895. doi: 10.1126/science.3283939

Felsenfeld, G., and Groudine, M. (2003). Controlling the double helix. *Nature* 421, 448–453. doi: 10.1038/nature01411

Francis, D. D., Champagne, F. A., Liu, D., and Meaney, M. J. (1999). Maternal care, gene expression, and the development of individual differences in stress reactivity. *Ann. N.Y. Acad. Sci.* 896, 66–84. doi: 10.1111/j.1749-6632.1999.tb08106.x

Freyschuss, B., and Grandien, K. (1996). The 5′ flank of the rat estrogen receptor gene: structural characterization and evidence for tissue- and species-specific promoter utilization. *J. Mol. Endocrinol.* 17, 197–206. doi: 10.1677/jme.0.0170197

Graff, J., and Tsai, L. H. (2013). Histone acetylation: molecular mnemonics on the chromatin. *Nat. Rev. Neurosci.* 14, 97–111. doi: 10.1038/nrn3427

Kato, J., Hirata, S., Koh, T., Yamada-Mouri, N., Hosh, K., and Okinaga, S. (1998). The multiple untranslated first exons and promoters system of the oestrogen receptor gene in the brain and peripheral tissues of the rat and monkey and the developing rat cerebral cortex. *J. Steroid Biochem. Mol. Biol.* 65, 281–293. doi: 10.1016/S0960-0760(97)00184-2

Kawata, M. (1995). Roles of steroid hormones and their receptors in structural organization in the nervous system. *Neurosci. Res.* 24, 1–46. doi: 10.1016/0168-0102(96)81278-8

Keverne, E. B., and Curley, J. P. (2008). Epigenetics, brain evolution and behaviour. *Front. Neuroendocrinol.* 29, 398–412. doi: 10.1016/j.yfrne.2008.03.001

Koehler, K. F., Helguero, L. A., Haldosen, L. A., Warner, M., and Gustafsson, J. A. (2005). Reflections on the discovery and significance of estrogen receptor beta. *Endocr. Rev.* 26, 465–478. doi: 10.1210/er.2004-0027

Kos, M., Reid, G., Denger, S., and Gannon, F. (2001). Minireview: genomic organization of the human ERalpha gene promoter region. *Mol. Endocrinol.* 15, 2057–2063. doi: 10.1210/mend.15.12.0731

Kouzarides, T. (2007). Chromatin modifications and their function. *Cell* 128, 693–705. doi: 10.1016/j.cell.2007.02.005

Kurian, J. R., Olesen, K. M., and Auger, A. P. (2010). Sex differences in epigenetic regulation of the estrogen receptor-alpha promoter within the developing preoptic area. *Endocrinology*. 151, 2297–2305. doi: 10.1210/en.2009-0649

Larsson, K., and Heimer, L. (1964). Mating behaviour of male rats after lesions in the preoptic area. *Nature* 202, 413–414. doi: 10.1038/202413a0

Leong, H., Sloan, J. R., Nash, P. D., and Greene, G. L. (2005). Recruitment of histone deacetylase 4 to the N-terminal region of estrogen receptor alpha. *Mol. Endocrinol.* 19, 2930–2942. doi: 10.1210/me.2005-0178

Liu, D., Diorio, J., Day, J. C., Francis, D. D., and Meaney, M. J. (2000). Maternal care, hippocampal synaptogenesis and cognitive development in rats. *Nat. Neurosci.* 3, 799–806. doi: 10.1038/77702

Martin, C., and Zhang, Y. (2005). The diverse functions of histone lysine methylation. *Nat. Rev. Mol. Cell Biol.* 6, 838–849. doi: 10.1038/nrm1761

Matsuda, K. I., Mori, H., and Kawata, M. (2012). Epigenetic mechanisms are involved in sexual differentiation of the brain. *Rev. Endocr. Metab. Disord.* 13, 163–171. doi: 10.1007/s11154-012-9202-z

Matsuda, K. I., Mori, H., Nugent, B. M., Pfaff, D. W., McCarthy, M. M., and Kawata, M. (2011). Histone deacetylation during brain development is essential for permanent masculinization of sexual behavior. *Endocrinology* 152, 2760–2767. doi: 10.1210/en.2011-0193

Matsuda, K. I., Ochiai, I., Nishi, M., and Kawata, M. (2002). Colocalization and ligand-dependent discrete distribution of the estrogen receptor (ER)alpha and ERbeta. *Mol. Endocrinol.* 16, 2215–2230. doi: 10.1210/me.2002-0110

Matsuda, K. I., Sakamoto, H., and Kawata, M. (2008). Androgen action in the brain and spinal cord for the regulation of male sexual behaviors. *Curr. Opin. Pharmacol.* 8, 747–751. doi: 10.1016/j.coph.2008.08.010

McCarthy, M. M. (2008). Estradiol and the developing brain. *Physiol. Rev.* 88, 91–124 doi: 10.1152/physrev.00010.2007

McCarthy, M. M., and Crews, D. (2008). Epigenetics–new frontiers in neuroendocrinology. *Front. Neuroendocrinol.* 29, 341–343. doi: 10.1016/j.yfrne.2008.01.002

Moore, C. L. (1992). The role of maternal stimulation in the development of sexual behavior and its neural basis. *Ann. N.Y. Acad. Sci.* 662, 160–177. doi: 10.1111/j.1749-6632.1992.tb22859.x

Mori, H., Matsuda, K. I., Tsukahara, S., and Kawata, M. (2010). Intrauterine position affects estrogen receptor alpha expression in the ventromedial nucleus of the hypothalamus via promoter DNA methylation. *Endocrinology* 151, 5775–5581. doi: 10.1210/en.2010-0646

Murray, E. K., Hien, A., de Vries, G. J., and Forger, N. G. (2009). Epigenetic control of sexual differentiation of the bed nucleus of the stria terminalis. *Endocrinology* 150, 4241–4247. doi: 10.1210/en.2009-0458

Musatov, S., Chen, W., Pfaff, D. W., Kaplitt, M. G., and Ogawa, S. (2006). RNAi-mediated silencing of estrogen receptor {alpha} in the ventromedial nucleus of hypothalamus abolishes female sexual behaviors. *Proc. Natl. Acad. Sci. U.S.A.* 103, 10456–10460. doi: 10.1073/pnas.0603045103

Nakao, M. (2001). Epigenetics: interaction of DNA methylation and chromatin. *Gene* 278, 25–31. doi: 10.1016/S0378-1119(01)00721-1

Numan, M. A. (1996). Lesion and neuroanatomical tract-tracing analysis of the role of the bed nucleus of the stria terminalis in retrieval behavior and other aspects of maternal responsiveness in rats. *Dev. Psychobiol.* 29, 23–51.

Numan, M., and Woodside, B. (2010). Maternity: neural mechanisms, motivational processes, and physiological adaptations. *Behav. Neurosci.* 124, 715–741. doi: 10.1037/a0021548

Ogawa, S., Eng, V., Taylor, J., Lubahn, D. B., Korach, K. S., and Pfaff, D. W. (1998a). Roles of estrogen receptor-alpha gene expression in reproduction-related behaviors in female mice. *Endocrinology* 139, 5070–5081.

Ogawa, S., Lubahn, D. B., Korach, K. S., and Pfaff, D. W. (1997). Behavioral effects of estrogen receptor gene disruption in male mice. *Proc. Natl. Acad. Sci. U.S.A.* 94, 1476–1481. doi: 10.1073/pnas.94.4.1476

Ogawa, S., Taylor, J. A., Lubahn, D. B., Korach, K. S., and Pfaff, D. W. (1996). Reversal of sex roles in genetic female mice by disruption of estrogen receptor gene. *Neuroendocrinology* 64, 467–470. doi: 10.1159/000127154

Ogawa, S., Washburn, T. F., Taylor, J., Lubahn, D. B., Korach, K. S., and Pfaff, D. W. (1998b). Modifications of testosterone-dependent behaviors by estrogen receptor-alpha gene disruption in male mice. *Endocrinology* 139, 5058–5069.

Parker, M. G. (1995). Structure and function of estrogen receptors. *Vitam. Horm.* 51, 267–287. doi: 10.1016/S0083-6729(08)61041-9

Pei, M., Matsuda, K. I., Sakamoto, H., and Kawata, M. (2006). Intrauterine proximity to male fetuses affects the morphology of the sexually dimorphic nucleus of the preoptic area in the adult rat brain. *Eur. J. Neurosci.* 23, 1234–1240. doi: 10.1111/j.1460-9568.2006.04661.x

Pena, C. J., Neugut, Y. D., and Champagne, F. A. (2013). Developmental timing of the effects of maternal care on gene expression and epigenetic regulation of hormone receptor levels in female rats. *Endocrinology* 154, 4340–4351. doi: 10.1210/en.2013-1595

Prior, K. M., Meaney, M. J., and Cameron, N. M. (2013). Variations in maternal care associated with differences in female rat reproductive behavior in a group-mating environment. *Dev. Psychobiol.* 55, 838–848. doi: 10.1002/dev.21075

Ribeiro, A. C., Musatov, S., Shteyler, A., Simanduyev, S., and Arrieta-Cruz, I. (2012). siRNA silencing of estrogen receptor-alpha expression specifically in medial preoptic area neurons abolishes maternal care in female mice. *Proc. Natl. Acad. Sci. U.S.A.* 109, 16324–16329. doi: 10.1073/pnas.1214094109

Rissman, E. F., Wersinger, S. R., Taylar, J. A., and Lubahn, D. B. (1997). Estrogen receptor function as revealed by knockout studies: neuroendocrine and behavioral aspects. *Horm. Behav.* 31, 232–243. doi: 10.1006/hbeh.1997.1390

Sakamoto, H., Takahashi, H., Matsuda, K. I., Nishi, M., and Takanami, K. (2012). Rapid signaling of steroid hormones in the vertebrate nervous system. *Front. Biosci. (Landmark Ed)* 17, 996–1019. doi: 10.2741/3970

Sano, K., Tsuda, M. C., Musatov, S., Sakamoto, T., and Ogawa, S. (2013). Differential effects of site-specific knockdown of estrogen receptor alpha in the medial amygdala, medial pre-optic area, and ventromedial nucleus of the hypothalamus on sexual and aggressive behavior of male mice. *Eur. J. Neurosci.* 37, 1308–1319. doi: 10.1111/ejn.12131

Schwarz, J. M., Nugent, B. M., and McCarthy, M. M. (2010). Developmental and hormone-induced epigenetic changes to estrogen and progesterone receptor genes in brain are dynamic across the life span. *Endocrinology* 151, 4871–4781. doi: 10.1210/en.2010-0142

Scordalakes, E. M., and Rissman, E. F. (2003). Aggression in male lacking functional estrogen receptor α. *Behav. Neurosci.* 44, 427–434. doi: 10.1037/0735-7044.117.1.38

Spiteri, T., Musatov, S., Ogawa, S., Ribeiro, A., Pfaff, D. W., and Agmo, A. (2010a). Estrogen-induced sexual incentive motivation, proceptivity and receptivity depend on a functional estrogen receptor alpha in the ventromedial nucleus of the hypothalamus but not in the amygdala. *Neuroendocrinology* 91, 142–154. doi: 10.1159/000255766

Spiteri, T., Musatov, S., Ogawa, S., Ribeiro, A., Pfaff, D. W., and Agmo, A. (2010b). The role of the estrogen receptor α in the medial amygdala and ventromedial nucleus of the hypothalamus in social recognition, anxiety and aggression. *Behav. Brain Res.* 210, 211–220. doi: 10.1016/j.bbr.2010.02.033

Spiteri, T., Ogawa, S., Musatov, S., Pfaff, D. W., and Agmo, A. (2012). The role of the estrogen receptor alpha in the medial preoptic area in sexual incentive motivation, proceptivity and receptivity, anxiety, and wheel running in female rats. *Behav Brain Res.* 230, 11–20. doi: 10.1016/j.bbr.2012.01.048

Tetel, M. J., and Pfaff, D. W. (2010). Contributions of estrogen receptor,-α, and estrogen receptor-β to the regulation of behavior. *Biochim. Biophys. Acta* 1800, 1084–1089. doi: 10.1016/j.bbagen.2010.01.008

Vasudevan, N., and Pfaff, D. W. (2008). Non-genomic actions of estrogens and their interaction with genomic actions in the brain. *Front. Neuroendocrinol.* 29, 238–257. doi: 10.1016/j.yfrne.2007.08.003

vom Saal, F. S. (1984). The intrauterine position phenomenon: effects on physiology, aggressive behavior and population dynamics in house mice. *Prog. Clin. Biol. Res.* 169, 135–179.

vom Saal, F. S. (1989). Sexual differentiation in litter-bearing mammals: influence of sex of adjacent fetuses in utero. *J. Anim. Sci.* 67, 1824–1840.

vom Saal, F. S., and Bronson, F. H. (1980). Sexual characteristics of adult female mice are correlated with their blood testosterone levels during prenatal development. *Science* 208, 597–599. doi: 10.1126/science.7367881

Wersinger, S. R., Sannen, K., Villalba, C., Lubahn, D. B., Rissman, E. F., and De Vries, G. J. (1997). Masculine sexual behavior is disrupted in male and female mice lacking a functional estrogen receptor α gene. *Horm. Behav.* 32, 176–183.

Wilson, M. E., Westberry, J. M., and Prewitt, A. K. (2008). Dynamic regulation of estrogen receptor-alpha gene expression in the brain: a role for promoter methylation? *Front. Neuroendocrinol.* 29, 375–385. doi: 10.1016/j.yfrne.2008.03.002

Yokosuka, M., Okamura, H., and Hayashi, S. (1997). Postnatal development and sex difference in neurons containing estrogen receptor-alpha immunoreactivity in the preoptic brain, the diencephalon, and the amygdala in the rat. *J. Comp. Neurol.* 389, 81–93.

Zhang, Y., and Reinberg, D. (2001). Transcription regulation by histone methylation: interplay between different covalent modifications of the core histone tails. *Genes Dev.* 15, 2343–2360. doi: 10.1101/gad.927301

Modification of female and male social behaviors in estrogen receptor beta knockout mice by neonatal maternal separation

Mumeko C. Tsuda[1], Naoko Yamaguchi[2], Mariko Nakata[1] and Sonoko Ogawa[1]*

[1] *Laboratory of Behavioral Neuroendocrinology, University of Tsukuba, Tsukuba, Japan*
[2] *Department of Pharmacology, School of Medicine, Aichi Medical University, Nagakute, Japan*

Correspondence:
Sonoko Ogawa, Laboratory of Behavioral Neuroendocrinology, University of Tsukuba, Research Building D-409, 1-1-1 Tennodai, Tsukuba, Ibaraki, 305-8577, Japan
e-mail: ogawa@kansei.tsukuba.ac.jp

Maternal separation (MS) is an animal model mimicking the effects of early life stress on the development of emotional and social behaviors. Recent studies revealed that MS stress increased social anxiety levels in female mice and reduced peri-pubertal aggression in male mice. Estrogen receptor (ER) β plays a pivotal role in the regulation of stress responses and anxiety-related and social behaviors. Behavioral studies using ERβ knockout (βERKO) mice reported increased social investigation and decreased social anxiety in βERKO females, and elevated aggression levels in βERKO males compared to wild-type (WT) mice. In the present study, using βERKO and WT mice, we examined whether ERβ contributes to MS effects on anxiety and social behaviors. βERKO and WT mice were separated from their dam daily (4 h) from postnatal day 1–14 and control groups were left undisturbed. First, MS and ERβ gene deletion individually increased anxiety-related behaviors in the open field test, but only in female mice. Anxiety levels were not further modified in βERKO female mice subjected to MS stress. Second, βERKO female mice showed higher levels of social investigation compared with WT in the social investigation test and long-term social preference test. However, MS greatly reduced social investigation duration and elevated number of stretched approaches in WT and βERKO females in the social investigation test, suggesting elevated levels of social anxiety in both genotypes. Third, peri-pubertal and adult βERKO male mice were more aggressive than WT mice as indicated by heightened aggression duration. On the other hand, MS significantly decreased aggression duration in both genotypes, but only in peri-pubertal male mice. Altogether, these results suggest that βERKO mice are sensitive to the adverse effects of MS stress on subsequent female and male social behaviors, which could then have overrode the ERβ effects on female social anxiety and male aggression.

Keywords: estrogen receptor β, stress, anxiety, aggression, adolescence, social anxiety, social preference, sex differences

INTRODUCTION

Childhood exposure to an adverse environment is frequently associated with an increased risk in developing emotional and social adjustment disorders (Agid et al., 1999; Heim and Nemeroff, 2001). Maternal separation (MS) is an animal model widely used to gain an understanding in the effects of early life stress on subsequent behaviors (see reviews Sanchez et al., 2001; Millstein and Holmes, 2007; Veenema, 2012). A large number of literature report effects of MS on emotionality and anxiety-related behaviors, but the effects on social behaviors are less understood. MS procedures used in our laboratory involves the removal of pups from their mother for 3–4 h each day during the dark phase of the light/dark cycle for the first two weeks of life. With this particular MS procedure, we previously reported sex-specific effects of MS on anxiety-related and social behaviors. Specifically, MS in C57BL/6J female mice increased anxiety-related behaviors in the open field test, increased social anxiety levels toward unfamiliar opponent mice in the social investigation test, and decreased social preference toward male opponent mice in the long-term social preference test compared to non-separated mice (Tsuda and Ogawa, 2012). In C57BL/6J male mice, MS was found to greatly suppress aggression levels during the peri-pubertal period without disrupting social investigative behaviors (Tsuda et al., 2011). Taken together, our MS paradigm demonstrated that early life stress could have detrimental effects on the development of female and male social behaviors.

It is well known that estrogen can regulate a variety of behavioral and physiological functions involving reproduction (Ogawa et al., 1998, 1999, 2000; Nomura et al., 2006), cognition (Luine et al., 1998; Luine, 2008), emotionality (Fink et al., 1998), and stress responses (Critchlow et al., 1963; Bohler et al., 1990). Estrogen's various effects are mediated by two nuclear receptors, estrogen receptor α (ERα) and ERβ (Green et al., 1986; Kuiper et al., 1996). Areas such as the bed nucleus of the stria terminalis, amygdala, medial preoptic nucleus, and locus coeruleus express both forms of ER, however the supraoptic nucleus and paraventricular nucleus of the hypothalamus (PVN) exclusively contains ERβ and nearly no ERα (Shughrue et al., 1996, 1997; Mitra et al., 2003). The expression of ERβ in the above-mentioned brain regions suggests for a potential involvement in the regulation of anxiety-related and social behaviors, as well stress responses.

Numerous studies have provided evidence for the potential role of ERβ in the regulation of anxiety levels as well as social behaviors (Handa et al., 2012). Studies using ERβ null mice (βERKO) have reported increased anxiety-related behaviors in βERKO female mice compared to their wild-type counterparts in the open field, elevated plus maze, and light-dark transition tests (Krezel et al., 2001; Imwalle et al., 2005; Tomihara et al., 2009). These results are indicative that ERβ has anxiolytic effects in nonsocial tests. On the other hand, reduced anxiety-related behaviors are observed in βERKO female mice in social conditions. In social recognition tests, βERKO female mice persistently showed high levels of social investigation and reduced number of stretched approaches (an index for anxiety levels) to a repeatedly presented conspecific (Choleris et al., 2003), suggesting reduced social anxiety. Therefore, depending on the context of the test, i.e., nonsocial vs. social, there are differential effects of ERβ on anxiety-related behaviors. Besides the involvement with anxiety behaviors, ERβ has also been shown to be a key player in the regulation of aggressive behaviors. For example, βERKO male mice exhibit increased levels of aggression, depending on their social experience and age (Ogawa et al., 1999; Nomura et al., 2002a, 2006), suggesting that ERβ may play an inhibitory role in the regulation of male aggressive behavior.

During the neonatal period, various factors might contribute to the effects of MS on subsequent behavioral and neuroendocrine functions. Genetic factors such as ERβ may be a possible candidate because of its known role in regulating stress responses, anxiety-related behaviors, and social behaviors. High levels of ERβ are detected in the PVN between postnatal days 1–9 (Zhang et al., 2004; Zuloaga et al., 2014), which coincides with the postnatal development of the hypothalamic-pituitary-adrenal (HPA) axis, the major regulatory system that controls reactions to stress (Schmidt et al., 2003). Furthermore, MS stress causes lasting alternations in HPA activity, in which MS rats and mice display augmented HPA function under basal and stressful conditions (Wigger and Neumann, 1999; Kalinichev et al., 2002; Parfitt et al., 2004). Therefore, it is possible that ERβ is involved in MS effects on the development of the HPA axis and any subsequent behaviors. To assess whether MS stress differentially affects mice lacking functional ERβ, we investigated the effects of MS on female and male anxiety-related behaviors in the open field test, female social behaviors in the social investigation and social preference tests, and male peri-pubertal and adult aggression of βERKO mice subjected to neonatal MS stress.

MATERIALS AND METHODS

ANIMALS

Adult female heterozygous (HZ) mice were mated with either βERKO or wild-type (WT) male mice. This specific mating scheme was necessary to obtain enough number of WT and βERKO pups in each treatment group. βERKO male mice were viable mating partners because they display normal male sexual behavior similar to WT mice (Ogawa et al., 1999). βERKO, WT, and HZ mice used for mating were obtained from βERKO breeding colonies maintained at the University of Tsukuba. Original HZ breeding pairs were obtained from the National Institute of Environmental Health Sciences (Research Triangle Park, NC, USA) and completely backcrossed to C57BL/6J mice (Krege et al., 1998). During the last week of gestation, pregnant HZ females were individually housed in plastic cages (29 × 19 × 12 cm) with nesting material and monitored daily for parturition. The day of parturition was defined as postnatal day (PND) 0. Stimuli mice used for behavioral testing were either C57BL/6J or ICR/Jcl from CLEA (Tokyo, Japan). All mice were maintained on a 12:12 light/dark cycle (lights off at 1200) and at a constant temperature (23 ± 2°C) throughout the study. Food and water were provided *ad libitum*. All procedures in this study were conducted with approval from the Animal Care and Use Committee and the Recombinant DNA Use Committee at the University of Tsukuba and strictly followed the National Institutes of Health guidelines.

MATERNAL SEPARATION PROCEDURES

MS procedures were followed as previously described in detail in Tsuda and Ogawa (2012). Briefly, on PND 1, each litter was culled to six pups (2–4 females in each litter) and assigned to either a control or MS group. From PND 1 to 14, MS pups were removed together into a small container placed on a warmer maintained a constant temperature of 36°C and separated from their dam for 4 h each day between 1500 and 1900. Control pups remained with their dam. On PND 21, all pups were ear punched, weaned and group-housed with littermates of the same sex. Tail samples were collected at this time for genotyping (Krege et al., 1998). Only βERKO and WT mice obtained from the respective HZ × βERKO and HZ × WT mating schemes were used for behavioral testing.

EXPERIMENTAL GROUPS

At 12 weeks of age, female offspring were ovariectomized (OVX) under general anesthesia with isoflurane inhalation (Dainippon Sumitomo Pharma, Japan) and single-housed at this time. At 13 weeks of age, anxiety-related behaviors in WT (control = 7; *MS* = 7) and βERKO (control = 7; *MS* = 11) female mice were measured in the open-field test (OFT). Following OFT, female mice were tested for social investigative behaviors toward an unfamiliar female opponent in the social investigation test (SIT) and social preference for female and male stimuli in a long-term social preference test (SPT) at 14–15 weeks of age.

Male mice were single-housed one week before testing and left as gonadally intact. At 13 weeks of age, WT (control = 9; *MS* = 6) and βERKO (control = 5; *MS* = 8) male mice were tested for anxiety-related behaviors in OFT. Following OFT, male mice were examined for adult male aggression at 14 weeks of age. A separate cohort of male mice was used to investigate peri-pubertal male aggression in WT (control = 10; *MS* = 9) and βERKO (control = 8; *MS* = 9) mice at 5 and 6 weeks of age. All behavior tests, unless otherwise noted, were tested during the dark phase (1400–1800, at least 2 h after lights off).

OPEN-FIELD TEST (OFT)

The open-field arena (60 × 60 × 30 cm) was illuminated to 5 lux and the floor was hypothetically divided into 25 equal square sections, 9 inner sections (center area) and 16 outer sections (peripheral area). Mice were placed in the corner and activity was monitored for 10 min on a Macintosh computer using Image OFC 2.03 (O'Hara & Co., Ltd., Tokyo, Japan), modified software based on the public domain NIH Image program (developed at the U.S. National Institutes of Health and available on the internet at http://rsb.info.nih.gov/nih-image/). Total moving distance was analyzed as a measure of activity and time spent in the center area was used as an index of anxiety.

SOCIAL INVESTIGATION TEST (SIT)

SIT apparatus (SOSI Type1, O'Hara & Co., Ltd., Tokyo, Japan) and methods are described in detail in Tsuda and Ogawa (2012). Social investigative behaviors of female mice were assessed against a cylinder containing an unfamiliar OVX female C57BL/6J mouse placed in the center of their home cage for 15 min. Cylinders used to introduce stimulus mice were made of clear Plexiglas and were perforated near the bottom (Mouse Cylinder SIOT1, O'Hara & Co., Ltd., Tokyo, Japan). All tests were video recorded and scored off-line using a digital event recorder program (Recordia 1.0b, O'Hara & Co., Ltd., Tokyo, Japan). All mice were analyzed for measurements of social investigation duration and number of stretched approaches. Detailed description of behaviors are presented in Tsuda and Ogawa (2012). One control WT female was excluded from analysis due to no activity during testing.

LONG-TERM SOCIAL PREFERENCE TEST (SPT)

Female mice were tested in a long-term SPT (AMAZENG TYPE1, O'Hara & Co., Ltd., Tokyo, Japan) as previously described in detail by our laboratory (Tsuda and Ogawa, 2012). The apparatus consisted of a large plastic cage (test mice) connected to two smaller cages (stimuli mice) by a tunnel. Wire mesh between tunnel and small cage prevented physical contact. Social preference between an OVX ICR/Jcl female and a gonadally intact ICR/Jcl male mouse was continuously measured for 5 days. The time experimental mice spent in each tunnel were recorded on a Windows computer using the Time BAP software (O'Hara & Co., Ltd., Tokyo, Japan). Cumulative duration spent in each tunnel during the 12 h dark phase was analyzed and averaged for the testing period. One MS WT and one control βERKO female mouse displayed a strong preference (>85%) for the same smaller cage during both baseline and testing periods and were excluded from analysis. Throughout SPT, all mice were provided with food and water *ad libitum*.

AGGRESSIVE BEHAVIOR TEST

Male aggression was assessed in a resident-intruder paradigm for 2 consecutive days at 5 and 6 weeks of age (peri-pubertal mice) or 3 consecutive days at 14 weeks of age (adult mice) under red lighting. Resident mice were tested in their home-cage against a weight-matched, group-housed, gonadally intact, olfactory bulbectomized (OBX) C57BL/6J intruder male mouse for 15 min. Resident mice encountered a different intruder mouse in each aggression test. OBX intruder males rarely display aggression but are capable of eliciting aggression from resident mice. Therefore, OBX stimuli mice eliminate possible confounding effects of social defeat experience. All tests were videotaped and scored for the number of aggressive bouts, cumulative duration of aggressive bouts, and latency to the first aggressive bout using the Recordia 1.0 b program. Data for each week were averaged for each mouse. An aggressive bout was defined as a series of behavioral interactions consisting of at least one of the following: chasing, boxing, tail rattling, wrestling, biting, and offensive lateral attack. If more than 3 s elapsed between aggressive bouts, they were scored as two separate bouts.

STATISTICS

OFT, SIT, and adult male aggression data were analyzed by a Two-Way ANOVA for main effects of treatment, genotype, and their interactions within each sex. Long-term SPT data were analyzed with either a Two-Way ANOVA for treatment and genotype differences in the combined time spent with both stimuli mice or a paired t-test to compare the differences in time spent investigating between paired stimulus mice. Peri-pubertal male aggression data were analyzed by a Three-Way ANOVA for repeated measurements for the main effects of treatment, genotype, age, and their interactions. Significant ANOVA interactions were followed by Bonferroni *post-hoc* tests and significant main effects were analyzed as a separate ANOVA for each main effect. Significant differences were considered when $p < 0.05$. All data were analyzed using SPSS 14.0J (SPSS, Chicago, IL) statistical package. All data are presented as mean ± standard error of the mean (SEM).

RESULTS

ANXIETY-RELATED BEHAVIORS

Females

In OFT, there were significant main effects of MS and genotype on the time spent in center area ([treatment: $F_{(1, 28)} = 5.06$, $p < 0.05$; genotype: $F_{(1, 28)} = 8.24$, $p < 0.01$], **Figure 1A**) and also a marginally significant interaction of treatment and genotype [$F_{(1, 28)} = 3.57$, $p = 0.07$]. *Post-hoc* analysis revealed that MS reduced the time spent in the center area only in WT mice compared to the control group ($p < 0.05$), and the center time of βERKO only differed from WT in the control group ($p < 0.05$). These results indicate that MS stress and ERβ deficiency may independently increase anxiety-related behaviors in female mice.

On the other hand, only genotype differences were found in the total moving distance ([$F_{(1, 28)} = 4.69, p < 0.05$], **Figure 1B**), in which βERKO mice were more active than WT regardless of treatment. Although βERKO female mice moved more during OFT, it is notable that in the control group, βERKO mice also spent less time in the center area. This may indicate an abnormal response of βERKO female mice to a novel environment in the OFT.

Males

In both behavioral measurements of time spent in the center area and total moving distance, no significant effects of treatment or genotype were found in male mice (**Figures 1C,D**). Therefore, neither MS nor ERβ gene deletion affected anxiety levels measured in OFT in male mice.

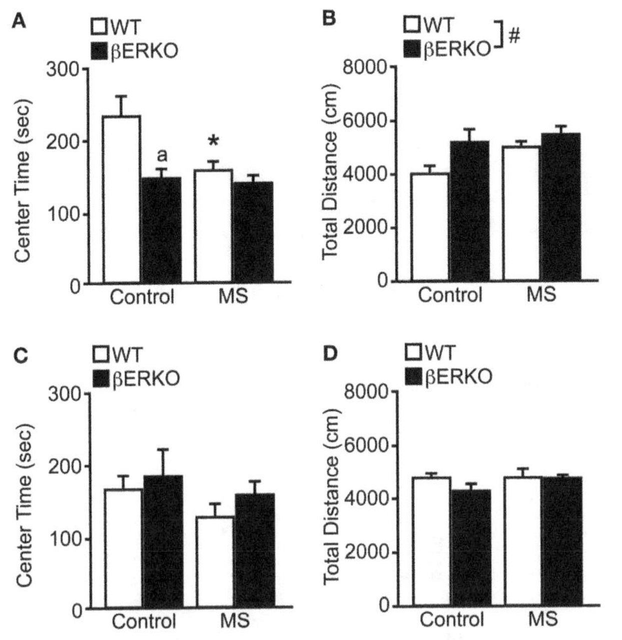

FIGURE 1 | MS effects on anxiety-related behaviors measured in the OFT in female and male WT and βERKO mice. (A,B) Female and **(C,D)** male WT and βERKO mice. **(A,C)** The total time spent in the center area and **(B,D)** total moving distance in the entire arena measured during OFT. All data are presented as mean ± s.e.m. $^{*}p < 0.05$ vs. control of same genotype; $^{a}p < 0.05$ vs. WT of same treatment group; $^{\#}p < 0.05$.

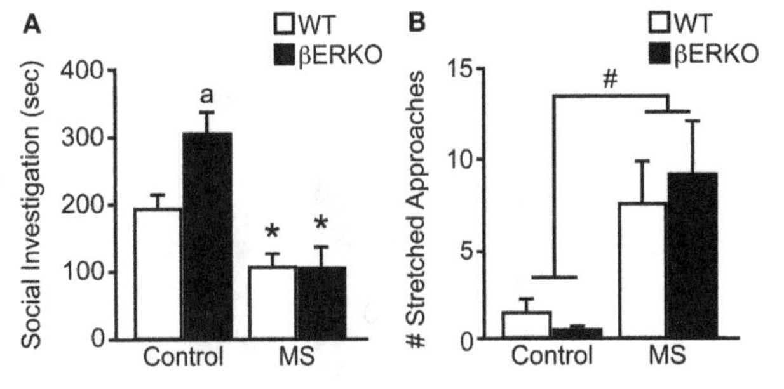

FIGURE 2 | Genotype and MS effects on social investigative behaviors during SIT. (A) Cumulative social investigation duration and **(B)** number of stretched approaches toward an unfamiliar female opponent mouse in SIT. All data are presented as mean ± s.e.m. $^{*}p < 0.05$ vs. control of same genotype; $^{a}p < 0.05$ vs. WT of same treatment group; $^{\#}p < 0.05$.

FEMALE SOCIAL INVESTIGATIVE BEHAVIORS

Similar to our previously reported findings (Tsuda and Ogawa, 2012), MS increased social anxiety levels toward unfamiliar female stimuli mice in SIT. Specifically, MS greatly reduced social investigation duration ([treatment: $F_{(1,\ 28)} = 19.77$, $p < 0.001$], **Figure 2A**) and significantly increased the number of stretched approaches ([treatment: $F_{(1,\ 28)} = 8.62$, $p < 0.01$], **Figure 2B**). Although no significant effect of genotype was found in either behavioral parameter, there was a marginally significant interaction of treatment and genotype in social investigation duration [$F_{(1,\ 28)} = 3.09$, $p < 0.08$]. *Post-hoc* analysis showed that control βERKO female mice spent more time sniffing the stimuli-containing cylinder compared to control WT mice ($p < 0.05$). However, MS greatly diminished social investigation duration in βERKO compared to control group ($p < 0.05$) and eliminated any genotype differences. Moreover, MS-induced reduction in social investigation duration was much greater in βERKO (61.88%) mice than WT mice (45.61%), suggesting that MS effects on social investigative behaviors were more apparent and possibly more adverse in mice that lack ERβ gene function.

FEMALE SOCIAL PREFERENCE

There was a significant interaction of treatment and genotype on the total time females spent in the two tunnels connected to female and male stimuli mice in long-term SPT ([treatment: n.s.; genotype: n.s.; treatment × genotype: $F_{(1,\ 28)} = 9.05$, $p < 0.01$]; **Figure 3A**). Control βERKO females spent more time in the tunnels compared to control WT ($p < 0.05$). In WT female mice, MS did not affect the total time spent in the tunnels whereas MS greatly reduced it in βERKO mice ($p < 0.05$). Altogether, lack of ERβ increased social interest toward unfamiliar opponents in female mice, but this phenotype was suppressed (or attenuated) when βERKO females experienced neonatal MS stress.

While control WT females displayed no preference for either stimuli sex, control βERKO [$t_{(5)} = 2.54$, $p = 0.06$] mice displayed a preference for female over male stimuli (**Figure 3B**). In MS groups, WT female mice showed a preference for female over male [$t_{(6)} = 2.88$, $p < 0.05$], but βERKO mice failed to show any preference for either stimuli mice. Greatly reduced total time spent in tunnels found in βERKO mice that underwent MS stress (**Figure 3A**) was actually due to the decreased time spent with the female opponent mouse.

PERI-PUBERTAL MALE AGGRESSION

Peri-pubertal male aggressive behaviors were greatly suppressed by MS stress in both βERKO and WT mice at 5 and 6 weeks of age. There was a significant main effect of MS and age on the number of aggressive bouts ([treatment: $F_{(1,\ 29)} = 11.03$, $p < 0.01$; age: $F_{(1,\ 29)} = 23.95$, $p < 0.0001$]; **Figure 4A**), cumulative duration of aggression ([treatment: $F_{(1,\ 29)} = 10.37$, $p < 0.01$; age: $F_{(1,\ 29)} = 10.82$, $p < 0.01$]; **Figure 4B**), and latency to the first aggressive bout ([treatment: $F_{(1,\ 29)} = 3.14$, $p = 0.09$; age: $F_{(1,\ 29)} = 17.45$, $p < 0.01$]; **Figure 4C**), in which aggression levels were greater at 6 weeks of age compared to 5 weeks. However, no effect of genotype or interactions was found in all three behavioral measurements.

Further detailed analysis within each week revealed that consistent with previously reported findings (Nomura et al., 2002a), control βERKO males were more aggressive compared to their WT counterparts at 5 weeks of age, as indicated by higher numbers of aggressive bouts ($p < 0.05$), increased cumulative duration of aggression ($p < 0.05$), shorter latency to the first aggressive bout ($p < 0.05$). There were no longer genotype differences in control mice at 6 weeks of age, possibly due to higher aggression levels in WT male mice at this age. During each week of testing, MS greatly reduced the levels of aggression in both genotypes. Particularly, MS βERKO males showed significantly lower number of aggressive bouts (5 weeks, $p < 0.01$; 6 weeks, $p < 0.05$) and cumulative duration of aggression (5 weeks,

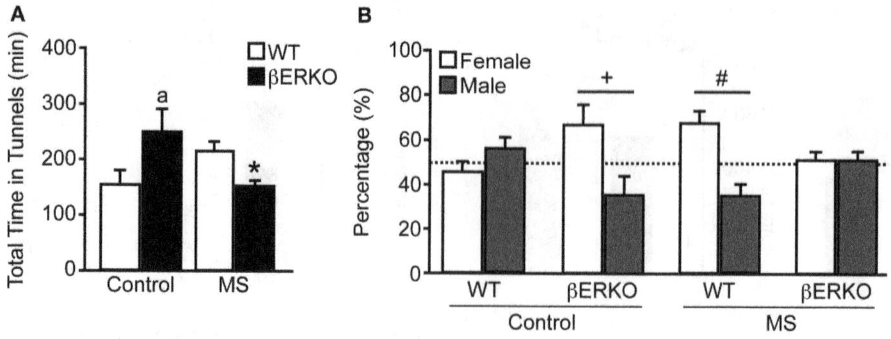

FIGURE 3 | Effects of MS and genotype on social preference during long-term SPT. (A) Total time spent in both tunnels and **(B)** percent of time spent in each tunnel connected to unfamiliar female and male stimuli cages. All data are presented as mean ± s.e.m. $*p < 0.05$ vs. control of same genotype; $^{a}p < 0.05$ vs. WT of same treatment group; $^{\#}p < 0.05$; $^{+}p = 0.06$.

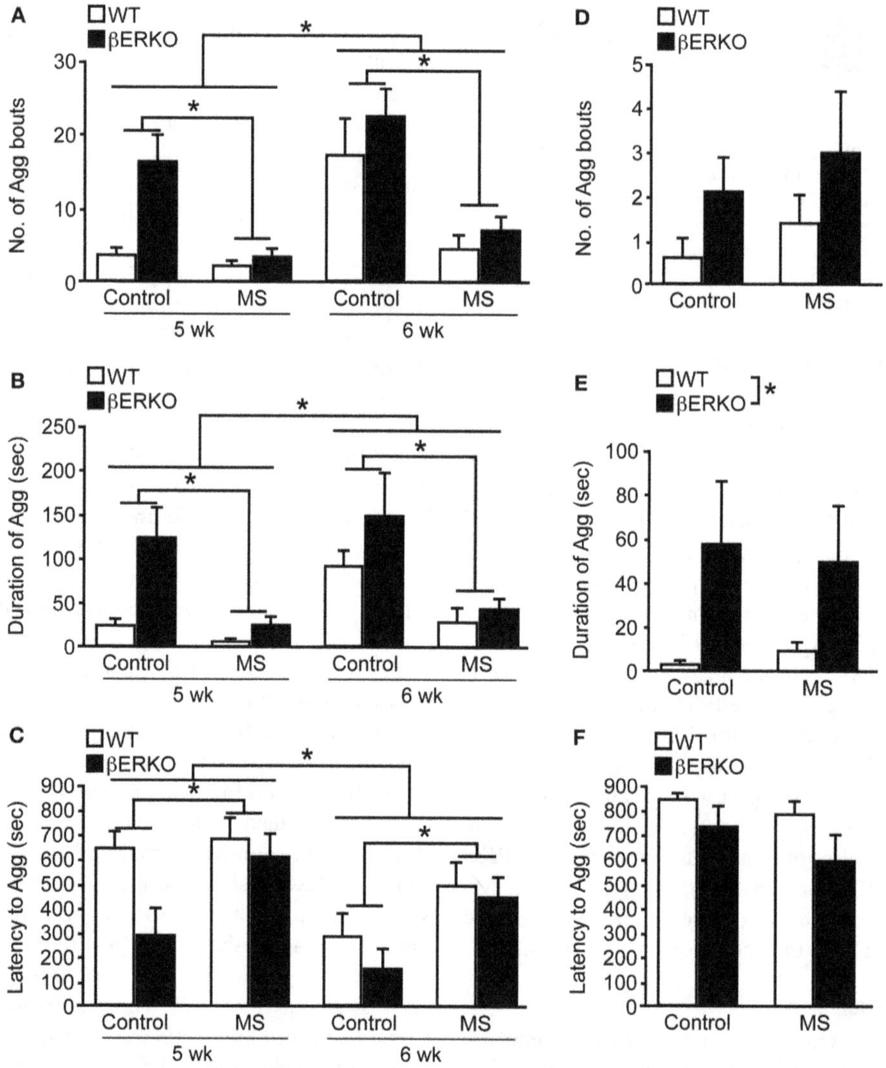

FIGURE 4 | MS effects on peri-pubertal and adult male aggression. (A–C) Peri-pubertal and **(D–F)** adult WT and βERKO male mice. **(A,D)** Number of aggressive bouts, **(B,E)** cumulative duration of aggression, and **(C,F)** latency to the first aggressive bout. All data are presented as mean ± s.e.m. $*p < 0.05$.

$p < 0.01$; 6 weeks, $p < 0.05$) compared to control males at both 5 and 6 weeks of age. In WT mice, MS males also showed significantly lower number of aggressive bouts compared to control males at 6 weeks ($p < 0.05$), but no MS effect was detected at 5 weeks possibly due to low levels of aggression in the control group.

ADULT MALE AGGRESSION

In contrast to peri-pubertal male aggression, there were no effects of MS found in all three behavioral measurements (**Figures 4D–F**) of adult male aggression. On the other hand, regardless of treatment, βERKO males were found to display significantly higher levels of aggression than WT mice as measured by cumulative duration of aggression ([$F_{(1, 24)} = 5.61$, $p < 0.05$], **Figure 4E**). Latency to the first aggressive bout was also marginally shorter in βERKO compared to WT mice ([$F_{(1, 24)} = 3.34, p = 0.08$], **Figure 4F**).

DISCUSSION

The present study provides two major findings. First, we confirmed that MS stress and ERβ gene deletion could individually modify female anxiety-related and social behaviors and male aggression. Specifically, MS increased female anxiety levels in OFT and social anxiety levels in SIT, and reduced peri-pubertal male aggression. On the other hand, ERβ gene knockout elevated anxiety in OFT and increased investigative behaviors in SIT and SPT of females and heightened adult and peri-pubertal male aggression. Second, social behavior alterations found during SIT and SPT in βERKO females and aggression tests in βERKO males were overruled by MS stress, but not anxiety-related behaviors in OFT (**Table 1**). These results suggest that social behaviors of βERKO mice are vulnerable to MS and can be modified by the adverse effects of early life stress.

SEX-DEPENDENT EFFECTS OF MS AND GENOTYPE ON ANXIETY-RELATED BEHAVIORS

Anxiety-related behaviors measured during OFT in female mice demonstrated that MS increased anxiety levels in a novel environment, which supports our previously published findings in OVX C57BL/6J female mice (Tsuda and Ogawa, 2012). Furthermore, control βERKO females also displayed enhanced anxiety levels compared to WT in OFT. These findings are consistent with previous studies that reported elevated anxiety-related behaviors in gonadally intact and OVX βERKO female mice in the elevated plus maze, OFT (Krezel et al., 2001; Imwalle et al., 2005) and light-dark transition tests (Tomihara et al., 2009), which suggests an ERβ involvement in anxiolysis in females. Given that both MS stress and ERβ gene deletion increased anxiety-related behaviors in OFT, βERKO females subjected to MS did not show amelioration or augmentation in anxiety levels. It may be possible that there is a threshold for anxiety beyond which no further increase can be measured in OFT. Therefore, it is possible that lack of ERβ during neonatal MS stress may have further contributed to already heightened levels of anxiety, but this effect was not measurable in OFT. Whether anxiety levels of βERKO females are indeed more susceptible to MS need to be further investigated using light-dark box transition, elevated zero maze, and/or elevated plus maze tests, which are widely used to examine anxiety levels in mice.

Few studies to date address sex differences of MS effects. As gonadally intact, studies report a stronger effect of MS in males rather than females (Wigger and Neumann, 1999; Kalinichev et al., 2002; Kundakovic et al., 2013) or no sex differences in anxiety levels measured in OFT and elevated plus maze (Rhees et al., 2001; Millstein and Holmes, 2007; Veenema et al., 2007). However, Romeo et al., found that MS increased anxiety in males, but decreased anxiety in diestrus (low estrogen) females (Romeo et al., 2003), suggesting endogenous estrogen levels may influence MS effects in females. In our study, females were tested as OVX to eliminate confounding effects of endogenous estrogen. It was never the intention to directly compare female and male littermates since hormonal conditions differ, but rather to examine whether MS affected female and male mice differently. Indeed, our findings demonstrated that MS effects on anxiety levels were stronger in females than males in OFT. The differential effects of MS in females may be due to differences in estrogen levels at the time of testing, i.e., no estrogen increases anxiety (OVX), low levels of estrogen (diestrus) decreases anxiety, and high levels of estrogen (estrus) has no effect in OFT. Interestingly, ERβ involvement in regulating anxiety levels may also depend on estrogen levels. High doses of estrogen were anxiogenic in both WT and βERKO females, but low doses of estrogen were anxiolytic only

Table 1 | Summary table describing effects of ERβ gene deletion, MS, and interaction of ERβ gene deletion and MS on anxiety-related and social behaviors in female and male mice.

	ERβ gene deletion	MS	ERβ gene deletion × MS
FEMALES			
Open-field test	↑ Anxiety	↑ Anxiety	↑ Anxiety
Social investigation test	↑ Social investigation	↓ Social investigation	↓ Social investigation
	↓ Social anxiety	↑ Social anxiety	↑ Social anxiety
Social preference test	↑ Female preference	↑ Female preference	No preference
MALES			
Open-field test	↔ Anxiety	↔ Anxiety	↔ Anxiety
Peri-pubertal aggression	↑ Aggression	↓ Aggression	↓ Aggression
Adult aggression	↑ Aggression	↔ Aggression	↑ Aggression

Arrows denote differences relative to control WT mice.

in WT and not βERKO females (Tomihara et al., 2009), which suggests that low doses of estrogen may decrease anxiety through ERβ activation. Therefore, MS effects on female anxiety may be associated or dependent on estrogen levels at the time of testing and may involve ERβ's estrogenic action.

EFFECTS OF MS AND GENOTYPE ON FEMALE SOCIAL BEHAVIORS

In SIT, control βERKO females displayed a substantial increase in social investigation levels toward an unfamiliar female stimuli mouse, suggesting heightened social reactivity in βERKO mice. Previous studies have described βERKO females to persistently display high levels of social investigation and reduced counts of stretched approaches toward familiar stimuli mice in social recognition and binary choice tests, suggesting that loss of ERβ function induces a hyper-reactive and low social anxiety phenotype in female mice (Choleris et al., 2003, 2006). However, this behavioral phenotype of βERKO females was eliminated with neonatal MS stress experience. MS reduced social investigation duration and increased number of stretched approaches toward an unfamiliar stimulus mouse in SIT in WT, supporting our previously published observations of elevated social anxiety in C57BL/6J female mice (Tsuda and Ogawa, 2012). Moreover, these same behavioral alterations induced by MS stress were found in MS βERKO female mice, suggesting MS overturned the socially hyper-reactive phenotype of control βERKO mice.

Both control βERKO and MS WT mice significantly preferred a female mouse to a male mouse in SPT, whereas control WT exhibited no social preference. However, MS βERKO females displayed no preference for either mouse and also spent less time in the tunnels connected to the stimuli cages. Enhanced female preference found in control βERKO may be correlated with high social reactivity to a female opponent observed in SIT. We previously reported that the distinct preference for female stimuli to male stimuli or an empty cage during SPT in C57BL/6J MS female mice might have been due to increased social anxiety toward male opponents (Tsuda and Ogawa, 2012). In Tsuda and Ogawa (2012), MS females displayed more social anxiety-like behaviors to male stimuli in SIT and showed no preference between a male mouse and an empty cage in long-term SPT. It is possible that the MS-induced increase in social anxiety may have been more prominent in βERKO females and contributed to the loss of social preference to both male and female stimuli in SPT. Future studies need to assess if MS effects on social anxiety levels differ between female and male opponents in βERKO mice and also evaluate if increased social anxiety in MS βERKO females contribute to a social phobia phenotype.

Heightened social anxiety levels in MS female mice were associated with increased neuronal activity (FosB expression) in the PVN, medial amygdala, and central amygdala following exposure to an unfamiliar social stimuli, while no baseline differences were found between treatment groups (Tsuda and Ogawa, 2012). Increased FosB induction in these regions was also found to be dependent on stimulus gender. Higher number of FosB cells was induced in the PVN with male stimuli exposure and in the medial amygdala with female stimuli exposure. These particular brains regions express ERβ, oxytocin, vasopressin, and corticotropin-releasing hormone, which are involved in the regulation of stress responses and social behavior (Shughrue et al., 1997; Ferguson et al., 2001, 2002; Mitra et al., 2003; Bielsky et al., 2004; Merchenthaler et al., 2004; Neumann, 2008; Milner et al., 2010). Elevated FosB induction in these brain regions possibly indicates a functional alteration of these neuroendocrine correlates in MS females. Furthermore, ERβ is co-localized and regulates oxytocin, vasopressin, and corticotropin-releasing hormone levels in these brain regions (Nomura et al., 2002b; Miller et al., 2004; Murakami et al., 2011). Thus, it is possible that MS induced alterations in female social behaviors are associated with changes in ERβ, oxytocin, vasopressin, corticotropin-releasing hormone in the amygdala and PVN and these neuroendocrine modifications are dependent on the regulatory role of ERβ.

EFFECTS OF MS AND GENOTYPE ON PERI-PUBERTAL AND ADULT MALE AGGRESSION

Consistent with our previous study (Tsuda et al., 2011), MS disrupted the development of peri-pubertal male aggression by suppressing levels of aggressive behavior in WT mice at 5 and 6 weeks of age. However, MS did not affect male aggression assessed in adulthood. This result is surprising since the two other studies that examined MS effects on adult male aggression in mice reported decreased male aggressive behaviors (Veenema et al., 2007; Hohmann et al., 2013). Differences in results may have been due to differences in procedures of MS and aggressive behavior testing. In particular, Veenema et al. (2007) and Hohmann et al. (2013) conducted MS during the light phase of the circadian cycle, but our MS was performed during the dark phase. Therefore, the data obtained in the present study make it difficult to directly compare results, but differences in the effects of MS between these studies demonstrates an intriguing effect of circadian phase as a potential variable to determine MS effects on adult male aggression.

Nomura et al. (2002a) reported higher levels of aggression in βERKO male mice compared to WT in pubertal (5 weeks of age) and young adult (12 weeks of age) mice, but not in adult (19 weeks of age) mice. Similarly, the present study demonstrated increased aggression levels in pubertal (4–5 weeks of age) and young adult (14 weeks of age) control βERKO male mice compared to their WT counterparts. Moreover, lack of ERβ may have advanced the pubertal onset of aggression in male mice. Control βERKO males displayed high levels of aggression already at 5 weeks of age, whereas WT males began to exhibit aggression at 6 weeks of age. Despite the strong aggressive behavior phenotype of βERKO males, neonatal MS stress remarkably suppressed aggression levels in βERKO mice, but only in peri-pubertal males and not young adult males. These results suggest that neonatal MS stress can suppress or attenuate the aggressive phenotype of βERKO male mice, at least during the pubertal period.

ERβ activation via estrogen increases oxytocin, but decreases vasopressin gene expression in the PVN of male mice (Nomura et al., 2002b). Oxytocin and vasopressin are reported to inhibit and facilitate, respectively, male aggression (Ferris, 2005). Furthermore, elevated aggression levels in pubertal βERKO male mice were associated with increased serum testosterone levels (Nomura et al., 2002a) and testosterone levels are known to be positively correlated with aggression in male rodents (Burge and Edwards, 1971). This regulatory role of ERβ on oxytocin and vasopressin expression in the PVN and plasma testosterone levels provides a potential mechanism of elevated aggression levels in βERKO male mice. On the contrary, we recently reported that lower levels of aggression in MS peri-pubertal males were associated with increased and decreased oxytocin and vasopressin positive cells in the PVN, respectively, and reduced serum testosterone levels in 4- to 6- weeks old male mice (Tsuda et al., 2011). MS induced changes in oxytocin, vasopressin, and testosterone may have outweighed or suppressed the phenotype of these hormones found in control βERKO males, resulting in less aggressive βERKO mice. To gain a stronger understanding of the possible neuroendocrine mechanisms in which MS may override ERβ effects on pubertal male aggression, MS effects on ERβ activity during the postnatal period need to be determined. Additionally, whether βERKO males subjected to MS stress display alterations in oxytocin, vasopressin, and serum testosterone levels similar to that of MS WT mice need to be evaluated to comprehend the reduced levels of aggression in pubertal male mice.

CONCLUSIONS

The present findings demonstrated that ERβ gene deletion and MS could individually modify anxiety and social behaviors in mice. However, behavioral phenotypes of βERKO mice were overturned by MS stress in exception to nonsocial anxiety. βERKO mice could be more sensitive to the stressful effects of MS because ERβ also functions to attenuate HPA reactivity to stress (Lund et al., 2005, 2006). The lack of ERβ's inhibitory function during MS may have increased vulnerability to the stressful effects of MS on female social behaviors and male aggression, but there are still other possible mechanisms that need to be investigated. The postnatal period is a critical time of brain development and factors such as genetics and environmental conditions are significantly influential. Findings in the present study demonstrate that there is a potential role for ERβ in MS effects on certain social behaviors and contribute to our understanding of MS effects on female and male social behaviors. The combination of ERβ gene deletion and neonatal MS stress possibly involves a variety of changes in neuroendocrine systems modulating female and male social behaviors in a complex manner that further investigation is needed to fully understand the effects of early life stress on social behaviors.

AUTHOR CONTRIBUTIONS

Mumeko C. Tsuda and Sonoko Ogawa conceived and designed the experiments; Mumeko C. Tsuda performed the experiments; Mumeko C. Tsuda, Naoko Yamaguchi, and Mariko Nakata analyzed the data, Mumeko C. Tsuda and Sonoko Ogawa contributed materials, reagents, and mice, and Mumeko C. Tsuda and Sonoko Ogawa wrote the manuscript.

ACKNOWLEDGMENTS

The authors would like to thank Junko Hirama and Kazuyo Nagata for their technical assistance throughout this study. This research was supported by Grant-in-Aid for Scientific Research (KAKEN #23240057), and University of Tsukuba Research Project to Sonoko Ogawa. Mumeko C. Tsuda was a recipient of the Japan Society for Promotion of Science research fellowship for young scientists.

REFERENCES

Agid, O., Shapira, B., Zislin, J., Ritsner, M., Hanin, B., Murad, H., et al. (1999). Environment and vulnerability to major psychiatric illness: a case control study of early parental loss in major depression, bipolar disorder and schizophrenia. *Mol. Psychiatry* 4, 163–172. doi: 10.1038/sj.mp.4000473

Bielsky, I. F., Hu, S. B., Szegda, K. L., Westphal, H., and Young, L. J. (2004). Profound impairment in social recognition and reduction in anxiety-like behavior in vasopressin V1a receptor knockout mice. *Neuropsychopharmacology* 29, 483–493. doi: 10.1038/sj.npp.1300360

Bohler, H. C., Zoeller, R. T., King, J. C., Rubin, B. S., Weber, R., and Merriam, G. R. (1990). Corticotropin releasing hormone mRNA is elevated on the afternoon of proestrus in the parvocellular paraventricular nuclei of the female rat. *Brain Res. Mol. Brain Res.* 8, 259–262. doi: 10.1016/0169-328X(90)90025-9

Burge, K. G., and Edwards, D. A. (1971). The adrenal gland and the pre and post castrational aggressive behavior of male mice. *Physiol. Behav.* 7, 885–888. doi: 10.1016/0031-9384(71)90058-8

Choleris, E., Gustafsson, J. A., Korach, K. S., Muglia, L. J., Pfaff, D. W., and Ogawa, S. (2003). An estrogen-dependent four-gene micronet regulating social recognition: a study with oxytocin and estrogen receptor-alpha and -beta knockout mice. *Proc. Natl. Acad. Sci. U.S.A.* 100, 6192–6197. doi: 10.1073/pnas.0631699100

Choleris, E., Ogawa, S., Kavaliers, M., Gustafsson, J. A., Korach, K. S., Muglia, L. J., et al. (2006). Involvement of estrogen receptor alpha, beta and oxytocin in social discrimination: a detailed behavioral analysis with knockout female mice. *Genes Brain Behav.* 5, 528–539. doi: 10.1111/j.1601-183X.2006.00203.x

Critchlow, V., Liebelt, R. A., Bar-Sela, M., Mountcastle, W., and Lipscomb, H. S. (1963). Sex difference in resting pituitary-adrenal function in the rat. *Am. J. Physiol.* 205, 807–815.

Ferguson, J. N., Aldag, J. M., Insel, T. R., and Young, L. J. (2001). Oxytocin in the medial amygdala is essential for social recognition in the mouse. *J. Neurosci.* 21, 8278–8285.

Ferguson, J. N., Young, L. J., and Insel, T. R. (2002). The neuroendocrine basis of social recognition. *Front. Neuroendocrinol.* 23:200–224. doi: 10.1006/frne.2002.0229

Ferris, C. F. (2005). Vasopressin/oxytocin and aggression. *Novartis Found. Symp.* 268, 190–198. discussion: 198–200, 242–253. doi: 10.1002/0470010703.ch13

Fink, G., Sumner, B. E., McQueen, J. K., Wilson, H., and Rosie, R. (1998). Sex steroid control of mood, mental state and memory. *Clin. Exp. Pharmacol. Physiol.* 25, 764–775. doi: 10.1111/j.1440-1681.1998.tb02151.x

Green, S., Walter, P., Kumar, V., Krust, A., Bornert, J. M., Argos, P., et al. (1986). Human oestrogen receptor cDNA: sequence, expression and homology to v-erb-A. *Nature* 320, 134–139. doi: 10.1038/320134a0

Handa, R. J., Ogawa, S., Wang, J. M., and Herbison, A. E. (2012). Roles for oestrogen receptor b in adult brain function. *J. Neuroendocrinol.* 24, 160–173. doi: 10.1111/j.1365-2826.2011.02206.x

Heim, C., and Nemeroff, C. B. (2001). The role of childhood trauma in the neurobiology of mood and anxiety disorders: preclinical and clinical studies. *Biol. Psychiatry* 49, 1023–1039. doi: 10.1016/S0006-3223(01)01157-X

Hohmann, C. F., Hodges, A., Beard, N., and Aneni, J. (2013). Effects of brief stress exposure during early postnatal development in balb/CByJ mice: I. Behavioral characterization. *Dev. Psychobiol.* 55, 283–293. doi: 10.1002/dev.21027

Imwalle, D. B., Gustafsson, J. A., and Rissman, E. F. (2005). Lack of functional estrogen receptor beta influences anxiety behavior and serotonin content in female mice. *Physiol. Behav.* 84, 157–163. doi: 10.1016/j.physbeh.2004.11.002

Kalinichev, M., Easterling, K. W., Plotsky, P. M., and Holtzman, S. G. (2002). Long-lasting changes in stress-induced corticosterone response and anxiety-like behaviors as a consequence of neonatal maternal separation in Long-Evans rats. *Pharmacol. Biochem. Behav.* 73, 131–140. doi: 10.1016/S0091-3057(02)00781-5

Krege, J. H., Hodgin, J. B., Couse, J. F., Enmark, E., Warner, M., Mahler, J. F., et al. (1998). Generation and reproductive phenotypes of mice lacking estrogen receptor beta. *Proc. Natl. Acad. Sci. U.S.A.* 95, 15677–15682. doi: 10.1073/pnas.95.26.15677

Krezel, W., Dupont, S., Krust, A., Chambon, P., and Chapman, P. F. (2001). Increased anxiety and synaptic plasticity in estrogen receptor beta -deficient mice. *Proc. Natl. Acad. Sci. U.S.A.* 98, 12278–12282. doi: 10.1073/pnas.221451898

Kuiper, G. G., Enmark, E., Pelto-Huikko, M., Nilsson, S., and Gustafsson, J. A. (1996). Cloning of a novel receptor expressed in rat prostate and ovary. *Proc. Natl. Acad. Sci. U.S.A.* 93, 5925–5930. doi: 10.1073/pnas.93.12.5925

Kundakovic, M., Lim, S., Gudsnuk, K., and Champagne, F. A. (2013). Sex-specific and strain-dependent effects of early life adversity on behavioral and epigenetic outcomes. *Front. Psychiatry* 4:78. doi: 10.3389/fpsyt.2013.00078

Luine, V. N. (2008). Sex steroids and cognitive function. *J. Neuroendocrinol.* 20, 866–872. doi: 10.1111/j.1365-2826.2008.01710.x

Luine, V. N., Richards, S. T., Wu, V. Y., and Beck, K. D. (1998). Estradiol enhances learning and memory in a spatial memory task and effects levels of monoaminergic neurotransmitters. *Horm. Behav.* 34, 149–162. doi: 10.1006/hbeh.1998.1473

Lund, T. D., Hinds, L. R., and Handa, R. J. (2006). The androgen 5alpha-dihydrotestosterone and its metabolite 5alpha-androstan-3beta, 17beta-diol inhibit the hypothalamo-pituitary-adrenal response to stress by acting through estrogen receptor beta-expressing neurons in the hypothalamus. *J. Neurosci.* 26, 1448–1456. doi: 10.1523/JNEUROSCI.3777-05.2006

Lund, T. D., Rovis, T., Chung, W. C., and Handa, R. J. (2005). Novel actions of estrogen receptor-beta on anxiety-related behaviors. *Endocrinology* 146, 797–807. doi: 10.1210/en.2004-1158

Merchenthaler, I., Lane, M. V., Numan, S., and Dellovade, T. L. (2004). Distribution of estrogen receptor alpha and beta in the mouse central nervous system: *in vivo* autoradiographic and immunocytochemical analyses. *J. Comp. Neurol.* 473, 270–291. doi: 10.1002/cne.20128

Miller, W. J., Suzuki, S., Miller, L. K., Handa, R., and Uht, R. M. (2004). Estrogen receptor (ER)beta isoforms rather than ERalpha regulate corticotropin-releasing hormone promoter activity through an alternate pathway. *J. Neurosci.* 24, 10628–10635. doi: 10.1523/JNEUROSCI.5540-03.2004

Millstein, R. A., and Holmes, A. (2007). Effects of repeated maternal separation on anxiety- and depression-related phenotypes in different mouse strains. *Neurosci. Biobehav. Rev.* 31, 3–17. doi: 10.1016/j.neubiorev.2006.05.003

Milner, T. A., Thompson, L. I., Wang, G., Kievits, J. A., Martin, E., Zhou, P., et al. (2010). Distribution of estrogen receptor β containing cells in the brains of bacterial artificial chromosome transgenic mice. *Brain Res.* 1351, 74–96. doi: 10.1016/j.brainres.2010.06.038

Mitra, S. W., Hoskin, E., Yudkovitz, J., Pear, L., Wilkinson, H. A., Hayashi, S., et al. (2003). Immunolocalization of estrogen receptor beta in the mouse brain: comparison with estrogen receptor alpha. *Endocrinology* 144, 2055–2067. doi: 10.1210/en.2002-221069

Murakami, G., Hunter, R. G., Fontaine, C., Ribeiro, A., and Pfaff, D. (2011). Relationships among estrogen receptor, oxytocin and vasopressin gene expression and social interaction in male mice. *Eur. J. Neurosci.* 34, 469–477. doi: 10.1111/j.1460-9568.2011.07761.x

Neumann, I. D. (2008). Brain oxytocin: a key regulator of emotional and social behaviours in both females and males. *J. Neuroendocrinol.* 20, 858–865. doi: 10.1111/j.1365-2826.2008.01726.x

Nomura, M., Andersson, S., Korach, K. S., Gustafsson, J. A., Pfaff, D. W., and Ogawa, S. (2006). Estrogen receptor-beta gene disruption potentiates estrogen-inducible aggression but not sexual behaviour in male mice. *Eur. J. Neurosci.* 23, 1860–1868. doi: 10.1111/j.1460-9568.2006.04703.x

Nomura, M., Durbak, L., Chan, J., Smithies, O., Gustafsson, J. A., Korach, K. S., et al. (2002a). Genotype/age interactions on aggressive behavior in gonadally intact estrogen receptor beta knockout (betaERKO) male mice. *Horm. Behav.* 41, 288–296. doi: 10.1006/hbeh.2002.1773

Nomura, M., McKenna, E., Korach, K. S., Pfaff, D. W., and Ogawa, S. (2002b). Estrogen receptor-beta regulates transcript levels for oxytocin and arginine vasopressin in the hypothalamic paraventricular nucleus of male mice. *Brain Res. Mol. Brain Res.* 109, 84–94. doi: 10.1016/S0169-328X(02)00525-9

Ogawa, S., Chan, J., Chester, A. E., Gustafsson, J. A., Korach, K. S., and Pfaff, D. W. (1999). Survival of reproductive behaviors in estrogen receptor beta gene-deficient (betaERKO) male and female mice. *Proc. Natl. Acad. Sci. U.S.A.* 96, 12887–12892. doi: 10.1073/pnas.96.22.12887

Ogawa, S., Chester, A. E., Hewitt, S. C., Walker, V. R., Gustafsson, J. A., Smithies, O., et al. (2000). Abolition of male sexual behaviors in mice lacking estrogen receptors alpha and beta (alpha beta ERKO). *Proc. Natl. Acad. Sci. U.S.A.* 97, 14737–14741. doi: 10.1073/pnas.250473597

Ogawa, S., Eng, V., Taylor, J., Lubahn, D. B., Korach, K. S., and Pfaff, D. W. (1998). Roles of estrogen receptor-alpha gene expression in reproduction-related behaviors in female mice. *Endocrinology* 139, 5070–5081.

Parfitt, D. B., Levin, J. K., Saltstein, K. P., Klayman, A. S., Greer, L. M., and Helmreich, D. L. (2004). Differential early rearing environments can accentuate or attenuate the responses to stress in male C57BL/6 mice. *Brain Res.* 1016, 111–118. doi: 10.1016/j.brainres.2004.04.077

Rhees, R. W., Lephart, E. D., and Eliason, D. (2001). Effects of maternal separation during early postnatal development on male sexual behavior and female reproductive function. *Behav. Brain Res.* 123, 1–10. doi: 10.1016/S0166-4328(00)00381-8

Romeo, R. D., Mueller, A., Sisti, H. M., Ogawa, S., McEwen, B. S., and Brake, W. G. (2003). Anxiety and fear behaviors in adult male and female C57BL/6 mice are modulated by maternal separation. *Horm. Behav.* 43, 561–567. doi: 10.1016/S0018-506X(03)00063-1

Sanchez, M. M., Ladd, C. O., and Plotsky, P. M. (2001). Early adverse experience as a developmental risk factor for later psychopathology: evidence from rodent and primate models. *Dev. Psychopathol.* 13, 419–449. doi: 10.1017/S0954579401003029

Schmidt, M. V., Enthoven, L., van der Mark, M., Levine, S., de Kloet, E. R., and Oitzl, M. S. (2003). The postnatal development of the hypothalamic-pituitary-adrenal axis in the mouse. *Int. J. Dev. Neurosci.* 21, 125–132. doi: 10.1016/S0736-5748(03)00030-3

Shughrue, P. J., Komm, B., and Merchenthaler, I. (1996). The distribution of estrogen receptor-beta mRNA in the rat hypothalamus. *Steroids* 61, 678–681. doi: 10.1016/S0039-128X(96)00222-X

Shughrue, P., Scrimo, P., Lane, M., Askew, R., and Merchenthaler, I. (1997). The distribution of estrogen receptor-beta mRNA in forebrain regions of the estrogen receptor-alpha knockout mouse. *Endocrinology* 138, 5649–5652.

Tomihara, K., Soga, T., Nomura, M., Korach, K. S., Gustafsson, J. A., Pfaff, D. W., et al. (2009). Effect of ER-beta gene disruption on estrogenic regulation of anxiety in female mice. *Physiol. Behav.* 96, 300–306. doi: 10.1016/j.physbeh.2008.10.014

Tsuda, M. C., and Ogawa, S. (2012). Long-lasting consequences of neonatal maternal separation on social behaviors in ovariectomized female mice. *PLoS ONE* 7:e33028. doi: 10.1371/journal.pone.0033028.g005

Tsuda, M. C., Yamaguchi, N., and Ogawa, S. (2011). Early life stress disrupts peripubertal development of aggression in male mice. *Neuroreport* 22, 259–263. doi: 10.1097/WNR.0b013e328344495a

Veenema, A. H. (2012). Toward understanding how early-life social experiences alter oxytocin- and vasopressin-regulated social behaviors. *Horm. Behav.* 61, 304–312. doi: 10.1016/j.yhbeh.2011.12.002

Veenema, A. H., Bredewold, R., and Neumann, I. D. (2007). Opposite effects of maternal separation on intermale and maternal aggression in C57BL/6 mice: link to hypothalamic vasopressin and oxytocin immunoreactivity. *Psychoneuroendocrinology* 32, 437–450. doi: 10.1016/j.psyneuen.2007.02.008

Wigger, A., and Neumann, I. D. (1999). Periodic maternal deprivation induces gender-dependent alterations in behavioral and neuroendocrine responses to emotional stress in adult rats. *Physiol. Behav.* 66, 293–302. doi: 10.1016/S0031-9384(98)00300-X

Zhang, J. Q., Su, B. Y., and Cai, W. Q. (2004). Immunolocalization of estrogen receptor beta in the hypothalamic paraventricular nucleus of female mice during pregnancy, lactation and postnatal development. *Brain Res.* 997, 89–96. doi: 10.1016/j.brainres.2003.10.039

Zuloaga, D. G., Zuloaga, K. L., Hinds, L. R., Carbone, D. L., and Handa, R. J. (2014). Estrogen receptor β expression in the mouse forebrain: age and sex differences. *J. Comp. Neurol.* 522, 358–371. doi: 10.1002/cne.23400

7

Behavioral relevance of species-specific vasotocin anatomy in gregarious finches

Aubrey M. Kelly and James L. Goodson*

Department of Biology, Indiana University, Bloomington, IN, USA

***Correspondence:**
James L. Goodson, Department of Biology, Indiana University, 1001 East Third St., Bloomington, IN 47405, USA
e-mail: jlgoodso@indiana.edu

Despite substantial species differences in the vasotocin/vasopressin (VT/VP) circuitry of the medial bed nucleus of the stria terminalis (BSTm) and lateral septum (LS; a primary projection target of BSTm VT/VP cells), functional consequences of this variation are poorly known. Previous experiments in the highly gregarious zebra finch (Estrildidae: *Taeniopygia guttata*) demonstrate that BSTm VT neurons promote gregariousness in a male-specific manner and reduce anxiety in both sexes. However, in contrast to the zebra finch, the less gregarious Angolan blue waxbill (Estrildidae: *Uraeginthus angolensis*) exhibits fewer VT-immunoreactive cells in the BSTm as well as differences in receptor distribution across the LS subnuclei, suggesting that knockdown of VT production in the BSTm would produce behavioral effects in Angolan blue waxbills that are distinct from zebra finches. Thus, we here quantified social contact, gregariousness (i.e., preference for the larger of two groups), and anxiety-like behavior following bilateral antisense knockdown of VT production in the BSTm of male and female Angolan blue waxbills. We find that BSTm VT neurons promote social contact, but not gregariousness (as in male zebra finches), and that antisense effects on social contact are significantly stronger in male waxbills than in females. Knockdown of BSTm VT production has no effect on anxiety-like behavior. These data provide novel evidence that species differences in the VT/VP circuitry arising in the BSTm are accompanied by species-specific effects on affiliation behaviors.

Keywords: affiliation, sociality, songbird, anxiety, medial bed nucleus of the stria terminalis, vasopressin, *Uraeginthus angolensis*, sex differences

INTRODUCTION

In most tetrapod species, the vasotocin/vasopressin (VT/VP) circuitry of the medial bed nucleus of the stria terminalis (BSTm) and lateral septum (LS) is seasonally variable, regulated by steroid hormones, and sexually differentiated (males > females)—often to an extreme degree in each of these respects (Goodson and Bass, 2001; De Vries and Panzica, 2006; Goodson and Thompson, 2010). This circuitry is absent in fishes (Goodson and Bass, 2000; Goodson et al., 2003; Greenwood et al., 2008), but is present in virtually all tetrapods, suggesting the presence of conserved behavioral functions. As reviewed below, these conserved functions appear to include a variety of affiliation functions. However, substantial species differences are observed in the numbers of VT/VP cells in the BSTm, and in the densities and topographical distributions of receptors across LS subnuclei, suggesting the presence of functional differences as well (e.g., see Insel et al., 1991; Wang, 1995; Bester-Meredith et al., 1999; Goodson et al., 2009b; Kabelik et al., 2010).

Importantly, although VT/VP cells of the BSTm exhibit direct projections to the ventral hippocampus, medial preoptic nucleus, periaqueductal gray, lateral habenula, and LS (De Vries and Al-Shamma, 1990; Absil et al., 2002; De Vries and Panzica, 2006; Goodson and Thompson, 2010), each of these sites likely also receives peptide in a paracrine manner from other VT/VP cell groups. For instance, magnocellular neurons of the hypothalamus release peptide volumetrically from soma and dendrites (Landgraf and Neumann, 2004; Ludwig and Leng, 2006), and PVN VP neurons modulate LS physiology in the absence of direct innervation (Disturnal et al., 1986). Indeed, binding of endogenous VP in the LS modulates behavior in Syrian hamsters (*Mesocricetus auratus*) (e.g., Irvin et al., 1990; Albers and Cooper, 1995) despite the fact that this species exhibits a complete lack of VP cells in the BSTm (Bolborea et al., 2010). Given these observations, it is difficult to link peptide effects in any given target zone specifically to one VT/VP cell group or another, and thus direct manipulations of the cells are required to establish function.

To date, the majority of evidence regarding behavioral functions of BSTm VT/VP neurons has come from immediate early gene studies, which show that these neurons respond primarily to affiliation-related stimuli, particularly in males and in the context of reproduction. For example, BSTm VT/VP cells increase their transcriptional activity (as measured by Fos induction, a proxy marker of neural activity) selectively in response to (1) positive but not negative social stimuli in a variety of estrildid finch species (Goodson and Wang, 2006); (2) copulation but not aggressive interactions in mice (Ho et al., 2010); and (3) appetitive sexual behavior but not agonistic behavior in chickens (Xie et al., 2011). The percent of BSTm VT cells expressing Fos also correlates with the intensity of male sexual behavior in brown anoles (*Anolis sagrei*), but not with the intensity of male-male aggression (Kabelik et al., 2013). Thus, VT/VP neurons of the BSTm appear to be sensitive to social valence, and in fact, these neurons are differentially responsive to same-sex stimuli in flocking and territorial finches (Goodson and Wang, 2006). Additionally, male zebra finches (*Taeniopygia guttata*) that reliably court females have significantly more VT-immunoreactive (-ir) neurons in the BSTm than males that fail to court females (Goodson et al., 2009a), and overnight cohabitation with a female increases VP mRNA in the BSTm of male prairie voles (*Microtus ochrogaster*) (Wang et al., 1994).

Consistent with the affiliation-related responses of the BSTm VT/VP neurons, we recently showed that antisense knockdown of VT production in these cells increases same-sex aggression in male zebra finches, but not females, and reduces courtship singing in males (Kelly and Goodson, 2013). These experiments suggest the hypothesis that the phylogenetically widespread sex difference in BSTm VT/VP production serves to promote male affiliative behavior in a context that is tied to reproduction, while concomitantly offsetting the tendency for males to be more aggressive than females (Kelly and Goodson, 2013). This hypothesis is strongly supported by a variety of other data. For instance, less aggressive (long attack latency) male mice show a denser VP-ir innervation of the LS and more VP-ir neurons in the BSTm than do more aggressive males that exhibit short attack latencies (Compaan et al., 1993). Similarly, in sparrows, the density of VT immunolabeling in the BSTm correlates negatively with both individual and species differences in aggression (Goodson et al., 2012c), and infusions of VT into the LS decrease resident-intruder aggression in both sparrows and finches (Goodson, 1998a,b). Because VT/VP production in the BSTm is typically observed only during the breeding season, these findings suggest that VT/VP circuitry of the BSTm-LS modulates male behavior primarily in the context of reproduction.

In addition to reproductive functions, BSTm VT neurons also promote gregariousness in male zebra finches, and modulate anxiety in both males and females (Kelly et al., 2011). However, unlike seasonally breeding bird species, opportunistically breeding finch species do not exhibit seasonal fluctuation in VT-ir cell numbers in the BSTm, and VT-ir cell numbers in adult zebra finches are not regulated by steroid hormones (Kabelik et al., 2010). Thus, the involvement of BSTm VT neurons in non-reproductive behaviors such as grouping likely evolved after the evolutionary loss of seasonal reproduction and seasonal VT expression, effectively allowing VT circuitry that modulates reproductive affiliation to be co-opted for non-reproductive aspects of affiliation, as well (Goodson, 2013). Notably, available evidence suggests that VP production in the human BSTm may likewise be uncoupled from reproductive state, given that VP neurons have even been detected in a post-menopausal woman receiving anti-estrogen treatment (Fliers et al., 1986), suggesting the possibility of functional parallels between humans and opportunistic finches (see Rilling et al., 2012; Goodson, 2013).

Although the findings reviewed above suggest that the anatomy and functions of the BSTm-LS circuitry are highly conserved and are strongly tied to reproduction, there is nonetheless variation among species in VT/VP cell numbers in the BSTm and in the densities of V1a and OT receptors (V1aRs and OTRs; which tend to bind promiscuously) in the LS. For example, the monogamous mouse, *Peromyscus californicus*, exhibits more VP-ir labeling in the BSTm and greater VP receptor densities in the LS than the polygamous mouse, *Peromyscus leucopus* (Bester-Meredith et al., 1999), and conversely, the monogamous prairie vole exhibits fewer VP-ir cells in the BSTm but a higher density of VP-ir fibers in the LS than the polygamous meadow vole (*Microtus pennsylvanicus*) (Wang, 1995).

BSTm cell numbers and peptide binding sites also differ across finch species, and importantly, this variation mirrors convergent and divergent patterns of social evolution (Goodson et al., 2012a). Relevant studies have used five estrildid finch species that differ selectively in grouping behavior (i.e., all five species are monogamous, biparental, and exhibit similar breeding ecologies), and include two species that have independently evolved a highly gregarious and colonial social structure, two species that have independently evolved territoriality, and one species that is modestly gregarious year-round. These studies demonstrate that all three gregarious species exhibit higher densities of OT-like binding sites in the dorsal (pallial) LS than do the territorial species, whereas this pattern tends to reverse in the ventral (subpallial) LS. Notably, the moderately gregarious Angolan blue waxbill (*Uraeginthus angolensis*) exhibits high binding densities in both dorsal and ventral LS subdivisions (Goodson et al., 2009b). A similar binding pattern is observed for a linear V1aR antagonist (Goodson et al., 2006). However, unlike the iodinated OTR antagonist, which appears to bind selectively to the avian OTR, the linear V1aR radioligand appears to be promiscuous (Leung et al., 2011).

These species also differ in VT-ir cell numbers in the BSTm, at least based on standard immunohistochemistry, with the two highly gregarious species having more cells than the moderately gregarious species and the two territorial species (Goodson and Wang, 2006). However, because VT/VP neurons in the BSTm are often weakly immunoreactive and sometimes not visible without the use of colchicine to block axonal peptide transport (Sofroniew, 1985), species differences reported in finches must be interpreted cautiously. In fact, VT-ir cell numbers observed following central colchicine infusions in the violet-eared waxbill [*Uraeginthus granatina*; data collected in conjunction with those reported in Goodson et al. (2012b)] and Angolan blue waxbill (present study) are far greater than reported in (Goodson and Wang, 2006), although only in males. However, relative to zebra finches, these cells are very weakly immunoreactive. In contrast, BSTm VT neurons in zebra finches are more strongly immunoreactive and do not appear to change following infusions of colchicine (Goodson and Kelly, unpubl. obs.).

We here use antisense oligonucleotides to knock down production of VT in the BSTm of male and female Angolan blue waxbills in order to determine whether these species differences in VT anatomy are associated with functional differences between Angolan blue waxbills and zebra finches.

MATERIALS AND METHODS

ANIMALS

Experiments were conducted in a humane manner and were in compliance with all federal and institutional regulations. Wild-caught Angolan blue waxbills were obtained from a commercial importer and were housed in mixed-sex cages (10–12 individuals) containing wicker nests. Because it is not possible to sex all blue waxbills based on plumage, the provision of nests allowed us to observe behaviors that aided in the sexing of subjects. Subjects remained in these cages until 5 days prior to pre-testing, at which time they were transferred to same-sex cages. Birds were housed on a 14L:10D photoperiod with full spectrum lighting and were provided finch seed mix, cuttlebone, grit, and water *ad libitum*. Liberal servings of mealworms were also provided. Subjects exhibited modest gonadal recrudescence at the beginning of studies. A total of 31 male and 27 female Angolan blue waxbills were available for the present experiments. Four males and 7 females were used for pilot surgeries and antisense validation, and of these, 1 male and 4 females exhibited accurate cannula placements and were used for the within-subjects validation experiment described below. The remaining birds were used for behavioral experiments, but due to attrition, the final *n*'s for analyses are 21 males and 9 females. Although a portion of this attrition was due to inaccurate cannula placements, we found the blue waxbills (which weigh only ~9 g) to be extremely sensitive to anesthesia, and thus mortality during surgeries was high, particularly for females.

SURGERIES, INFUSIONS, AND HISTOLOGY

Subjects were stereotaxically fitted with a bilateral 26-ga cannula device (1.5 mm tip separation; Plastics One, Akron, OH) aimed at the dorsolateral aspect of the BSTm (see **Figure 1A**). Cannulae were referenced to the anterior pole of the cerebellum, and were then moved 2.8 mm rostral and advanced 3.0 mm into the brain. Cannulae were affixed to the skull using dental acrylic and veterinary-grade cyanoacrylate glue. The skin was closed with cyanoacrylate glue, and subjects were allowed at least 5 days to recover. Infusions began 2.5 days prior to behavioral testing. Subjects were bilaterally infused at 12 h intervals with either 1 μg VT antisense oligonucleotides or scrambled oligonucleotides in 0.25 μl of isotonic saline. Injectors extended 1 mm beyond the tip of the guide cannula. Testing was initiated following the 5th infusion (delivered AM) and completed in the morning following the 6th infusion (delivered PM). Subjects were euthanized by an overdose of isoflurane vapor and transcardially perfused with 0.1 M phosphate-buffered saline, followed by 0.4% paraformaldehyde. Brains were post-fixed overnight, transferred to 30% sucrose for 2 days, and then sectioned on a cryostat at 40 μm for verification of cannula placement.

ANTISENSE VALIDATION

The antisense construct used here has previously been validated in zebra finches, using a within-subjects design in which subjects were infused unilaterally into the dorsolateral BSTm with scrambled oligonucleotides, and with antisense oligonucleotides into the contralateral hemisphere (sides counterbalanced across subjects). This design was used because large individual differences in VT-ir cell numbers preclude the use of between-subjects approaches to validation (i.e., by comparing treatment groups). The sequence for the zebra finch VT LNA antisense was CT+CTGC CAT GG+CT+CA, and the sequence for the zebra finch VT LNA scrambled oligonucleotide construct was AG+C GTA TCT TG+CC+CC (see GenBank accession number ABQF01053428 for sequence data on the gene encoding zebra finch VT). In this previous experiment, antisense infusions produced an average reduction of VT-ir neuron numbers by 55% relative to the control hemisphere (Kelly et al., 2011).

We here used this same within-subjects design to verify efficacy of the VT antisense oligonucleotides in the Angolan blue waxbill, using 4 males and 7 females in which we piloted BSTm coordinates, of which 1 male and 4 females exhibited accurate placements in the dorsolateral BSTm. Following the 5th infusion of oligonucleotides (when behavioral testing would normally occur), subjects were infused with colchicine (3% in 0.25 μl saline) to block axonal transport of peptide, increasing our ability to visualize VT-producing cells. Histology was conducted as described above, and tissue was immunofluorescently labeled for VT as previously described (Kelly et al., 2011) using a rabbit VP antibody (ImmunoStar, Hudson, WI).

BEHAVIORAL TESTING

Group size preference (gregariousness) and social contact were quantified in a two-choice paradigm. In this test, subjects were

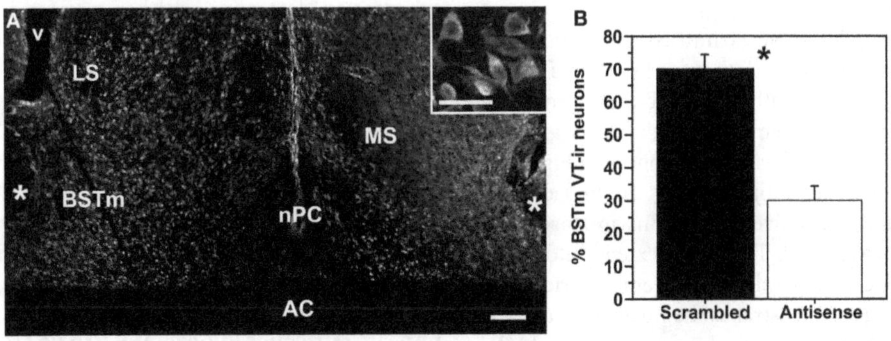

FIGURE 1 | (A) Representative knockdown of VT production as shown in a colchicine-treated pilot subject that received infusions of scrambled oligonucleotides in the left hemisphere and VT antisense oligonucleotides in the right hemisphere. *Inset*: Magnified view of VT-ir neurons in the BSTm. Scale bar = 100 μm; 50 μm for inset. Abbreviations: AC, anterior commissure; LS, lateral septum; MS, medial septum; nPC, nucleus of the pallial commissure; v, ventrical. **(B)** Data from a within-subjects validation experiment, showing the percent of total BSTm VT-ir neurons that were observed in hemispheres infused with scrambled (control) and antisense oligonucleotides. $^*p = 0.01$.

placed into a 1 m wide cage that was divided into 7 zones by perches. The perches at each end of the cage were approximately 4 cm from the cage wall, and were adjoined by a 0.5 m wide cage containing 2 stimulus birds at one end and 10 stimulus birds at the other (sides counterbalanced across subjects). Subject location was recorded every 15 s for 4 min [see Goodson et al. (2009b); Kelly et al. (2011)], with sides changed at 2 min. "Social contact" was operationally defined as the percent of test time that the subject spent in the two zones closest to the stimulus cages combined, and "gregariousness" was operationally defined as the percentage of that contact time that was spent next to the larger group.

Anxiety-like behavior was assessed using tests of novelty-suppressed feeding and exploration. For novelty-suppressed feeding, food was removed from the subjects' cage prior to lights-on, and 10 min after lights-on subjects were placed into a small, unfamiliar test cage (31 cm W × 20 cm H × 36 cm D) with a novel object (a purple nitrile glove) placed above a food dish. The latency to feed was quantified during a 90 min video-recorded trial. For exploration tests, subjects were placed into an unfamiliar cage (1.3 m W × 0.43 m H × 0.36 m D) containing 3 clusters of tree branches, and the number of hops/flights and number of visits to the branch clusters were recorded during a 3 min period.

STATISTICS

With the exception of antisense validation data, which were analyzed by paired *t*-tests, data were not normally distributed and were therefore analyzed using Mann-Whitney tests, comparing subjects that received scrambled oligonucleotides and subjects that received antisense oligonucleotides, with data presented as post-testing minus pre-testing values. Because antisense knockdown of BSTm VT production produces sex-specific effects on social behavior in zebra finches (Kelly et al., 2011; Kelly and Goodson, 2013), data for gregariousness and social contact were analyzed separately for each sex. However, because VT knockdown increases anxiety in both male and female zebra finches (Kelly et al., 2011), anxiety data were analyzed for the sexes combined as well as separately.

RESULTS

ANTISENSE VALIDATION

As shown in **Figure 1**, pilot subjects infused unilaterally with scrambled oligonucleotides and contralaterally with antisense oligonucleotides exhibit significantly fewer VT-ir neurons in the BSTm of the antisense-treated hemisphere ($t = 4.61$; $p = 0.01$; $n = 5$), with a mean reduction of ~57%. The photo in **Figure 1** is from a colchicine-infused male subject, and as can be seen, large numbers of weakly immunoreactive VT neurons are observed in the BSTm and other areas as well. These cells extend into the LS, lateral BST, medial telencephalon (along the lateral ventricle), and hippocampus, extending as far rostral as the nucleus accumbens. This is not observed in females, which show only scattered VT-ir neurons in the BSTm following colchicine infusions. Importantly, we have observed this sex difference in a much larger sample of tissue from another *Uraeginthus* species, the violet-eared waxbill, collected in conjunction with an experiment focused on vasoactive intestinal polypeptide, in which all subjects were treated with colchicine (Goodson et al., 2012b). Virtually all of the 11 males in that study showed extensive distributions of VT-ir neurons as just described, whereas the 10 females showed either no VT-ir neurons in extrahypothalamic areas outside of the BSTm, or very few in relation to males (Goodson and Kelly, unpubl. obs.).

BSTm VT ANTISENSE KNOCKDOWN REDUCES SOCIAL CONTACT, BUT HAS NO EFFECT ON GREGARIOUSNESS

Males infused with VT antisense oligonucleotides exhibited less social contact compared to control males (Mann-Whitney $U = 25.5$; $p = 0.04$). Effects were more pronounced in the first 2 min of testing (Mann-Whitney $U = 24.5$; $p = 0.03$) relative to the second 2 min after the stimulus cages containing large and small conspecifics were rotated (Mann-Whitney $U = 33.0$; $p = 0.13$; **Figures 2A–C**). In contrast, antisense infusions produced no overall effect on social contact time in females (Mann-Whitney $U = 7.0$; $p = 0.46$), although antisense did reduce social contact in the first 2 min of testing (Mann-Whitney $U = 2.0$; $p = 0.04$), but not in the second 2 min (Mann-Whitney $U = 7.5$; $p = 0.54$; **Figures 2D–F**).

We observed no significant effects of VT antisense infusions on gregariousness in males or females regardless of whether the data were analyzed with the first 2 min and second 2 min pooled or separately (all $p > 0.17$). However, these analyses were of limited power due to empty cells, resulting from the fact that numerous subjects did not exhibit contact time with the large group in pre-testing, post-testing, or both ($n = 4$ females and $n = 12$ males eliminated from the analysis). Thus, we reanalyzed data for gregariousness by adding the second zone at each end of the test cage, effectively increasing the contact zone, and thus increasing the number of subjects included in the analysis ($n = 8$ scramble control males, $n = 8$ antisense males, $n = 4$ scramble control females, $n = 4$ antisense females). This modified analysis yielded no significant effects (all $p > 0.08$).

BSTm VT NEURONS PROMOTE SOCIAL CONTACT IN A SEXUALLY DIFFERENTIATED MANNER

Although antisense infusions produced significant effects on social contact in both males and females as described above, the effects in males appeared to be much more pronounced. Thus, in order to determine whether male and female subjects differed in their response to antisense infusions, we subtracted the median social contact score of scrambled control subjects from the score of each subject that received antisense (performed separately for males and females). The resultant "antisense effect size" did not differ between males and females in the first 2 min (Mann-Whitney $U = 11$; $p = 0.11$), but did differ in the second 2 min after rotation of the stimulus cages (Mann-Whitney $U = 6.5$; $p = 0.03$), and for the total 4 min test period (Mann-Whitney $U = 8$; $p = 0.05$; **Figures 3A–C**).

BSTm VT ANTISENSE KNOCKDOWN HAS NO EFFECT ON ANXIETY-LIKE BEHAVIOR

Subjects that received VT antisense oligonucleotides did not differ from subjects that received scrambled oligonucleotides in their latency to feed in the novelty-suppressed feeding paradigm or for exploration measures in the novel environment (all $p > 0.15$

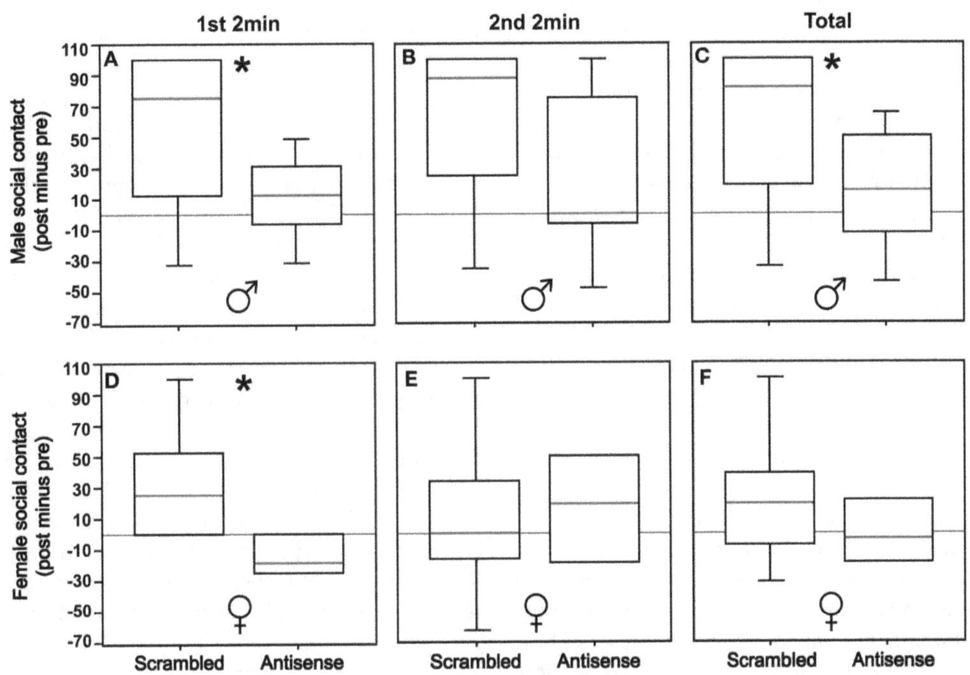

FIGURE 2 | (A,B) Knockdown of VT production in the BSTm reduces social contact in males in the first 2 min of testing ($^*p = 0.03$), but not in the second 2 min of testing following the rotation of the stimulus cages containing 2 or 10 same-sex birds ($p = 0.13$). **(C)** With the first and second test periods combined, there is an overall reduction in social contact in males ($^*p = 0.04$). **(D,E)** Knockdown of VT production in the BSTm reduces social contact in females in the first 2 min of testing ($p = 0.04$), but not in the second 2 min of testing ($p = 0.54$). **(F)** With the first and second test periods combined, there is no overall effect on social contact in females ($^*p = 0.46$). Data are shown as post-treatment minus pre-surgical values. Box plots show the median (red line), 75th and 25th percentile (box), and 95% confidence interval (whiskers).

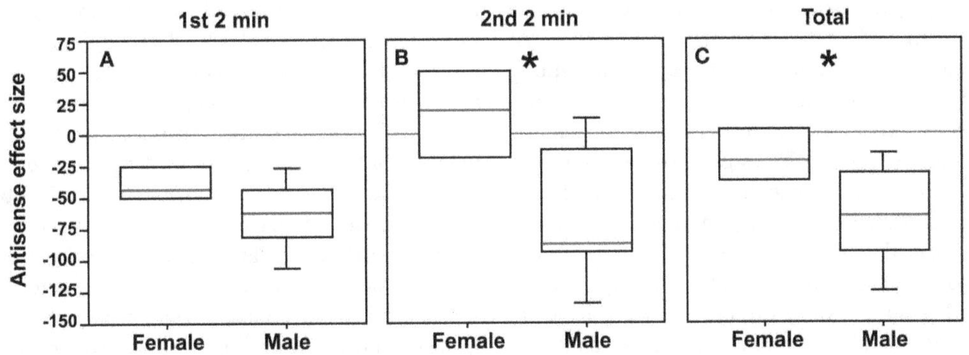

FIGURE 3 | In order to determine whether male and female subjects differ in their response to antisense infusions, the median social contact score (post-minus pre-surgical values, as shown in Figure 2) of scrambled control subjects was subtracted from the score of each subject that received antisense, yielding a measure of "antisense effect size." (A) Although there is no significant difference between sexes during the first 2 min, strong differences are observed for the second 2 min ($^*p = 0.03$; **B)** and for the total test period ($^*p = 0.05$; **C)**.

regardless of whether data were analyzed with sexes separated or combined).

DISCUSSION

SPECIES DIFFERENCES IN VT NEURONAL FUNCTION

In most tetrapod vertebrates, VT/VP immunoreactivity in the BSTm and LS is expressed only during the breeding season (Goodson and Bass, 2001; De Vries and Panzica, 2006), suggesting that the primary functions of this circuitry are tied to reproduction. Indeed, BSTm VT/VP neurons exhibit strong responses to sexual stimuli in male mice, chickens, and finches (Goodson et al., 2009a; Ho et al., 2010; Xie et al., 2011), and knockdown of BSTm VT production profoundly reduces courtship singing in male zebra finches while concomitantly increasing aggression (Kelly and Goodson, 2013). Similarly, VT-ir cells are more numerous in male zebra finches that reliably court females than males that fail to court females (Goodson et al., 2009a). However, in contrast to seasonally breeding species, several estrildid finch species that breed semi-opportunistically do not exhibit temporal fluctuations in VT immunoreactivity (Kabelik et al., 2010), and thus VT circuitry arising in the BSTm of these species is available to modulate non-reproductive affiliation behaviors as well. In fact, antisense experiments show that this circuitry modulates same-sex gregariousness (i.e., non-reproductive affiliation) in male but not female zebra finches (Kelly et al., 2011; Kelly and Goodson, 2013). In contrast, we here show that BSTm VT cells do not modulate gregariousness in the less gregarious Angolan blue waxbill, but do promote social contact, most strongly in males. Furthermore, whereas knockdown of BSTm VT production produces robust increases in anxiety in both male and female zebra finches (Kelly et al., 2011; Kelly and Goodson, 2013), no effects on anxiety are observed for the Angolan blue waxbill.

These species differences may be interpreted in multiple ways. First, because zebra finches typically form very large groups (Zann, 1996), we hypothesize that redundant neural systems have evolved to ensure that individuals in this species always maintain social contact. If this is so, then knockdown of VT production may not be sufficient to reduce social contact in zebra finches (i.e., due to redundant neural systems), but is sufficient to reduce preferences for larger groups, while in the less social blue waxbill it reduces social contact altogether. By this interpretation, BSTm VT neurons may promote affiliation similarly in both zebra finches and blue waxbills, but with species-specific effects due to interactions with other neural systems that modulate social behavior. A problem for this interpretation is that whereas knockdown of BSTm VT production reduces gregariousness in male zebra finches by ~80%, social contact is actually *increased*, albeit only modestly (~25%) (Kelly et al., 2011). This observation suggests that gregariousness and social contact are not on a single continuum, although interpretation of the social contact data in zebra finches is difficult (and the relevant finding may be anomalous), given that central infusions of OTR and V1aR antagonists have no detectable impact on social contact, yet produce profound reductions in gregariousness (Goodson et al., 2009b; Kelly et al., 2011). Hence the hypothesis that BSTm VT neurons promote affiliation similarly in zebra finches and waxbills cannot be rejected with confidence.

Whereas the above interpretation places the divergent antisense effects in finches and waxbills on a continuum, an alternative possibility is that the divergent effects are truly qualitative and rooted in significant species differences in VT anatomy. As discussed earlier, gregarious estrildid species (including zebra finches and Angolan blue waxbills) exhibit higher densities of OT-like binding sites in the dorsal (pallial) LS than territorial species, where this pattern tends to reverse in the ventral (subpallial) LS. However, unlike zebra finches, Angolan blue waxbills exhibit high binding densities in both dorsal and ventral LS subdivisions (Goodson et al., 2009b). Similar binding differences are observed for linear V1aR antagonist (Goodson et al., 2006), although this antagonist does not appear to bind selectively to the avian V1aR (Leung et al., 2011). As previously shown using standard immunocytochemistry, zebra finches also exhibit many more VT-ir neurons in the BSTm than do Angolan blue waxbills, and these cells tend to be much more strongly immunoreactive (Goodson and Wang, 2006). However, as shown here, blue waxbills treated with colchicine exhibit larger numbers of weakly immunoreactive neurons in the BSTm than previously reported, and at least in males this cell group is very large and extends into adjacent areas such as the LS and lateral BST. In contrast, colchicine infusions do not alter the basic pattern of immunolabeling in zebra finches (Goodson and Kelly, unpubl. obs.). Given these significant species differences in VT anatomy and receptor distributions, the differential social effects of VT knockdown in zebra finches (reduction of gregariousness) and Angolan blue waxbills (reduction of social contact) may reflect truly qualitative variation in the way in which VT modulates behavior in these species.

The hypothesis that differences in VT anatomy are reflected in qualitative differences in behavioral function is strongly supported by the findings that whereas antisense knockdown of BSTm VT production dramatically increases anxiety-like responses to novelty in both male and female zebra finches (Kelly et al., 2011; Kelly and Goodson, 2013), antisense infusions have no discernable impact on anxiety-like behavior in the blue waxbill. Studies in rodents likewise suggest an involvement of septal VP in anxiety that is species- and/or context-specific, although it remains to be determined whether these effects are attributable to VP release from neurons in the BSTm. For example, in individually housed male Wistar rats, septal infusions of V1aR antagonists and V1aR antisense reduce anxiety in the elevated plus maze (EPM), suggesting that endogenous VT release into the septum is anxiogenic (Landgraf et al., 1995; Liebsch et al., 1996). Interestingly, another study in *group-housed* male Wistar rats showed that retrodialysis of VP into the septum increases activity in the open arms of the EPM, suggesting that septal VP is *anxiolytic* (Appenrodt et al., 1998). Hence, it is possible that social housing conditions (individual vs. group) may modulate the relationship between septal VP release and anxiety. Findings in lab mice are likewise mixed. For instance, re-expression of V1aR in the LS of V1aR knockout mice does not alter anxiety-like behavior in the EPM, light/dark box, or open field tests, although overexpression of V1aR in the LS of wild type mice does weakly increase anxiety-like behavior, but only in the light/dark box (Bielsky et al., 2005). Hence, endogenous VP release into the LS likely exerts little or no effects on anxiety in male mice, but modulates anxiety in male rats in a manner that appears to vary in relation to social and/or other contextual factors (which may be lab-specific). Combined with the findings from zebra finches and Angolan blue waxbills, it is clear that VT/VP modulates anxiety-like behavior in very species-specific (and likely context-specific) ways, although it remains to be determined whether these differential effects on anxiety are integrated with the expression of social behavior.

SEX DIFFERENCES IN VT NEURONAL FUNCTION

In most tetrapod vertebrate species, males exhibit significantly more VT/VP neurons in the BSTm than do females and significantly denser projections to basal forebrain areas such as the LS (Goodson and Bass, 2001; De Vries and Panzica, 2006), although this sexual dimorphism is quite subtle in zebra finches (Kabelik et al., 2010), even following colchicine infusions (Goodson and Kelly, unpubl. obs.). Similarly, no sex differences in VT-ir cell numbers have been detected in several other estrildid finch species, including two in the genus *Uraeginthus*—the Angolan blue waxbill and violet-eared waxbill (Goodson and Wang, 2006). However, violet-eared waxbills treated with colchicine as part of another experiment (Goodson et al., 2012b) show profound sex differences in VT-ir cell numbers in the BSTm and other extrahypothalamic areas (Goodson and Kelly, unpubl. obs.), and limited data from the present experiments demonstrate a comparable condition in the Angolan blue waxbill

Although zebra finches show only modest dimorphism in VT anatomy (Kabelik et al., 2010), antisense experiments reveal large sex differences in function. For instance, knockdown of VT production in the BSTm reduces preferences for the larger of two groups (gregariousness) by 80% in males while having no effect in females, and produces large male-specific increases in aggression (Kelly et al., 2011; Kelly and Goodson, 2013). In contrast, the differential effects of VT knockdown in male and female waxbills are quantitative in nature, not dichotomous. The combined findings therefore suggest that the degree of sex differences in function is not wholly dependent upon the degree of sexual dimorphism in VT anatomy. Sex differences in receptor distributions could potentially account for this surprising result, although no sex differences have been described to date in finches (Goodson et al., 2006, 2009b). Fos responses to simple social stimuli are also similar in male and female zebra finches (Goodson and Wang, 2006), but a recent study using more complex stimuli shows that BSTm VT neurons exhibit Fos responses in zebra finches that vary not only across sexes, but across different personality types as well (Kelly and Goodson, unpubl. obs.). Hence, sex differences in VT function may rely on a combination of sex-specific neuronal responses and sexually differentiated VT production. Given that BSTm VT neurons are strongly regulated by steroid hormones (Goodson and Bass, 2001; De Vries and Panzica, 2006), sex differences in VT response and function may be hormone-dependent.

Finally, the fact that male waxbills express extrahypothalamic VT-ir cells not only the BSTm, but also in adjacent areas, suggests that antisense effects in males may rely to some extent on VT knockdown in areas such as the LS and lateral BST [although importantly, BSTm infusions do not impact VT production in the paraventricular hypothalamus; (Kelly et al., 2011)]. However, the lack of VT production in these additional sites in females clarifies the situation considerably, given that antisense effects in female Angolan blue waxbills are qualitatively similar to males, albeit weaker. Thus, it is clear that VT neurons in the BSTm promote social contact in Angolan blue waxbills, although the possible contributions of cells outside of the BSTm in males cannot be excluded.

CONCLUSIONS

Anatomical features of VT/VP circuits arising in the BSTm vary across species, suggesting that BSTm VT neurons may exert species-specific effects on behavior. We here show that knockdown of VT production in the BSTm reduces social contact in the modestly gregarious Angolan blue waxbill, without effects on anxiety-like behavior or group size preferences (gregariousness). Effects are observed in both sexes, but are stronger in males. In contrast, VT knockdown in the highly social zebra finch dramatically increases anxiety-like behavior in both males and females and produces a profound male-specific decrease in gregariousness that is accompanied by a much more modest increase in social contact (Kelly et al., 2011; Kelly and Goodson, 2013). These species differences may be rooted in one or more factors, including species differences in VT production, VT receptor distributions, VT interactions with other neurochemical systems, and/or patterns of VT neuronal response to environmental stimuli. However, despite the presence of species differences, BSTm VT neurons appear to generally increase aspects of affiliation (including courtship), particularly in males.

REFERENCES

Absil, P., Papello, M., Viglietti-Panzica, C., Balthazart, J., and Panzica, G. (2002). The medial preoptic nucleus receives vasotocinergic inputs in male quail: a tract-tracing and immunocytochemical study. *J. Chem. Neuroanat.* 24, 27–39. doi: 10.1016/S0891-0618(02)00017-0

Albers, H. E., and Cooper, T. T. (1995). Effects of testosterone on the behavioral response to arginine vasopressin microinjected into the central gray and septum. *Peptides* 16, 269–273. doi: 10.1016/0196-9781(94)00188-X

Appenrodt, E., Schnabel, R., and Schwarzberg, H. (1998). Vasopressin administration modulates anxiety-related behavior in rats. *Physiol. Behav.* 64, 543–547. doi: 10.1016/S0031-9384(98)00119-X

Bester-Meredith, J. K., Young, L. J., and Marler, C. A. (1999). Species differences in paternal behavior and aggression in *Peromyscus* and their associations with vasopressin immunoreactivity and receptors. *Horm. Behav.* 36, 25–38. doi: 10.1006/hbeh.1999.1522

Bielsky, I. F., Hu, S. B., Ren, X., Terwilliger, E. F., and Young, L. J. (2005). The V_{1a} vasopressin receptor is necessary and sufficient for normal social recognition: a gene replacement study. *Neuron* 47, 503–513. doi: 10.1016/j.neuron.2005.06.031

Bolborea, M., Ansel, L., Weinert, D., Steinlechner, S., Pevet, P., and Klosen, P. (2010). The bed nucleus of the stria terminalis in the Syrian hamster (*Mesocricetus auratus*): absence of vasopressin expression in standard and wild-derived hamsters and galanin regulation by seasonal changes in circulating sex steroids. *Neuroscience* 165, 819–830. doi: 10.1016/j.neuroscience.2009.11.006

Compaan, J. C., Buijs, R. M., Pool, C. W., De Ruiter, A. J., and Koolhaas, J. M. (1993). Differential lateral septal vasopressin innervation in aggressive and nonaggressive male mice. *Brain Res. Bull.* 30, 1–6. doi: 10.1016/0361-9230(93)90032-7

De Vries, G. J., and Al-Shamma, H. A. (1990). Sex differences in hormonal responses of vasopressin pathways in the rat brain. *J. Neurobiol.* 21, 686–693. doi: 10.1002/neu.480210503

De Vries, G. J., and Panzica, G. C. (2006). Sexual differentiation of central vasopressin and vasotocin systems in vertebrates: different mechanisms, similar endpoints. *Neuroscience* 138, 947–955. doi: 10.1016/j.neuroscience.2005.07.050

Disturnal, J. E., Veale, W. L., and Pittman, Q. L. (1986). The ventral septal area: electrophysiological evidence for putative arginine vasopressin projections onto thermoresponsive neurons. *Neuroscience* 19, 795–802. doi: 10.1016/0306-4522(86)90299-X

Fliers, E., Guldenaar, S. E., van de Wal, N., and Swaab, D. F. (1986). Extrahypothalamic vasopressin and oxytocin in the human brain; presence of vasopressin cells in the bed nucleus of the stria terminalis. *Brain Res.* 375, 363–367. doi: 10.1016/0006-8993(86)90759-6

Goodson, J. L. (1998a). Territorial aggression and dawn song are modulated by septal vasotocin and vasoactive intestinal polypeptide in male field sparrows (*Spizella pusilla*). *Horm. Behav.* 34, 67–77. doi: 10.1006/hbeh.1998.1467

Goodson, J. L. (1998b). Vasotocin and vasoactive intestinal polypeptide modulate aggression in a territorial songbird, the violet-eared waxbill (Estrildidae: *Uraeginthus granatina*). *Gen. Comp. Endocrinol.* 111, 233–244. doi: 10.1006/gcen.1998.7112

Goodson, J. L. (2013). Deconstructing sociality, social evolution and relevant nonapeptide functions. *Psychoneuroendocrinology* 38, 465–478. doi: 10.1016/j.psyneuen.2012.12.005

Goodson, J. L., and Bass, A. H. (2000). Vasotocin innervation and modulation of vocal-acoustic circuitry in the teleost Porichthys notatus. *J. Comp. Neurol.* 422, 363–379. doi: 10.1002/1096-9861

Goodson, J. L., and Bass, A. H. (2001). Social behavior functions and related anatomical characteristics of vasotocin/vasopressin systems in vertebrates. *Brain Res. Rev.* 35, 246–265. doi: 10.1016/S0165-0173(01)00043-1

Goodson, J. L., Evans, A. K., and Bass, A. H. (2003). Putative isotocin distributions in sonic fish: relation to vasotocin and vocal-acoustic circuitry. *J. Comp. Neurol.* 462, 1–14. doi: 10.1002/cne.10679

Goodson, J. L., Evans, A. K., and Wang, Y. (2006). Neuropeptide binding reflects convergent and divergent evolution in species-typical group sizes. *Horm. Behav.* 50, 223–236. doi: 10.1016/j.yhbeh.2006.03.005

Goodson, J. L., Kelly, A. M., and Kingsbury, M. A. (2012a). Evolving nonapeptide mechanisms of gregariousness and social diversity in birds. *Horm. Behav.* 61, 239–250. doi: 10.1016/j.yhbeh.2012.01.005

Goodson, J. L., Kelly, A. M., Kingsbury, M. A., and Thompson, R. R. (2012b). An aggression-specific cell type in the anterior hypothalamus of finches. *Proc. Natl. Acad. Sci. U.S.A.* 109, 13847–13852. doi: 10.1073/pnas.1207995109

Goodson, J. L., Wilson, L. C., and Schrock, S. E. (2012c). To flock or fight: neurochemical signatures of divergent life histories in sparrows. *Proc. Natl. Acad. Sci. U.S.A.* 109(Suppl. 1), 10685–10692. doi: 10.1073/pnas.1203394109

Goodson, J. L., Rinaldi, J., and Kelly, A. M. (2009a). Vasotocin neurons in the bed nucleus of the stria terminalis preferentially process social information and exhibit properties that dichotomize courting and non-courting phenotypes. *Horm. Behav.* 55, 197–202. doi: 10.1016/j.yhbeh.2008.10.007

Goodson, J. L., Schrock, S. E., Klatt, J. D., Kabelik, D., and Kingsbury, M. A. (2009b). Mesotocin and nonapeptide receptors promote estrildid flocking behavior. *Science* 325, 862–866. doi: 10.1126/science.1174929

Goodson, J. L., and Thompson, R. R. (2010). Nonapeptide mechanisms of social cognition, behavior and species-specific social systems. *Curr. Opin. Neurobiol.* 20, 784–794. doi: 10.1016/j.conb.2010.08.020

Goodson, J. L., and Wang, Y. (2006). Valence-sensitive neurons exhibit divergent functional profiles in gregarious and asocial species. *Proc. Natl. Acad. Sci. U.S.A.* 103, 17013–17017. doi: 10.1073/pnas.0606278103

Greenwood, A. K., Wark, A. R., Fernald, R. D., and Hofmann, H. A. (2008). Expression of arginine vasotocin in distinct preoptic regions is associated with dominant and subordinate behaviour in an African cichlid fish. *Proc. Biol. Sci.* 275, 2393–2402. doi: 10.1098/rspb.2008.0622

Ho, J. M., Murray, J. H., Demas, G. E., and Goodson, J. L. (2010). Vasopressin cell groups exhibit strongly divergent responses to copulation and male-male interactions in mice. *Horm. Behav.* 58, 368–377. doi: 10.1016/j.yhbeh.2010.03.021

Insel, T. R., Gelhard, R., and Shapiro, L. E. (1991). The comparative distribution of forebrain receptors for neurohypophyseal peptides in monogamous and polygamous mice. *Neuroscience* 43, 623–630. doi: 10.1016/0306-4522(91)90321-E

Irvin, R. W., Szot, P., Dorsa, D. M., Potegal, M., and Ferris, C. F. (1990). Vasopressin in the septal area of the golden hamster controls scent marking and grooming. *Physiol. Behav.* 48, 693–699. doi: 10.1016/0031-9384(90)90213-N

Kabelik, D., Alix, V. C., Burford, E. R., and Singh, L. J. (2013). Aggression-and sex-induced neural activity across vasotocin populations in the brown anole. *Horm. Behav.* 63, 437–446. doi: 10.1016/j.yhbeh.2012.11.016

Kabelik, D., Morrison, J. A., and Goodson, J. L. (2010). Cryptic regulation of vasotocin neuronal activity but not anatomy by sex steroids and social stimuli in opportunistic desert finches. *Brain Behav. Evol.* 75, 71–84. doi: 10.1159/000297522

Kelly, A. M., and Goodson, J. L. (2013). Functional significance of a phylogenetically widespread sexual dimorphism in vasotocin/vasopressin production. *Horm. Behav.* 64, 840–846. doi: 10.1016/j.yhbeh.2013.09.006

Kelly, A. M., Kingsbury, M. A., Hoffbuhr, K., Schrock, S. E., Waxman, B., Kabelik, D., et al. (2011). Vasotocin neurons and septal V_{1a}-like receptors potently modulate songbird flocking and responses to novelty. *Horm. Behav.* 60, 12–21. doi: 10.1016/j.yhbeh.2011.01.012

Landgraf, R., Gerstberger, R., Montkowski, A., Probst, J. C., Wotjak, C. T., Holsboer, F., et al. (1995). V_1 vasopressin receptor antisense oligodeoxynucleotide into septum reduces vasopressin binding, social discrimination abilities, and anxiety-related behavior in rats. *J. Neurosci.* 15, 4250–4258.

Landgraf, R., and Neumann, I. D. (2004). Vasopressin and oxytocin release within the brain: a dynamic concept of multiple and variable modes of neuropeptide communication. *Front. Neuroendocrinol.* 25, 150–176. doi: 10.1016/J.Yfrne.2004.05.001

Leung, C. H., Abebe, D. F., Earp, S. E., Goode, C. T., Grozhik, A. V., Mididoddi, P., et al. (2011). Neural distribution of vasotocin receptor mRNA in two species of songbird. *Endocrinology* 152, 4865–4881. doi: 10.1210/en.2011-1394

Liebsch, G., Wotjak, C. T., Landgraf, R., and Engelmann, M. (1996). Septal vasopressin modulates anxiety-related behaviour in rats. *Neurosci. Lett.* 217, 101–104. doi: 10.1016/S0304-3940(96)13069-X

Ludwig, M., and Leng, G. (2006). Dendritic peptide release and peptide-dependent behaviours. *Nat. Rev. Neurosci.* 7, 126–136. doi: 10.1038/nrn1845

Rilling, J. K., Demarco, A. C., Hackett, P. D., Thompson, R., Ditzen, B., Patel, R., et al. (2012). Effects of intranasal oxytocin and vasopressin on cooperative behavior and associated brain activity in men. *Psychoneuroendocrinology* 37, 447–461. doi: 10.1016/j.psyneuen.2011.07.013

Sofroniew, M. V. (1985). Vasopressin-and neurophysin-immunoreactive neurons in the septal region, medial amygdala and locus coeruleus in colchicine-treated rats. *Neuroscience* 15, 347–358. doi: 10.1016/0306-4522(85)90217-9

Wang, Z. (1995). Species differences in the vasopressin-immunoreactive pathways in the bed nucleus of the stria terminalis and medial amygdaloid nucleus in prairie voles (*Microtus ochrogaster*) and meadow voles (*Microtus pennsylvanicus*). *Behav. Neurosci.* 109, 305–311. doi: 10.1037//0735-7044.109.2.305

Wang, Z., Smith, W., Major, D. E., and De Vries, G. J. (1994). Sex and species differences in the effects of cohabitation on vasopressin messenger RNA expression in the bed nucleus of the stria terminalis in prairie voles (*Microtus ochrogaster*) and meadow voles (*Microtus pennsylvanicus*). *Brain Res.* 650, 212–218. doi: 10.1016/0006-8993(94)91784-1

Xie, J., Kuenzel, W. J., Sharp, P. J., and Jurkevich, A. (2011). Appetitive and consummatory sexual and agonistic behaviour elicits FOS expression in aromatase and vasotocin neurones within the preoptic area and bed nucleus of the stria terminalis of male domestic chickens. *J. Neuroendocrinol.* 23, 232–243. doi: 10.1111/j.1365-2826.2011.02108.x

Zann, R. A. (1996). *The Zebra Finch: A Synthesis of Field and Laboratory Studies.* Oxford: Oxford University Press.

8

Sexual attractiveness of male chemicals and vocalizations in mice

Akari Asaba, Tatsuya Hattori, Kazutaka Mogi and Takefumi Kikusui*

Department of Animal Science and Biotechnology, Graduate School of Veterinary Medicine, Azabu University, Kanagawa, Japan

Correspondence:
Takefumi Kikusui, Department of Animal Science and Biotechnology, Graduate School of Veterinary Medicine, Azabu University, 1-17-71 Fuchinobe, Chuoh-ku, Sagamihara, Kanagawa-ken 252-5201, Japan
e-mail: kikusui@azabu-u.ac.jp

Male-female interaction is important for finding a suitable mating partner and for ensuring reproductive success. Male sexual signals such as pheromones transmit information and social and sexual status to females, and exert powerful effects on the mate preference and reproductive biology of females. Likewise, male vocalizations are attractive to females and enhance reproductive function in many animals. Interestingly, females' preference for male pheromones and vocalizations is associated with their genetic background, to avoid inbreeding. Moreover, based on acoustic cues, olfactory signals have significant effects on mate choice in mice, suggesting mate choice involves multisensory integration. In this review, we synopsize the effects of both olfactory and auditory cues on female behavior and neuroendocrine functions. We also discuss how these male signals are integrated and processed in the brain to regulate behavior and reproductive function.

Keywords: mouse, pheromones, ultrasonic vocalizations, neural circuit, reproduction, multisensory integration

INTRODUCTION

Animals have evolved specific communication strategies to find a suitable mating partner and ensure reproductive success. These adaptive strategies are widely observed in the animal kingdom in a species-specific manner. In each species, sex-specific behavioral and sexual signals, such as chemical and auditory cues, transmit information about social and sexual status to the sexual counterpart, and this information is thought to be involved in mating success. In the majority of sexual encounters, females select their partners, or male compete with one another to obtain a chance to reproduce. The former is referred to as the "female mate choice." This is probably because females have a smaller copulation potential and fewer reproductive outcomes than males and these sex biases in the level of parental investment create a condition that favors mating choice (Trivers, 1972). Therefore, male signals play a critical role in the females' choice of the best partner and in reproductive physiology. To date, many theoretical and empirical research studies have addressed the "good genes" hypothesis of mate choice, where females choose a mate based on the quality of genes that their offspring would inherit from the sire (Kokko et al., 2003; Neff and Pitcher, 2005; Andersson, 2006; Andersson and Simmons, 2006). In other words, a female's preference for male traits can provide genetic benefits to the offspring that inherit favorable alleles from the father (Mead and Arnold, 2004).

According to this hypothesis, three female strategies have been identified for mate preference. First, females prefer masculine males with a higher social rank to males with a lower social rank. Usually male social rank is related to circulating testosterone levels, with higher-ranking males having a higher testosterone level than lower-ranking males. Therefore, females prefer males with stronger testosterone-controlled signals, such as male chemosignals (Xiao et al., 2004), hair color (West and Packer, 2002), body masculinity (Roney and Simmons, 2008), and vocalizations (Pasch et al., 2011), which are also related to social rank. Second, females prefer healthy male individuals. For example, female mice can discriminate parasitized from unparasitized males via their odor (Kavaliers and Colwell, 1993), and are more attracted to the odor of unparasitized males (Kavaliers and Colwell, 1995a,b). Third, females prefer males that exhibit genetic-related signals that help them avoid inbreeding and increase genetic diversity, which also increases disease resistance (Potts et al., 1991; Penn and Potts, 1998b). Therefore, females receive variable information about the social and health status, and genetic background of individual males by the quality and quantity of their signals.

Furthermore, many reports show that male signals enhance reproductive function in recipient females. Especially, male mouse odors contain chemical cues called pheromones that exert powerful effects on the preference and reproductive biology of female mice. For example, in biological function, male urine is chiefly responsible for estrus synchronization (the Whitten effect; Whitten, 1958), puberty acceleration in young females (the Vandenberg effect; Vandenbergh, 1969), and pregnancy block (the Bruce effect; Bruce, 1959). In addition, male courtship vocalizations enhance reproductive function in avian and mammal species (Shelton, 1980; McComb, 1987; Leboucher et al., 1998; Delgadillo et al., 2012). Thus, male signals are used both as social cues for mate preference and as a way to stimulate female reproduction. This notion is logical because when a female encounters a "better male (masculine/dominant male)," she has to approach the male (preference) and copulate with him (reproduction) to increase her chances of obtaining offspring with greater fitness. It has actually been suggested that dominant males tend to sire more litters than subordinate males (DeFries and McClearn, 1970; Oakeshott, 1974), probably by the effects of dominant male signals in the preference and reproduction.

Male mice emit song-like "ultrasonic vocalizations (USVs)" both in the presence of females and when stimulated by a female's urinary pheromones (Nyby et al., 1977; Holy and Guo, 2005). Recent studies have revealed that USVs are attractive to female mice and that females prefer the USVs of males that are different from their parents (Hammerschmidt et al., 2009; Musolf et al., 2010; Asaba et al., 2014), similar to the pheromonal effects. Therefore, in a natural context, female mice usually use chemical and auditory cues that carry male-specific information required for mating. This means that laboratory mice are useful model for understanding female strategies of mate choice using multiple sensory stimulations. Here, we review discoveries about the effect of male pheromones and vocalizations on mate choice and their role in reproductive and neuroendocrine functions in female mice. Subsequently, we shed light on how multisensory stimuli from males are integrated in the brain and how this information regulates female behaviors and reproductive functions.

ATTRACTIVENESS OF MALE PHEROMONES

Females attend to male odors that contain various types of information, such as a male's dominance status. Dominance-associated traits in males, such as aggressiveness and territoriality, have long been viewed as ecologically significant. Since social subordinations suppress gonadal function in mice, emission of male-specific pheromones (Bronson, 1979), which are synthesized under the control of testosterone, are likely diminished in subordinates compared to those of dominant males. Actually, male social status is assessed through changes in testosterone-dependent volatiles in urine that are attractive to females (Jemiolo et al., 1985, 1991; Novotny et al., 1990). Moreover, peripubertal period (Postnatal day 21–38) exposure to male odors also accelerates the expression of mate odor preference in female (Jouhanneau et al., 2014).

The control of pheromones secretion by testosterone in the urine is not only for attracting females, but also for increasing reproductive function in females. Urine from dominant males is far more effective at promoting puberty acceleration in young female mice compared to urine from subordinate males and castrated males (Lombardi and Vandenbergh, 1977). Treatment with testosterone restored the ability of castrated males to induce these effects (Dominic, 1965; Lombardi et al., 1976), demonstrating that testosterone-dependent pheromones are responsible for female puberty acceleration. In addition, male pheromones have pivotal roles in inducing estrus synchronization (Novotny et al., 1990; Dulac and Torello, 2003) and terminating pregnancy in females (Bruce, 1960; Spironello Vella and deCatanzaro, 2001), whereas the urine from castrated males cannot induce these effects.

Several instances have been identified in which a single pheromone compound can evoke certain effects on female sexual behaviors and reproduction as described above. These pheromones could be classically divided into "releaser pheromones," which affect rapid mating behavior, and "primer pheromones," which affect long-term physiological processes. Indeed, many identified pheromones have multiple behavioral and physiological functions (Novotny, 2003), suggesting that the distinction between releaser and primer pheromones is not meaningful at the stimulus level. Below, we review male pheromones that are reportedly attractive to females or that increase the reproductive function of female mice (**Figure 1**).

	Pheromones		Source	Sensory organs	Effects
non-Volatile	ESP1	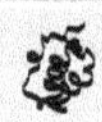	Male tear fluids from extraorbital lacrimal grand	VNO	Sexual receptivity (Lordosis)
	MUPs Darcin	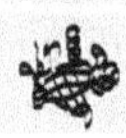	Male major urinary protein	VNO	Female sexual attention
Volatile	α- and β-farnesense	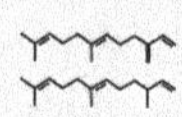	Male preputial grand	MOE ? VNO ?	Estrus induction and synchronization Puberty acceleration Attract female mice
	SBT 2-sec-butyl-4,5-dihydrothiazole	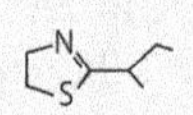	Male bladder urine	VNO	Estrus induction and synchronization Puberty acceleration Attract female mice
	DHB 2,3-deydro-exo-brevicomin	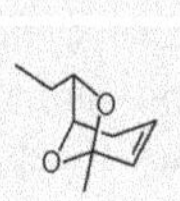	Male bladder urine	VNO	Estrus induction and synchronization Puberty acceleration Attract female mice
	MTMT (methylthio)methanethiol	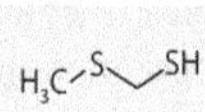	Male urine	MOE	Attract female mice
	Z5-14:OH ((Z)-5-tetradecen-1-ol)	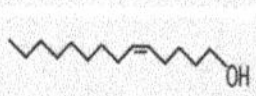	Male preputial gland	MOE	Attract female mice
	Estorogens (E2)	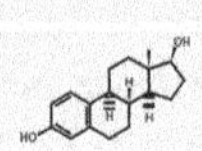	male urine	?	Bruce effect Puberty acceleration

FIGURE 1 | Table of male pheromones that affect female mice. VNO, vomeronasal organ; MOE, main olfactory epithelium.

In rodents, pheromones are perceived by two separate olfactory systems, the main olfactory system (MOS) and the vomeronasal system (VNS), which convey chemical information to the central brain area. These two systems have separate sensory neural populations in the nasal cavity. It has traditionally been demonstrated that pheromonal molecules are mainly perceived through the vomeronasal organ (VNO) (Tirindelli et al., 2009). Non-volatile molecules contained in the urine or on the body's surface are transferred to the VNO when an animal's nares directly contact a stimulus on the opponent mouse. This behavior is commonly observed when mice show sexual or aggressive behavior. Therefore, the VNS is thought to mediate the detection of most species- and sex-specific cues involved in the control of mating and aggressive behavior (Stowers et al., 2002; Dulac and Torello, 2003). The MOS, on the other hand, mainly detects airborne scents, that is, volatile chemical components and small airborne peptides, via receptors in the main olfactory epithelium (MOE). Airborne volatiles are essential for detecting scents at a distance, which can alert animals to both the presence and location of a scent's source. In order to detect non- or low volatile components through the VNS, an animal must approach and make nasal contact with the source of the scent. In this review, we also describe the sensory organs responsible for detecting each of the identified compounds in the social odors (**Figure 1**) and their neural pathways below.

EXOCRINE GLAND-SECRETING PEPTIDE1 (ESP1)

ESP1 is secreted into tear fluids from the extraorbital lacrimal glands (Kimoto et al., 2005) in adult male mice, and it promotes female sexual behaviors, such as lordosis (Haga et al., 2010). When female mice make close nasal contacts with either the facial area of an adult male or soiled bedding, non-volatile ESP1 binds to the specific vomeronasal receptor, V2Rp5, which is one of the V2R family receptor involved in female sexual behavior (Oboti et al., 2014). The ligand-receptor interaction results in sex-specific signal transmission through the accessory olfactory bulb (AOB) and medial amygdala (MeA), to the ventromedial hypothalamic nuclei (VMH), which serve as a center for female lordosis behavior (Haga et al., 2010).

DARCIN

The single atypical major urinary protein (MUP) named darcin is present in adult male urine (Roberts et al., 2010). Darcin can promote female attraction and induces the spatial learning of other chemical cues, allowing both females and competitor males to find sites of previous social interactions (Roberts et al., 2012). Because darcin is a non-volatile chemical like ESP1, female mice have to make direct contact with male urine to promote attraction to the chemicals and to enhance the conditioned place preference. Darcin may be perceived by the VNO, however, the receptors and neural pathways for darcin have not been identified.

α- AND β-FARNESENSE

α- and β-farnesense induce territorial avoidance among male mice (Novotny et al., 1990; Jemiolo et al., 1992). The urine of dominant males has a higher concentration of these molecules compared to the urine of subordinate males. These molecules are conspicuously absent in bladder urine (Harvey et al., 1989), suggesting that α- and β-farnesense are synthesized in and secreted from the testes, or the preputial gland, probably by testosterone-dependent manner (Novotny et al., 1990). α- and β-farnesense also attract females (Jemiolo et al., 1991; Mucignat-Caretta et al., 1995), and can effectively induce estrus (Brennan and Peele, 2003; Dulac and Torello, 2003). These small ligands bind to MUPs in the urine, and this mixture shows puberty-accelerating pheromonal activity in recipient females (Novotny et al., 1999b). Thus, these molecules have complex functions in recipient females.

2-SEC-BUTYL-4,5-DIHYDROTHIAZOLE (SBT) AND 3,4-DEYDRO-EXO-BREVICOMIN (DHB)

SBT and DHB are the volatile urinary constituents in male mice; castration drastically reduces their concentration, while testosterone supplementation restores their concentrations to normal levels (Novotny et al., 1985). Although merely presenting a mixture of SBT and DHB has no primer pheromone effects on recipient females, the addition of these compounds to urine from castrated males can be attractive to females (Jemiolo et al., 1985) and can induce estrus synchronization (Jemiolo et al., 1986). It is possible that peptide molecules in male urine act as transporters that transmit SBT or DHB to the VNO, where these two compounds bind to receptors located in the vomeronasal epithelium. Actually, these compounds also bind to MUPs and increase puberty-accelerating pheromonal activity in recipient females (Novotny et al., 1999b).

OTHER CANDIDATE MALE PHEROMONES

(Methylthio)methanethiol (MTMT) is found in only male mouse urine and are attractive to females (Alema et al., 1988; Lin et al., 2005). The specific mitral cells in the main olfactory bulb (MOB) that respond to MTMT were not stimulated by any other urinary compound. Thus, MTMT is highly volatile, and it may advertise the presence of a male from a distance, perhaps as a signal to attract females. (Z)-5-tetradecen-1-ol (Z5-14:OH) was recently identified as a natural ligand for a mouse odorant receptor, and is excreted from the preputial gland into male mouse urine under the control of testosterone and enhances the attractiveness of urine to female mice (Yoshikawa et al., 2013). This compound could act as a natural ligand for the specific chemosensory receptor Olfr288 in the MOE.

ESTRADIOL (IN MALE URINE)

The occurrence of the Bruce effect and the Vandenberg effect in female mice is generally thought to depend on detection and processing of urinary odors from male through the VNS (Leinders-Zufall et al., 2004). Castration of male mice reduced these effects and treatment with either testosterone (Dominic, 1965; Lombardi et al., 1976) or estrogens (Thorpe and deCatanzaro, 2012) restores the ability of castrated males to induce these effects. Intact male mouse urine consistently contains substantial quantities of unconjugated estrogens, and the levels rise when males are in the presence of females (deCatanzaro et al., 2006). It was proposed that estradiol excreted in the male's urine may be ingested nasally by female (Guzzo et al., 2012; Baum and Bakker, 2013), and this circulating estradiol may directly influence blastocyst implantation (the Bruce effect) and maturation of the reproductive tract (the Vandenergh effect). Recently, it has been found that activation of VNO neurons was observed in response to sulfated steroids such as androgens, estrogens, and glucocorticoids (Nodari et al., 2008; Guzzo et al., 2010). Thus, estrogens in male urine can transmit information of the status of male mouse to females, acting either as a pheromone or as an endocrine stimulator. However, other female urine that also contains estradiol would not cause pregnancy block. Thus, some additional male pheromonal cues (such as MHC described below) plays a critical role in the Bruce effect.

PHEROMONAL CUES FOR AVOIDING INBREEDING

Mice have a remarkable ability to detect individual genetic differences by their odors. In particular, mice can detect differences in urine odor type from mice with different major histocompatibility complexes (MHCs) under laboratory (Beauchamp et al., 1985; Penn and Potts, 1998b) and semi-natural conditions (Potts et al., 1991). The genes of the MHC are the most polymorphic coding loci known among vertebrates, and their products, MHC molecules, play a central role in immunological self/non-self recognition (Janeway et al., 2001). Interestingly, MHC genes also influence individual odor differences (Penn and Potts, 1998b). When given a choice via mating or two-choice assays, female mice prefer males with MHCs that are different from their own (Yamazaki et al., 1976). It has been suggested that the peptide ligand of MHC class I molecules are release into urine and can elicit an MHC-haplotype-specific behavioral response after uptake into the nose by sniffing (Overath et al., 2014). As a result, mice can increase the MHC-heterozygosity of their progeny. MHC-dependent mating preferences may function to increase disease resistance, since MHC-heterozygous offspring have less inbreeding and fewer hereditary diseases (Potts and Wakeland, 1993; Brown and Eklund, 1994; Apanius et al., 1997). Interestingly, MHC-related chemicals may be responsible for the Bruce effect (Leinders-Zufall et al., 2004). MHC-related chemicals are important for forming olfactory memories in the context of pregnancy block.

Recent studies revealed that females also use variant MUP profiles to recognize the urine scent marks of individual males (Hurst et al., 2005; Cheetham et al., 2007). These MUP patterns in the urine act like an individual "bar code" that signals the identity of the scent marks' owner (Beynon and Hurst, 2003). In wild house mice, females use self-referent matching of MUP patterns to avoid inbreeding, but there is little evidence that MHC sharing influences mate choice (Sherborne et al., 2007). Indeed, MUPs have been implicated as chemical signals that allow the recognition of genetic heterozygosity (a sign of phenotypic vigor) and enable the avoidance of inbreeding. Furthermore, MUPs help distinguish individuals of the same or different species.

Collectively, it appears that MHC-related chemicals and MUPs contribute non-volatile proteins or peptides of mouse scent signals, permitting individual recognition, for which mice have specific receptors in the VNO (Leinders-Zufall et al., 2004). MUPs show individual expression consistent with a role in sexual signaling, and these MHC and MUP signals may provide information regarding an individual's genetic identity that could be used in mate selection.

PHEROMONAL EFFECTS ON FEMALE NEUROENDOCRINE FUNCTION

As mentioned above, male pheromones can modulate female behaviors, but they also stimulate female reproductive abilities. Regulating these reproductive effects involves male pheromone signatures, which are formed in part by neural circuitry within the olfactory system and hypothalamic-pituitary-gonadal (HPG) axis. Modification of the HPG axis, which is regulated by male pheromones, stimulates the release of luteinizing hormone (LH) and prolactin (PRL), two hormones that are important for female reproductive function (Halpern, 1987; Mak et al., 2007). These pituitary hormones subsequently act on the gonads. Actually, gonadotropin-releasing hormone (GnRH) neurons, which are the key hormone regulators of LH secretion, originate in the olfactory system in the early neonatal period, and migrate into the hypothalamus, suggesting a tight connection between olfaction and reproduction (Wray, 2010). In fact, pheromones from opposite sex conspecifics induce sexually dimorphic responses in GnRH neurons in mice (Yoon et al., 2005), and, neuropeptide kisspeptin which play an important role in modulating GnRH neurons, are activated by male odor in female mice (Bakker et al., 2010). Compared to the MOS, the VNS provides a neural pathway that directly links olfactory sensations to the hypothalamus, and the modulation of LH and PRL release through this pathway seems to provide the endocrine basis for the "primer" effect of pheromones.

These hypothalamic areas are involved in reproductive endocrinology and sexual behavior in females. In particular, the GnRH-LH axis has a key role in the "releaser" effect, in that it regulates pheromone-mediated sexual behavior. GnRH itself can reverse the effects induced by surgical removal of the VNO, which diminishes sexual behavior, including mount attempts in males (Fernandez-Fewell and Meredith, 1995) and lordosis responses in females, highlighting the crucial role of this hormone in the regulation of female sexual behavior (Mackay-Sim and Rose, 1986). Therefore, pheromones can enhance sexual behavior via stimulating GnRH release. Another pathway for modulating sexual behavior is through the activation of the HPG axis. Explicitly, primer pheromones increase activity of the GnRH-LH axis, which stimulates estrogen release from the ovaries (Kerbeshian et al., 1994). Circulating gonadal hormones, especially estradiol and progesterone, enhance female sexual behavior (Lydon et al., 1995), and probably exert rapid non-genomic effects. Specifically, estrogen can rapidly stimulate GnRH neurons in the preoptic area (POA) via estrogen receptor β (ERβ), implying that either circulating estrogen or *de novo* synthesized estrogen in the brain can rapidly stimulate female sexual behavior through GnRH neurons. There is no clear evidence showing that pheromones induce *de novo* estrogen synthesis in the hypothalamus, thus future research should establish whether male pheromones are able to enhance *de novo* synthesis of estrogen in the POA via stimulating aromatase in the neurons.

ATTRACTIVENESS OF MALE VOCALIZATIONS

Females might use vocalization to assist in mate selection (McComb, 1991; Rehsteiner et al., 1998). In many species, vocal displays associated with sexual encounters are often mediated by testosterone released from the testes (Floody, 1981; Moore et al., 2005; Bass and Remage-Healey, 2008). Thus, testosterone levels strongly influence vocal performance in some species because vocalizations accurately reflect a male's social status and resource holding potential (Parker, 1974; Galeotti et al., 1997). For example, in birds, males that had calls with high vocal performance scores were considered more successful breeders than males with low performance scores (Ballentine et al., 2004; Illes et al., 2006; Janicke et al., 2008). Similarly, in deer, there is strong relationship between the time invested in vocal display and their mating success (McElligott et al., 1999).

Male mouse USVs are also under androgenic control (Dizinno and Whitney, 1977; Nunez et al., 1978; James et al., 2006). Female mice move toward male USVs, suggesting that the USVs of male mice are attractive to female mice (Hammerschmidt et al., 2009). Likewise, in neotropical singing mice, testosterone plays a strong role in modulating vocal performance in males, increasing the duration and complexity of trills (Pasch et al., 2011). Females in neotropical singing mice spend more time near speakers that generate high-performance trills resembling the vocalizations of testosterone-treated males (Pasch et al., 2011). Moreover, dominant males emit more USVs toward a female than male of lower rank in C57/BL6 mice (Wang et al., 2011). Thus, testosterone levels strongly influence vocal performance because vocalizations reflect a male's social status in mice. These findings indicate that the vocalization of male mice function to show females their masculine phenotype, which is under the control of testosterone, similar to the vocalization of other species.

MALE VOCALIZATIONS FOR AVOIDING INBREEDING

The characteristics of male mouse USVs differ across inbred strains (Panksepp et al., 2007; Kikusui et al., 2011; Sugimoto et al., 2011). A cross-fostering study revealed that the sequences of male USVs are under strong genetic control (Kikusui et al., 2011). Research using transgenic mouse models suggests that USV profiles are genetically regulated in males (Wang et al., 2008; Ey et al., 2012; Hammerschmidt et al., 2012; Roy et al., 2012; Mahrt et al., 2013). Although the song characteristics of male USVs are highly variable, the biological significance of these repertoires has not been identified. To demonstrate that female mice can discriminate different male USVs, we recently conducted playback experiments to assess the responses of female mice to USVs of male mice from different strains. We found that inbred female mice could discriminate the different male USV characteristics, and that they preferred the USVs of mice that were from different strains than their parents (Asaba et al., 2014). Similarly, wild-derived female mice showed a greater preference for USVs produced by unfamiliar males compared to the USVs produced by familiar males (Musolf et al., 2010; Hoffmann et al., 2012), implying that female mice can use male USVs to select a mating partner.

As mentioned above, a cross-fostering study in male mice revealed that USV sequences are under strong genetic control (Kikusui et al., 2011). It is of interest whether the preference for male USVs in females is genetically controlled or experience-dependent. We conducted the same cross fostering experiment in female mice and found that these preferences are based on early social experiences, unlike the male USV characteristics, which are genetically controlled (Asaba et al., 2014).

These findings suggest that the preference for USVs of males from a different strain contributes to disassortative mating, which is an important mate choice strategy for avoiding inbreeding and facilitating the heterozygosity of offspring. As described above, MHCs and MUPs have a pivotal role in disassortative mating, in that mice avoid individuals with similar MHCs and MUPs using chemical cues. Our recent findings suggest that another social signal, male mouse songs, have an important role in courtship by potentially facilitating mate attraction or mate choice.

MALE VOCALIZATIONS ENHANCE FEMALE ESTROGENS AND MATING BEHAVIOR

Although it is unclear whether the neural circuits for ultrasonic songs are responsible for reproductive outcomes in mice, other reports show that male courtship vocalizations trigger female sexual and endocrine responses in avian and mammal species. The effects of male vocalizations on female reproduction are well documented in songbirds. Songs presented to females via audio playback are sufficient to enhance female reproduction, such as LH secretion, follicle growth, egg laying, and nest-building behavior (Brockway, 1965; Kroodsma, 1976; Hinde and Steele, 1978; Morton et al., 1985; Leboucher et al., 1998; Bentley et al., 2000). Additionally, in mammals, playback vocalizations of males advance the onset of seasonal ovulatory activity in red deer (McComb, 1987). Similarly, the auditory signals emitted by bucks are strong enough to stimulate the secretion of LH from the pituitary, sexual behavior, and ovulation in female goats (Shelton, 1980; Delgadillo et al., 2012). These reproductive effects induced by male vocalizations are mediated by the development of ovarian follicles and the consequent production of estradiol, which is a key hormone for displaying sexual behavior.

MULTISENSORY INTEGRATION FOR FEMALE BEHAVIOR

The social environments of animals are very complex, and correspondingly place great information processing demands on the brain. Individuals are faced with complex and multisensory signals from which they have to extract functionally relevant cues. As mentioned above, there is behavioral evidence that supports the value of each sensory signal separately, but how these sensory signals are integrated in a natural context has not been elucidated. In male-female communication, it is normal for females to be simultaneously exposed to olfactory and acoustic cues emitted by males. One possible mechanism for sensory integration is that the exposure of female mice to chemical and acoustic cues from males activates a common neural circuit involved in reproductive function and behavior.

Earlier work has shown that adult females have an innate interest in male USVs (Pomerantz et al., 1983), but that females habituate rapidly to the pure playback of male USVs in the absence of real males (Hammerschmidt et al., 2009; Shepard and Liu, 2011). When females were exposed to living males, they showed a reinstated preference for these vocalizations upon retest, suggesting that chemical or physical contact with males is important for maintaining the response to vocal cues (Shepard and Liu, 2011). Behaviorally, female mice discriminate among males not only using olfactory cues, but also using USVs, and it has been shown that females prefer unfamiliar individuals to familiar kin (Bowers and Alexander, 1967; Hammerschmidt et al., 2009; Musolf et al., 2010; Shepard and Liu, 2011). We demonstrated that olfactory signals have significant effects on mate choice when paired with acoustic cues in mice. The preference for USVs appeared when females were exposed to male-soiled bedding or to ESP1 before USV preference tests (Asaba et al., 2014). Interestingly, both auditory (USV) and odorant (MHC) preferences for mate choice were imprinted during the developmental period of female mice (Penn and Potts, 1998a). This implies that the integrated sensory system for mate choice has plastic qualities that are dependent upon social experiences during the pre-weaning period.

Multisensory information is also important for inducing maternal behavior in mother-infant communication (Levy and Keller, 2009). Maternal retrieving behavior is regulated by multisensory information from pup olfactory and auditory cues (Okabe et al., 2013). In electrophysiological studies, exposure to pup odors enhances the neuronal responses to pup USVs in the auditory cortex in the mother, indicating that sensory information from the pup, including both acoustic and chemical signals, affects the function of the auditory cortex (AuC) (Cohen et al., 2011). It is hypothesized that male odors enhance the processing circuits for acoustic information, or vice versa, which may be the neural mechanisms underlying female mate choice. Multimodal sensory systems for mate choice may explain the cross-modal information processing involved in this behavior. Below, we provide a detailed examination of the possible neural circuits involved in the sensory integration of chemical and audible cues.

OLFACTORY PATHWAY

While no behavioral or neural evidence supports the existence of multimodal sensory processing in mice, the basic anatomy and physiology of the pheromone-processing circuits are well defined and available. The two major olfactory systems, the MOS and VNS, convey chemical information to the central nervous system (**Figure 2**). VNO receptors extend axons to glomeruli located in the AOB. AOB mitral cells, which are second-order neurons, extend axons to the MeA (Kevetter and Winans, 1981). In turn, neurons in the MeA project to hypothalamic targets that control female proceptive (approach) and receptive (lordosis) behaviors (Brennan and Zufall, 2006). Therefore, one characteristic of the VNS is that it sends information directly to the behavioral and endocrine center of the hypothalamus, which is not involved in the cortex-thalamic sensory processing pathways.

In contrast, the MOS has traditionally been recognized as the detection system for non-pheromonal odorants present in the environment. As mentioned earlier, the MOS detects airborne scents, that is, volatile chemical components and small airborne peptides, via receptors in the MOE, and these scents can be detected at some distance from their source. Receptor neurons in the MOE extend axons to mitral cells in the MOB. The mitral cells of the MOB project to several higher centers including the anterior olfactory nucleus (AON), the olfactory tubercle (OT), the piriform cortex (Pir), and the cortical amygdala (Kevetter and Winans, 1981). Recently, studies have shown that a subpopulation of MOB mitral cells projects directly to the MeA (Pro-Sistiaga et al., 2007; Kang et al., 2009; Thompson et al., 2012). The AOB and MOB pathways converge in several cortical and sub-cortical amygdaloid targets, suggesting that these locations are where chemosignals involved in social communication are integrated.

Although the MOS is thought to detect volatile odorants and the VNS is thought to be specialized for the detection of non-volatile pheromones, recent findings suggest that the MOS is also involved in pheromone detection (Alema et al., 1988; Boehm et al., 2005; Lin et al., 2005; Yoon et al., 2005; Spehr et al., 2006). As mentioned above, adult male mice produce several male-specific volatiles in their urine under the control of testosterone (Schwende et al., 1986; Alema et al., 1988; Novotny et al., 1999a; Lin et al., 2005), and these chemicals can be detected through the MOE and VNO. Therefore, the recognition and assessment of conspecifics though scents involves an important interaction between the MOS and VNS that controls sexual attraction. A functional magnetic resonance imaging (fMRI) study revealed that MOB activation in female mice occurred slightly earlier than activation in the AOB in response to male urinary volatiles (Xu et al., 2005). These results suggest that the VNO responses to volatile pheromones are typically preceded by MOE detection, which then leads the animal to make nasal contact with a non-volatile pheromone, thus activating the VNO. Once animals are in close nasal contact with the scent source, the VNO pump is activated to gain additional information through the VNS. Therefore, detecting airborne scents through the MOS may be necessary to activate scent delivery to the VNO (Hurst and Beynon, 2004; Keller et al., 2006).

Once the sex information of an individual is encoded, it is transmitted to the limbic system. The MeA in the limbic system is one of the most important regions for integrating this information since it receives axons from both the MOS and VNS (Pro-Sistiaga et al., 2007; Kang et al., 2009; Thompson et al., 2012). The MeA sends the information to the hypothalamic nuclei, including the VMH and bed nucleus of the stria terminalis (BNST), both of which are involved in sexual or aggressive behavior (Brennan and Zufall, 2006). Therefore, the chemical information within social stimuli perceived by the MOS and VNS acts in simple and stereotyped neural circuits that lead to behavioral and neuroendocrinological outcomes.

ESTROGEN MODULATES CHEMICAL NEURAL PATHWAYS

Olfactory sensitivity and preferences are modulated by sex hormones. The neural mechanisms underlying the action of estrogens on the olfactory system are intricately organized. Studies in humans suggest that estrogens enhance olfactory sensitivity by acting on the reception and perception of chemicals. For example, the composition of mucus in the olfactory epithelium is altered by the menstrual cycle (Mair et al., 1978). Similarly, estrogens enhance olfactory sensitivity and olfactory preferences through peripheral and central mechanisms in rodents (Pietras and Moulton, 1974; Moffatt, 2003). In fact, the olfactory sensitivity of female mice changes throughout the estrous cycle, and ovariectomized animals are sensitive to treatment with exogenous steroids (Caroom and Bronson, 1971). Indeed, after exposing

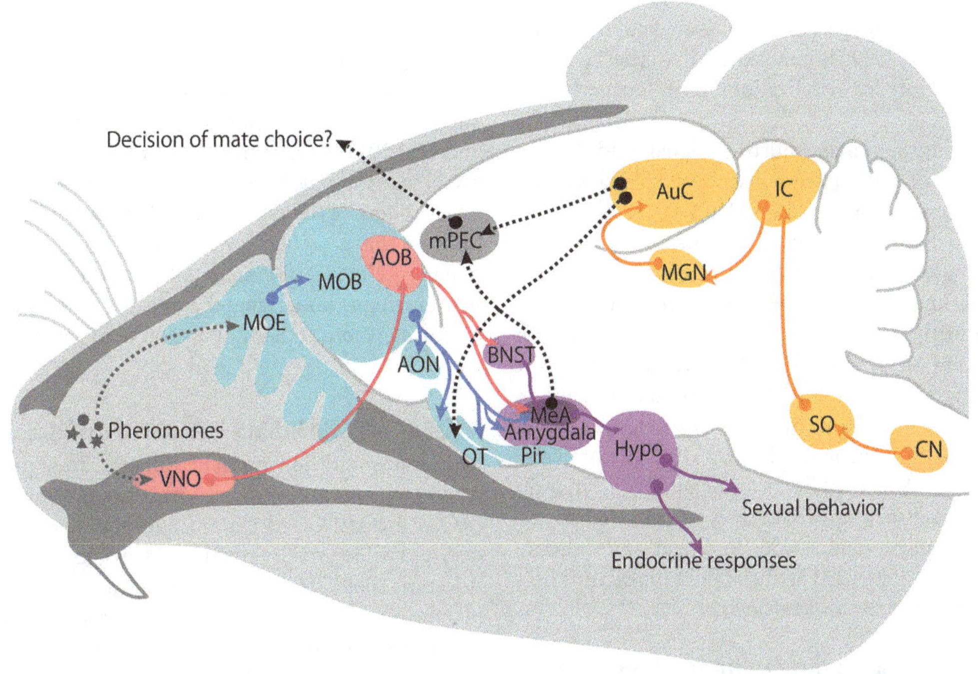

FIGURE 2 | Proposed schematic of female neural pathways for male chemical and vocalization signals. The vomeronasal pathway is shown in pink, main olfactory pathway in blue, intracortical projection in purple, auditory pathway in yellow, and the hypothetical integrate pathway is represented with a gray dotted line. Abbreviations: accessory olfactory bulb (AOB), anterior olfactory nucleus (AON), auditory cortex (AuC), bed nucleus of the stria terminalis (BNST), cochlear nucleus (CN), Hypothalamus (Hypo), inferior colliculus (IC), medial amygdala (MeA), medial geniculate nucleus (MGN), main olfactory bulb (MOB), main olfactory epithelium (MOE), medial prefrontal cortex (mPFC), olfactory tubercle (OT), piriform cortex (Pir), superior olivary nucleus (SO), vomeronasal organ (VNO).

estradiol-treated females to soiled male bedding, more VNO neurons were activated in estradiol-treated females compared to in oil-treated females (Halem et al., 1999). However, male urine activated mitral and granule cells in the AOB of female mice independently of estrogens. In the central portion of the VNS, namely the BNST and medial POA, neuronal cFos responses to male pheromones, an indicator of neural activation, were observed equally in females regardless of estrogen treatment, implying that estrogen effects mainly occur in VNO sensory neurons. Therefore, the effects of estrogens on the sensitivity to male pheromones and on neuronal responses to male pheromones probably work in concert to maximize the likelihood of mating and reproduction in reproductively permissive environments (Moffatt, 2003).

Steroid hormone receptors, especially estrogen receptors, are widely distributed in the MOS and VNS. Estrogen receptor α (ERα) is located in the MOB and AOB (Merchenthaler et al., 2004). In the subsequent region that receive axons from the MOB and AOB, both ERα and ERβ are expressed in the cortical and medial divisions of the amygdala, which is the key brain region involved in the integration of chemical information from the MOB and AOB (Mitra et al., 2003). ERα and ERβ are also found in the POA and BNST, suggesting that estrogens can act on the central neural circuits of olfaction. Interestingly, the distribution of estradiol-induced progestin receptors is similar to ERs, and estradiol-induced progestin receptors colocalize with ERs in the amygdala, hypothalamus, and POA (Moffatt et al., 1998). Regarding female sexual behavior, combined treatment with estrogen and progesterone enhances female lordosis behavior (Pfaff, 1994); therefore, neurons in the olfactory pathway that express ERs and progesterone receptors can be involved in female sexual behavior induced by chemical stimulation.

AUDITORY PATHWAY

Regarding ultrasonic neural circuits in mice, it is not clear which neural circuits are responsible for the behavioral and reproductive outcomes. However, neural circuits for audible sounds have been identified. Encoded sound information is transmitted from the cochlea to the central nervous system (**Figure 2**). The auditory nerve enters the brainstem at the pons-medulla junction and sends its axons to the cochlear nucleus (CN). The secondary auditory neurons in the CN send their axons decussately in the ventral pons and ascend to the superior olivary complex (SO). The SO is important for detecting the interaural level and time differences necessary for sound localization. Third-order neurons of the SO send axons via the lateral lemniscus to the inferior colliculus (IC) of the midbrain, which is important for binaural information processing and is a major site of auditory information integration. Fourth-order neurons continue to the medial geniculate body (MGN), which is the thalamic relay where sensory information is filtered before it is transmitted to the cortex. The axons of fifth-order MGN neurons synapse with neurons of the AuC on the superior temporal gyrus (Charitidi, 2011). Given that the primary AuC is involved in auditory object recognition and is a known site of neuronal plasticity (Nelken, 2004; Weinberger, 2004; Nelken and Bar-Yosef, 2008; Miranda and Liu, 2009; Romanski and Averbeck, 2009), the learning and memory of vocalizations likely occur in this region.

Although the evolution of male courtship signals and the corresponding sensitivity of auditory responses in females are found in a variety of species (White et al., 1992; Vyas et al., 2009), there is no clear evidence pinpointing the neural circuits responsible for the female preference for male ultrasonic songs in mice. Furthermore, less is known about how neurons respond to multisensory stimuli during the imprinting of female preference for mate choice. A recent study showed that neural activity in the mouse OT regarding MOS is also responsive to auditory input, that is, a subpopulation of neurons in the OT displayed responses to a 2.8-kHz pure tone (Wesson and Wilson, 2010). Anatomically, neurons in the primary AuC send fibers to the olfactory Pir, indicating that auditory sensory information is transmitted to the olfactory cortex (Budinger et al., 2006; Budinger and Scheich, 2009). However, these studies used artificial pure tones, thus how natural male signals merge remains unclear.

ESTROGEN MODULATES AUDITORY NEURAL PATHWAYS

Estrogens also modulate the physiological and reproductive behavioral responses to sensory signals, including auditory stimuli, in many species (Maney and Pinaud, 2011). For example, in humans, fluctuations in auditory perception (Haggard and Gaston, 1978; Cowell et al., 2011) and in electrophysiological measures of auditory function (Walpurger et al., 2004; Al-Mana et al., 2010) during the menstrual cycle highlight the effects of estrogen on auditory processing. When estradiol levels are exogenously modified, alterations in auditory perception, auditory brainstem latencies, auditory thresholds, and sound localization are observed (Haggard and Gaston, 1978; Jerger and Johnson, 1988; Wharton and Church, 1990; Coleman et al., 1994; Caruso et al., 2003). Direct evidence from animal electrophysiological and behavioral studies shows that hearing plasticity and communication skills are enhanced by estradiol (Sisneros et al., 2004; Remage-Healey et al., 2008, 2012; Tremere et al., 2009). Estradiol can rapidly modulate neural responses in the auditory association cortex of the zebra finch by suppressing inhibitory transmission (Tremere et al., 2009). Additionally, in mice, estrogen antagonists alter the auditory feedback mechanisms in mice (Thompson et al., 2006).

These estrogen effects are mediated by both ERα and ERβ, which belong to the nuclear receptor superfamily and act as transcription factors. Regarding auditory processing circuits, both ERα and ERβ are expressed in the peripheral organs and central auditory systems in mice (Stenberg et al., 1999; Charitidi and Canlon, 2010; Charitidi et al., 2010). Specifically, ERα and ERβ were found predominantly in the CN, the nucleus of the trapezoid body, the lateral- and medio-ventral periolivary nuclei, the dorsal lateral lemniscus, and the IC.

However, it is not evident whether male mice USVs play a role in female reproductive function or not; several studies revealed that estradiol is necessary for reacting to vocalizations. In mice, female preference for the vocalizing male was absent after ovariectomy, and was recovered via treatment with ovarian hormones (Pomerantz et al., 1983), indicating that female USV preference depends on the gonadal estrogens. Previous studies using a choice test showed that female USV preference was not altered by the estrus state (Hammerschmidt et al., 2009; Shepard and Liu, 2011); however, our recent study demonstrated that the preference for male USVs from a different mouse strain depended on the phase of the estrus cycle (Asaba et al., 2014). These results indicate that a certain level of estrogen is necessary for eliciting female preference for male vocalizations. The mechanisms and neural circuits underlying the role of estrogen in song preference, including where and how it acts on neurons, is the target of future research.

NEURAL MECHANISMS FOR MATE CHOICE

In humans and non-human primates, the anterior medial prefrontal cortex (mPFC) and rostral anterior cingulate cortex (ACC) are related to certain components of social interpretation and behavioral interaction (Damasio, 1996; Stuss et al., 2002; Adolphs, 2009). These brain regions are active during judgments of kinship and close others later in life (Krienen et al., 2010). Regarding auditory preference, the choice of listening to one type of music over another likely reflects limbic, decision-making brain regions, such as the prefrontal cortex in humans (Levitin and Tirovolas, 2009). In rodent models, the lesion studies suggest that regions along the frontal midline including the mPFC and ACC have a critical role in behavioral decision-making (Kvitsiani et al., 2013). Interestingly, Jouhaneau and Bagady (1984) demonstrated that Swiss albino mice exposed to a certain type of music during postnatal days 10–20 demonstrated a preference for that kind of music when given a choice during adulthood, indicating that there is a sensitive period for forming auditory preferences even in mice. Moreover, the acoustic environment during the critical period for auditory preference shapes the mPFC response in C57BL/6 mice. Furthermore, this preference can be altered by epigenetic modification to the mPFC (Yang et al., 2012), suggesting that the mPFC has a pivotal role in imprinting auditory preferences in mice. We recently found that the female preference for male USVs is formed during the juvenile period while in the presence of the father mouse (Asaba et al., 2014). Therefore, the mPFC may be responsible for the plasticity of the vocalization preference in female mice.

In contrast, there is little evidence showing mPFC involvement in pheromone-induced mate preference. As mentioned above, chemical information perceived in the VNO is transmitted to the MeA and ends in the hypothalamus. Therefore, there is no direct connection between the VNS and mPFC. However, even in the pheromonal circuits underlying the olfactory-limbic-hypothalamus pathway, there is anatomical evidence of a connection between the amygdala and prefrontal cortex (McDonald et al., 1996; Marek et al., 2013), especially for emotional behavior.

There is one example of prefrontal cortex involvement in odorant preference. The male-derived volatiles become attractive if they are associated with non-volatile attractive pheromones, suggesting that non-volatile pheromones can stimulate the reward circuit via the VNS and act as an unconditioned stimulus. When

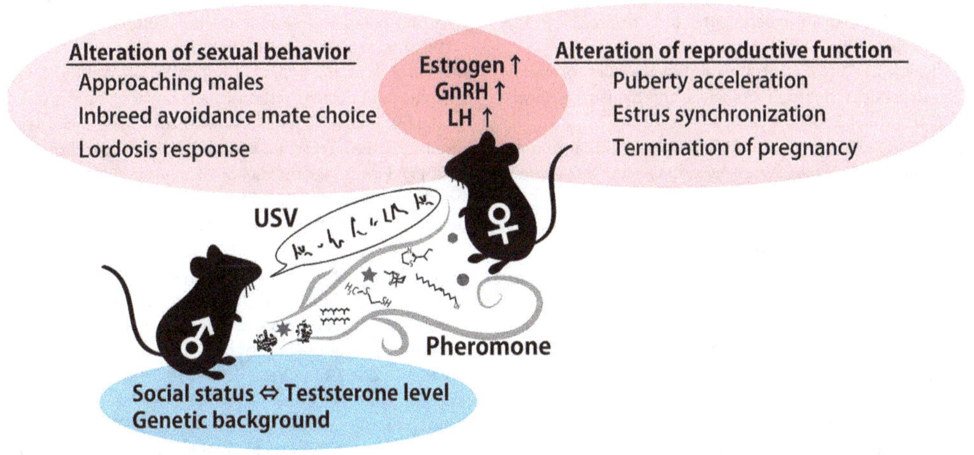

FIGURE 3 | A schematic illustration of the effect of male cues. Testosterone-controlled male pheromones alter female sexual behavior and reproductive function by increasing estrogen and GnRH. In addition, genetic background-dependent male USVs and pheromones contribute to inbreeding avoidance. Abbreviations: gonadotropin-releasing hormone (GnRH), luteinizing hormone (LH), ultrasonic vocalization (USV).

female mice were exposed to the non-volatile pheromones, the basolateral amygdala and the shell of the nucleus accumbens were activated. In contrast, exploring the volatile pheromones conditioned with non-volatile pheromones activated the basolateral amygdala, prefrontal cortex, and ventral tegmental area (Moncho-Bogani et al., 2005). Therefore, the prefrontal cortex can be involved in the reward circuit via stimulation by male pheromones in females, resulting in female mate-preference behavior (McDonald et al., 1996; Moncho-Bogani et al., 2005). Collectively, one feasible neural mechanism for the sensory integration of chemical and auditory cues involved in female mate preference is the mPFC, which is activated by both pheromones and auditory cues. Future studies are needed to clarify this hypothesis.

SUMMARY

As described above, female preference for male traits can provide genetic benefits to offspring that inherit favorable alleles from their father. Therefore, female reproductive functions can be activated if the female encounters a masculine male in order to obtain offspring with greater fitness. It is generally agreed that dominant males tend to sire more litters than subordinate males (DeFries and McClearn, 1970; Oakeshott, 1974). Female usually use pheromones and ultrasonic vocalizations, and these signals carry the male-specific information required to support these phenomena. The summarized roles of pheromones and USVs in males to female cues are shown in **Figure 3**. Although it is unclear which neural circuits are involved in USVs preference and the stimulation of reproductive outcomes in females, the behavioral and reproductive effect of pheromones and vocalizations are similar, suggesting that a common neural pathway integrates both types of information. Moreover, both signals characteristically contribute to inbreeding avoidance by imprinting during the developmental period. Imprinted sound preference is associated with mPFC activation in mice, as is a conditioned preference to pheromones. These results imply that male signals are integrated and processed in the mPFC to regulate behavioral decision-making processes. This idea is schematically represented in **Figure 2**. Understanding how females integrate sensory information from males, that is, pheromonal and auditory cues, in natural settings from a neuroscience and adaptive behavior perspective is of great interest.

ACKNOWLEDGMENTS

This work was financially supported by Grants-in-Aid for Scientific Research from the Ministry of Education, Culture, Sports, Science, and Technology of Japan (#14760187, #23248049, and #23132510 to Takefumi Kikusui, and #23780301 to Kazutaka Mogi), Innovative Areas No. 25118007 "The Evolutionary Origin and Neural Basis of the Empathetic Systems," and Promotion and Mutual Aid Corporation for Private Schools of Japan, Grant-in-Aid for Matching Fund Subsidy for Private Universities.

REFERENCES

Adolphs, R. (2009). The social brain: neural basis of social knowledge. *Annu. Rev. Psychol.* 60, 693–716. doi: 10.1146/annurev.psych.60.110707.163514

Alema, G. S., Maccari, S., Micci, M. A., and Patacchioli, F. R. (1988). Hippocampal serotonin in the regulation of the hypothalamo-pituitary-adrenocortical axis (HPAA) stress response. *Pharmacol. Res. Commun.* 20, 429–430. doi: 10.1016/S0031-6989(88)80027-4

Al-Mana, D., Ceranic, B., Djahanbakhch, O., and Luxon, L. M. (2010). Alteration in auditory function during the ovarian cycle. *Hear. Res.* 268, 114–122. doi: 10.1016/j.heares.2010.05.007

Andersson, M. (2006). "Condition-dependent indicators in sexual selection: development of theory and tests," in *Essays in Animal Behaviour, Celebrating 50 Years of Animal Behaviour*, eds J. R. Lucas and L. W. Simmons (Massachusetts: Academic Press), 253–267.

Andersson, M., and Simmons, L. (2006). Sexual selection and mate choice. *Trends Ecol. Evol.* 21, 296. doi: 10.1016/j.tree.2006.03.015

Apanius, V., Penn, D., Slev, P. R., Ruff, L. R., and Potts, W. K. (1997). The nature of selection on the major histocompatibility complex. *Crit. Rev. Immunol.* 17, 179–224. doi: 10.1615/CritRevImmunol.v17.i2.40

Asaba, A., Okabe, S., Nagasawa, M., Kato, M., Koshida, N., Osakada, T., et al. (2014). Developmental social environment imprints female preference for male song in mice. *PLoS ONE* 9:e87186. doi: 10.1371/journal.pone.0087186

Bakker, J., Pierman, S., and Gonzalez-Martinez, D. (2010). Effects of aromatase mutation (ArKO) on the sexual differentiation of kisspeptin neuronal numbers and their activation by same versus opposite sex urinary pheromones. *Horm. Behav.* 57, 390–395. doi: 10.1016/j.yhbeh.2009.11.005

Ballentine, B., Hyman, J., and Nowicki, S. (2004). Vocal performance influences female response to male bird song: an experimental test. *Behav. Ecol.* 15, 163–168. doi: 10.1093/beheco/arg090

Bass, A. H., and Remage-Healey, L. (2008). Central pattern generators for social vocalization: Androgen-dependent neurophysiological mechanisms. *Horm. Behav.* 53, 659. doi: 10.1016/j.yhbeh.2007.12.010

Baum, M. J., and Bakker, J. (2013). Roles of sex and gonadal steroids in mammalian pheromonal communication. *Front. Neuroendocrinol.* 34, 268–284. doi: 10.1016/j.yfrne.2013.07.004

Beauchamp, G. K., Yamazaki, K., Wysocki, C. J., Slotnick, B. M., Thomas, L., and Boyse, E. A. (1985). Chemosensory recognition of mouse major histocompatibility types by another species. *Proc. Natl. Acad. Sci. U.S.A.* 82, 4186–4188. doi: 10.1073/pnas.82.12.4186

Bentley, G. E., Wingfield, J. C., Morton, M. L., and Ball, G. F. (2000). Stimulatory effects on the reproductive axis in female songbirds by conspecific and heterospecific male song. *Horm. Behav.* 37, 179–189. doi: 10.1006/hbeh.2000.1573

Beynon, R. J., and Hurst, J. L. (2003). Multiple roles of major urinary proteins in the house mouse, Mus domesticus. *Biochem. Soc. Trans.* 31, 142–146. doi: 10.1042/BST0310142

Boehm, U., Zou, Z., and Buck, L. B. (2005). Feedback loops link odor and pheromone signaling with reproduction. *Cell* 123, 683–695. doi: 10.1016/j.cell.2005.09.027

Bowers, J. M., and Alexander, B. K. (1967). Mice: individual recognition by olfactory cues. *Science* 158, 1208–1210. doi: 10.1126/science.158.3805.1208

Brennan, P. A., and Peele, P. (2003). Towards an understanding of the pregnancy-blocking urinary chemosignals of mice. *Biochem. Soc. Trans.* 31, 152–155. doi: 10.1042/BST0310152

Brennan, P. A., and Zufall, F. (2006). Pheromonal communication in vertebrates. *Nature* 444, 308–315. doi: 10.1038/nature05404

Brockway, B. F. (1965). Stimulation of ovarian development and egg laying by male courtship vocalization in budgerigars (Melopsittacus undulatus). *Anim. Behav.* 13, 575–578. doi: 10.1016/0003-3472(65)90123-5

Bronson, F. H. (1979). The reproductive ecology of the house mouse. *Q. Rev. Biol.* 54, 265–299. doi: 10.1086/411295

Brown, J. L., and Eklund, A. (1994). Kin recognition and the major histocompatibility complex: an integrative review. *Am. Nat.* 143, 435–461. doi: 10.1086/285612

Bruce, H. M. (1959). An exteroceptive block to pregnancy in the mouse. *Nature* 184, 105.

Bruce, H. M. (1960). A block to pregnancy in the mouse caused by proximity of strange males. *J. Reprod. Fertil.* 1, 96–103. doi: 10.1530/jrf.0.0010096

Budinger, E., Heil, P., Hess, A., and Scheich, H. (2006). Multisensory processing via early cortical stages: connections of the primary auditory cortical field with other sensory systems. *Neuroscience* 143, 1065–1083. doi: 10.1016/j.neuroscience.2006.08.035

Budinger, E., and Scheich, H. (2009). Anatomical connections suitable for the direct processing of neuronal information of different modalities via the rodent primary auditory cortex. *Hear. Res.* 258, 16–27. doi: 10.1016/j.heares.2009.04.021

Caroom, D., and Bronson, F. H. (1971). Responsiveness of female mice to preputial attractant: effects of sexual experience and ovarian hormones. *Physiol. Behav.* 7, 659–662. doi: 10.1016/0031-9384(71)90126-0

Caruso, S., Maiolino, L., Agnello, C., Garozzo, A., Di Mari, L., and Serra, A. (2003). Effects of patch or gel estrogen therapies on auditory brainstem response in surgically postmenopausal women: a prospective, randomized study. *Fertil. Steril.* 79, 556–561. doi: 10.1016/S0015-0282(02)04763-5

Charitidi, K. (2011). *The Role of Estrogen Receptors in the Auditory System.* Stockholm: Karolinska Institutet.

Charitidi, K., and Canlon, B. (2010). Estrogen receptors in the central auditory system of male and female mice. *Neuroscience* 165, 923–933. doi: 10.1016/j.neuroscience.2009.11.020

Charitidi, K., Frisina, R. D., Vasilyeva, O. N., Zhu, X., and Canlon, B. (2010). Expression patterns of estrogen receptors in the central auditory system change in prepubertal and aged mice. *Neuroscience* 170, 1270–1281. doi: 10.1016/j.neuroscience.2010.08.010

Cheetham, S. A., Thom, M. D., Jury, F., Ollier, W. E. R., Beynon, R. J., and Hurst, J. L. (2007). The genetic basis of individual-recognition signals in the mouse. *Curr. Biol.* 17, 1771–1777. doi: 10.1016/j.cub.2007.10.007

Cohen, L., Rothschild, G., and Mizrahi, A. (2011). Multisensory integration of natural odors and sounds in the auditory cortex. *Neuron* 72, 357–369. doi: 10.1016/j.neuron.2011.08.019

Coleman, J. R., Campbell, D., Cooper, W. A., Welsh, M. G., and Moyer, J. (1994). Auditory brainstem responses after ovariectomy and estrogen replacement in rat. *Hear. Res.* 80, 209–215. doi: 10.1016/0378-5955(94)90112-0

Cowell, P. E., Ledger, W. L., Wadnerkar, M. B., Skilling, F. M., and Whiteside, S. P. (2011). Hormones and dichotic listening: evidence from the study of menstrual cycle effects. *Brain Cogn.* 76, 256–262. doi: 10.1016/j.bandc.2011.03.010

Damasio, A. R. (1996). The somatic marker hypothesis and the possible functions of the prefrontal cortex. *Philos. Trans. R. Soc. Lond. B Biol. Sci.* 351, 1413–1420. doi: 10.1098/rstb.1996.0125

deCatanzaro, D., Beaton, E. A., Khan, A., and Vella, E. (2006). Urinary oestradiol and testosterone levels from novel male mice approach values sufficient to disrupt early pregnancy in nearby inseminated females. *Reproduction* 132, 309–317. doi: 10.1530/rep.1.00965

DeFries, J., and McClearn, G. (1970). Social dominance and Darwinian fitness in the laboratory mouse. *Am. Nat.* 408–411. doi: 10.1086/282675

Delgadillo, J. A., Vielma, J., Hernandez, H., Flores, J. A., Duarte, G., Fernandez, I. G., et al. (2012). Male goat vocalizations stimulate the estrous behavior and LH secretion in anestrous goats that have been previously exposed to bucks. *Horm. Behav.* 62, 525–530. doi: 10.1016/j.yhbeh.2012.08.014

Dizinno, G., and Whitney, G. (1977). Androgen influence on male mouse ultrasounds during courtship. *Horm. Behav.* 8, 188–192. doi: 10.1016/0018-506X(77)90035-6

Dominic, C. J. (1965). The origin of the pheromones causing pregnancy block in mice. *J. Reprod. Fertil.* 10, 469–472. doi: 10.1530/jrf.0.0100469

Dulac, C., and Torello, A. T. (2003). Molecular detection of pheromone signals in mammals: from genes to behaviour. *Nat. Rev. Neurosci.* 4, 551–562. doi: 10.1038/nrn1140

Ey, E., Yang, M., Katz, A. M., Woldeyohannes, L., Silverman, J. L., Leblond, C. S., et al. (2012). Absence of deficits in social behaviors and ultrasonic vocalizations in later generations of mice lacking neuroligin4. *Genes Brain Behav.* 11, 928–941. doi: 10.1111/j.1601-183X.2012.00849.x

Fernandez-Fewell, G. D., and Meredith, M. (1995). Facilitation of mating behavior in male hamsters by LHRH and AcLHRH5-10: interaction with the vomeronasal system. *Physiol. Behav.* 57, 213–221. doi: 10.1016/0031-9384(94)00276-B

Floody, O. R. (1981). The hormonal control of ultrasonic communication in rodents. *Am. Zool.* 21, 129–142.

Galeotti, P., Saino, N., Sacchi, R., and Moller, A. P. (1997). Song correlates with social context, testosterone and body condition in male barn swallows. *Anim. Behav.* 53, 687–700. doi: 10.1006/anbe.1996.0304

Guzzo, A. C., Berger, R. G., and deCatanzaro, D. (2010). Excretion and binding of tritium-labelled oestradiol in mice (Mus musculus): implications for the Bruce effect. *Reproduction* 139, 255–263. doi: 10.1530/REP-09-0382

Guzzo, A. C., Jheon, J., Imtiaz, F., and deCatanzaro, D. (2012). Oestradiol transmission from males to females in the context of the Bruce and Vandenbergh effects in mice (Mus musculus). *Reproduction* 143, 539–548. doi: 10.1530/REP-11-0375

Haga, S., Hattori, T., Sato, T., Sato, K., Matsuda, S., Kobayakawa, R., et al. (2010). The male mouse pheromone ESP1 enhances female sexual receptive behaviour through a specific vomeronasal receptor. *Nature* 466, 118–122. doi: 10.1038/nature09142

Haggard, M., and Gaston, J. B. (1978). Changes in auditory perception in the menstrual cycle. *Br. J. Audiol.* 12, 105–118. doi: 10.3109/03005367809078862

Halem, H. A., Cherry, J. A., and Baum, M. J. (1999). Vomeronasal neuroepithelium and forebrain Fos responses to male pheromones in male and female mice. *J. Neurobiol.* 39, 249–263.

Halpern, M. (1987). The organization and function of the vomeronasal system. *Annu. Rev. Neurosci.* 10, 325–362. doi: 10.1146/annurev.ne.10.030187.001545

Hammerschmidt, K., Radyushkin, K., Ehrenreich, H., and Fischer, J. (2009). Female mice respond to male ultrasonic 'songs' with approach behaviour. *Biol. Lett.* 5, 589. doi: 10.1098/rsbl.2009.0317

Hammerschmidt, K., Reisinger, E., Westekemper, K., Ehrenreich, L., Strenzke, N., and Fischer, J. (2012). Mice do not require auditory input for the normal development of their ultrasonic vocalizations. *BMC Neurosci.* 13:40. doi: 10.1186/1471-2202-13-40

Harvey, S., Jemiolo, B., and Novotny, M. (1989). Pattern of volatile compounds in dominant and subordinate male mouse urine. *J. Chem. Ecol.* 15, 2061–2072. doi: 10.1007/BF01207438

Hinde, R. A., and Steele, E. (1978). The influence of daylength and male vocalization on the estrogen-dependent behavior of female canaries and budgerigars, with discussion of data from other species. *Adv. Stud. Behav.* 8, 40–73.

Hoffmann, F., Musolf, K., and Penn, D. J. (2012). Spectrographic analyses reveal signals of individuality and kinship in the ultrasonic courtship vocalizations of wild house mice. *Physiol. Behav.* 105, 766–771. doi: 10.1016/j.physbeh.2011.10.011

Holy, T. E., and Guo, Z. (2005). Ultrasonic songs of male mice. *PLoS Biol.* 3:e386. doi: 10.1371/journal.pbio.0030386

Hurst, J. L., and Beynon, R. J. (2004). Scent wars: the chemobiology of competitive signalling in mice. *Bioessays* 26, 1288–1298. doi: 10.1002/bies.20147

Hurst, J. L., Thom, M. D., Nevison, C. M., Humphries, R. E., and Beynon, R. J. (2005). MHC odours are not required or sufficient for recognition of individual scent owners. *Proc. Biol. Sci.* 272, 715–724. doi: 10.1098/rspb.2004.3004

Illes, A. E., Hall, M. L., and Vehrencamp, S. L. (2006). Vocal performance influences male receiver response in the banded wren. *Proc. Biol. Sci.* 273, 1907. doi: 10.1098/rspb.2006.3535

James, P. J., Nyby, J. G., and Saviolakis, G. A. (2006). Sexually stimulated testosterone release in male mice (Mus musculus): roles of genotype and sexual arousal. *Horm. Behav.* 50, 424–431. doi: 10.1016/j.yhbeh.2006.05.004

Janeway, C. A., Travers, P., Walport, M., and Shlomchik, M. J. (2001). *Immunobiology.* New York, NY: Garland Science.

Janicke, T., Hahn, S., Ritz, M. S., and Peter, H. (2008). Vocal performance reflects individual quality in a nonpasserine. *Anim. Behav.* 75, 91–98. doi: 10.1016/j.anbehav.2007.04.007

Jemiolo, B., Alberts, J., Sochinski-Wiggins, S., Harvey, S., and Novotny, M. (1985). Behavioural and endocrine responses of female mice to synthetic analogues of volatile compounds in male urine. *Anim. Behav.* 33, 1114–1118. doi: 10.1016/S0003-3472(85)80170-6

Jemiolo, B., Harvey, S., and Novotny, M. (1986). Promotion of the Whitten effect in female mice by synthetic analogs of male urinary constituents. *Proc. Natl. Acad. Sci. U.S.A.* 83:4576. doi: 10.1073/pnas.83.12.4576

Jemiolo, B., Xie, T., and Novotny, M. (1992). Urine marking in male mice: responses to natural and synthetic chemosignals. *Physiol. Behav.* 52, 521. doi: 10.1016/0031-9384(92)90341-X

Jemiolo, B., Xie, T. M., and Novotny, M. (1991). Socio-sexual olfactory preference in female mice: attractiveness of synthetic chemosignals. *Physiol. Behav.* 50, 1119–1122. doi: 10.1016/0031-9384(91)90570-E

Jerger, J., and Johnson, K. (1988). Interactions of age, gender, and sensorineural hearing loss on ABR latency. *Ear Hear.* 9, 168–176. doi: 10.1097/00003446-198808000-00002

Jouhaneau, J., and Bagady, A. (1984). Effect of early auditory stimulation on the choice of acoustical environment by adult Swiss albino mice (Mus musculus). *J. Comp. Psychol.* 98, 318–326. doi: 10.1037/0735-7036.98.3.318

Jouhanneau, M., Cornilleau, F., and Keller, M. (2014). Peripubertal exposure to male odors influences female puberty and adult expression of male-directed odor preference in mice. *Horm. Behav.* 65, 128–133. doi: 10.1016/j.yhbeh.2013.12.006

Kang, N., Baum, M. J., and Cherry, J. A. (2009). A direct main olfactory bulb projection to the 'vomeronasal' amygdala in female mice selectively responds to volatile pheromones from males. *Eur. J. Neurosci.* 29, 624–634. doi: 10.1111/j.1460-9568.2009.06638.x

Kavaliers, M., and Colwell, D. D. (1993). Aversive responses of female mice to the odors of parasitized males: neuromodulatory mechanisms and implications for mate choice. *Ethology* 95, 202–212. doi: 10.1111/j.1439-0310.1993.tb00471.x

Kavaliers, M., and Colwell, D. D. (1995a). Discrimination by female mice between the odours of parasitized and non-parasitized males. *Proc. Biol. Sci.* 261, 31–35.

Kavaliers, M., and Colwell, D. D. (1995b). Odours of parasitized males induce aversive responses in female mice. *Anim. Behav.* 50, 1161–1169.

Keller, M., Douhard, Q., Baum, M. J., and Bakker, J. (2006). Destruction of the main olfactory epithelium reduces female sexual behavior and olfactory investigation in female mice. *Chem. Senses* 31, 315–323. doi: 10.1093/chemse/bjj035

Kerbeshian, M. C., LePhuoc, H., and Bronson, F. H. (1994). The effects of running activity on the reproductive axes of rodents. *J. Comp. Physiol. A* 174, 741–746. doi: 10.1007/BF00192723

Kevetter, G. A., and Winans, S. S. (1981). Connections of the corticomedial amygdala in the golden hamster. II. Efferents of the "olfactory amygdala." *J. Comp. Neurol.* 197, 99–111. doi: 10.1002/cne.901970108

Kikusui, T., Nakanishi, K., Nakagawa, R., Nagasawa, M., Mogi, K., and Okanoya, K. (2011). Cross fostering experiments suggest that mice songs are innate. *PLoS ONE* 6:e17721. doi: 10.1371/journal.pone.0017721

Kimoto, H., Haga, S., Sato, K., and Touhara, K. (2005). Sex-specific peptides from exocrine glands stimulate mouse vomeronasal sensory neurons. *Nature* 437, 898–901. doi: 10.1038/nature04033

Kokko, H., Brooks, R., Jennions, M. D., and Morley, J. (2003). The evolution of mate choice and mating biases. *Proc. R. Soc. B Biol. Sci.* 270, 653. doi: 10.1098/rspb.2002.2235

Krienen, F. M., Tu, P. C., and Buckner, R. L. (2010). Clan mentality: evidence that the medial prefrontal cortex responds to close others. *J. Neurosci.* 30, 13906–13915. doi: 10.1523/JNEUROSCI.2180-10.2010

Kroodsma, D. E. (1976). Reproductive development in a female songbird: differential stimulation by quality of male song. *Science* 192, 574–575. doi: 10.1126/science.192.4239.574

Kvitsiani, D., Ranade, S., Hangya, B., Taniguchi, H., Huang, J. Z., and Kepecs, A. (2013). Distinct behavioural and network correlates of two interneuron types in prefrontal cortex. *Nature* 498, 363–366. doi: 10.1038/nature12176

Leboucher, G., Depraz, V., Kreutzer, M., and Nagle, L. (1998). Male song stimulation of female reproduction in canaries: features relevant to sexual displays are not relevant to nest-building or egg-laying. *Ethology* 104, 613–624. doi: 10.1111/j.1439-0310.1998.tb00096.x

Leinders-Zufall, T., Brennan, P., Widmayer, P., S, P. C., Maul-Pavicic, A., Jager, M., et al. (2004). MHC class I peptides as chemosensory signals in the vomeronasal organ. *Science* 306, 1033–1037. doi: 10.1126/science.1102818

Levitin, D. J., and Tirovolas, A. K. (2009). Current advances in the cognitive neuroscience of music. *Ann. N.Y. Acad. Sci.* 1156, 211–231. doi: 10.1111/j.1749-6632.2009.04417.x

Levy, F., and Keller, M. (2009). Olfactory mediation of maternal behavior in selected mammalian species. *Behav. Brain Res.* 200, 336–345. doi: 10.1016/j.bbr.2008.12.017

Lin, D. Y., Zhang, S. Z., Block, E., and Katz, L. C. (2005). Encoding social signals in the mouse main olfactory bulb. *Nature* 434, 470–477. doi: 10.1038/nature03414

Lombardi, J. R., and Vandenbergh, J. G. (1977). Pheromonally induced sexual maturation in females: regulation by the social environment of the male. *Science* 196, 545–546. doi: 10.1126/science.557838

Lombardi, J. R., Vandenbergh, J. G., and Whitsett, J. M. (1976). Androgen control of the sexual maturation pheromone in house mouse urine. *Biol. Reprod.* 15, 179–186. doi: 10.1095/biolreprod15.2.179

Lydon, J. P., DeMayo, F. J., Funk, C. R., Mani, S. K., Hughes, A. R., Montgomery, C. A., et al. (1995). Mice lacking progesterone receptor exhibit pleiotropic reproductive abnormalities. *Genes Dev.* 9, 2266–2278. doi: 10.1101/gad.9.18.2266

Mackay-Sim, A., and Rose, J. D. (1986). Removal of the vomeronasal organ impairs lordosis in female hamsters: effect is reversed by luteinising hormone-releasing hormone. *Neuroendocrinology* 42, 489–493. doi: 10.1159/000124492

Mahrt, E. J., Perkel, D. J., Tong, L., Rubel, E. W., and Portfors, C. V. (2013). Engineered deafness reveals that mouse courtship vocalizations do not require auditory experience. *J. Neurosci.* 33, 5573–5583. doi: 10.1523/JNEUROSCI.5054-12.2013

Mair, R. G., Bouffard, J. A., Engen, T., and Morton, T. H. (1978). Olfactory sensitivity during the menstrual cycle. *Sens. Processes* 2, 90–98.

Mak, G. K., Enwere, E. K., Gregg, C., Pakarainen, T., Poutanen, M., Huhtaniemi, I., et al. (2007). Male pheromone-stimulated neurogenesis in the adult female brain: possible role in mating behavior. *Nat. Neurosci.* 10, 1003–1011. doi: 10.1038/nn1928

Maney, D. L., and Pinaud, R. (2011). Estradiol-dependent modulation of auditory processing and selectivity in songbirds. *Front. Neuroendocrinol.* 32, 287–302. doi: 10.1016/j.yfrne.2010.12.002

Marek, R., Strobel, C., Bredy, T. W., and Sah, P. (2013). The amygdala and medial prefrontal cortex: partners in the fear circuit. *J. Physiol.* 591, 2381–2391. doi: 10.1113/jphysiol.2012.248575

McComb, K. (1987). Roaring by red deer stags advances the date of oestrus in hinds. *Nature* 330, 648–649. doi: 10.1038/330648a0

McComb, K. E. (1991). Female choice for high roaring rates in red deer, Cervus elaphus. *Anim. Behav.* 41, 79–88. doi: 10.1016/S0003-3472(05)80504-4

McDonald, A. J., Mascagni, F., and Guo, L. (1996). Projections of the medial and lateral prefrontal cortices to the amygdala: a Phaseolus vulgaris leucoagglutinin study in the rat. *Neuroscience* 71, 55–75. doi: 10.1016/0306-4522(95)00417-3

McElligott, A. G., O'Neill, K. P., and Hayden, T. J. (1999). Cumulative long-term investment in vocalization and mating success of fallow bucks, Dama dama. *Anim. Behav.* 57, 1159–1167. doi: 10.1006/anbe.1999.1076

Mead, L. S., and Arnold, S. J. (2004). Quantitative genetic models of sexual selection. *Trends Ecol. Evol.* 19, 264–271. doi: 10.1016/j.tree.2004.03.003

Merchenthaler, I., Lane, M. V., Numan, S., and Dellovade, T. L. (2004). Distribution of estrogen receptor alpha and beta in the mouse central nervous system: *in vivo* autoradiographic and immunocytochemical analyses. *J. Comp. Neurol.* 473, 270–291. doi: 10.1002/cne.20128

Miranda, J. A., and Liu, R. C. (2009). Dissecting natural sensory plasticity: hormones and experience in a maternal context. *Hear. Res.* 252, 21–28. doi: 10.1016/j.heares.2009.04.014

Mitra, S. W., Hoskin, E., Yudkovitz, J., Pear, L., Wilkinson, H. A., Hayashi, S., et al. (2003). Immunolocalization of estrogen receptor beta in the mouse brain: comparison with estrogen receptor alpha. *Endocrinology* 144, 2055–2067. doi: 10.1210/en.2002-221069

Moffatt, C. A. (2003). Steroid hormone modulation of olfactory processing in the context of socio-sexual behaviors in rodents and humans. *Brain Res. Brain Res. Rev.* 43, 192–206. doi: 10.1016/S0165-0173(03)00208-X

Moffatt, C. A., Rissman, E. F., Shupnik, M. A., and Blaustein, J. D. (1998). Induction of progestin receptors by estradiol in the forebrain of estrogen receptor-alpha gene-disrupted mice. *J. Neurosci.* 18, 9556–9563.

Moncho-Bogani, J., Martinez-Garcia, F., Novejarque, A., and Lanuza, E. (2005). Attraction to sexual pheromones and associated odorants in female mice involves activation of the reward system and basolateral amygdala. *Eur. J. Neurosci.* 21, 2186–2198. doi: 10.1111/j.1460-9568.2005.04036.x

Moore, F. L., Boyd, S. K., and Kelley, D. B. (2005). Historical perspective: hormonal regulation of behaviors in amphibians. *Horm. Behav.* 48, 373–383. doi: 10.1016/j.yhbeh.2005.05.011

Morton, M. L., Pereyra, M. E., and Baptista, L. F. (1985). Photoperiodically induced ovarian growth in the white-crowned sparrow *Zonotrichia leucophrys gambelii* and its augmentation by song. *Comp. Biochem. Physiol. A Physiol.* 80, 93–97. doi: 10.1016/0300-9629(85)90684-X

Mucignat-Caretta, C., Caretta, A., and Cavaggioni, A. (1995). Acceleration of puberty onset in female mice by male urinary proteins. *J. Physiol.* 486(pt 2), 517–522.

Musolf, K., Hoffmann, F., and Penn, D. J. (2010). Ultrasonic courtship vocalizations in wild house mice, Mus musculus musculus. *Anim. Behav.* 79, 757–764. doi: 10.1016/j.anbehav.2009.12.034

Neff, B. D., and Pitcher, T. E. (2005). Genetic quality and sexual selection: an integrated framework for good genes and compatible genes. *Mol. Ecol.* 14, 19–38. doi: 10.1111/j.1365-294X.2004.02395.x

Nelken, I. (2004). Processing of complex stimuli and natural scenes in the auditory cortex. *Curr. Opin. Neurobiol.* 14, 474–480. doi: 10.1016/j.conb.2004.06.005

Nelken, I., and Bar-Yosef, O. (2008). Neurons and objects: the case of auditory cortex. *Front. Neurosci.* 2, 107–113. doi: 10.3389/neuro.01.009.2008

Nodari, F., Hsu, F. F., Fu, X., Holekamp, T. F., Kao, L. F., Turk, J., et al. (2008). Sulfated steroids as natural ligands of mouse pheromone-sensing neurons. *J. Neurosci.* 28, 6407–6418. doi: 10.1523/JNEUROSCI.1425-08.2008

Novotny, M., Harvey, S., and Jemiolo, B. (1990). Chemistry of male dominance in the house mouse, Mus domesticus. *Experientia* 46, 109–113. doi: 10.1007/BF01955433

Novotny, M., Harvey, S., Jemiolo, B., and Alberts, J. (1985). Synthetic pheromones that promote inter-male aggression in mice. *Proc. Natl. Acad. Sci. U.S.A.* 82:2059. doi: 10.1073/pnas.82.7.2059

Novotny, M. V. (2003). Pheromones, binding proteins and receptor responses in rodents. *Biochem. Soc. Trans.* 31, 117–122. doi: 10.1042/BST0310117

Novotny, M. V., Jemiolo, B., Wiesler, D., Ma, W., Harvey, S., Xu, F., et al. (1999a). A unique urinary constituent, 6-hydroxy-6-methyl-3-heptanone, is a pheromone that accelerates puberty in female mice. *Chem. Biol.* 6, 377–383.

Novotny, M. V., Ma, W., Wiesler, D., and Zidek, L. (1999b). Positive identification of the puberty-accelerating pheromone of the house mouse: the volatile ligands associating with the major urinary protein. *Proc. Biol. Sci.* 266, 2017–2022.

Nunez, A. A., Nyby, J., and Whitney, G. (1978). The effects of testosterone, estradiol, and dihydrotestosterone on male mouse (Mus musculus) ultrasonic vocalizations. *Horm. Behav.* 11, 264–272. doi: 10.1016/0018-506X(78)90030-2

Nyby, J., Wysocki, C. J., Whitney, G., and Dizinno, G. (1977). Pheromonal regulation of male mouse ultrasonic courtship (Mus musculus). *Anim. Behav.* 25, 333–341. doi: 10.1016/0003-3472(77)90009-4

Oakeshott, J. (1974). Social dominance, aggressiveness and mating success among male house mice (Mus musculus). *Oecologia* 15, 143–158. doi: 10.1007/BF00345742

Oboti, L., Pérez-Gómez, A., Keller, M., Jacobi, E., Birnbaumer, L., Leinders-Zufall, T., et al. (2014). A wide range of pheromone-stimulated sexual and reproductive behaviors in female mice depend on G protein G (alpha) o. *BMC Biol.* 12:31. doi: 10.1186/1741-7007-12-31

Okabe, S., Nagasawa, M., Kihara, T., Kato, M., Harada, T., Koshida, N., et al. (2013). Pup odor and ultrasonic vocalizations synergistically stimulate maternal attention in mice. *Behav. Neurosci.* 127, 432. doi: 10.1037/a0032395

Overath, P., Sturm, T., and Rammensee, H. (2014). Of volatiles and peptides: in search for MHC-dependent olfactory signals in social communication. *Cell. Mol. Life Sci.* 71, 2429–2442. doi: 10.1007/s00018-014-1559-6

Panksepp, J. B., Jochman, K. A., Kim, J. U., Koy, J. J., Wilson, E. D., Chen, Q., et al. (2007). Affiliative behavior, ultrasonic communication and social reward are influenced by genetic variation in adolescent mice. *PLoS ONE* 2:e351. doi: 10.1371/journal.pone.0000351

Parker, G. A. (1974). Assessment strategy and the evolution of fighting behaviour. *J. Theor. Biol.* 47, 223–243. doi: 10.1016/0022-5193(74)90111-8

Pasch, B., George, A. S., Campbell, P., and Phelps, S. M. (2011). Androgen-dependent male vocal performance influences female preference in Neotropical singing mice. *Anim. Behav.* 82, 177–183. doi: 10.1016/j.anbehav.2011.04.018

Penn, D., and Potts, W. (1998a). MHC–disassortative mating preferences reversed by cross–fostering. *Proc. Biol. Sci.* 265, 1299.

Penn, D., and Potts, W. (1998b). How do major histocompatibility complex genes influence odor and mating preferences? *Adv. Immunol.* 69, 411–436.

Pfaff, D. (1994). Cellular and molecular mechanisms of female reproductive behaviors. *Physiol. Reprod.* 107–220.

Pietras, R. J., and Moulton, D. G. (1974). Hormonal influences on odor detection in rats: changes associated with the estrous cycle, pseudopregnancy, ovariectomy, and administration of testosterone propionate. *Physiol. Behav.* 12, 475–491. doi: 10.1016/0031-9384(74)90125-5

Pomerantz, S. M., Nunez, A. A., and Bean, N. J. (1983). Female behavior is affected by male ultrasonic vocalizations in house mice. *Physiol. Behav.* 31, 91–96. doi: 10.1016/0031-9384(83)90101-4

Potts, W. K., Manning, C. J., and Wakeland, E. K. (1991). Mating patterns in seminatural populations of mice influenced by MHC genotype. *Nature* 352, 619–621. doi: 10.1038/352619a0

Potts, W. K., and Wakeland, E. K. (1993). Evolution of MHC genetic diversity: a tale of incest, pestilence and sexual preference. *Trends Genet.* 9, 408–412. doi: 10.1016/0168-9525(93)90103-O

Pro-Sistiaga, P., Mohedano-Moriano, A., Ubeda-Banon, I., Del Mar Arroyo-Jimenez, M., Marcos, P., Artacho-Perula, E., et al. (2007). Convergence of olfactory and vomeronasal projections in the rat basal telencephalon. *J. Comp. Neurol.* 504, 346–362. doi: 10.1002/cne.21455

Rehsteiner, U., Geisser, H., and Reyer, H. (1998). Singing and mating success in water pipits: one specific song element makes all the difference. *Anim. Behav.* 55, 1471–1481. doi: 10.1006/anbe.1998.0733

Remage-Healey, L., Dong, S. M., Chao, A., and Schlinger, B. A. (2012). Sex-specific, rapid neuroestrogen fluctuations and neurophysiological actions in the songbird auditory forebrain. *J. Neurophysiol.* 107, 1621–1631. doi: 10.1152/jn.00749.2011

Remage-Healey, L., Maidment, N. T., and Schlinger, B. A. (2008). Forebrain steroid levels fluctuate rapidly during social interactions. *Nat. Neurosci.* 11, 1327–1334. doi: 10.1038/nn.2200

Roberts, S. A., Davidson, A. J., McLean, L., Beynon, R. J., and Hurst, J. L. (2012). Pheromonal induction of spatial learning in mice. *Science* 338, 1462–1465. doi: 10.1126/science.1225638

Roberts, S. A., Simpson, D. M., Armstrong, S. D., Davidson, A. J., Robertson, D. H., McLean, L., et al. (2010). Darcin: a male pheromone that stimulates female memory and sexual attraction to an individual male's odour. *BMC Biol.* 8:75. doi: 10.1186/1741-7007-8-75

Romanski, L. M., and Averbeck, B. B. (2009). The primate cortical auditory system and neural representation of conspecific vocalizations. *Annu. Rev. Neurosci.* 32, 315–346. doi: 10.1146/annurev.neuro.051508.135431

Roney, J. R., and Simmons, Z. L. (2008). Women's estradiol predicts preference for facial cues of men's testosterone. *Horm. Behav.* 53, 14–19. doi: 10.1016/j.yhbeh.2007.09.008

Roy, S., Watkins, N., and Heck, D. (2012). Comprehensive analysis of ultrasonic vocalizations in a mouse model of fragile X syndrome reveals limited, call type specific deficits. *PLoS ONE* 7:e44816. doi: 10.1371/journal.pone.0044816

Schwende, F., Wiesler, D., Jorgenson, J., Carmack, M., and Novotny, M. (1986). Urinary volatile constituents of the house mouse, Mus musculus, and their endocrine dependency. *J. Chem. Ecol.* 12, 277–296. doi: 10.1007/BF01045611

Shelton, M. (1980). Goats: influence of various exteroreceptive factors on initiation of estrus and ovulation. *Int. Goat Sheep Res.* 1, 156–162.

Shepard, K. N., and Liu, R. C. (2011). Experience restores innate female preference for male ultrasonic vocalizations. *Genes Brain Behav.* 10, 28–34. doi: 10.1111/j.1601-183X.2010.00580.x

Sherborne, A. L., Thom, M. D., Paterson, S., Jury, F., Ollier, W. E. R., Stockley, P., et al. (2007). The Genetic Basis of Inbreeding Avoidance in House Mice. *Curr. Biol.* 17, 2061–2066. doi: 10.1016/j.cub.2007.10.041

Sisneros, J. A., Forlano, P. M., Deitcher, D. L., and Bass, A. H. (2004). Steroid-dependent auditory plasticity leads to adaptive coupling of sender and receiver. *Science* 305, 404–407. doi: 10.1126/science.1097218

Spehr, M., Kelliher, K. R., Li, X. H., Boehm, T., Leinders-Zufall, T., and Zufall, F. (2006). Essential role of the main olfactory system in social recognition of major histocompatibility complex peptide ligands. *J. Neurosci.* 26, 1961–1970. doi: 10.1523/JNEUROSCI.4939-05.2006

Spironello Vella, E., and deCatanzaro, D. (2001). Novel male mice show gradual decline in the capacity to disrupt early pregnancy and in urinary excretion of testosterone and 17 beta-estradiol during the weeks immediately following castration. *Horm. Metab. Res.* 33, 681–686. doi: 10.1055/s-2001-18690

Stenberg, A. E., Wang, H., Sahlin, L., and Hultcrantz, M. (1999). Mapping of estrogen receptors alpha and beta in the inner ear of mouse and rat. *Hear. Res.* 136, 29–34. doi: 10.1016/S0378-5955(99)00098-2

Stowers, L., Holy, T. E., Meister, M., Dulac, C., and Koentges, G. (2002). Loss of sex discrimination and male-male aggression in mice deficient for TRP2. *Science* 295, 1493–1500. doi: 10.1126/science.1069259

Stuss, D. T., Alexander, M. P., Floden, D., Binns, M. A., Levine, B., McIntosh, A. R., et al. (2002). "Fractionation and localization of distinct frontal lobe processes: evidence from focal lesions in humans," in *Principles of Frontal Lobe Function*, eds D. T. Stuss and R. T. Knight (New York, NY: Oxford University Press), 392–407.

Sugimoto, H., Okabe, S., Kato, M., Koshida, N., Shiroishi, T., Mogi, K., et al. (2011). A role for strain differences in waveforms of ultrasonic vocalizations during male–female interaction. *PLoS ONE* 6:e22093. doi: 10.1371/journal.pone.0022093

Thompson, J. A., Salcedo, E., Restrepo, D., and Finger, T. E. (2012). Second-order input to the medial amygdala from olfactory sensory neurons expressing the transduction channel TRPM5. *J. Comp. Neurol.* 520, 1819–1830. doi: 10.1002/cne.23015

Thompson, S. K., Zhu, X., and Frisina, R. D. (2006). Estrogen blockade reduces auditory feedback in CBA mice. *Otolaryngol. Head. Neck. Surg.* 135, 100–105. doi: 10.1016/j.otohns.2006.02.004

Thorpe, J. B., and deCatanzaro, D. (2012). Oestradiol treatment restores the capacity of castrated males to induce both the Vandenbergh and the Bruce effects in mice (Mus musculus). *Reproduction* 143, 123–132. doi: 10.1530/REP-11-0251

Tirindelli, R., Dibattista, M., Pifferi, S., and Menini, A. (2009). From pheromones to behavior. *Physiol. Rev.* 89, 921–956. doi: 10.1152/physrev.00037.2008

Tremere, L. A., Jeong, J. K., and Pinaud, R. (2009). Estradiol shapes auditory processing in the adult brain by regulating inhibitory transmission and plasticity-associated gene expression. *J. Neurosci.* 29, 5949–5963. doi: 10.1523/JNEUROSCI.0774-09.2009

Trivers, R.L. (1972). "Parental investment and sexual selection," in *Sexual Selection and the Descent of Man*, ed B. Campbell (Chicago, IL: Aldine), 136–179.

Vandenbergh, J. G. (1969). Male odor accelerates female sexual maturation in mice. *Endocrinology* 84, 658–660. doi: 10.1210/endo-84-3-658

Vyas, A., Harding, C., Borg, L., and Bogdan, D. (2009). Acoustic characteristics, early experience, and endocrine status interact to modulate female zebra finches' behavioral responses to songs. *Horm. Behav.* 55, 50–59. doi: 10.1016/j.yhbeh.2008.08.005

Walpurger, V., Pietrowsky, R., Kirschbaum, C., and Wolf, O. T. (2004). Effects of the menstrual cycle on auditory event-related potentials. *Horm. Behav.* 46, 600–606. doi: 10.1016/j.yhbeh.2004.07.002

Wang, F., Zhu, J., Zhu, H., Zhang, Q., Lin, Z., and Hu, H. (2011). Bidirectional control of social hierarchy by synaptic efficacy in medial prefrontal cortex. *Science* 334, 693–697. doi: 10.1126/science.1209951

Wang, H., Liang, S., Burgdorf, J., Wess, J., and Yeomans, J. (2008). Ultrasonic vocalizations induced by sex and amphetamine in M2, M4, M5 muscarinic and D2 dopamine receptor knockout mice. *PLoS ONE* 3:e1893. doi: 10.1371/journal.pone.0001893

Weinberger, N. M. (2004). Specific long-term memory traces in primary auditory cortex. *Nat. Rev. Neurosci.* 5, 279–290. doi: 10.1038/nrn1366

Wesson, D. W., and Wilson, D. A. (2010). Smelling sounds: olfactory-auditory sensory convergence in the olfactory tubercle. *J. Neurosci.* 30, 3013–3021. doi: 10.1523/JNEUROSCI.6003-09.2010

West, P. M., and Packer, C. (2002). Sexual selection, temperature, and the lion's mane. *Science* 297, 1339–1343. doi: 10.1126/science.1073257

Wharton, J. A., and Church, G. T. (1990). Influence of menopause on the auditory brainstem response. *Audiology* 29, 196–201. doi: 10.3109/00206099009072850

White, T. D., Schmitz, B., and Narins, P. M. (1992). Directional dependence of auditory sensitivity and frequency selectivity in the leopard frog. *J. Acoust. Soc. Am.* 92, 1953–1961. doi: 10.1121/1.405243

Whitten, W. K. (1958). Modification of the oestrous cycle of the mouse by external stimuli associated with the male; changes in the oestrous cycle determined by vaginal smears. *J. Endocrinol.* 17, 307–313. doi: 10.1677/joe.0.0170307

Wray, S. (2010). From nose to brain: development of gonadotrophin-releasing hormone-1 neurones. *J. Neuroendocrinol.* 22, 743–753. doi: 10.1111/j.1365-2826.2010.02034.x

Xiao, K., Kondo, Y., and Sakuma, Y. (2004). Sex-specific effects of gonadal steroids on conspecific odor preference in the rat. *Horm. Behav.* 46, 356–361. doi: 10.1016/j.yhbeh.2004.05.008

Xu, F., Schaefer, M., Kida, I., Schafer, J., Liu, N., Rothman, D. L., et al. (2005). Simultaneous activation of mouse main and accessory olfactory bulbs by odors or pheromones. *J. Comp. Neurol.* 489, 491–500. doi: 10.1002/cne.20652

Yamazaki, K., Boyse, E., Mike, V., Thaler, H., Mathieson, B., Abbott, J., et al. (1976). Control of mating preferences in mice by genes in the major histocompatibility complex. *J. Exp. Med.* 144:1324. doi: 10.1084/jem.144.5.1324

Yang, E. J., Lin, E. W., and Hensch, T. K. (2012). Critical period for acoustic preference in mice. *Proc. Natl. Acad. Sci. U.S.A.* 109(Suppl. 2), 17213–17220. doi: 10.1073/pnas.1200705109

Yoon, H., Enquist, L. W., and Dulac, C. (2005). Olfactory inputs to hypothalamic neurons controlling reproduction and fertility. *Cell* 123, 669–682. doi: 10.1016/j.cell.2005.08.039

Yoshikawa, K., Nakagawa, H., Mori, N., Watanabe, H., and Touhara, K. (2013). An unsaturated aliphatic alcohol as a natural ligand for a mouse odorant receptor. *Nat. Chem. Biol.* 9, 160–162. doi: 10.1038/nchembio.1164

9

Sexually dimorphic nuclei in the spinal cord control male sexual functions

***Hirotaka Sakamoto* ***

Laboratory of Neuroendocrinology, Ushimado Marine Institute, Graduate School of Natural Science and Technology, Okayama University, Okayama, Japan

***Correspondence:**
Hirotaka Sakamoto, Laboratory of Neuroendocrinology, Ushimado Marine Institute, Graduate School of Natural Science and Technology, Okayama University, 130-17 Kashino, Ushimado, Setouchi, Okayama 701-4303, Japan
e-mail: hsakamo@okayama-u.ac.jp

Lower spinal cord injuries frequently cause sexual dysfunction in men, including erectile dysfunction and an ejaculation disorder. This indicates that the important neural centers for male sexual function are located within the lower spinal cord. It is interesting that the lumbar spinal segments contain several neural circuits, showing a clear sexually dimorphism that, in association with neural circuits of the thoracic and sacral spinal cord, are critical in expressing penile reflexes during sexual behavior. To date, many sex differences in the spinal cord have been discovered. Interestingly, most of these are male dominant. Substantial evidence of sexually dimorphic neural circuits in the spinal cord have been reported in many animal models, but major issues remain unknown. For example, it is not known how the different circuits cooperatively function during male sexual behavior. In this review, therefore, the anatomical and functional significance of the sexually dimorphic nuclei in the spinal cord corresponding to the expression of male sexual behavior is discussed.

Keywords: sexual dimorphism, spinal cord, male sexual function, steroid hormones, neuroanatomy

INTRODUCTION

Sexual function and behavior significantly differ in sexes in adulthood, suggesting that the neural circuits also differ between sexes. However, it is difficult to correlate evidence gene expression levels with results of behavioral modifications. It is possible that the sexual differences are affected by a variety of extrinsic and intrinsic factors (Kawata, 1995; Morris et al., 2004; Sakamoto, 2012). Masculine sexual behavior is complex and modulated by intrinsic as well as extrinsic factors, including sensory inputs, autonomic regulations and their circumstances (Rosen and Sachs, 2000; Coolen, 2005). Spinal cord injuries located at the lower levels frequently cause sexual dysfunction in men, including erectile dysfunction and an ejaculation disorder (Sipski, 1998; Brown et al., 2006). This indicates that the important neural centers for male sexual function are located within the lower spinal cord. It is likely that the lumbar spinal segments contain several neural circuits, showing a clear sexually dimorphism that, in association with neural circuits of the thoracic (sympathetic) and sacral (parasympathetic) spinal cord. They play an important role in eliciting penile responses (i.e., erection and ejaculation) (Breedlove and Arnold, 1983a,b; Breedlove, 1985; Morris et al., 2004; Matsuda et al., 2008; Sakamoto, 2012) (see **Figure 1**). Substantial evidence of sexually dimorphic neural circuits in the spinal cord have been reported in many animal models, but major issues remain unknown, such as how they cooperatively function during male sexual behavior. In this review, the anatomical and functional significance of the sexually dimorphic nuclei in the spinal cord corresponding to the expression of male sexual behavior is discussed.

LUMBAR SPINOTHALAMIC (LSt) NEURONS

Several studies have identified that a male-dominant sexual dimorphism in the lumbar spinal cord is observed in rats (**Figure 1**). These neurons are located within the third and fourth lumbar segments of the spinal cord dorsolateral to the central canal in lamina X and express galanin (Newton, 1992), cholecystokinin (Phan and Newton, 1999), and enkephalin (Nicholas et al., 1999), possibly projecting to medial portion of the parvocellular subparafascicular thalamic nucleus (mSPFp) (Ju et al., 1987; Truitt et al., 2003). Therefore, they are a male-dominant sexually dimorphic nucleus, and so-called lumbar spinothalamic (LSt) neurons (Ju et al., 1987; Truitt et al., 2003). In rats, the increased Fos expression can be considered as a marker for neural activation. The activation of these LSt neurons is triggered by stimuli associated with ejaculation specifically, but mounts or intromission did not trigger Fos expression in LSt neurons. It is suggested that a specific subpopulation of LSt neurons signals information associated with ejaculation in rats (Truitt et al., 2003). A specific population of LSt neurons in the lumbar segments (L3–L4 level) of the spinal cord acts as a "spinal ejaculation generator" because ablation of these neurons by the selective toxins resulted in a complete disruption of ejaculatory behavior in rats (Truitt and Coolen, 2002). In contrast, other components of male sexual behavior remain intact, suggesting that this population of LSt neurons plays an important role in generation of ejaculation and is part of a spinal ejaculation generator (Truitt and Coolen, 2002). Furthermore, these LSt neurons convey the sexual information to the thalamus (Ju et al., 1987; Truitt et al., 2003), and integrate the information within the neural connections between LSt and autonomic/somatic centers in the spinal cord (Xu et al.,

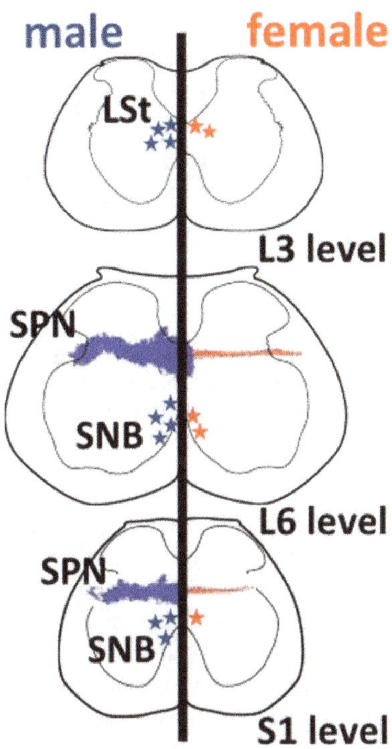

FIGURE 1 | Schematic drawings of neural sexual dimorphisms in the rodent lumbar spinal cord. The spinal levels are indicated on the lower right. Anatomical features in males and in females are shown on the left and right hemispheres, respectively. Sexually dimorphic cell numbers and axonal projections in the spinal cord are shown by stars and fine dots (males in blue; females in red), respectively. The density of the symbols is proportional to the relative density of the sexual dimorphisms in the spinal cord. L, lumbar; S, sacral; LSt, lumbar spinothalamic neurons; SNB, spinal nucleus of the bulbocavernosus; SPN, sacral parasympathetic nucleus.

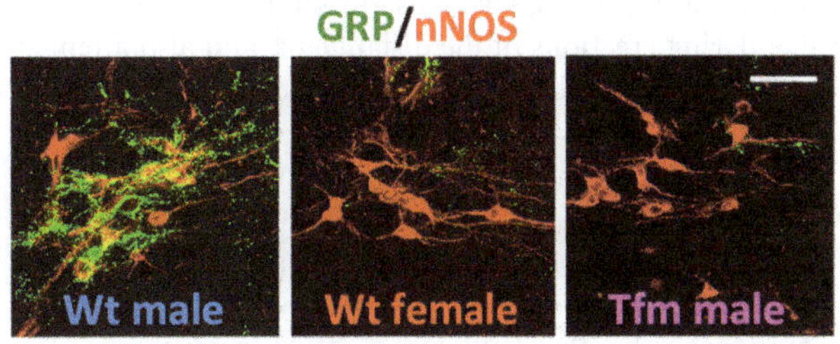

FIGURE 2 | A newly discovered sexual dimorphism in the lumbar spinal cord of rats that controls male sexual function. Co-immunofluorescence for gastrin-releasing peptide (GRP) (green) and neuronal nitric oxide synthase (nNOS) (red) confirmed that GRP-containing axons surrounding the autonomic sacral parasympathetic nucleus (SPN) neurons are significantly prominent in male rats, but vestigial or absent in females. In addition, testicular feminization mutation (Tfm) male rats display an entirely feminine pattern of GRP-containing fibers in the SPN autonomic nucleus. Wt, wild-type. Scale bar, 50 μm. The figure was reproduced from Sakamoto et al. (2008) with permission.

2005, 2006; Sun et al., 2009). However, the central and molecular mechanisms, including the neuropeptides involved, that directly regulate erection and ejaculation remain unclear.

THE GASTRIN-RELEASING PEPTIDE (GRP) SYSTEM IN THE LUMBAR SPINAL CORD

Using immunohistochemistry for gastrin-releasing peptide (GRP) in rats, we newly identified a collection of neurons containing GRP in the lumbar spinal region (L3–L4 level), showing a clear male-dominant sexual dimorphism (Sakamoto et al., 2008; Sakamoto, 2011) (**Figure 2**). These GRP-expressing neurons send axons onto the more caudal segments of the lumbosacral spinal cord (L5–L6 and S1 levels), including the autonomic sacral parasympathetic nucleus (SPN) as well as the somatic spinal nucleus of the bulbocavernosus (SNB) (Sakamoto et al., 2008). Double immunofluorescence of GRP and neuronal nitric oxide synthase (nNOS), a marker for autonomic preganglionic (SPN) neurons (Vizzard et al., 1995) clearly showed that GRP-expressing fibers densely projected into the SPN (Sakamoto et al., 2008). These GRP-expressing fibers surrounding cell bodies and dendrites of the SPN neurons were observed in only males but vestigial or absent in females (Sakamoto et al., 2008) (**Figure 2**).

It is reported that the autonomic SPN neurons play a pivotal role in controls of penile function and express high levels of nNOS (Studeny and Vizzard, 2005). In rats, these GRP neurons located in the lumbar spinal cord also express androgen receptor (AR) but do not express estrogen receptor alpha subtype (ERα) (Sakamoto et al., 2008; Sakamoto and Kawata, 2009). Using genetically male (XY) rats carrying the testicular feminization mutation (*Tfm*) of the *AR* gene, we examine whether androgens direct sexual differentiation of these GRP neurons. These mutant males develop testes embryologically and secrete testosterone prenatally. However, their AR protein is dysfunctional, they develop a complete feminine exterior phenotype, including a clitoris rather than a penis. We found that the spinal cord of genetic male rats, carrying the *Tfm* allele for *AR* hyperfeminine characteristics, have even fewer GRP-positive neurons in this region than do wild-type females (**Figure 2**). In this species, GRP-containing presynaptic boutons have also been shown by electron microscopic immunohistochemistry to innervate nNOS-positive dendrites in the autonomic SPN of the lower lumbar and upper sacral spinal cord (Sakamoto et al., 2008).

Substantial evidence indicated that the presence of a GRP receptor (GRPR) in the lumbar and sacral spinal cord of rats based on specific binding of GRP (Sakamoto et al., 2008). The higher expressions of GRPR at the mRNA and protein levels in SPN neurons were also obvious from the immunochemical and PCR analyses in rats (Sakamoto et al., 2008, 2009). Furthermore, the rat homolog of GRPR agonists ($rGRP_{20-29}$) (Ladenheim et al., 1996) is able to restore a lot of the spinal reflexes of the penis that are lost after orchiectomy (Sakamoto et al., 2008). The agonists were mostly effective in reinstating ejaculatory reflex *per se*, resulting in a greater frequency of ejaculation in treated castrates than in gonadally intact control males (Sakamoto et al., 2008). To probe whether GRPR activation of penile reflexes is mediated by the spinal cord, we also administered RC-3095, a specific GRPR antagonist (Pinski et al., 1992; Roesler et al., 2004), intrathecally to the lumbosacral spinal cord of gonadally intact males. The antagonistic treatment significantly inhibited penile reflexes, including simple erections, dorsal flips of the penis, and cup-like flaring erections of the distal glans, and also attenuated the spontaneous ejaculation rate (Sakamoto et al., 2008). These results indicate that the GRP/GRPR system controlling masculine reproductive function is within the lower spinal cord (Sakamoto et al., 2008).

The identification of this male-specific neural system using a specific neuropeptide, GRP, that controls sexual function offers new approaches for the development of pharmacological treatments to relief the male reproductive dysfunction (Sakamoto, 2011). In addition to the parasympathetic nucleus, LSt neurons in the spinal cord project to the sympathetic neurons of the intermediolateral column in the thoracic spinal cord, which is crucial for the emission phase of ejaculation (Coolen, 2005; Kozyrev et al., 2012). The local administration of the specific blocker for GRPR, RC-3095 significantly attenuated bursts in response to dorsal penile nerve stimuli of the bulbocavernosus muscles that are innervated by the SNB motoneurons during ejaculation (Kozyrev et al., 2012). This supports our hypothesis that GRP in the spinal cord plays a pivotal role in the regulation of penile reflexes during masculine copulatory behavior in rodents. Clinically, the next question is now: Does the spinal GRP system exist and function in the human spinal cord? Future attention should be focused on comparative studies for the spinal GRP system using other vertebrates, including humans and/or primates.

ONUF'S NUCLEUS (SNB)

Onufrowicz (1899) reported that a sexually dimorphic nucleus is located in the motor pools of the sacral spinal cord in most mammals, that innervates the penile functions involved in sexual behavior; so-called Onuf's nucleus. In humans, Onuf's nucleus are composed of a discrete group of motoneurons located in the ventral motor pool of the sacral spinal cord that play an important role in the micturition and defecatory as well as in rhythmic contractions of perineal muscles during orgasm (Onufrowicz, 1899). The number of motoneurons in Onuf's nucleus in humans is a sexually dimorphic: greater in men than that in women (Onufrowicz, 1899; Sato et al., 1978; Nakagawa, 1980; Forger and Breedlove, 1986). In rats, the SNB is located in the lumbosacral spinal cord; it is homologous to Onuf's nucleus in humans in that it innervates the striated perineal muscles attached to the base of the penis (Breedlove and Arnold, 1980; Forger and Breedlove, 1986; Sengelaub and Forger, 2008) (**Figures 1, 3**). Although the dorsolateral nucleus (DLN) innervating the ischiocavernosus and external urethral sphincter is also sexually dimorphic, the retrodorsolateral (RDLN) motoneurons that innervate foot muscles show no sexual difference and are relatively unresponsive to androgens (Jordan et al., 2002; Ottem et al., 2007) (**Figure 3**). Male rats have more and larger SNB as well as DLN motoneurons than females, a dimorphism that results from differences in perinatal androgen signaling through an AR-mediated mechanism (Breedlove and Arnold, 1980) (**Figure 3**). This male-dominant sex difference in SNB first found in rats has been extended to many mammalian species, including mice, cats, gerbils, dogs, hyenas, and monkeys (Ueyama et al., 1984, 1985; Forger and Breedlove, 1986; Wee et al., 1988; Ulibarri et al., 1995; Forger et al., 1996). The sex-related difference in the number of SNB motoneurons develops perinatally in rats. Prior to birth, the number of motoneurons in the SNB increases and reaches a maximum in both sexes; at this time, functional neuromuscular junctions have been established in the SNB system. However, in female rats, these components (both motoneurons and muscles) die near the time of birth unless the animals are exposed to testosterone during the critical period (androgen surge) (Nordeen et al., 1985). If an androgen surge occurs, it results in higher expression of AR in both the perineal muscles and spinal motoneurons. In male rats, testosterone primarily prevents the muscle from dying, which secondarily prevents the death of motoneurons in the spinal cord. Testosterone is thought to induce the muscle to produce a neurotrophic factor that protects the muscle, and the same factor or an additional factor then protects the motoneurons from developmental cell death. However, it is unclear which downstream genes first respond to testosterone. In the SNB system, testosterone may alter the expression of trophic factor genes to spare both the muscle and innervating motoneurons. Ciliary neurotrophic factor (CNTF) is a candidate trophic factor for the perineal neuromuscular junction because receptors for CNTF are expressed in the motoneurons and in their target muscles (Davis et al., 1991; Ip et al., 1993), and injection of CNTF into the perineum of newborn rats spares the SNB system in normal females (Forger et al., 1993).

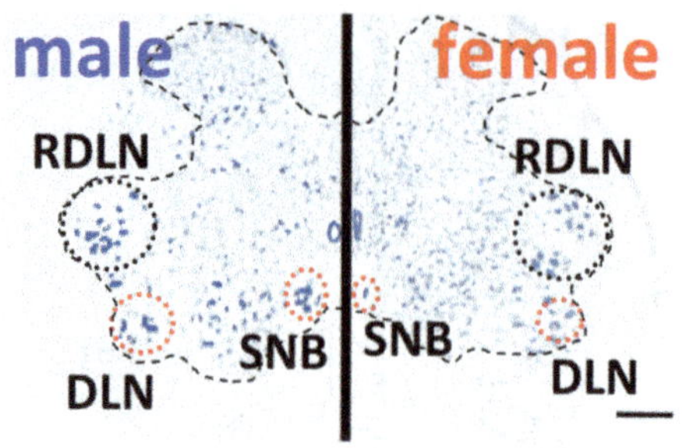

FIGURE 3 | Spinal nucleus of the bulbocavernosus (SNB) motoneurons are more numerous in male than in female rats. The dorsolateral nucleus (DNL) is also male-dominant sexually dimorphic, but the retrodorsolateral (RDLN) nucleus is similar in both male and females. Scale bar, 200 μm.

INTERACTION OF THE GRP SYSTEM WITH BOTH THE AUTONOMIC AND SOMATIC NUCLEI IN THE SPINAL CORD

Orchiectomy of adult male rats results in the shrinkage of soma size and dendritic arborization of SNB motoneurons as well as in a reduction in the number of synaptic inputs, all of which can be prevented by testosterone replacement for castrates (Breedlove and Arnold, 1981; Kurz et al., 1986; Matsumoto et al., 1988; Goldstein et al., 1990; Yang et al., 2004). In female rats, a long-term testosterone treatment to castrates also increase the SNB motoneuronal cell size, however, the increase did not reach to the level observed in males (Breedlove and Arnold, 1981; Sengelaub and Forger, 2008). The GRP system in the lumbosacral spinal cord also showed similar results; regarding the lower sensitivity to androgens in adult females (Sakamoto et al., 2008, 2009) and the AR signaling cascades that are necessary to maintain the GRP and SNB systems in the lumbosacral spinal cord in adult males (Sengelaub and Forger, 2008; Forger, 2009; Sakamoto and Kawata, 2009). It is interesting that the GRP and SNB systems, which are localized at the same lower spinal cord, might interact directly or indirectly to modulate the male sexual function. Furthermore, the sexually dimorphic distribution of GRP-containing fibers in the lumbosacral spinal cord (L5–L6 and S1) is controlled by circulating testosterone levels (Sakamoto et al., 2009) and mirroring changes in SNB motoneurons in male rats (Kurz et al., 1986; Matsumoto et al., 1988; Matsumoto, 2001). Recently, it has been reported using a mouse line specifically lacking *AR* in the nervous system (AR^{NesCre}) that the number of SNB motoneurons is unrelated to both AR^{NesCre} mutation status (Raskin et al., 2012), although adult AR^{NesCre} males exhibit higher levels of circulating testosterone than controls (Raskin et al., 2009). In the SNB, the central AR participates in the developmental regulation of both soma size and dendritic length but not in the survival of SNB motoneurons (Raskin et al., 2012). Immunohistochemical studies in the lumbosacral spinal cord also demonstrated the expression of AR in the cellular nuclei of SNB motoneurons in controls but not in AR^{NesCre} males (Raskin et al., 2012). However, loss of *AR* expression in the nervous system caused a significant decrease in the number of GRP-immunoreactive neurons compared with that in control littermates (Sakamoto et al., 2014). Consequently, the intensity of GRP axonal projections to the lower spinal cord (L5–L6 and S1 level) was greater in control males than that in AR^{NesCre} males (Sakamoto et al., 2014). Taken together, these results suggested that nervous system AR participates in both morphological differentiation and adult activation of SNB motoneurons, but not directly in the survival of SNB motoneurons during neonatal development (Raskin et al., 2012). In contrast, ARs expressed in the nervous system play critical roles in the development as well as in the maintenance of GRP neurons in the lumbosacral spinal cord in males. The *AR*-deletion mutation may attenuate sexual behavior and activity of mutant males *via* spinal GRP system-mediated neural mechanisms (Raskin et al., 2009; Sakamoto et al., 2014).

High-voltage electron microscopy (HVEM) is a powerful methodology for studying chemical neuroanatomy at the ultrastructural level, and the results with this method can be easily linked to the conventional light and electron microscopies (Sakamoto and Kawata, 2012). We combined an immunohistochemistry with a retrograde labeling technique utilizing a cholera toxin beta subunit-horseradish peroxidase conjugate under the HVEM. Three-dimensional (3-D) analysis by HVEM provided clear solid visualization of synaptic contacts from the spinal GRP system to the SNB motoneurons in male rats (Sakamoto et al., 2010; Sakamoto and Kawata, 2012). By means of a double labeling with immunohistochemistry and retrograde tracing, we observed that the many GRP-immunoreactive axons directly contact dendrites of the SNB motoneurons on a single section (Sakamoto et al., 2010; Sakamoto and Kawata, 2012). The molecular and neural regulations of male sexual behavior by the GRP system at the spinal cord level are revealed by HVEM at the 3-D ultrastructural level (Sakamoto et al., 2010; Sakamoto and Kawata, 2012). Because the bulbocavernosus muscles are considered to be a homologous to Onuf's nucleus in humans, they play an important role in the rhythmic contractions of perineal muscles during ejaculation also in rats (Sachs, 1982). Therefore, these 3-D results taken together suggested that GRP-containing afferents to SNB motoneurons may control penile reflexes during sexual behavior through the identified GRP-SNB synapses (Sakamoto et al., 2010). Nevertheless, the functional synchronization of these two neural systems in the lower spinal cord is required for normal penile reflexes (Sakamoto, 2011). Using HVEM, we further demonstrated that the terminals of GRP neurons may form 3-D multiple synapses with the dendrites of SPN neurons revealed by a double immunohistochemical study (Oti et al., 2012). Using a viral trans-synaptic retrograde tracing technique, Dobberfuhl et al. (2014) recently reported that after the pseudorabies virus (PRV) injection into the levator ani muscle, about a half of PRV-positive neurons in the medial gray at the upper lumbar spinal cord level expressed GRP. Interestingly, very few PRV-labeled spinal interneurons were found in the medial region of the upper lumbar spinal cord in preadolescent pups. These results indicate the presence of either direct or indirect synaptic contacts from GRP-containing neurons to SPN (autonomic) neurons and/or to SNB (somatic) motoneurons, and these neural circuits might develop during puberty. It has also been reported that GRPRs are expressed in both the SPN and SNB (Sakamoto et al., 2008). Thus, a spinal GRP/GRPR system could generate an ejaculatory behavior by synchronizing autonomic and somatic centers; e.g., the SPN and SNB in the lumbosacral spinal cord. A set of these findings supports the hypothesis that the GRP/GRPR system may regulate male sexual behavior *via* afferents to both SPN and SNB neurons, and coordinate autonomic and somatic functions in response to penile reflexes during male copulatory behavior.

AFFERENTS FROM THE SPINAL GRP SYSTEM TO THE BRAIN

Truitt and Coolen (2002) reported a potential ejaculation generator in the spinal cord in rats. Because LSt neurons project to the brain thalamus and are involved in the relay of ejaculation-related sensory information and/or sexual arousal to evoke ejaculation, the discovery of the "spinal ejaculation generator" provides an excellent target for further understanding of the neural processes controlling ejaculatory behavior. Namely, the characterization of hormonal dynamics involved in the modulation of either LSt neuronal function or the activation of LSt neuronal target cites is required for a better understanding of the molecular mechanisms underlying the expression of male sexual behavior. GRP and galanin might be possible candidates for neuromodulator(s) regulating LSt neuronal activity (Truitt et al., 2003; Sakamoto et al., 2008). In fact, local injection of galanin into the mSPFp significantly attenuated male copulatory behavior in rats (Coolen, 2005), suggesting that LSt signaling might play an important role in the refractory period after ejaculation. On the other hand, similar microinjection of galanin into neighboring thalamic areas did not affect any components of male sexual behavior (Coolen, 2005). Since the detailed molecular mechanisms of ejaculatory behavior in the central nervous system remains unknown, further investigation of the LSt-mSPFp interaction is required to draw a firm conclusion.

CONCLUSIONS

Further understanding of the neural and molecular basis of the sexual dimorphism in the central nervous system will progress our understanding of the expression of the sexually different behavior. The expression of sexual behavior in vertebrates is properly affected by the interactions between endocrine and psychological factors. During the ontogeny, therefore, it is important to know how, when, and where sex steroid hormones (estrogens and/or androgens) behave in the sexual differentiation of the brain and spinal cord *via* the genomic and/or non-genomic actions. The sexually differentiated nervous system is influenced by the region- and temporal-specific sex steroid milieu, suggesting a significance of sex differences observed in many neurobiological dysfunctions. Although this agenda is especially difficult and controversial when applied to humans because of the highly social species, interdisciplinary studies at the molecular, behavioral, and social levels might be able to make demonstration of the hormonally orchestrated sexual dimorphism in the nervous system and related clinical disorders in humans.

ACKNOWLEDGMENTS

This work was supported in part by Grants-in-Aid for Scientific Research (KAKENHI) [Grant-in-Aid for Young Scientists (A): no. 24680039, no. 21680031, and Grant-in-Aid for Challenging Exploratory Research: no. 23659758] from the Ministry of Education, Science, Sports, Culture and Technology, Japan, by the Research Grant from the Senri Life Science Foundation, Japan, and by the Naito Memorial Grant for Natural Science Researches, Japan.

REFERENCES

Breedlove, S. M. (1985). Hormonal control of the anatomical specificity of motoneuron-to-muscle innervation in rats. *Science* 227, 1357–1359. doi: 10.1126/science.3975621

Breedlove, S. M., and Arnold, A. P. (1980). Hormone accumulation in a sexually dimorphic motor nucleus of the rat spinal cord. *Science* 210, 564–566. doi: 10.1126/science.7423210

Breedlove, S. M., and Arnold, A. P. (1981). Sexually dimorphic motor nucleus in the rat lumbar spinal cord: response to adult hormone manipulation, absence in androgen-insensitive rats. *Brain Res.* 225, 297–307. doi: 10.1016/0006-8993(81)90837-4

Breedlove, S. M., and Arnold, A. P. (1983a). Hormonal control of a developing neuromuscular system. I. Complete demasculinization of the male rat spinal nucleus of the bulbocavernosus using the anti-androgen flutamide. *J. Neurosci.* 3, 417–423.

Breedlove, S. M., and Arnold, A. P. (1983b). Hormonal control of a developing neuromuscular system. II. Sensitive periods for the androgen-induced masculinization of the rat spinal nucleus of the bulbocavernosus. *J. Neurosci.* 3, 424–432.

Brown, D. J., Hill, S. T., and Baker, H. W. (2006). Male fertility and sexual function after spinal cord injury. *Prog. Brain Res.* 152, 427–439. doi: 10.1016/S0079-6123(05)52029-6

Coolen, L. M. (2005). Neural control of ejaculation. *J. Comp. Neurol.* 493, 39–45. doi: 10.1002/cne.20784

Davis, S., Aldrich, T. H., Valenzuela, D. M., Wong, V. V., Furth, M. E., Squinto, S. P., et al. (1991). The receptor for ciliary neurotrophic factor. *Science* 253, 59–63. doi: 10.1126/science.1648265

Dobberfuhl, A. D., Oti, T., Sakamoto, H., and Marson, L. (2014). Identification of CNS neurons innervating the levator ani and ventral bulbospongiosus muscles in male rats. *J. Sex. Med.* 11, 664–677. doi: 10.1111/jsm.12418

Forger, N. G. (2009). The organizational hypothesis and final common pathways: sexual differentiation of the spinal cord and peripheral nervous system. *Horm. Behav.* 55, 605–610. doi: 10.1016/j.yhbeh.2009.03.008

Forger, N. G., and Breedlove, S. M. (1986). Sexual dimorphism in human and canine spinal cord: role of early androgen. *Proc. Natl. Acad. Sci. U.S.A.* 83, 7527–7531. doi: 10.1073/pnas.83.19.7527

Forger, N. G., Frank, L. G., Breedlove, S. M., and Glickman, S. E. (1996). Sexual dimorphism of perineal muscles and motoneurons in spotted hyenas. *J. Comp. Neurol.* 375, 333–343. doi: 10.1002/(SICI)1096-9861(19961111)375:2%3C333::AID-CNE11%3E3.0.CO;2-W

Forger, N. G., Roberts, S. L., Wong, V., and Breedlove, S. M. (1993). Ciliary neurotrophic factor maintains motoneurons and their target muscles in developing rats. *J. Neurosci.* 13, 4720–4726.

Goldstein, L. A., Kurz, E. M., and Sengelaub, D. R. (1990). Androgen regulation of dendritic growth and retraction in the development of a sexually dimorphic spinal nucleus. *J. Neurosci.* 10, 935–946.

Ip, N. Y., McClain, J., Barrezueta, N. X., Aldrich, T. H., Pan, L., Li, Y., et al. (1993). The alpha component of the CNTF receptor is required for signaling and defines potential CNTF targets in the adult and during development. *Neuron* 10, 89–102. doi: 10.1016/0896-6273(93)90245-M

Jordan, C. L., Christensen, S. E., Handa, R. J., Anderson, J. L., Pouliot, W. A., and Breedlove, S. M. (2002). Evidence that androgen acts through NMDA receptors to affect motoneurons in the rat spinal nucleus of the bulbocavernosus. *J. Neurosci.* 22, 9567–9572.

Ju, G., Melander, T., Ceccatelli, S., Hokfelt, T., and Frey, P. (1987). Immunohistochemical evidence for a spinothalamic pathway co-containing cholecystokinin- and galanin-like immunoreactivities in the rat. *Neuroscience* 20, 439–456. doi: 10.1016/0306-4522(87)90103-5

Kawata, M. (1995). Roles of steroid hormones and their receptors in structural organization in the nervous system. *Neurosci. Res.* 24, 1–46. doi: 10.1016/0168-0102(96)81278-8

Kozyrev, N., Lehman, M. N., and Coolen, L. M. (2012). Activation of gastrin-releasing peptide receptors in the lumbosacral spinal cord is required for ejaculation in male rats. *J. Sex. Med.* 9, 1303–1318. doi: 10.1111/j.1743-6109.2012.02688.x

Kurz, E. M., Sengelaub, D. R., and Arnold, A. P. (1986). Androgens regulate the dendritic length of mammalian motoneurons in adulthood. *Science* 232, 395–398. doi: 10.1126/science.3961488

Ladenheim, E. E., Taylor, J. E., Coy, D. H., Moore, K. A., and Moran, T. H. (1996). Hindbrain GRP receptor blockade antagonizes feeding suppression by peripherally administered GRP. *Am. J. Physiol.* 271, R180–R184.

Matsuda, K. I., Sakamoto, H., and Kawata, M. (2008). Androgen action in the brain and spinal cord for the regulation of male sexual behaviors. *Curr. Opin. Pharmacol.* 8, 747–751. doi: 10.1016/j.coph.2008.08.010

Matsumoto, A. (2001). Androgen stimulates neuronal plasticity in the perineal motoneurons of aged male rats. *J. Comp. Neurol.* 430, 389–395. doi: 10.1002/1096-9861(20010212)430:3<389::AID-CNE1038>3.0.CO;2-3

Matsumoto, A., Micevych, P. E., and Arnold, A. P. (1988). Androgen regulates synaptic input to motoneurons of the adult rat spinal cord. *J. Neurosci.* 8, 4168–4176.

Morris, J. A., Jordan, C. L., and Breedlove, S. M. (2004). Sexual differentiation of the vertebrate nervous system. *Nat. Neurosci.* 7, 1034–1039. doi: 10.1038/nn1325

Nakagawa, S. (1980). Onuf's nucleus of the sacral cord in a South American monkey (Saimiri): its location and bilateral cortical input from area 4. *Brain Res.* 191, 337–344. doi: 10.1016/0006-8993(80)91285-8

Newton, B. W. (1992). A sexually dimorphic population of galanin-like neurons in the rat lumbar spinal cord: functional implications. *Neurosci. Lett.* 137, 119–122. doi: 10.1016/0304-3940(92)90312-U

Nicholas, A. P., Zhang, X., and Hokfelt, T. (1999). An immunohistochemical investigation of the opioid cell column in lamina X of the male rat lumbosacral spinal cord. *Neurosci. Lett.* 270, 9–12. doi: 10.1016/S0304-3940(99)00446-2

Nordeen, E. J., Nordeen, K. W., Sengelaub, D. R., and Arnold, A. P. (1985). Androgens prevent normally occurring cell death in a sexually dimorphic spinal nucleus. *Science* 229, 671–673. doi: 10.1126/science.4023706

Onufrowicz, B. (1899). Notes on the arrangement and function of the cell groups in the sacral region of the spinal cord. *J. Nerv. Ment. Dis.* 26, 498–504. doi: 10.1097/00005053-189908000-00006

Oti, T., Satoh, K., Saito, K., Murata, K., Kawata, M., Sakamoto, T., et al. (2012). Three-dimensional evaluation of the spinal local neural network revealed by the high-voltage electron microscopy: a double immunohistochemical study. *Histochem. Cell Biol.* 138, 693–697. doi: 10.1007/s00418-012-0976-6

Ottem, E. N., Beck, L. A., Jordan, C. L., and Breedlove, S. M. (2007). Androgen-dependent regulation of brain-derived neurotrophic factor and tyrosine kinase B in the sexually dimorphic spinal nucleus of the bulbocavernosus. *Endocrinology* 148, 3655–3665. doi: 10.1210/en.2007-0308

Phan, D. C., and Newton, B. W. (1999). Cholecystokinin-8-like immunoreactivity is sexually dimorphic in a midline population of rat lumbar neurons. *Neurosci. Lett.* 276, 165–168. doi: 10.1016/S0304-3940(99)00819-8

Pinski, J., Yano, T., Groot, K., Cai, R. Z., Radulovic, S., and Schally, A. V. (1992). Endocrine effects of new bombesin/gastrin-releasing peptide antagonists in rats. *Am. J. Physiol.* 263, E712–E717.

Raskin, K., de Gendt, K., Duittoz, A., Liere, P., Verhoeven, G., Tronche, F., et al. (2009). Conditional inactivation of androgen receptor gene in the nervous system: effects on male behavioral and neuroendocrine responses. *J. Neurosci.* 29, 4461–4470. doi: 10.1523/JNEUROSCI.0296-09.2009

Raskin, K., Marie-Luce, C., Picot, M., Bernard, V., Mailly, P., Hardin-Pouzet, H., et al. (2012). Characterization of the spinal nucleus of the bulbocavernosus neuromuscular system in male mice lacking androgen receptor in the nervous system. *Endocrinology* 153, 3376–3385. doi: 10.1210/en.2012-1001

Roesler, R., Lessa, D., Venturella, R., Vianna, M. R., Luft, T., Henriques, J. A., et al. (2004). Bombesin/gastrin-releasing peptide receptors in the basolateral amygdala regulate memory consolidation. *Eur. J. Neurosci.* 19, 1041–1045. doi: 10.1111/j.0953-816X.2004.03175.x

Rosen, R. C., and Sachs, B. D. (2000). Central mechanisms in the control of penile erection: current theory and research. *Neurosci. Biobehav. Rev.* 24, 503–505. doi: 10.1016/S0149-7634(00)00018-X

Sachs, B. D. (1982). Role of striated penile muscles in penile reflexes, copulation, and induction of pregnancy in the rat. *J. Reprod. Fertil.* 66, 433–443. doi: 10.1530/jrf.0.0660433

Sakamoto, H. (2011). The gastrin-releasing peptide system in the spinal cord mediates masculine sexual function. *Anat. Sci. Int.* 86, 19–29. doi: 10.1007/s12565-010-0097-z

Sakamoto, H. (2012). Brain-spinal cord neural circuits controlling male sexual function and behavior. *Neurosci. Res.* 72, 103–116. doi: 10.1016/j.neures.2011.11.002

Sakamoto, H., Arii, T., and Kawata, M. (2010). High-voltage electron microscopy reveals direct synaptic inputs from a spinal gastrin-releasing peptide system to neurons of the spinal nucleus of bulbocavernosus. *Endocrinology* 151, 417–421. doi: 10.1210/en.2009-0485

Sakamoto, H., and Kawata, M. (2009). Gastrin-releasing peptide system in the spinal cord controls male sexual behaviour. *J. Neuroendocrinol.* 21, 432–435. doi: 10.1111/j.1365-2826.2009.01847.x

Sakamoto, H., and Kawata, M. (2012). Ultrahigh voltage electron microscopy links neuroanatomy and neuroscience/neuroendocrinology. *Anat. Res. Int.* 2012:948704. doi: 10.1155/2012/948704

Sakamoto, H., Matsuda, K.-I., Zuloaga, D. G., Hongu, H., Wada, E., Wada, K., et al. (2008). Sexually dimorphic gastrin releasing peptide system in the spinal cord controls male reproductive functions. *Nat. Neurosci.* 11, 634–636. doi: 10.1038/nn.2126

Sakamoto, H., Saito, K., Marie-Luce, C., Raskin, K., Oti, T., Satoh, K., et al. (2014). Androgen regulates development of the sexually dimorphic gastrin-releasing peptide neuron system in the lumbar spinal cord: evidence from a mouse line lacking androgen receptor in the nervous system. *Neurosci. Lett.* 558, 109–114. doi: 10.1016/j.neulet.2013.10.068

Sakamoto, H., Takanami, K., Zuloaga, D. G., Matsuda, K. I., Jordan, C. L., Breedlove, S. M., et al. (2009). Androgen regulates the sexually dimorphic gastrin-releasing peptide system in the lumbar spinal cord that mediates male sexual function. *Endocrinology* 150, 3672–3679. doi: 10.1210/en.2008-1791

Sato, M., Mizuno, N., and Konishi, A. (1978). Localization of motoneurons innervating perineal muscles: a HRP study in cat. *Brain Res.* 140, 149–154. doi: 10.1016/0006-8993(78)90244-5

Sengelaub, D. R., and Forger, N. G. (2008). The spinal nucleus of the bulbocavernosus: firsts in androgen-dependent neural sex differences. *Horm. Behav.* 53, 596–612. doi: 10.1016/j.yhbeh.2007.11.008

Sipski, M. L. (1998). Sexual functioning in the spinal cord injured. *Int. J. Impot. Res.* 10(Suppl. 2), S128–S130. discussion: S138–S140.

Studeny, S., and Vizzard, M. A. (2005). Corticotropin-releasing factor (CRF) expression in postnatal and adult rat sacral parasympathetic nucleus (SPN). *Cell Tissue Res.* 322, 339–352. doi: 10.1007/s00441-005-0014-2

Sun, X. Q., Xu, C., Leclerc, P., Benoit, G., Giuliano, F., and Droupy, S. (2009). Spinal neurons involved in the control of the seminal vesicles: a transsynaptic labeling study using pseudorabies virus in rats. *Neuroscience* 158, 786–797. doi: 10.1016/j.neuroscience.2008.10.008

Truitt, W. A., and Coolen, L. M. (2002). Identification of a potential ejaculation generator in the spinal cord. *Science* 297, 1566–1569. doi: 10.1126/science.1073885

Truitt, W. A., Shipley, M. T., Veening, J. G., and Coolen, L. M. (2003). Activation of a subset of lumbar spinothalamic neurons after copulatory behavior in male but not female rats. *J. Neurosci.* 23, 325–331.

Ueyama, T., Mizuno, N., Nomura, S., Konishi, A., Itoh, K., and Arakawa, H. (1984). Central distribution of afferent and efferent components of the pudendal nerve in cat. *J. Comp. Neurol.* 222, 38–46. doi: 10.1002/cne.902220104

Ueyama, T., Mizuno, N., Takahashi, O., Nomura, S., Arakawa, H., and Matsushima, R. (1985). Central distribution of efferent and afferent components of the pudendal nerve in macaque monkeys. *J. Comp. Neurol.* 232, 548–556. doi: 10.1002/cne.902320411

Ulibarri, C., Popper, P., and Micevych, P. E. (1995). Motoneurons dorsolateral to the central canal innervate perineal muscles in the Mongolian gerbil. *J. Comp. Neurol.* 356, 225–237. doi: 10.1002/cne.903560207

Vizzard, M. A., Erdman, S. L., and De Groat, W. C. (1995). Increased expression of neuronal nitric oxide synthase (NOS) in visceral neurons after nerve injury. *J. Neurosci.* 15, 4033–4045.

Wee, B. E., Weaver, D. R., and Clemens, L. G. (1988). Hormonal restoration of masculine sexual behavior in long-term castrated B6D2F1 mice. *Physiol. Behav.* 42, 77–82. doi: 10.1016/0031-9384(88)90263-6

Xu, C., Giuliano, F., Yaici, E. D., Conrath, M., Trassard, O., Benoit, G., et al. (2006). Identification of lumbar spinal neurons controlling simultaneously the prostate and the bulbospongiosus muscles in the rat. *Neuroscience* 138, 561–573. doi: 10.1016/j.neuroscience.2005.11.016

Xu, C., Yaici, E. D., Conrath, M., Blanchard, P., Leclerc, P., Benoit, G., et al. (2005). Galanin and neurokinin-1 receptor immunoreactive [corrected] spinal neurons controlling the prostate and the bulbospongiosus muscle identified by transsynaptic labeling in the rat. *Neuroscience* 134, 1325–1341. doi: 10.1016/j.neuroscience.2005.06.002

Yang, L. Y., Verhovshek, T., and Sengelaub, D. R. (2004). Brain-derived neurotrophic factor and androgen interact in the maintenance of dendritic morphology in a sexually dimorphic rat spinal nucleus. *Endocrinology* 145, 161–168. doi: 10.1210/en.2003-0853

10

Genetic mapping of escalated aggression in wild-derived mouse strain MSM/Ms: association with serotonin-related genes

Aki Takahashi[1,2], Toshihiko Shiroishi[2,3] and Tsuyoshi Koide[1,2]*

[1] Mouse Genomics Resource Laboratory, National Institute of Genetics (NIG), Mishima, Japan
[2] Department of Genetics, SOKENDAI, Mishima, Japan
[3] Mammalian Genetics Laboratory, National Institute of Genetics (NIG), Mishima, Japan

***Correspondence:**
Tsuyoshi Koide, Mouse Genomics Resource Laboratory, National Institute of Genetics, 1111 Yata, Mishima, Shizuoka 411-8540, Japan
e-mail: tkoide@nig.ac.jp

The Japanese wild-derived mouse strain MSM/Ms (MSM) retains a wide range of traits related to behavioral wildness, including high levels of emotionality and avoidance of humans. In this study, we observed that MSM showed a markedly higher level of aggression than the standard laboratory strain C57BL/6J. Whereas almost all MSM males showed high frequencies of attack bites and pursuit in the resident-intruder test, only a few C57BL/6J males showed aggressive behaviors, with these behaviors observed at only a low frequency. Sexually mature MSM males in their home cages killed their littermates, or sometimes female pair-mates. To study the genetic and neurobiological mechanisms that underlie the escalated aggression observed in MSM mice, we analyzed reciprocal F1 crosses and five consomic strains of MSM (Chr 4, 13, 15, X and Y) against the background of C57BL/6J. We identified two chromosomes, Chr 4 and Chr 15, which were involved in the heightened aggression observed in MSM. These chromosomes had different effects on aggression: whereas MSM Chr 15 increased agitation and initiation of aggressive events, MSM Chr 4 induced a maladaptive level of aggressive behavior. Expression analysis of mRNAs of serotonin receptors, serotonin transporter and *Tph2*, an enzyme involved in serotonin synthesis in seven brain areas, indicated several differences among MSM, C57BL/6J, and their consomic strains. We found that *Tph2* expression in the midbrain was increased in the Chr 4 consomic strain, as well as in MSM, and that there was a strong positive genetic correlation between aggressive behavior and *Tph2* expression at the mRNA level. Therefore, it is possible that increased expression of the *Tph2* gene is related to escalated aggression observed in MSM.

Keywords: escalated aggression, wild mouse, MSM/Ms (MSM), genetic mapping, quantitative trait loci (QTLs), chromosome, tryptophan hydroxylase 2 (*Tph2*)

INTRODUCTION

Aggression is one of the most conserved behavioral traits in the animal kingdom. It is observed in insects, fish, crustaceans, reptiles, amphibians, birds, and mammals, including humans. However, there are also large differences in the level of aggression between individuals from the same species. These differences can be caused by both environmental and genetic factors. Mouse strains can differ substantially in their levels of aggressive behavior (Ginsberg and Allee, 1942; Scott, 1942), and selective breeding on a certain aspect of aggressive behavior has successfully produced strains of mice that exhibit high and low levels of aggression (Lagerspetz, 1964; Ebert and Hyde, 1976; van Oortmerssen and Bakker, 1981; Gariepy et al., 1996; Sandnabba, 1996). The identification of several knockout mice that show either increased or decreased aggressive behaviors (for reviews, see Miczek et al., 2001; Nelson and Chiavegatto, 2001; Takahashi et al., 2012) indicates that many genes affect aggression. Genetic mapping that involves quantitative trait locus (QTL) analysis has been used to understand the genetic mechanisms that produce the diversity of aggression in natural populations. Four studies have identified genetic loci related to inter-male aggressive behavior in mice (Brodkin et al., 2002; Roubertoux et al., 2005; Nehrenberg et al., 2010; Dow et al., 2011). Comparative analysis of two substrains of BALB/c, which exhibit different levels of aggression, identified variations in the copy number of several sections of DNA between these substrains (Velez et al., 2010). However, identification of the genes or genetic mechanisms that are involved in the individual differences in aggression remains challenging.

The neurobiological mechanisms that control aggression are widely conserved, and the involvement of the serotonin (5-HT) system in aggressive behavior has been confirmed for species from fly to human (for review, see Olivier et al., 1995; Miczek et al., 2007; Yanowitch and Coccaro, 2011). Therefore, it is likely that the 5-HT system is one of the most important endophenotypes for escalated aggression. However, there are numerous receptors for 5-HT, and the effects triggered by their activation can be complex. Pharmacological studies have shown that each receptor type differs in its involvement in aggressive behavior, and that its effect can also vary depending on the brain region (for review, see Takahashi et al., 2010a). Expression analysis of animals that showed escalated aggression after either alcohol consumption or steroid treatment indicated altered expression of some 5-HT receptors specifically in certain brain areas, such as the prefrontal cortex and amygdala (Ambar and Chiavegatto, 2009; Chiavegatto et al., 2010). Thus, it is necessary to examine which receptor type in which brain area is responsible for the individual differences in aggressive behavior.

It has been unclear whether results from studies of laboratory mice are representative of their wild conspecifics. For example, it has been shown that the level of emotionality is attenuated and behavioral patterns are changed in laboratory strains compared with those in wild mice (Holmes et al., 2000; Furuse et al., 2002; Fernandes et al., 2004; Takahashi et al., 2006). The aggressive behavior of wild rodents is also more intense and more diversified than that of laboratory rodents (de Boer et al., 2003). In this study, we examined aggressive behavior in a wild-derived strain of mice, MSM/Ms, and compared it with that of a commonly used laboratory strain, C57BL/6J (B6). MSM originated from Japanese wild mice (*Mus musculus molossinus*) that were captured in 1978; they have been subjected to brother-sister mating and established as an inbred strain (Moriwaki et al., 2009). Behavioral analysis has shown that MSM retains a wide range of behavioral wildness (Koide et al., 2000; Takahashi et al., 2006; Goto et al., 2013). Given the availability of the complete genome sequence of MSM (Takada et al., 2013) and a panel of consomic strains of MSM and B6 (Takada et al., 2008), we considered MSM to be a good model for genetic analysis of aggressive behavior.

In this study, we aimed to identify (1) the genetic basis of escalated aggressive behavior and (2) the involvement of the 5-HT system in the escalated aggression of MSM. For the genetic analysis, we first characterized the aggressive behavior of MSM in comparison with that of B6 in a standard test for territorial aggression (resident-intruder test) and in the daily housing condition. Then, we analyzed a selected set of consomic strains of MSM against a background of B6 to identify the chromosomes that are involved in the escalated aggression of MSM. To examine the involvement of the 5-HT system as one of the intermediate phenotypes (endophenotypes) of the individual differences in aggression, we also examined the mRNA expression of genes for the receptors, synthesizing enzyme and transporter of 5-HT in several brain areas of the consomic strains, MSM and B6.

MATERIALS AND METHODS

SUBJECTS AND HOUSING

The MSM/Ms (MSM) strain was established and bred at the National Institute of Genetics (NIG). C57BL/6JJcl (B6) mice were purchased from CLEA Japan and bred at NIG. For F1 analysis, we made reciprocal crosses of B6 and MSM (3–4 pairs for each line) to make (B×M)F1 progeny (MSM father) and (M×B)F1 (MSM mother) progeny at NIG. A panel of B6-ChrNMSM consomic strains were established and has been maintained at NIG. The process used to establish this panel was described previously (Takada et al., 2008; Takada and Shiroishi, 2012); briefly, MSM was backcrossed into B6 over 10 generations, and all consomic strains have the same genetic background as B6 except for one pair of chromosomes, which have been substituted for the corresponding MSM chromosome.

Each resident male was housed in pairs with a female of the same strain in transparent polycarbonate cage (22 × 32 × 13.5 cm) with wood chips as bedding material. Intruder males were group-housed at 3–6 per cage in the absence of females. All animals were maintained at NIG with controlled humidity and temperature (50 ± 10%, 23 ± 2°C) under a 12/12-h light/dark cycle (lights on at 6:00 AM). Food and water were freely available. All of the behavioral testing was conducted during the dark period of the photo-cycle (from 6:00 PM to 10:00 PM). All procedures were approved (permit numbers 23-10, 24-10 and 25-10) by the Institutional Committee for Animal Care and Use of the NIG.

BREEDING RECORDS

To follow the aggression of MSM and B6 strains in the rearing conditions, we examined their breeding records in the NIG for the previous six years. These records contain information on all the animals from after they were weaned from their parents (at about 3–4 weeks old) until they were used for other studies (at 9–10 weeks old) or used for breeding to produce the next generation. Animals that had been severely injured (lost their tails or had some signs of wounding) or died from attacks by a littermate were recorded as having been subjected to "injurious aggression." Animals with severe injuries were euthanized once we found evidence of injurious aggression, given that such injuries often result in death within a few days. Given that these records were limited to only the animals in the maintenance colony, we could not follow the animals after they were used for other studies (after 9–10 weeks old). Therefore, there is a limitation in these breeding records insofar as there is the possibility of overlooking incidents of aggression that occur later in the life of these animals.

RESIDENT-INTRUDER TEST

Resident males at the age of 7 weeks were housed in pairs with females of the same strain to enhance territorial aggression. In the case of consomic strains, B6 females were sometimes used as the pair-mate if females of the same genotype were not available. After 3 weeks of being housed with a female, the residents were studied for their territorial aggression to an intruder male by using the resident-intruder test. Animals were 10 weeks of age when their aggression was assessed (10–12 weeks in the analysis of consomic strains). Males of a different litter but the same strain were used as the intruders to estimate the aggression in B6 and MSM strains. For reciprocal F1s and consomic strains, we used B6 males as the intruders. The female and pups were removed, and an intruder male was introduced into the home cage of the resident male. Their behaviors were observed for 5 min after the first attack bite, or the intruder was removed after 5 min if no attack occurred. This encounter occurred twice, with a 48-h interval. All behaviors of the animals during the test were videotaped for subsequent behavioral analysis. During the video analysis, the frequency of attack bites and the durations of sideways threats, tail rattles, pursuit, and non-aggressive behaviors (walking, rearing, self-grooming and contact) were quantified as operationally defined and illustrated previously (Grant and Mackintosh, 1963; Miczek and O'Donnell, 1978). The occurrence and duration of those behaviors were recorded by a trained observer using free software established by Akira Tanave (TanaMove0.07, http://www.nig.ac.jp/labs/MGRL/tanaMove.html).

QUANTIFICATION OF mRNA EXPRESSION IN EACH BRAIN AREA

Total RNA isolation and cDNA synthesis

Animals were euthanized by CO_2 inhalation, and their brains were rapidly removed and placed on ice. Seven brain areas (olfactory bulb, prefrontal cortex, striatum, hippocampus, hypothalamus, midbrain, and cerebellum) were dissected by a surgical knife on ice. Briefly, the olfactory bulb was first dissected at the rostral tip of the prefrontal cortex, then the brain was inverted upside-down and the hypothalamus—defined as the area between optic chiasm and mammillary body—was dissected. Next, the midbrain and the cerebellum were obtained. The midbrain area was defined as a coronal section that includes both the superior and the inferior colliculus, and thus both the dorsal raphe and the median raphe nuclei were included in this area. Finally, the brain was sagittally split by the midline, and the prefrontal cortex was dissected from both hemispheres by cutting the 1 mm rostral tip of the frontal cortex at approximately a 45° angle. The whole hippocampal structure was also taken out from both hemispheres, and the striatum was dissected using scissors. These samples were homogenized on ice in Trizol (Invitrogen, USA). Total RNA was extracted and the quantity and quality were checked using a spectrophotometer (NanoDrop, USA). The RNA purity was assessed by determining the OD ratio (260/280 nm > 2) and the 28S/18S rRNA ratio by denaturing RNAs and separating them in a 1% agarose gel with ethidium bromide staining. After DNase treatment (TURBO DNA-free™ kit, Ambion, USA), cDNA was synthesized from each brain area using Primescript Reverse Transcriptase (TaKaRa Bio, Japan). All cDNA samples were stored at −20°C until analysis by real-time PCR.

Real-time PCR

The primers used in this study are listed in Table S1. Whereas some primers were chosen by referring to previous work (Chiavegatto et al., 2010), others were selected from the open-access website Primer 3 (v. 0.4.0). Given the extensive polymorphism between B6 and MSM (0.82%), we checked the genome database of MSM (http://molossinus.lab.nig.ac.jp/msmdb/index.jsp) to select primers that were not specific to regions with polymorphisms between B6 and MSM. The expression level of mRNA transcript was quantified using a Thermal Cycler Dice® Real Time System (TP800, TaKaRa Bio, Japan) using SYBR Premix Ex Taq II, Perfect Real Time (TaKaRa Bio, Japan). We used the second derivative maximum (SDM) method to quantifying the expression level of mRNA.

Eight to fifteen animals in each strain at around 11–12 weeks of age were used for this analysis. Each male was housed with a female for 3 weeks and then experienced two aggressive encounters separated by a 48-h interval. Their brains were removed five days after the last aggressive encounter.

HPLC measurement of brain 5-HT contents

The midbrain and prefrontal cortex were sampled from males of B6 ($n = 7$), consomic strains of Chr 4 ($n = 8$) and Chr 15 ($n = 6$) that have experiences of about 3 weeks of pair-housing with a female. Animals were euthanized by CO_2 inhalation, and their brains were rapidly removed, dissected on ice, and frozen at −80°C. Then, tissue samples were weighed and homogenized in 20 μl/mg of ice-cold buffer (0.2 M perchloric acid and 100 μM EDTA-2Na). Samples were centrifuged at 20,000 g for 15 min at 0°C. Supernatants were collected, and the pH was adjusted to be pH 0.3 by adding sodium acetate. Supernatants were filtered through 0.45 μm pore size Cosmonice Filter (Nakalai tesque, Kyoto, Japan) and immediately frozen and stored at −80°C until analysis.

Samples were measured using a high performance liquid chromatography (HPLC) system equipped with an electrochemical detector (ECD-300, Eicom Co., Kyoto, Japan) and ODS column [EICOMPAC PP-ODS II (4.6 × 30 mm) at 25°C (Eicom Co.)]. To measure 5-HT, a mobile phase with 100 mM PBS (pH 5.4), 500 mg/L sodium n-Dodecyl Sulfate (SDS), 13.4 uM EDTA-2Na and 2% methanol in HPLC grade water was used. Samples were diluted by 10%, and 10 μl samples were injected into the HPLC.

STATISTICAL ANALYSIS

Fisher's exact test was used to compare the proportion of animals that showed aggressive behaviors during the 5-min encounter in B6 with those in MSM, F1s, and consomic strains. A repeated-measures Two-Way ANOVA was performed to examine the strain difference in aggressive and non-aggressive behaviors over the two encounters. For the analysis of consomic strains, One-Way ANOVA was conducted using the average value of the first and second encounters owing to the low occurrence of aggressive behavior in the consomic strains. One-Way ANOVA was performed to examine strain differences in the expression of mRNA. When a significant F value was obtained, the Tukey-Kramer test and Dunnett's test were conducted as *post-hoc* tests for F1 analysis and consomic analysis, respectively ($\alpha = 0.05$). For genetic correlation analysis, Pearson's correlations were calculated using the mean score for each strain in all consomic strains and B6. For brain 5-HT contents analysis, outliers that were defined as having datapoints greater than 2 standard deviations away from the mean were excluded from statistical analysis. T-test with Bonferroni correction was conducted to compare strain difference of 5-HT contents between B6 and consomic strains.

RESULTS

BREEDING RECORDS OF MSM

Although the records kept during the breeding of the MSM strain are incomplete (see Materials and Methods), we found an interesting trend in the differences between strains in terms of their aggression toward same-sex littermates in the home cage. As mentioned above, animals that had been severely injured or died after an attack by another littermate were recorded as having suffered from "injurious aggression." From the records of MSM, injurious aggression was observed in 13.6% of the housing cages (24 out of 177 cages) that contained multiple male littermates (on average, three males per cage). This injurious aggression was observed after the age of 7 weeks old, when the males are sexually mature. In contrast, injurious aggression was never noted in any of the 265 cages that housed B6 animals. In addition, none of the females of either the MSM or B6 strains showed injurious aggression toward their same-sex cage mates. However, MSM males sometimes attacked their female pair-mates. Females in 9 out of 62 breeding pairs of MSM (14.5%) were injured or killed.

RESIDENT-INTRUDER TEST OF MSM

Mice of the MSM strain showed higher levels of inter-male aggression than their B6 counterparts in the resident-intruder test. Whereas 14 resident males out of 16 pairs (87.5%) of MSM showed attack bites at the first encounter, only 2 residents out of 19 pairs (10.5%) of B6 showed aggressive behaviors (**Table 1**).

Table 1 | Resident-intruder test in MSM and B6 males.

	B6		MSM	
	1st	2nd	1st	2nd
NUMBER OF ANIMALS				
Total resident males	19	19	16	16
Males that showed attack bites	2	4	14^{+}	15^{+}
% aggressive males	10.5 %	21.1 %	87.5 %	93.8 %
DETAILED BEHAVIORS				
Attack bites (f)	3.4 ± 2.3	5.7 ± 2.7	42.9 ± 6.0**	33.8 ± 6.1**
Sideways threats (d)	2.9 ± 2.0	5.7 ± 4.0	6.2 ± 1.7	4.0 ± 0.9
Tail rattles (d)	1.2 ± 0.8	2.5 ± 1.4	8.8 ± 1.4*	8.1 ± 3.5
Pursuit (d)	0.8 ± 0.7	0.7 ± 0.5	70.3 ± 10.2**	50.1 ± 8.9**
Walking (d)	124.8 ± 8.8	102.5 ± 7.4	57.4 ± 5.8**	62.1 ± 8.0**
Rearing (d)	43.1 ± 3.9	34.6 ± 4.6	18.5 ± 3.9**	18.7 ± 4.1*
Grooming (d)	7.8 ± 1.8	8.6 ± 2.0	6.3 ± 3.7	9.3 ± 4.9
Contact (d)	44.7 ± 5.5	39.6 ± 6.3	21.7 ± 12.7	11.9 ± 10.1*
Attack latency	287.9 ± 9	263.5 ± 18	172.7 ± 23**	99.2 ± 24**

Significant strain differences between B6 and MSM are indicated as $^{+}p < 0.05$ by Fisher's exact test, and $^{*}p < 0.05$ and $^{**}p < 0.01$ by the Tukey-Kramer test. (f): frequency, (d): duration.

Fisher's exact test showed that the number of animals that showed aggressive behavior was significantly higher in MSM than in B6 during both first and second encounters. We then analyzed the detailed behaviors during the 5-min encounter from the video recordings. Repeated-measures Two-Way ANOVA showed significant strain differences in aggressive behaviors, including attack bites, pursuit and attack latency [$F_{(1, 33)} > 43.456$, $p < 0.0001$], as well as non-aggressive behaviors including walking, rearing and contact [$F_{(1, 33)} = 4.847$, $p < 0.035$] (**Table 1**). Compared with B6 mice, MSM mice showed a significantly higher frequency of attack bites and longer pursuit (**Figure 1**), as well as shorter attack latency. In contrast, B6 showed more non-aggressive behaviors (walking, rearing and contact) than MSM. A significant strain × encounter interaction was observed only for walking [$F_{(1, 33)} = 4.247$, $p = 0.0473$] and B6 showed a significant decrease of walking in the second encounter compared with that in the first encounter, but there was no change in MSM.

Aggressive behaviors of the reciprocal F1 heterozygotes, (B×M)F1 and (M×B)F1, were also examined and compared with those of their parental strains, B6 and MSM (**Figure 2**). Males of (M×B)F1, which have MSM as a mother, showed high territorial aggression similar to that of MSM in terms of the proportion of aggressive males, the frequency of attack bites, the duration of tail rattles, and short attack latency. In contrast, the males of (B×M)F1, which have MSM as a father, showed an intermediate level of aggression between B6 and MSM in these indices (**Figure 2** left, **Table 2**). On the other hand, the frequency of pursuit (a characteristic behavior of MSM) in both (B×M)F1 and (M×B)F1 was similar to the level of B6 at both first and second encounters (**Figure 2** right). Furthermore, breeding records showed that there was no injurious aggression in either F1 groups during daily housing condition.

ANALYSIS OF B6/MSM CONSOMIC STRAINS

This study examined five strains (that correspond to chromosomes Chr 4, Chr 13, Chr 15, Chr X, and Chr Y) of twenty-nine consomic strains. We chose these strains in this analysis because a previous study that used the social interaction test indicated that a subset of male pairs in the consomic strains of Chr 4, 13, 15, and

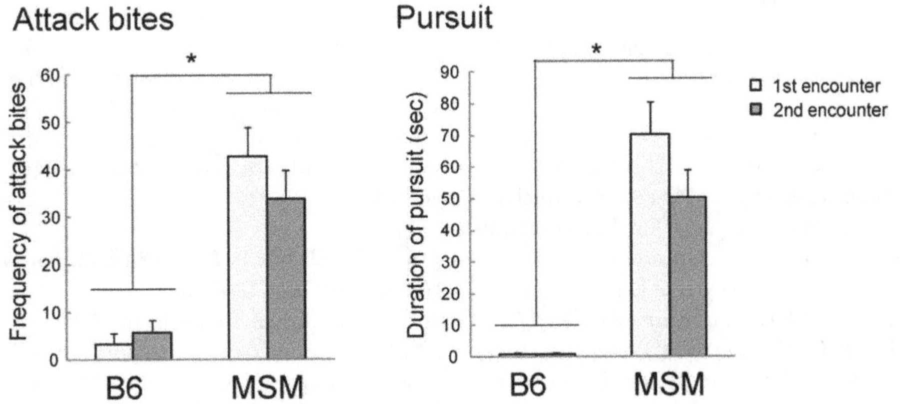

FIGURE 1 | Aggressive behaviors of MSM and B6 in the resident-intruder test. MSM showed significantly more attack bites and pursuit than B6 at both first and second encounters. *Significant strain difference between B6 and MSM ($p < 0.05$).

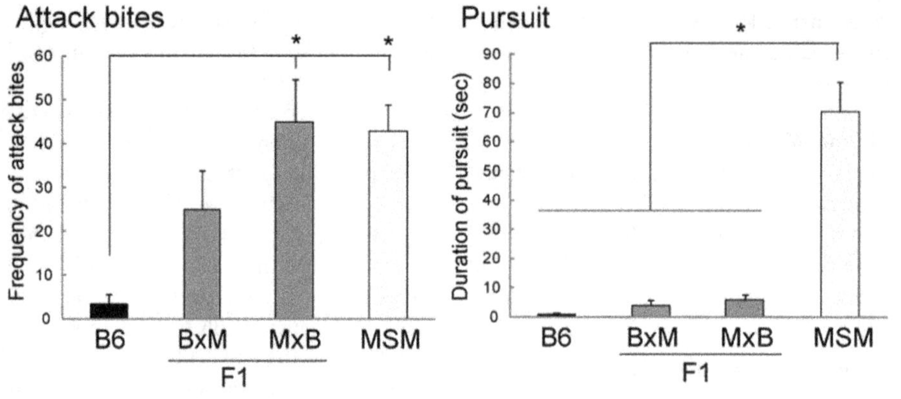

FIGURE 2 | Aggressive behaviors of reciprocal F1 crosses between B6 and MSM in the resident-intruder test. Whereas B×M represents F1 males that have a B6 mother, M×B represents those with an MSM mother. *Significant strain difference ($p < 0.05$).

Table 2 | Resident-intruder test in reciprocal F1 crosses.

	(B×M)F1		(M×B)F1	
	1st	**2nd**	**1st**	**2nd**
NUMBER OF ANIMALS				
Total resident males	10	10	10	10
Males that showed attack bites	6	8	9[a]	10[a]
% aggressive males	60 %	80 %	90 %	100 %
DETAILED BEHAVIORS				
Attack bites (f)	25.0 ± 8.9	31.6 ± 7.4[a]	44.9 ± 9.7[a]	42.8 ± 11.5[a]
Sideways threats (d)	8.2 ± 2.3	8.3 ± 1.6	13.5 ± 2.8[a]	11.4 ± 3.3
Tail rattles (d)	4.6 ± 1.6	12.3 ± 4.7	17.0 ± 6.1[a]	19.8 ± 7.5[a]
Pursuit (d)	4.0 ± 1.8[b]	7.6 ± 3.4[b]	5.9 ± 1.9[b]	4.4 ± 1.7[b]
Walking (d)	79.3 ± 5.2[a]	80.5 ± 7.0	73.5 ± 7.2[a]	55.7 ± 8.8[a]
Rearing (d)	50.3 ± 10.1[b]	36.4 ± 6.8	32.7 ± 7.5	16.7 ± 6.7
Grooming (d)	13.5 ± 5.5	9.8 ± 2.0	9.3 ± 4.8	9.5 ± 3.0
Contact (d)	48.1 ± 15.4	26.9 ± 11.0	43.0 ± 13.8	8.4 ± 5.8
Attack latency	197.0 ± 27[a]	111.9 ± 33[a]	89.4 ± 26[abc]	58.6 ± 14[a]

*Significant differences compared with B6 ([a]), MSM ([b]) (**Table 1**) and (B×M)F1 ([c]) by Tukey-Kramer test ($p < 0.05$). (f): frequency, (d): duration.*

17 showed attack bites during the test, whereas the other strains did not show any aggressive behavior (Takahashi et al., 2010c). In addition, we examined consomic strains of Chr X (XT, which has the telomeric half of Chr X from MSM) and Chr Y because some reports have mentioned the role of sex chromosomes in aggressive behavior (Selmanoff et al., 1975; Sluyter et al., 1996; Brodkin et al., 2002; Roubertoux et al., 2005). Unfortunately, Chr 17 and Chr XC (centromeric half of Chr X from MSM) consomic strains were not included in the analysis because we could not obtain a sufficient number of animals.

All of the consomic strains analyzed in this study showed a low level of aggressive behavior similar to that of B6 at the first encounter (**Table 3**). By contrast, we found that the consomic strain of Chr 15 showed a higher level of initiation of aggressive behavior than B6 at the second encounter. Fisher's exact test indicated that the proportion of animals that showed attack bites was significantly higher in the Chr 15 strain than in B6 ($p = 0.0317$, **Figure 3**). We then analyzed the detailed behaviors during the 5-min encounter. One-Way ANOVA revealed a significant main effect of strain in attack bites [$F_{(5,\ 121)} = 4.081$, $p = 0.0019$], tail rattles [$F_{(5,\ 121)} = 4.381$, $p = 0.0011$], sideways threats [$F_{(5,\ 121)} = 2.357$, $p = 0.0443$], and pursuit [$F_{(5,\ 121)} = 3.495$, $p = 0.0055$]. A *post-hoc* Dunnett's *t*-test showed that, compared with B6, the consomic strain of Chr 4 exhibited significantly higher levels of attack bites, tail rattles, sideways threats, and pursuit (**Figure 3**). In addition, the Chr 15 consomic strain showed a significantly higher level of tail rattles than B6 (**Figure 3**). In terms of non-aggressive behaviors, a significant main effect of strain was observed only for walking [$F_{(5,\ 121)} = 8.981$, $p < 0.0001$], and the Chr X consomic strain showed more walking than B6.

The escalation of aggression in the Chr 4 consomic strain was also observed in the daily housing condition according to the breeding record. During the 3 weeks of housing with a female before the test, we also checked the occurrence of injurious aggression toward a female pair-mate. The Chr 4 consomic strain showed injurious aggression toward females, and females in 8 out of 20 pairs were injured. This strain also showed injurious aggression toward male cage mates (11.9%, 15 out of 126 cages). On the other hand, we did not observe any cages with injurious aggression in the other consomic strains of Chr 13, Chr 15, Chr X, and Chr Y.

STRAIN DIFFERENCE IN THE mRNA EXPRESSION OF 5-HT RECEPTORS, ENZYME AND TRANSPORTER

To evaluate the difference in the 5-HT system between B6 and MSM, we examined the expression level of 5-HT receptor mRNAs in seven brain areas of B6 and MSM using quantitative real-time PCR (**Figure 4**). The mRNA expression of 5-HT_{1A} receptor was significantly higher in MSM than in B6 in the prefrontal cortex, hypothalamus, hippocampus, and striatum [$F_{(1,\ 11)} > 6.043$,

Table 3 | Resident-intruder test in five consomic mouse strains and B6.

	B6	Chr 4	Chr 13	Chr 15	Chr X	Chr Y
NUMBER OF ANIMALS						
Total resident males	32	20	18	23	18	15
Males that showed attack bites	5 (2)	9 (5)	4 (1)	13 (2)$^+$	2 (0)	1 (0)
% aggressive males	15.6 %	45.0 %	22.2 %	56.5 %	11.1 %	6.7 %
DETAILED BEHAVIORS						
Attack bites (f)	2.7 ± 1.2	14.8 ± 5.0*	5.8 ± 3.1	5.2 ± 1.5	1.2 ± 0.8	1.0 ± 1.0
Sideways threat (d)	2.6 ± 1.4	7.8 ± 2.4*	3.3 ± 1.9	4.1 ± 1.3	1.2 ± 0.9	0.6 ± 0.6
Tail rattles (d)	1.1 ± 0.5	9.7 ± 2.8*	5.8 ± 3.1	8.8 ± 2.5*	0.5 ± 0.3	0.8 ± 0.8
Pursuit (d)	0.4 ± 0.3	6.6 ± 3.4*	0.8 ± 0.6	0.4 ± 0.2	0.3 ± 0.3	0.0 ± 0.0
Walking (d)	108.0 ± 4.7	100.7 ± 6.6	123.1 ± 6.6	92.7 ± 4.1	140.9 ± 4.0*	106.1 ± 7.9
Rearing (d)	39.7 ± 2.4	37.4 ± 3.2	41.5 ± 3.2	37.6 ± 2.5	36.8 ± 2.2	37.1 ± 2.9
Grooming (d)	7.6 ± 0.9	9.1 ± 2.4	5.9 ± 0.8	11.0 ± 1.5	5.5 ± 1.0	6.4 ± 1.1
Contact (d)	44.1 ± 3.6	42.0 ± 5.8	43.0 ± 6.0	35.3 ± 3.6	32.5 ± 3.0	28.4 ± 4.8
Attack latency	278.3 ± 11.0	189.6 ± 27.1*	262.9 ± 20.3	219.8 ± 19.1*	276.2 ± 16.6	288.3 ± 11.7

Significant strain difference between B6 and MSM by Dunnett's t-test ($p < 0.05$) or Fisher's exact test ($^+p < 0.05$), (f): frequency, (d): duration. Numbers in parentheses are the numbers of males that showed attack bites at the first encounter. For the detailed behaviors, the averages of first and second encounters are indicated. For attack latency, the result of the second encounter is indicated.*

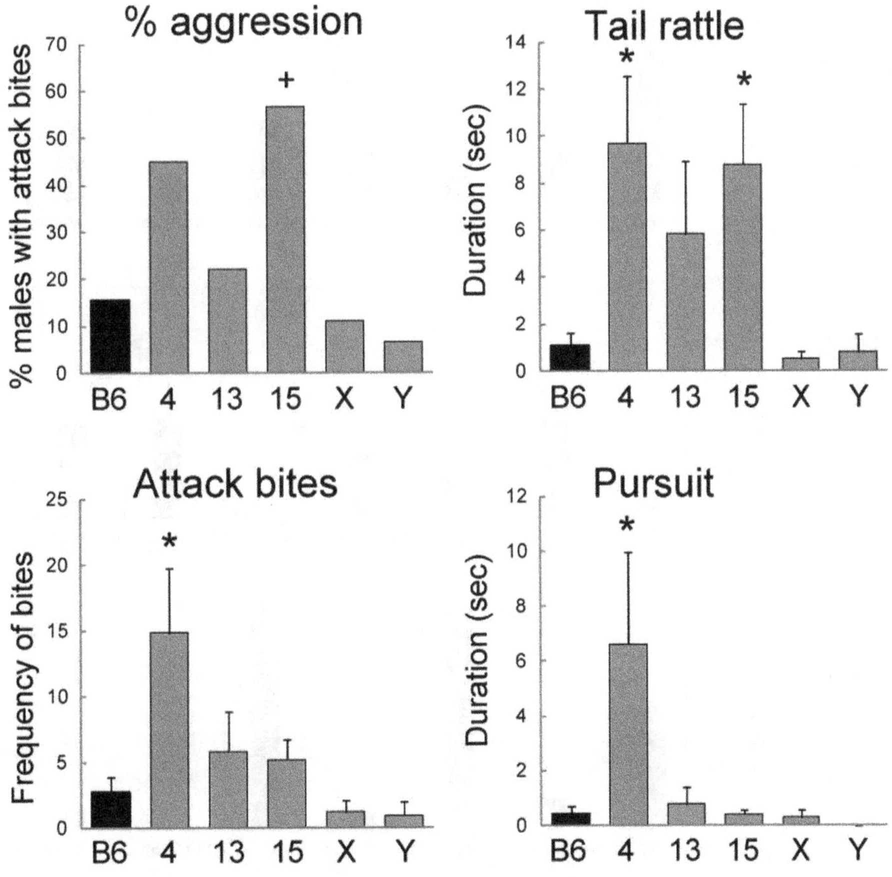

FIGURE 3 | Aggressive behaviors of consomic strains of MSM in the resident-intruder test. The numbers (4, 13, 15) and letters (X, Y) indicate the chromosome that was substituted for that of MSM in the B6 genetic background. Significant difference compared with B6 by Dunnett's test (*$p < 0.05$) or Fisher's exact test ($^+p < 0.05$).

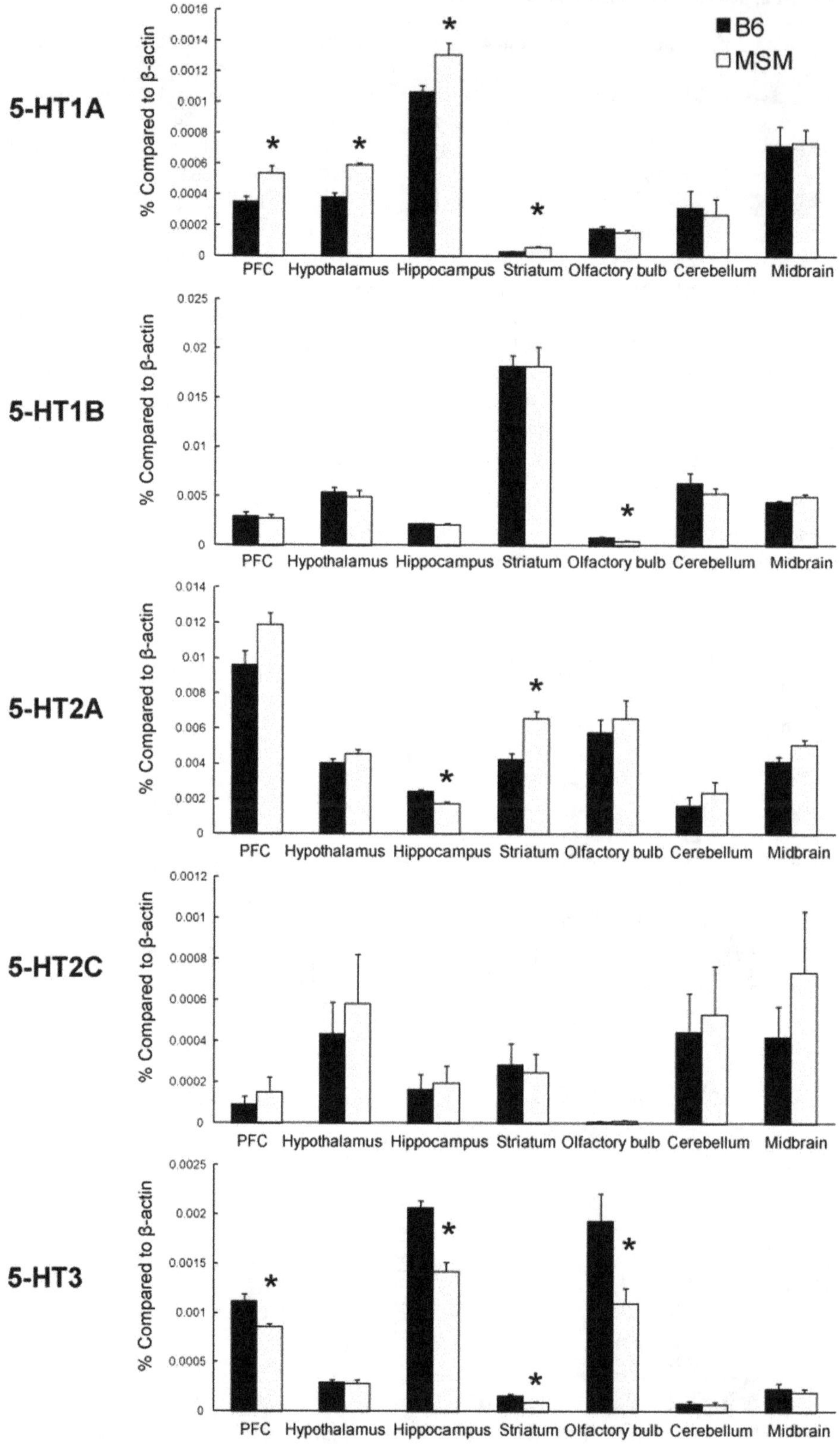

FIGURE 4 | Real-time quantitative PCR analysis of the mRNA expression of 5-HT receptors in seven brain areas of MSM and B6. *Significant strain difference between B6 and MSM ($p < 0.05$).

$p \leq 0.0318$], whereas there was no difference between the strains in levels of the same transcript in the olfactory bulb, cerebellum and midbrain. For 5-HT_{1B} mRNA, a significant difference in expression was observed only in olfactory bulb [$F_{(1, 11)} = 7.208$, $p = 0.0199$], with no differences observed in the six other areas tested. The expression difference in 5-HT_{2A} receptor mRNA was bidirectional: MSM showed lower 5-HT_{2A} mRNA in hippocampus [$F_{(1, 11)} = 20.235, p = 0.0009$], but a higher level in striatum [$F_{(1, 11)} = 17.120, p = 0.0017$], compared with B6. There was no significant strain difference in the expression of 5-HT_{2C} mRNA. On the other hand, 5-HT_{3A} mRNA expression was significantly lower in MSM than in B6 in the prefrontal cortex, hippocampus, striatum and olfactory bulb [$F_{(1, 11)} > 6.133$, $p \leq 0.0308$]. We also examined the mRNA expression of serotonin transporter (SERT) and Tph2 in the midbrain area (**Figure 5**). The Tph2 expression was significantly higher in MSM than in B6 [$F_{(1, 14)} = 10.901$, $p = 0.0052$]. The SERT expression was also higher in MSM, but the difference was not statistically significant [$F_{(1, 14)} = 3.770, p = 0.0726$].

To examine whether these strain differences observed in the expression of 5-HT-related mRNA correspond to heightened aggression in MSM, we then examined the expression of 5-HT receptors and Tph2 using five consomic strains, and its genetic correlation with aggressive behaviors (**Table 4**). This expression analysis showed that the Chr 4 consomic strain, which exhibited escalated and injurious aggressive behavior, had significantly increased *Tph2* mRNA expression in the midbrain (**Figure 6A**). This strain, but not MSM, also showed elevated expression of 5-HT_{2A} receptor in the prefrontal cortex relative to B6. On the other hand, the Chr 15 consomic strain, which showed a higher level of initiation of aggressive behavior than the other strains tested, did not show any significant difference in the expression of 5-HT receptor at the mRNA level. There was also a slight increase (124%) of Tph2 expression in the Chr 15 consomic strain, but this was not statistically significant. Significant positive genetic correlations were shown between *Tph2* mRNA expression and aggressive behaviors (% aggressive animals, bites and tail rattles, $r \geq 0.82, p < 0.05$; **Figure 6B**). In addition, a positive correlation was observed between 5-HT_{2A} expression in the prefrontal cortex and attack bites ($r = 0.81$, $p = 0.0527$). Although they were not statistically significant, moderate negative correlations were observed between 5-HT_{1A} or 5-HT_{3A} in the prefrontal cortex and aggressive behaviors (**Table 4**). However, there were no correlations between 5-HT receptor expression in the hippocampus and any aggressive behaviors.

To examine whether the increase of *Tph2* expression at the mRNA level can affect the brain 5-HT contents, we measured 5-HT contents in the midbrain and prefrontal cortex in B6, Chr 4, and Chr 15 consomic strains. Unexpectedly, we found that the 5-HT contents were decreased in the midbrain homogenate of Chr 4 consomic strain compared to B6 [$t_{(11)} = -2.669$, $p = 0.0436$; **Figure 7A**]. There was no change in 5-HT contents in the midbrain sample of Chr 15 consomic strain. By contrast, in the prefrontal cortex, both Chr 4 consomic [$t_{(11)} = 3.951$, $p = 0.0046$] and Chr 15 consomic strains [$t_{(9)} = 3.820$, $p = 0.0082$] showed increases in 5-HT contents compared to B6 (**Figure 7B**).

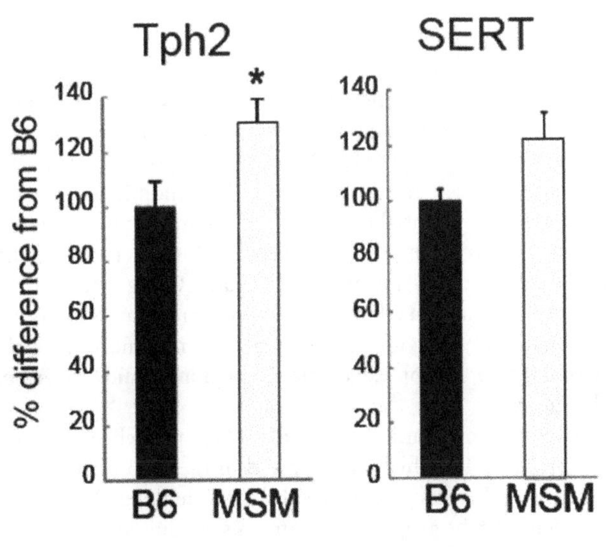

FIGURE 5 | mRNA expressions of tryptophan hydroxylase 2 (*Tph2*) and 5-HT transporter (*SERT*) in the midbrain of MSM and B6. *Significant strain difference between B6 and MSM ($p < 0.05$).

DISCUSSION

ESCALATED AGGRESSION IN MSM

This study revealed that a Japanese wild-derived mouse strain, MSM, has an escalated level of aggressive behavior compared with the commonly used laboratory strain B6. This aggressive behavior of MSM was characterized by frequent pursuit (chasing) behavior, in addition to attack bites. This pursuing contrasts with the behavior of not only B6 strain but other laboratory mouse lines, such as ICR and CFW (Takahashi et al., 2010b). Fierce chasing behavior with no respite was also observed in wild mice (Crowcroft, 1966). It can thus be postulated that MSM retains some patterns of aggressive behavior that are observed in wild mice. From the breeding records of MSM, we found that some MSM males showed a high level of injurious attacks (or killing) against cage mates. This injurious behavior was also directed toward female mates. Therefore, under the laboratory housing conditions, the aggression of male MSM mice appears to be maladaptive because there is a lack of inhibition of aggressive behavior of MSM even toward inappropriate targets (females). The expression of escalated aggressive behavior in MSM was observed after sexual maturation, suggesting that the sex steroids might have an important role in triggering their aggression.

GENETIC ANALYSIS OF ESCALATED AGGRESSIVE BEHAVIOR

The analysis of reciprocal F1s showed that there is a different mode of inheritance for some indices of escalated aggression observed in MSM. Given that we did not observe any injurious aggression and also no increase of pursuit in both F1 intercrosses, these phenotypes are considered as recessive traits. On the other hand, the frequency of attack bites and tail rattles, as well as the percentage of aggressive animals, were higher in the F1 intercrosses than in B6, whereas attack latency was lower in F1 intercrosses than in B6. Thus, these behaviors have either a

Table 4 | The expression of 5-HT receptors and Tph2 mRNAs in five consomic strains and their genetic correlations with aggressive behaviors.

	Prefrontal cortex			Hippocampus			Midbrain
	5-HT1A	5-HT2A	5-HT3A	5-HT1A	5-HT2A	5-HT3a	Tph2
mRNA EXPRESSION (% DIFFERENCE FROM B6)							
Chr 4	86 ± 9	150 ± 14*	98 ± 11	85 ± 9	97 ± 4	72 ± 10	146 ± 15*
Chr 13	108 ± 12	146 ± 27*	125 ± 27	164 ± 14*	79 ± 6	55 ± 6	117 ± 10
Chr 15	113 ± 16	91 ± 13	84 ± 13	83 ± 9	83 ± 8	68 ± 13	124 ± 11
Chr X	114 ± 12*	92 ± 14	126 ± 18	93 ± 13	82 ± 10	39 ± 9*	113 ± 14
Chr Y	106 ± 2	86 ± 9	106 ± 26	81 ± 8	99 ± 15	77 ± 11	98 ± 10
GENETIC CORRELATION							
% aggressive animals	−0.49	0.31	−0.69	−0.07	−0.21	0.03	0.82*
Attack bites	−0.46	0.81+	−0.31	0.00	0.12	0.06	0.85*
Tail rattles	−0.53	0.61	−0.49	0.15	−0.22	−0.05	0.90*
Pursuit	−0.32	0.72	−0.23	−0.20	0.31	0.07	0.74+

Significant strain differences between B6 and each consomic strain by Dunnett's t-test ($p < 0.05$) for mRNA expression. Genetic correlations were calculated by Pearson's correlations. *$p < 0.05$, $^{+}p < 0.10$.*

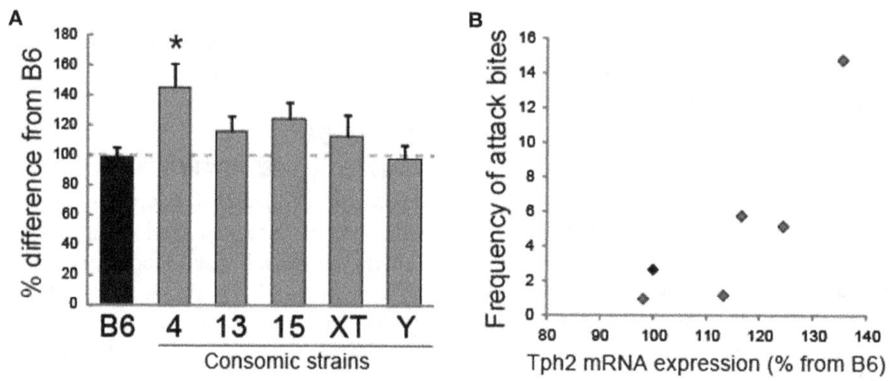

FIGURE 6 | Analysis of the abundances of *Tph2* transcripts in five consomic strains and B6. (A) Chr 4 consomic strains showed a significant increase of *Tph2* mRNA expression in the midbrain. *Significant difference compared with B6 ($p < 0.05$). **(B)** Positive genetic correlation between *Tph2* expression and the frequency of attack bites.

dominant or an additive mode of inheritance. Interestingly, we found differences between the reciprocal F1 crosses in these phenotypes: whereas (M×B)F1, which has MSM as a mother, showed a pronounced increase of aggression similar to that of MSM, (B×M)F1, which has MSM as a father, showed a level of aggression intermediate between that of B6 and MSM. The genetic differences between (M×B)F1 and (B×M)F1 are only in sex chromosomes and mitochondrial DNA; all autosomes are identically heterozygote. However, our analysis of consomic strains did not find any effect of the sex chromosomes on intermale aggression despite the sex chromosomes previously being implicated in aggressive behaviors by the analysis of both hybrid or congenic strains of Y (Selmanoff et al., 1975; Sluyter et al., 1996) as well as by QTL mapping (Brodkin et al., 2002; Roubertoux et al., 2005). Therefore, it is likely that genetic loci involved in escalated aggression of MSM are not localized on the sex chromosomes, or that they need to interact with other autosomal loci (Maxson et al., 1979) or with the specific maternal environment (Carlier et al., 1991) to exert their behavioral effects. Also, it has been reported that the difference in maternal behavior could change aggressive behavior of same-genotype offspring (Bester-Meredith and Marler, 2001; Cox et al., 2013). Another possible reason for differences between reciprocal F1s is the genomic imprinting, which causes preferential expression of the maternal or paternal allele, and it has reported that more than 1300 loci showed differential allelic expression in mouse brain (Gregg et al., 2010). Whether this maternal effect observed in the reciprocal F1s is due to the maternal behavior or the epigenetic modification in the maternal loci or a complex genetic interaction should be clarified in the future.

Analysis of consomic strains identified two chromosomes, Chr 4 and Chr 15, which are involved in these different aspects of aggressive behavior. Our results indicated that Chr 15 of MSM increased the proportion of animals that initiated aggressive behavior and the frequency of tail rattles. However, the frequencies of attack bites and pursuit were similar to those in B6, and there was no injurious aggression observed in Chr 15 consomic males. These findings suggest that there is genetic locus that

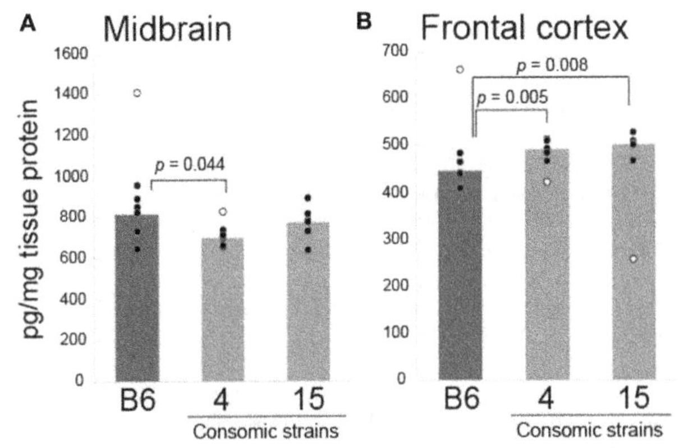

FIGURE 7 | Brain 5-HT content (pg/mg tissue) in the midbrain (A) and prefrontal cortex (B) in B6 and consomic strains of Chr 4 and Chr 15. Each circle indicates each individual's 5-HT content, and open circles indicate outliers that were excluded for statistical analysis. The *p*-values were calculated by *t*-test with Bonferroni correction.

increases agitation and the initiation of aggressive behaviors on Chr 15. On the other hand, we found that the consomic strain of Chr 4 showed a maladaptive level of aggression. The breeding records from daily housing conditions indicated that the Chr 4 consomic males showed injurious aggression toward both their same-sex littermates and their female mates. In the resident-intruder test, Chr 4 males showed increased frequencies of attack bite and a longer duration of pursuit. On the other hand, the proportion of animals that showed aggressive behavior was not significantly different from that in B6. This indicated that Chr 4 consomic animals showed exaggerated aggressive behavior after aggression had been triggered. Thus, a genetic locus on MSM Chr 4 might be responsible for the maladaptive aspect of aggression observed in MSM. Our findings indicate that there are different genetic bases for agitation and readily provoked aggressive behavior (Chr 15) and for escalated maladaptive aggressive behavior (Chr 4). A role for Chr 4 in controlling aggression is consistent with a report that strains of A/J and B6, which carry substitutions in Chr 4, also showed severe fighting in the housing cage (Singer et al., 2005). In addition, QTL analysis of the initiation of aggression of F2 mice derived from a cross between BALB/c and A/J strains toward an intruder dangled at a corner of test cage identified an aggression-related QTL on Chr 15 (Dow et al., 2011).

Compared with MSM, all tested consomic strains showed a low level of aggression at the first encounter compared with MSM. This indicates that the genetic effect of either Chr 4 or Chr 15 is not very large and that multiple loci contribute to the escalated aggression of MSM.

ESCALATED AGGRESSION AND THE 5-HT SYSTEM

Expression analysis of several 5-HT receptors, *Tph2* and a serotonin transporter showed several strain differences in mRNA expression between B6 and MSM. To examine which differences in the 5-HT system between B6 and MSM actually correlate with the level of aggressive behavior, we analyzed the mRNA expression in consomic mouse strains and calculated the genetic correlation between mRNA expression and aggressive behavior. The result showed highly positive correlations between the level of the 5-HT synthetic enzyme *Tph2* in the midbrain and several aggressive behaviors. Both MSM and the consomic strain of Chr 4 showed injurious aggression toward both male and female cage mates, and also showed large increase in *Tph2* expression compared with that in B6. The consomic strain of Chr 15 that showed high agitation toward male intruders also showed a modest increase in the abundance of *Tph2* mRNA.

Although Tph2 has been implicated in aggression because it directly affects the activity of 5-HT neurons, the relationship between Tph2 activity and the level of aggression seems to be complex. It has been shown that both male and female *Tph2* gene knockout mice, which have very low levels of 5-HT but normal 5-HT neuron development (Gutknecht et al., 2008), exhibited escalated aggressive behavior in both their daily housing conditions and the resident-intruder test (Alenina et al., 2009; Angoa-Pérez et al., 2012; Mosienko et al., 2012). Knock-in mice with an R439H point mutation in the *Tph2* gene, which causes an 80% reduction of enzymatic activity, consistently showed increased attack behavior compared with the wild type in a neutral test area (Beaulieu et al., 2008). These results consistently indicate that a reduction of Tph2 activity, and hence a reduction in brain 5-HT, corresponds to exaggerated aggressive behavior. On the other hand, strain comparison studies of Tph2 activity have shown a positive correlation between the activity of Tph2 and the level of aggression in several mouse strains (Kulikov and Popova, 1996; Kulikov et al., 2005). A single-nucleotide polymorphism in the gene that encodes Tph2 (C1473G) affects the activity of Tph2 (Zhang et al., 2004; Kulikov et al., 2005; Osipova et al., 2009), and congenic mice that have the C1473G-type locus from the CC57BR strain, which causes low Tph2 activity in the midbrain, showed a reduced level of aggression compared with the parental B6 strain (Osipova et al., 2009). Given these findings, it is possible that deviation of 5-HT function from its appropriate level in either direction may escalate the level of aggression. Our finding that MSM expresses increased levels of the mRNA that encode Tph2 seems to be consistent with the latter findings, namely, a positive correlation between the abundance of *Tph2* mRNA and aggressive behavior. However, when we measured the 5-HT contents in the brain, we found mixed results; Chr 4 consomic strain showed reduced 5-HT in the midbrain but increased 5-HT in the prefrontal cortex. By contrast, Chr 15 consomic strain showed increased 5-HT contents in the prefrontal cortex, but no change in the midbrain. This different pattern of change of 5-HT contents may correspond to the different type of aggression observed in Chr 4 and Chr 15 consomic strains. While it is unclear how these complex effects on 5-HT contents in each brain region were produced by increased *Tph2* mRNA expression, our data suggest that the expression of *Tph2* can be a good candidate for an endophenotype of escalated aggression observed in MSM. Given that MSM has the same genotype at the C1473G locus as B6 (Osipova et al., 2010) and that the *Tph2* gene is also localized on Chr 10, there should be no C1473G-related difference in Tph2 activity between B6 and MSM or the Chr 4 or Chr 15 consomic strain. Further investigation is thus required to examine the direct relationship between Tph2 expression and the increased aggression observed in MSM.

This study identified the involvement of two chromosomes, Chr 4 and Chr 15, in different aspects of escalated aggression in MSM. Our result of a correlation between *Tph2* and aggressive behaviors suggests that a difference in the expression of Tph2 in midbrain can be an endophenotype for the escalated aggression in MSM. The analysis of a panel of congenic strains for either Chr 4 or Chr 15, in which only small segment of chromosome was substituted with MSM, will lead to identify genes that are involved in the escalated aggression and their relationships to the 5-HT system.

ACKNOWLEDGMENTS

The authors would like to thank Kumiko Takahashi, Michiko Arii and Miyoko Umehara for the maintenance and breeding records of the consomic strains, MSM, and B6, and Akira Tanave for establishing behavioral analysis software. This research was funded by KAKENHI (22830130, 25116527, and 23683021).

REFERENCES

Alenina, N., Kikic, D., Todiras, M., Mosienko, V., Qadri, F., Plehm, R., et al. (2009). Growth retardation and altered autonomic control in mice lacking brain serotonin. *Proc. Natl. Acad. Sci. U.S.A.* 106, 10332–10337. doi: 10.1073/pnas.0810793106

Ambar, G., and Chiavegatto, S. (2009). Anabolic-androgenic steroid treatment induces behavioral disinhibition and downregulation of serotonin receptor messenger RNA in the prefrontal cortex and amygdala of male mice. *Genes Brain Behav.* 8, 161–173. doi: 10.1111/j.1601-183X.2008.00458.x

Angoa-Pérez, M., Kane, M. J., Briggs, D. I., Sykes, C. E., Shah, M. M., Francescutti, D. M., et al. (2012). Genetic depletion of brain 5HT reveals a common molecular pathway mediating compulsivity and impulsivity. *J. Neurochem.* 121, 974–984. doi: 10.1111/j.1471-4159.2012.07739.x

Beaulieu, J. M., Zhang, X., Rodriguiz, R. M., Sotnikova, T. D., Cools, M. J., Wetsel, W. C., et al. (2008). Role of GSK3 beta in behavioral abnormalities induced by serotonin deficiency. *Proc. Natl. Acad. Sci. U.S.A.* 105, 1333–1338. doi: 10.1073/pnas.0711496105

Bester-Meredith, J. K., and Marler, C. A. (2001). Vasopressin and aggression in cross-fostered California mice (*Peromyscus californicus*) and white-footed mice (*Peromyscus leucopus*). *Horm. Behav.* 40, 51–64. doi: 10.1006/hbeh.2001.1666

Brodkin, E. S., Goforth, S. A., Keene, A. H., Fossella, J. A., and Silver, L. M. (2002). Identification of quantitative trait loci that affect aggressive behavior in mice. *J. Neurosci.* 22, 1165–1170. Available online at: http://www.jneurosci.org/content/22/3/1165.full

Carlier, M., Roubertoux, P. L., and Pastoret, C. (1991). The Y chromosome effect on intermale aggression in mice depends on the maternal environment. *Genetics* 129, 231–236.

Chiavegatto, S., Quadros, I. M. H., Ambar, G., and Miczek, K. A. (2010). Individual vulnerability to escalated aggressive behavior by a low dose of alcohol: decreased serotonin receptor mRNA in the prefrontal cortex of male mice. *Genes Brain Behav.* 9, 110–119. doi: 10.1111/j.1601-183X.2009.00544.x

Cox, K. H., So, N. L., and Rissman, E. F. (2013). Foster dams rear fighters: strain-specific effects of within-strain fostering on aggressive behavior in male mice. *PLoS ONE* 8:e75037. doi: 10.1371/journal.pone.0075037

Crowcroft, P. (1966). *Mice All Over*. London: Foulis.

de Boer, S. F., van der Vegt, B. J., and Koolhaas, J. M. (2003). Individual variation in aggression of feral rodent strains: a standard for the genetics of aggression and violence? *Behav. Genet.* 33, 485–501. doi: 10.1023/A:1025766415159

Dow, H. C., Kreibich, A. S., Kaercher, K. A., Sankoorikal, G. M. V., Pauley, E. D., Lohoff, F. W., et al. (2011). Genetic dissection of intermale aggressive behavior in BALB/cJ and A/J mice. *Genes Brain Behav.* 10, 57–68. doi: 10.1111/j.1601-183X.2010.00640.x

Ebert, P. D., and Hyde, J. S. (1976). Selection for agonistic begavior in wild female *Mus musculus*. *Behav. Genet.* 6, 291–304. doi: 10.1007/BF01065725

Fernandes, C., Liu, L., Paya-Cano, J. L., Gregorová, S., Forejt, J., and Schalkwyk, L. C. (2004). Behavioral characterization of wild derived male mice (*Mus musculus musculus*) of the PWD/Ph inbred strain: high exploration compared to C57BL/6J. *Behav. Genet.* 34, 621–630. doi: 10.1007/s10519-004-5589-y

Furuse, T., Blizard, D. A., Moriwaki, K., Miura, Y., Yagasaki, K., Shiroishi, T., et al. (2002). Genetic diversity underlying capsaicin intake in the Mishima battery of mouse strains. *Brain Res. Bull.* 57, 49–55. doi: 10.1016/S0361-9230(01)00636-0

Gariepy, J. L., Lewis, M. H., and Cairns, R. B. (1996). "Neurobiology and aggression," in *Aggression and Violence: Genetic, Neurobiological and Biosocial Perspectives*, eds D. M. Stoff and R. B. Cairns (Mahwah, NJ: Lawrence Erlbaum Associates), 41–63.

Ginsberg, B. E., and Allee, W. C. (1942). Some effects of conditioning on social dominance and subordination in inbred strains of mice. *Physiol. Zool.* 15, 485–506.

Goto, T., Tanave, A., Moriwaki, K., Shiroishi, T., and Koide, T. (2013). Selection for reluctance to avoid humans during the domestication of mice. *Genes Brain Behav.* 12, 760–770. doi: 10.1111/gbb.12088

Grant, E. C., and Mackintosh, J. H. (1963). A comparison of the social postures of some common laboratory rodents. *Behaviour* 21, 246–259. doi: 10.1163/156853963X00185

Gregg, C., Zhang, J., Weissbourd, B., Luo, S., Schroth, G. P., Haig, D., et al. (2010) High-resolution analysis of parent-of-origin allelic expression in the mouse brain. *Science* 329, 643–648. doi: 10.1126/science.1190830

Gutknecht, L., Waider, J., Kraft, S., Kriegebaum, C., Holtmann, B., Reif, A., et al. (2008). Deficiency of brain 5-HT synthesis but serotonergic neuron formation in Tph2 knockout mice. *J. Neural. Transm.* 115, 1127–1132. doi: 10.1007/s00702-008-0096-6

Holmes, A., Parmigiani, S., Ferrari, P. F., Palanza, P., and Rodgers, R. J. (2000). Behavioral profile of wild mice in the elevated plus-maze test for anxiety. *Physiol. Behav.* 71, 509–516. doi: 10.1016/S0031-9384(00)00373-5

Koide, T., Moriwaki, K., Ikeda, K., Niki, H., and Shiroishi, T. (2000). Multi-phenotype behavioral characterization of inbred strains derived from wild stocks of *Mus musculus*. *Mamm. Genome* 11, 664–670. doi: 10.1007/s003350010129

Kulikov, A., and Popova, N. (1996). Association between intermale aggression and genetically-defined tryptophan hydroxylase activity in the mouse brain. *Aggressive Behav*, 22, 111–117. doi: 10.1002/(SICI)1098-2337(1996)22:2<111::AID-AB4>3.0.CO;2-R

Kulikov, A. V., Osipova, D. V., Naumenko, V. S., and Popova, N. K. (2005). Association between Tph2 gene polymorphism, brain tryptophan hydroxylase activity and aggressiveness in mouse strains. *Genes Brain Behav.* 4, 482–485. doi: 10.1111/j.1601-183X.2005.00145.x

Lagerspetz, K. (1964). Studies on the aggressive behaviour of mice. *Ann. Acad. Sci. Fenn. B* 131, 1–13.

Maxson, S. C., Ginsburg, B. E., and Trattner, A. (1979). Interaction of Y-chromosomal and autosomal gene(s) in the development of intermale aggression in mice. *Behav. Genet.* 9, 219–226. doi: 10.1007/BF01071302

Miczek, K. A., Faccidomo, S., Fish, E. W., and DeBold, J. F. (2007). "Neurochemistry and molecular neurobiology of aggressive behavior," in *Behavioral Neurochemistry, Neuroendocrinology and Molecular Neurobiology*, ed J. Blaustein (New York, NY: Springer), 285–336.

Miczek, K. A., Maxson, S. C., Fish, E. W., and Faccidomo, S. (2001). Aggressive behavioral phenotypes in mice. *Behav. Brain Res.* 125, 167–181. doi: 10.1016/S0166-4328(01)00298-4

Miczek, K. A., and O'Donnell, J. M. (1978). Intruder-evoked aggression in isolated and nonisolated mice: effects of psychomotor stimulants and L-dopa. *Psychopharmacology* 57, 47–55. doi: 10.1007/BF00426957

Moriwaki, K., Miyashita, N., Mita, A., Gotoh, H., Tsuchiya, K., Kato, H., et al. (2009). Unique inbred strain MSM/Ms established from the Japanese wild mouse. *Exp. Anim.* 58, 123–134. doi: 10.1538/expanim.58.123

Mosienko, V., Bert, B., Beis, D., Matthes, S., Fink, H., Bader, M., et al. (2012). Exaggerated aggression and decreased anxiety in mice deficient in brain serotonin. *Transl. Psychiatry* 2, e122. doi: 10.1038/tp.2012.44

Nehrenberg, D. L., Wang, S., Buus, R. J., Perkins, J., de Villena, F. P., and Pomp, D. (2010). Genomic mapping of social behavior traits in a F2 cross derived from mice selectively bred for high aggression. *BMC Genet.* 11, 113. doi: 10.1186/1471-2156-11-113

Nelson, R. J., and Chiavegatto, S. (2001). Molecular basis of aggression. *Trends Neurosci.* 24, 713–719. doi: 10.1016/S0166-2236(00)01996-2

Olivier, B., Mos, J., van Oorschot, R., and Hen, R. (1995). Serotonin receptors and animal models of aggressive behavior. *Pharmacopsychiatry* 28, 80–90. doi: 10.1055/s-2007-979624

Osipova, D. V., Kulikov, A. V., Mekada, K., Yoshiki, A., Moshkin, M. P., Kotenkova, E. V., et al. (2010). Distribution of the C1473G polymorphism in tryptophan hydroxylase 2 gene in laboratory and wild mice. *Genes Brain Behav.* 9, 537–543. doi: 10.1111/j.1601-183X.2010.00586.x

Osipova, D. V., Kulikov, A. V., and Popova, N. K. (2009). C1473G polymorphism in mouse tph2 gene is linked to tryptophan hydroxylase-2 activity in the brain, intermale aggression, and depressive-like behavior in the forced swim test. *J. Neurosci. Res.* 87, 1168–1174. doi: 10.1002/jnr.21928

Roubertoux, P. L., Guillot, P., Mortaud, S., Pratte, M., Jamon, M., Cohen-Salmon, C., et al. (2005). Attack behaviors in mice: from factorial structure to quantitative trait loci mapping. *Eur. J. Pharmacol.* 526, 172–185. doi: 10.1016/j.ejphar.2005.09.026

Sandnabba, N. K. (1996). Selective breeding for isolation-induced intermale aggression in mice: associated responses and environmental influences. *Behav. Genet.* 26, 477–488. doi: 10.1007/BF02359752

Scott, J. P. (1942). Genetic differences in the social behavior of inbred strains of mice. *J. Hered.* 33, 11–15.

Selmanoff, M. K., Jumonville, J. E., Maxson, S. C., and Ginsburg, B. E. (1975). Evidence for a Y chromosomal contribution to an aggressive phenotype in inbred mice. *Nature* 253, 529–530. doi: 10.1038/253529a0

Singer, J. B., Hill, A. E., Nadeau, J. H., and Lander, E. S. (2005). Mapping quantitative trait loci for anxiety in chromosome substitution strains of mice. *Genetics* 169, 855–862. doi: 10.1534/genetics.104.031492

Sluyter, F., van Oortmerssen, G. A., de Ruiter, A. J., and Koolhaas, J. M. (1996). Aggression in wild house mice: current state of affairs. *Behav. Genet.* 26, 489–496. doi: 10.1007/BF02359753

Takada, T., Ebata, T., Noguchi, H., Keane, T. M., Adams, D. J., Narita, T., et al. (2013) The ancestor of extant Japanese fancy mice contributed to the mosaic genomes of classical inbred strains. *Genome Res.* 23, 1329–1338. doi: 10.1101/gr.156497.113

Takada, T., Mita, A., Maeno, A., Sakai, T., Shitara, H., Kikkawa, Y., et al. (2008). Mouse inter-subspecific consomic strains for genetic dissection of quantitative complex traits. *Genome Res.* 18, 500–508. doi: 10.1101/gr.7175308

Takada, T., and Shiroishi, T. (2012). Complex quantitative traits cracked by the mouse inter-subspecific consomic strains. *Exp. Anim.* 61, 375–388. doi: 10.1538/expanim.61.375

Takahashi, A., Kato, K., Makino, J., Shiroishi, T., and Koide, T. (2006). Multivariate analysis of temporal descriptions of open-field behavior in wild-derived mouse strains. *Behav. Genet.* 36, 763–774. doi: 10.1007/s10519-005-9038-3

Takahashi, A., Quadros, I. M., de Almeida, R. M. M., and Miczek, K. A. (2010a). Brain serotonin receptors and transporters: initiation vs. termination of escalated aggression. *Psychopharmacology* 213, 183–212. doi: 10.1007/s00213-010-2000-y

Takahashi, A., Quadros, I. M., de Almeida, R. M. M., and Miczek, K. A. (2012). Behavioral and pharmacogenetics of aggressive behavior. *Curr. Top. Behav. Neurosci.* 12, 73–138. doi: 10.1007/7854_2011_191

Takahashi, A., Shimamoto, A., Boyson, C. O., DeBold, J. F., and Miczek, K. A. (2010b). $GABA_B$ receptor modulation of serotonin neurons in the dorsal raphe nucleus and escalation of aggression in mice. *J. Neurosci.* 30, 11771–11780. doi: 10.1523/JNEUROSCI.1814-10.2010

Takahashi, A., Tomihara, K., Shiroishi, T., and Koide, T. (2010c). Genetic mapping of social interaction behavior in B6/MSM consomic mouse strains. *Behav. Genet.* 40, 366–376. doi: 10.1007/s10519-009-9312-x

van Oortmerssen, G. A., and Bakker, T. C. (1981). Artificial selection for short and long attack latencies in wild *Mus musculus domesticus*. *Behav. Genet.* 11, 115–126. doi: 10.1007/BF01065622

Velez, L., Sokoloff, G., Miczek, K. A., Palmer, A. A., and Dulawa, S. C. (2010). Differences in aggressive behavior and DNA copy number variants between BALB/cJ and BALB/cByJ substrains. *Behav. Genet.* 40, 201–210. doi: 10.1007/s10519-009-9325-5

Yanowitch, R., and Coccaro, E. F. (2011). The neurochemistry of human aggression. *Adv. Genet.* 75, 151–169. doi: 10.1016/B978-0-12-380858-5.00005-8

Zhang, X., Beaulieu, J., Sotnikova, T. D., Gainetdinov, R. R., and Caron, M. G. (2004). Tryptophan hydroxylase-2 controls brain serotonin synthesis. *Science* 305, 217. doi: 10.1126/science.1097540

11

Neuroestrogen regulation of socio-sexual behavior of males

Takayoshi Ubuka* and *Kazuyoshi Tsutsui*

Department of Biology and Center for Medical Life Science, Waseda University, Shinjuku, Tokyo, Japan

Correspondence:
Kazuyoshi Tsutsui, Laboratory of Integrative Brain Sciences, Department of Biology, Waseda University, Center for Medical Life Science of Waseda University, 2-2 Wakamatsu-cho, Shinjuku-ku, Tokyo 162-8480, Japan
e-mail: k-tsutsui@waseda.jp

It is thought that estrogen (neuroestrogen) synthesized by the action of aromatase in the brain from testosterone activates male socio-sexual behaviors, such as aggression and sexual behavior in birds. We recently found that gonadotropin-inhibitory hormone (GnIH), a hypothalamic neuropeptide, inhibits socio-sexual behaviors of male quail by directly activating aromatase and increasing neuroestrogen synthesis in the preoptic area (POA). The POA is thought to be the most critical site of aromatization and neuroestrogen action for the regulation of socio-sexual behavior of male birds. We concluded that GnIH inhibits socio-sexual behaviors of male quail by increasing neuroestrogen concentration beyond its optimal concentration in the brain for expression of socio-sexual behavior. On the other hand, it has been reported that dopamine and glutamate, which stimulate male socio-sexual behavior in birds and mammals, inhibit the activity of aromatase in the POA. Multiple studies also report that the activity of aromatase or neuroestrogen is negatively correlated with changes in male socio-sexual behavior in fish, birds, and mammals including humans. Here, we review previous studies that investigated the role of neuroestrogen in the regulation of male socio-sexual behavior and reconsider the hypothesis that neuroestrogen activates male socio-sexual behavior in vertebrates. It is considered that basal concentration of neuroestrogen is required for the maintenance of male socio-sexual behavior but higher concentration of neuroestrogen may inhibit male socio-sexual behavior.

Keywords: neuroestrogen, aromatase, socio-sexual behavior, aggressive behavior, sexual behavior, gonadotropin-inhibitory hormone, glutamate, dopamine

INTRODUCTION

Originally it was considered that males display male-typical behavior because they are exposed to androgen secreted by the testis, whereas females display female-typical behavior because they are exposed to female sex hormones secreted by the ovary, such as 17β-estradiol (E2) and progesterone (Reviewed in Beach, 1948; Balthazart et al., 2004). However, it was later discovered that estrogen is able to activate male-typical behavior in castrated male rats (Beach, 1942). As the male-typical behavior activated by androgen can be blocked by concomitant antiestrogen treatment (Beyer and Vidal, 1971) and because the anterior hypothalamus can synthesize estrogens (neuroestrogen) from androgens by aromatization (Naftolin et al., 1972, 1975), it was hypothesized that central actions of androgen in males require its aromatization into neuroestrogen in the brain (aromatization hypothesis; Yahr, 1979). It was confirmed that aromatizable androgens such as testosterone or androstenedione can activate male sexual behavior in castrates, but non-aromatizable androgen such as 5α-dihydrotestosterone (5α-DHT) has little or no effect in mammals (McDonald et al., 1970; Whalen and Luttge, 1971) and birds (Adkins, 1977; Adkins et al., 1980; Harding et al., 1983). Aromatase inhibitors, such as Fadrozole (FAD) and Vorozole, inhibited or blocked the effect of testosterone on male sexual behavior in mammals (Christensen and Clemens, 1975; Beyer et al., 1976; Morali et al., 1977; Roselli et al., 2003) and birds (Adkins et al., 1980; Walters and Harding, 1988; Balthazart et al., 1990; Schlinger and Callard, 1990; Soma et al., 1999, 2000). It was further shown that male copulatory behavior was severely impaired in the aromatase knockout (ArKO) mouse (Fisher et al., 1998; Honda et al., 1998; Toda et al., 2001b; Matsumoto et al., 2003). Testosterone administration to castrated ArKO mice did not rescue copulatory behavior, but combined treatment with E2 and dihydrotestosterone (DHT) almost completely rescued it (Bakker et al., 2004).

It is widely accepted that the actions of neuroestrogen in the brain are mediated by estrogen receptor α (ERα) and β (ERβ) that belong to the nuclear receptor superfamily, leading to transcriptional regulation of the target genes (Tsai and O'Malley, 1994). It has been shown that E2 can increase cAMP in the uterus of ovariectomized mice within 15 s (Szego and Davis, 1967) suggesting non-genomic actions of E2. As genomic actions of estrogens take hours for changes in protein expression to occur, non-genomic actions of estrogens are defined as rapid effects occurring within seconds to minutes that are generally initiated at the plasma membrane, resulting in the activation of signal transduction pathways, such as kinase activation or calcium flux (Vasudevan and Pfaff, 2008). It is also becoming clear that that the activity of aromatase itself is rapidly regulated by non-genomic mechanism, such as direct phosphorylation of the enzyme (Balthazart et al., 2003; Roselli et al., 2009; Cornil et al., 2012). These results suggest that some factors in the brain may rapidly regulate socio-sexual behaviors of males by controlling the activity of aromatase and neuroestrogen synthesis. Candidates include glutamate and dopamine as they have been reported to rapidly inhibit the activity of aromatase in the brain (Balthazart et al., 2001a,b, 2002, 2006).

Gonadotropin-inhibitory hormone (GnIH) is a hypothalamic neuropeptide that inhibits gonadotropin secretion from the pituitary in birds and mammals (Tsutsui et al., 2000; Kriegsfeld et al., 2006; Ubuka et al., 2006, 2009a, 2012a; for reviews, see Tsutsui, 2009; Tsutsui et al., 2009, 2010; Ubuka and Bentley, 2011; Tsutsui and Ubuka, 2013; Ubuka et al., 2013c). GnIH expression is regulated by daily rhythm or melatonin (Ubuka et al., 2005), stress or glucocorticoid (Kirby et al., 2009; Son et al., 2014), and social environment (Tobari et al., 2014). In birds GnIH is synthesized in the paraventricular nucleus (PVN) in neurons that project to the median eminence (Tsutsui et al., 2000; Ubuka et al., 2003; Ukena et al., 2003). Abundant GnIH-immunoreactive (ir) fibers are observed in the preoptic area (POA) and the periaqueductal central gray (PAG) (Ubuka et al., 2008), where mRNA of the cognate G protein-coupled receptor (GPR147) for GnIH is expressed (Yin et al., 2005; Ubuka et al., 2008). As the POA and PAG are brain areas that regulate socio-sexual behaviors such as aggression and sexual behavior (Absil et al., 2001; Cornil et al., 2012), GnIH released in these brain areas may modify socio-sexual behaviors (Ubuka et al., 2012b, 2013b,c). The medial preoptic area (MPOA) is thought to play an important role in the regulation of male sexual behavior, because damage to the MPOA impairs sexual behavior (Klaric and Hendricks, 1986; Liu et al., 1997; Paredes et al., 1998), whereas MPOA stimulation enhances behavior (Malsbury, 1971; Paredes et al., 1990; Rodríguez-Manzo et al., 2000). The major efferent projections from the MPOA are to hypothalamic, midbrain, and brain stem nuclei that regulate autonomic or somatomotor patterns and motivational states (Simerly and Swanson, 1988).

Male socio-sexual behavior of birds is androgen dependent because it is reduced by castration and restored by androgen treatment (Selinger and Bermant, 1967; Mills et al., 1997), however there is no correlation between the order of aggressiveness and peripheral testosterone concentration (Tsutsui and Ishii, 1981). It is thought that the complete expression of testosterone action requires its aromatization into E2 in the brain, because socio-sexual behaviors of reproductively inactive male birds are only activated by aromatizable androgen, such as testosterone and androstenedione, or E2, but not by non-aromatizable androgen, such as DHT. Indeed the co-administration of aromatase inhibitors blocks testosterone-induced aggression in male quail (Tsutsui and Ishii, 1981; Schlinger and Callard, 1990). Ubuka et al. (2014) hypothesized that GnIH may inhibit socio-sexual behaviors of male quail by regulating aromatase activity and neuroestrogen synthesis in the brain. Their findings suggest that GnIH inhibits socio-sexual behaviors of male quail by directly activating aromatase and increasing neuroestrogen concentration in the POA beyond its optimal concentration (Ubuka et al., 2014; Ubuka and Tsutsui, 2014).

Here we review previous studies that investigated the role of neuroestrogen in the regulation of male socio-sexual behaviors and reconsider the hypothesis that neuroestrogen activates male socio-sexual behaviors in vertebrates. It is proposed that basal concentration of neuroestrogen is required for the maintenance of male socio-sexual behaviors but higher concentration of neuroestrogen may inhibit male socio-sexual behaviors in vertebrates.

MOLECULAR MECHANISMS REGULATING THE ACTIVITY OF AROMATASE AND MALE SOCIO-SEXUAL BEHAVIOR IN BIRDS AND MAMMALS

ACTION OF DOPAMINE IN MAMMALS

Dopamine facilitates sexual behavior in a number of species including humans (Bitran and Hull, 1987; Melis and Argiolas, 1995). Male estrogen receptor α knock-out (ERαKO) mice do not exhibit male-typical sexual behaviors (Wersinger et al., 1997), but treating ERαKO males with apomorphine, a non-selective dopamine agonist which activates both D1-like and D2-like dopamine receptors, stimulated male-typical copulatory behavior (Wersinger and Rissman, 2000a). Dopamine is thought to enhance sensorimotor integration by removing tonic inhibition (Chevalier and Deniau, 1990). Dopamine is not thought to directly elicit behavior, but it is thought to allow hormonally primed output pathways to have easier access to sexually relevant stimuli (Hull et al., 1999).

Three major integrative systems, the nigrostriatal system, the mesolimbic system, and the medial preoptic system, are thought to control sexual motivation and genital and somatomotor responses in male rats. Sensory input from a receptive female and/or copulation elicits the release of dopamine in each of these three integrative systems (Hull et al., 1999). The nigrostriatal system enhances both the readiness to respond to stimuli and motor integration; the mesolimbic system is critical for appetitive behavior and reinforcement, a motivational aspects of behavior but not only sexual motivation; and the medial preoptic system may focus the male's motivation on sexually relevant stimuli, coordinate the genital reflexes necessary for erection and ejaculation, and enhance species-typical motor patterns of copulation (Hull et al., 1999).

Dopaminergic input to the MPOA arises from the periventricular system, including cell bodies in the medial portion of the MPOA and the anterior portion of the incertohypothalamic tract (Simerly et al., 1986). The MPOA is one site where dopamine may promote sexual behavior, because dopamine agonists microinjected into the MPOA facilitate sexual behavior (Hull et al., 1986; Markowski et al., 1994), whereas microinjections of a dopamine antagonist impair copulation, genital reflexes, and sexual motivation to some extent (Pehek et al., 1988; Warner et al., 1991). Extracellular dopamine increases in the MPOA of male rats during precopulatory exposure to an estrous female and during copulation (Hull et al., 1995) and it is thought that both dopamine receptor subtypes (D1 and D2 receptors) are involved in the initiation and rate of copulatory behavior (Blackburn et al., 1992).

ACTION OF DOPAMINE IN BIRDS

Kleitz-Nelson et al. (2010a) developed an *in vivo* microdialysis system to measure dopamine release in the MPOA of quail. Males failed to copulate with a female in the absence of a pre-copulatory rise in dopamine. In contrast, males that showed a substantial increase in MPOA dopamine during pre-copulatory interactions copulated with females. As there was no difference in dopamine during periods when the quail were copulating as compared to when the female was present but the males were not copulating, dopamine action in the MPOA was thought to be linked to sexual motivation rather than copulatory behavior (Kleitz-Nelson et al., 2010a). Kleitz-Nelson et al. (2010b) investigated the role of D1 and D2 receptors on male sexual behavior by examining how intracerebroventricular (i.c.v.) injections and microinjections of D1 and D2 agonists and antagonists into the MPOA influenced sexual behavior in male quail. I.c.v. injections of D1 or D2 agonists and antagonists indicated that D1 receptors facilitated consummatory male sexual behavior, whereas D2 receptors inhibited both appetitive and consummatory behavior.

Immunohistochemical studies have demonstrated that there are dense networks of tyrosine hydroxylase (TH)-ir fibers in brain areas that contain aromatase-ir neurons, such as the sexually dimorphic MPOA or the bed nucleus striae terminalis (BNST) in quail. Double-labeling has confirmed that aromatase-ir cells are in close association with TH-ir fibers in quail (Balthazart et al., 1998). Therefore, the possible existence of a direct modulation of aromatase activity by dopamine and/or norepinephrine was systematically investigated by *in vitro* incubations of quail hypothalamic homogenates (Balthazart et al., 2002). Aromatase activity was quantified by the production of tritiated water from [1β-^{3}H] androstenedione (Baillien and Balthazart, 1997). Norepinephrine had no or very limited effects on aromatase activity. In contrast, dopamine and several D1 and/or D2 receptor agonists [apomorphine (for both D1/D2), SKF-38393 (for D1) and RU-24213 (for D2)] depressed aromatase activity. As the inhibitory effect of the agonists was not antagonized by the D1 antagonist SCH-23390 or the D2 antagonist spiperone, the inhibitory effects of dopamine or dopaminergic compounds were thought not to be mediated through binding to dopamine receptors. Instead dopamine was thought to act as an alternative substrate for aromatase to compete with testosterone and prevent its transformation into neuroestrogens (Balthazart et al., 2002). Accordingly, dopamine should be transported into the aromatase cells in the MPOA by dopamine transporter or internalization of dopamine receptors to inhibit the activity of aromatase existing in the cytosol (**Figure 1**).

REGULATION OF AROMATASE ACTIVITY BY PHOSPHORYLATION

Several consensus sites of phosphorylation are present in aromatase sequences in mammals and birds (Corbin et al., 1988; Harada, 1988; Harada et al., 1992; McPhaul et al., 1988; Means et al., 1989; Shen et al., 1994), so it was hypothesized that phosphorylation may regulate the aromatase activity (Balthazart et al., 2001a,b). Balthazart et al. (2001a) demonstrated that aromatase activity in quail hypothalamic homogenates was rapidly down-regulated by adding Ca^{2+}, Mg^{2+}, ATP, conditions that enhance protein phosphorylation, and this inhibition of aromatase activity was blocked by kinase inhibitors (Balthazart et al., 2001b).

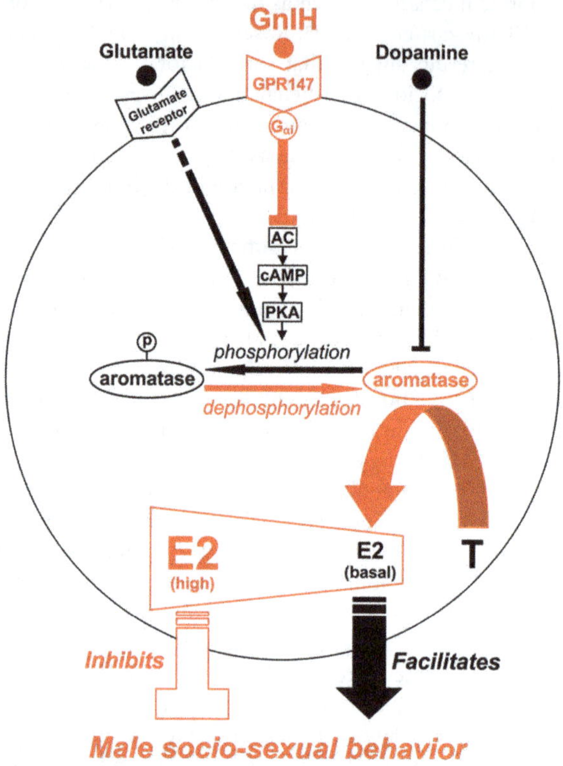

FIGURE 1 | Model of the intracellular mechanism of GnIH and its receptor (GPR147), glutamate and its receptor, dopamine that may control male socio-sexual behavior by regulating the activity of aromatase and neuroestrogen synthesis in the brain. GPR147 is expressed on aromatase immunoreactive cells in the brain. GPR147 is coupled to $G_{\alpha i}$ protein that inhibits the activity of adenylate cyclase (AC) and decreases cAMP production and the activity of protein kinase A (PKA). Inhibition of AC/cAMP/PKA pathway may thus decrease phosphorylated aromatase and increase dephosphorylated aromatase. 17β-estradiol (E2) synthesized from androgen such as testosterone (T) by aromatase in the brain especially in the preoptic area (POA) regulates male aggression. It has been previously demonstrated that aromatase activity is rapidly down-regulated by phosphorylation, and this down-regulation is blocked by kinase inhibitors. The administration of GnIH activates aromatase by decreasing phosphorylated aromatase, and stimulates neuroestrogen synthesis in the brain. Aromatase activity and estrogen concentration in the brain especially in the POA are low in the morning when the birds are active, but aromatase activity and E2 concentration gradually increased until the evening when the birds became inactive. E2 release in the POA also increased in the evening. Finally, centrally administered E2 at higher doses in the morning inhibited aggressive behavior. These results suggest that GnIH inhibits aggressive behavior by directly activating aromatase and increasing neuroestrogen synthesis in the brain beyond its optimum concentration for the expression of aggressive behavior. Glutamate was shown to decrease the activity of aromatase by phosphorylation, and dopamine may act as an alternative substrate for aromatase to compete with testosterone and prevent its transformation into estrogens. Glutamate and dopamine may thus facilitate male socio-sexual behavior by decreasing the activity of aromatase and maintaining the optimum concentration of neuroestrogen for the expression of male socio-sexual behavior.

ACTION OF GLUTAMATE IN BIRDS

Balthazart et al. (2006) further showed that aromatase activity in quail hypothalamic explants was decreased within minutes by glutamate agonists (kainate, AMPA or NMDA), possibly by enhancing intracellular Ca^{2+} concentration and phosphorylation of aromatase. Cornil et al. (2000) visualized the distribution of the major ionotropic glutamate receptors in the quail brain by using primary antibodies raised against rat glutamate receptor 1 and receptors 2–3 (GluR1, GluR2/3: AMPA subtype), glutamate receptors 5–7 (GluR5–7: kainate subtype), and NMDA receptors (NMDAR1). The four types of receptors were broadly distributed in the brain. In particular immunoreactive cells are identified within the major aromatase cell groups located in the MPOA, ventromedial hypothalamus, nucleus striae terminalis, and nucleus taeniae. Dense populations of glutamate receptor-ir cells were also present with a receptor subtype-specific distribution in broad areas of the telencephalon (Cornil et al., 2000).

ACTION OF GLUTAMATE IN MAMMALS

Dominguez et al. (2006) measured glutamate in microdialysate samples from the MPOA before, during, and after copulation by male rats. There was a slight rise in extracellular glutamate when the female was presented, a significant increase during periods of mounting and intromitting, and a very large increase in samples collected during ejaculation with a precipitous fall in the first post ejaculatory sample. Dominguez et al. (2006) also administered a mixture of glutamate uptake inhibitors into the MPOA before and during mating by retromicrodialysis. The mixture increased extracellular glutamate and increased the number of ejaculations in the 40 min test, decreased ejaculation latency, and decreased the post ejaculatory latency to resume copulation. These results strongly suggest that MPOA glutamate is a major facilitator of copulation and the post ejaculatory fall in glutamate regulates the post ejaculatory interval (Dominguez et al., 2006). The results obtained in several species suggest that glutamate facilitates male sexual behavior by decreasing the activity of aromatase by phosphorylation in the MPOA (**Figure 1**).

ACTION OF GNIH IN BIRDS

Ubuka et al. (2014) first measured daily changes in the frequency of aggressive behavior of male quail and tested the effect of i.c.v. administration of GnIH on the frequency of aggressive behavior of male quail in the morning when its natural expression is high. I.c.v. administration of GnIH rapidly inhibited the number of male-typical aggressive behaviors of quail.

As previous studies suggested that full expression of testosterone action in the brain requires its aromatization in birds (Yahr, 1979; Tsutsui and Ishii, 1981; Balthazart and Surlemont, 1990; Schlinger and Callard, 1990; Panzica et al., 1996; Balthazart et al., 2009, 2011), Ubuka et al. (2014) hypothesized that GnIH may inhibit aggressive behavior of male quail by regulating neuroestrogen synthesis in the brain. Abundant GnIH-ir neuronal fibers and aromatase-ir cells were observed in the POA, BNST, mediobasal hypothalamus (MBH), and PAG, where aromatase mRNA is distinctively expressed in the quail brain (Voigt et al., 2007). Merged image of GnIH-ir neuronal fibers and aromatase-ir cells showed close appositions of GnIH-ir neuronal fibers in the vicinity of aromatase-ir cells in these brain areas (Ubuka et al., 2014). *In situ* hybridization for GPR147 mRNA combined with aromatase immunohistochemistry in the POA further showed that almost all aromatase-ir cells observed in the POA expressed GPR147 mRNA.

The effect of GnIH administration on aromatase activity and E2 synthesis in the POA *in vitro* and *in vivo* was examined by Ubuka et al. (2014). GnIH increased the activity of aromatase and E2 in an organ cultured brain block including the POA in a dose dependent manner. Ubuka et al. (2014) have also shown that the administration of a GnIH receptor antagonist RF9 (Simonin et al., 2006; Pineda et al., 2010) or an aromatase inhibitor FAD (Steele et al., 1987; Wade et al., 1994) canceled the stimulatory action of GnIH on E2 synthesis. Together these results indicate that GnIH increases neuroestrogen concentration by increasing the activity of aromatase after binding to GPR147 expressed on aromatase cells in the POA (Ubuka et al., 2014).

It was previously demonstrated that aromatase activity in hypothalamic homogenates of male quail is rapidly down-regulated by phosphorylation, and this inhibition is blocked by kinase inhibitors (Balthazart et al., 2001a,b, 2003, 2006; Charlier et al., 2011a). In order to investigate if GnIH activates aromatase by dephosphorylation of phosphorylated aromatase, Ubuka et al. (2014) measured phosphorylated aromatase by the Phos-Tag SDS PAGE method (Kinoshita et al., 2006) in the brain block including the POA of birds that were centrally administered with GnIH or vehicle in the morning. I.c.v. administration of GnIH reduced phosphorylated aromatase in the POA 30 min after administration (Ubuka et al., 2014).

Aromatase activity is not only controlled in the long term (hours to days) by transcription of the aromatase gene by steroids, but also in the short term (minutes) by phosphorylation by neurotransmitters, such as glutamate (Balthazart et al., 2006). GnIH was shown to be the first neuropeptide that can stimulate aromatase activity in the medium term (minutes to hours) (Ubuka et al., 2014). GnIH receptor GPR147 has been shown to couple predominantly through the $G_{\alpha i}$ protein to inhibit cAMP production in mammals (Hinuma et al., 2000; Ubuka et al., 2009b, 2012c, 2013c; Son et al., 2012). Son et al. (2012) investigated the cell signaling process of GPR147 using LβT2 cells, a mouse gonadotrope cell line, and it was shown that GnIH inhibits gonadotropin-releasing hormone (GnRH) induced gonadotropin subunit gene transcriptions by inhibiting adenylate cyclase (AC)/cAMP/PKA dependent ERK phosphorylation. As mentioned above, the action of GnIH on E2 synthesis in the POA was prevented by concomitant administration of RF9, a potent GPR147 antagonist, or FAD, an aromatase inhibitor (Ubuka et al., 2014). Ubuka et al. (2014) further demonstrated that i.c.v. administration of GnIH reduces phosphorylated aromatase in the POA. Previous studies have shown that aromatase activity is inhibited by phosphorylation in hypothalamic and ovarian homogenates of quail (Balthazart et al., 2001a,b, 2003) and in various cell lines transfected with human aromatase (Charlier et al., 2011a). Accordingly, it is highly possible that GnIH stimulates neuroestrogen synthesis in the POA by activating aromatase through dephosphorylation after binding to GPR147 expressed on aromatase cells (**Figure 1**).

ENVIRONMENTAL OR SOCIAL FACTORS THAT MODULATE AROMATASE ACTIVITY IN MALE BIRDS

EFFECT OF DAILY RHYTHM

When sexually active male quail are paired in a relatively small cage they fight using sequential aggressive actions. They often threaten the opponent by stretching the neck and walking around (strutting), approach and chase, peck the opponent (pecking), grab the back of the opponent's head or neck with their beak (grabbing), attempt to mount the opponent (mounting), mounting the opponent and lowering their cloaca close to the opponent's cloaca (cloacal contact (CC)-like actions). The frequency of these actions represents the activity of aggressive or sexual behavior of male quail (Selinger and Bermant, 1967; Tsutsui and Ishii, 1981; Schlinger and Callard, 1990; Mills et al., 1997).

Ubuka et al. (2014) quantified strutting, pecking, grabbing, mounting, and CC-like actions in 5 min during the light hours around zietgeiber time (ZT) 3, 6, 9, and 12 h. All male quail used in the experiment were kept under long day photoperiods (16 h light, 8 h dark) to keep them sexually active. The frequency of strutting, pecking, and grabbing actions was significantly higher in the morning (ZT 3 h) and decreased in the afternoon (ZT 9 h) and the evening (ZT 12 h). The frequency of mounting and CC-like actions was also high in the morning and tended to decrease until the evening.

Aromatase activity was assessed by measuring the conversion of [^{3}H]androstenedione to [^{3}H]E2 using brain homogenates or organ cultured quail brain blocks (Ubuka et al., 2014). Aromatase activity in the brain block including the POA or BSTM was low in the morning (ZT 3 h) and increased in the evening (ZT 12 h). The change in aromatase activity in the other brain blocks showed similar trends. E2 content and release in the POA was also low in the morning (ZT 3 h) and increased in the evening (ZT 12 h) possibly by the action of activated aromatase by dephosphorylation. Ubuka et al. (2014) also measured daily changes in E2 and testosterone concentrations in the serum, because changes in aromatase activity or E2 concentration in the brain may have reflected changes in E2 or testosterone concentration in the circulation. However, there was no daily change in E2 and testosterone concentrations in the serum.

EFFECT OF SOCIAL INTERACTION

Cornil et al. (2005) measured aromatase activity in hypothalamic/preoptic area (HPOA) homogenates of male quail following visual access to or copulation with a female. Sexual interactions resulted in a decrease in aromatase activity that reached its maximum after 5 min (Cornil et al., 2005). The time course of the effect of copulation on aromatase activity was also measured specifically in the different populations in the brain expressing high levels of aromatase activity (Schumacher and Balthazart, 1987) of male quail that experienced varying durations of visual exposure to or copulation with a female by the Palkovits punch method (de Bournonville et al., 2013). Sexual interactions resulted in a rapid inhibition of aromatase activity in specific brain regions including the MPOA and the tuberal hypothalamus (de Bournonville et al., 2013). The rapid decrease in neuroestrogen concentration in the MPOA may be important during the motivational phase of the behavior to trigger physiological events essential to activate mate search and thus copulation.

EFFECT OF STRESS

Balthazart et al. (2009) showed that exposing male quail to acute restraint stress for 15 min or injecting corticosterone 30 min before brain collection results in a significant increase in aromatase activity in HPOA homogenates. Dickens et al. (2011) investigated the effects of acute stress on aromatase activity in both sexes by measuring enzyme activity in all aromatase-expressing brain nuclei before, during, and after 30 min of acute restraint stress. Acute stress rapidly increased aromatase activity in the male MPOA in 5 min. This elevated activity persisted as long as the stressor was present and returned to control levels within 30 min after stress cessation (Dickens et al., 2011). These results suggest that stress rapidly increases aromatase activity in the brain of birds.

AROMATASE ACTIVITY, NEUROESTROGEN CONCENTRATION AND SOCIO-SEXUAL BEHAVIOR OF MALE VERTEBRATES

STUDIES IN FISH

Huffman et al. (2013) tested the role of aromatase in mediating aggression and reproductive behavior of male *Astatotilapia burtoni*, an African cichlid fish that display plasticity in social behavior. They found that subordinate males have higher aromatase expression than dominant males in the magnocellular and gigantocellular regions of the POA that regulate social behavior. Intraperitoneal injections into dominant male fish with FAD decreased aggressive, but not reproductive behavior. Indeed FAD treated males had increased aromatase expression in the gigantocellular portion of the POA (Huffman et al., 2013). These results suggest aromatase expression in the POA is negatively correlated with dominance or aggression in male *A. burtoni*.

Black et al. (2005) investigated the effect of social environmental change on aggressive behavior and brain aromatase activity in a sex-changing fish, *Lythrypnus dalli*. Male removal from a socially stable group results in rapid increases in aggression in the dominant female, which will later become male. These dominant females, and recently sex-changed individuals, had lower brain aromatase activity compared with control females and the established males had the lowest brain aromatase activity. Within hours of male removal, dominant females' aggressive behavior was inversely related to brain aromatase activity (Black et al., 2005). These results suggest that high E2 concentration in the brain caused by higher aromatase activity may inhibit aggressive behavior so that E2 concentration and aromatase activity should be reduced to increase aggressiveness and dominance within the social group.

Lord et al. (2009) tested the effects of testosterone, E2, and FAD on approach responses toward females in male goldfish (*Carassius auratus*). Injections of testosterone stimulated approach responses toward the visual cues of females 30–45 min later. E2 produced the same effect 30–45 min and even 10–25 min after administration and treatment with FAD blocked the exogenous effect of testosterone. The authors suggest that the testosterone surge induced by sexual stimuli may rapidly prime males to mate by increasing sensitivity within visual pathways that guide approach responses toward females and/or by increasing the motivation to approach potential mates. These actions occur within traditional limbic circuits, and the aromatization of testosterone maybe important for the male approach response toward females (Lord et al., 2009).

STUDIES IN BIRDS

Historically studies in birds that have reported the involvement of aromatase in male sexual behavior and the stimulatory effect of E2 on male sexual behavior have used castrated male quail (Adkins, 1977) or reproductively inactivated male quail by photoperiodic manipulation (Adkins et al., 1980). Single doses of various steroids were administered peripherally to reproductively inactive birds for days or weeks to compare their effects (Adkins, 1977; Adkins et al., 1980; Tsutsui and Ishii, 1981; Wada, 1982; Schlinger and Callard, 1990). These studies are likely to have shown the genomic effects of E2 and other sex steroids on the brain that facilitated socio-sexual behaviors, which were attenuated by castration or photoperiodic manipulation.

Silverin et al. (2004) investigated the relationships among territorial aggression and brain aromatase activity in pied flycatcher, *Ficedula hypoleuca*, at the peak of the reproductive season. Aggressive behavior was measured during a simulated territorial intrusion in unpaired males holding primary territories. A significant correlation was observed between number of attacks/min displayed during the simulated territorial intrusion and aromatase activity in the anterior diencephalon but not in the posterior diencephalon and telencephalon (Silverin et al., 2004). These results suggest that aromatase activity in the anterior diencephalon is important for territorial aggression. Charlier et al. (2011b) exposed wild male white-crowned sparrows in the late breeding season to simulated territorial intrusion (STI) (song playback and live decoy) for 30 min. Although STI significantly increased aggressive behavior aromatase activity was not affected in the brain regions collected using the Palkovits punch technique. STI did not affect circulating levels of E2, but rapidly reduced E2 concentrations in the hippocampus, ventromedial nucleus of the hypothalamus and bed nucleus of the stria terminalis (Charlier et al., 2011b).

Many species also defend territories in the non-breeding season, when circulating testosterone levels are low. Castration of the western male song sparrow *Melospiza melodia morphna* had no effect on aggression in the non-breeding season, suggesting that autumnal territoriality is independent of gonadal hormones. Soma et al. (2000) treated wild, free-living non-breeding male song sparrows with FAD using micro-osmotic pumps. FAD greatly reduced aggressive behavior, and the effects of FAD were rescued by E2 replacement. These data indicate that E2 regulates male aggression despite low circulating levels of sex steroids or despite castration (Soma et al., 2000). Studies in diverse avian and mammalian species suggested that adrenal dehydroepiandrosterone (DHEA), an androgen precursor and prohormone, is important for aggressive behavior when gonadal testosterone is low and circulating DHEA can be converted into active sex steroids within the brain (Soma et al., 2014).

To investigate the physiological role of GnIH in the stimulation of E2 synthesis in the brain, Ubuka et al. (2014) analyzed the effects of i.c.v. administration of GnIH on E2 concentration in the brain and aggressiveness (peck frequency against the standard bird) of individual birds. I.c.v. administration of GnIH increased E2 concentration in the brain blocks including the POA or PAG, 30 min after administration. This was associated with a significant decrease in the frequency of pecking in the morning (ZT 2–4 h). As i.c.v. administration of GnIH stimulated E2 synthesis in the brain and inhibited the frequency of pecking actions, it was hypothesized that the high concentration of E2 in the brain may inhibit aggressive behavior. To test this hypothesis Ubuka et al. (2014) centrally administered various doses of E2 and measured five stereotypic actions of aggressive behavior in the morning (ZT 2–6 h). I.c.v. administration of E2 at 1 ng increased the frequency of CC-like action compared with vehicle administered birds. However, i.c.v. administrations of E2 at 10 ng, 100 ng, 1 μg, and 10 μg inhibited the frequency of pecking, grabbing, mounting, and CC-like actions compared with vehicle or 1 ng E2 administered birds (Ubuka et al., 2014). These results suggest that high concentrations of neuroestrogen inhibit socio-sexual behaviors of male quail although basal concentration of neuroestrogen facilitates socio-sexual behaviors (Ubuka and Tsutsui, 2014).

STUDIES IN RODENTS

Compaan et al. (1994) measured the brain aromatase activity in the POA, amygdaloid nuclei (Am), ventromedial hypothalamus (VMH), and parietal cortex (CTX) from two strains of adult male house mice, which were genetically selected for territorial aggression, based upon their attack latencies (short attack latency: SAL; long attack latency: LAL). Non aggressive LAL males had higher aromatase activity in the POA compared to aggressive SAL animals. The aromatase activity levels in both the VMH and Am did not differ significantly between strains. Aromatase activity was higher in POA than VMH in nonaggressive LAL males, whereas aromatase activity was higher in VMH than POA in aggressive SAL males. In both selection lines, the Am exhibited the highest levels of aromatase activity, as compared to the other investigated areas (Compaan et al., 1994).

Toda et al. (2001a,b) generated ArKO mice by targeting disruption of the CYP19 (aromatase) gene. They observed that ArKO males exhibited a complete loss of aggressive behavior in a resident-intruder paradigm. The behavior of ArKO males was partially reinstated when the mice received supplements of E2 soon after birth until the day of testing, but it was not restored when the supplementation was started at 7 days after birth (Toda et al., 2001a,b). These results suggest that neuroestrogen is required to construct neuronal infrastructure for aggressive behavior after birth and to maintain it in adult male mice.

Harada et al. (2009) also generated ArKO mice, which showed undetectable estrogen and enhanced androgen levels in blood. These ArKO mice exhibited enhanced appetite and displayed disorders in sexual motivation, sexual partnership preference, sexual performance, aggressive behavior, parental behavior, infanticide behavior and exploratory (anxiety) behavior. By introducing a transgene of human aromatase, controlled by the minimal promoter region, into the ArKO mouse they showed near recovery from behavioral disorders. This transgenic mouse line (ArKO/hArom) have a POA, hypothalamus and amygdala that are exposed to neuroestrogen only in the perinatal period, and then to enhanced androgens but no neuroestrogen exposure in adulthood, These results suggest that neuroestrogen acting in specific brain regions are important to organize sex-specific neural networks during the perinatal period (Harada et al., 2009).

STUDIES IN NON HUMAN PRIMATES

Phoenix (1974) studied the sexual and sex-related behavior of adult male rhesus monkeys castrated 3 years earlier in pair tests with receptive females. The performance before, and during, daily treatment with 1 mg/kg dihydrotestosterone propionate (DHTP), a non-aromatizable androgen, was compared. It was shown that DHTP effectively rendered the performance level of the castrates comparable to that of the intact controls (Phoenix, 1974). This result suggests that aromatization of androgen is not required for male sexual behavior in this monkey species.

Zumpe et al. (1996) tested the effect of medroxyprogesterone acetate (MPA) (that reduces androgen uptake by brain), FAD, and E2 on the sexual motivation and behavior of castrated and testosterone treated male cynomolgus monkeys, *Macaca fascicularis.* Sexual motivation reflected in mounting attempts and mounting attempt latencies was diminished by E2 treatment in males receiving both MPA and FAD, but ejaculatory activity was unchanged (Zumpe et al., 1996). These results suggest that although testosterone and basal concentration of neuroestrogen is required for sexual motivation of males, higher concentration of neuroestrogen may inhibit sexual motivation reflected in mounting attempts.

STUDIES IN HUMANS

Gooren (1985) reported that administration of tamoxifen, estrogen receptor antagonist, or testolactone, an aromatase inhibitor, had no effect on male human sexual function. Replacement of testosterone substitution therapy of agonadal men by DHT, non-aromatizable androgen, was not associated with any change of sexual functioning. Administration of DHT to eugonadal men led to a transient increase in nocturnal sexual dreams, erections and irritability. It was concluded that aromatization of testosterone is not required and that DHT maintains sexual functions in the adult male with an established sex life (Gooren, 1985).

Kyomen et al. (1999) performed a randomized, double-blind, placebo-controlled clinical trial to investigate the efficacy and safety of short-term estrogen therapy in decreasing aggressive behavior in elderly patients with moderate-to-severe dementia. They found that estrogen therapy was associated with lower total aggression scores and with decreased frequency of physical aggression over the 4-week trial and no adverse effects of estrogen were observed during the course of the study (Kyomen et al., 1999).

Orengo et al. (2002) investigated if testosterone and estrogen levels correlate with aggression in older men with dementia. Plasma total and free testosterone and estrogen levels and scores for behavioral disturbances, in particular aggression, were measured in elderly males who had a diagnosis of dementia. They found that free testosterone levels showed significant positive correlations with measures of aggression, but plasma estrogen levels showed significant negative correlations with measures of aggression (Orengo et al., 2002).

CONCLUSION AND POSSIBLE MECHANISM

In this review we give an account of studies that have investigated the role of neuroestrogen or estrogen on socio-sexual behavior of males. Many correlational studies in fish, birds, and mammals suggest that male aggression or sexual behavior and aromatase activities in the brain are negatively correlated. Basal activity of aromatase appears to be required for male socio-sexual behaviors especially during development when neuronal infrastructure for male socio-sexual behavior is constructed or organized in the brain. As administration of aromatase inhibitor such as FAD decreases socio-sexual behaviors of adult males in many animals, aromatase and neuroestrogen seem to be also important for the maintenance of neuronal infrastructure for male socio-sexual behavior in adulthood. However, neuroestrogen may not be important for the maintenance of male socio-sexual behavior in some monkeys and humans. We speculate that this may be because of the relative roles that a developed cerebrum plays in the socio-sexual behavior of primates. Higher concentrations of neuroestrogen or estrogen may inhibit aggressive behavior in adulthood that was experimentally shown in male quail and elderly human males with dementia.

Although dopamine and glutamate stimulate male socio-sexual behaviors in birds and mammals, it was shown that they inhibit aromatase activity in the POA that is thought to be the most critical site of aromatization and neuroestrogen action for the regulation of male socio-sexual behaviors. These results further suggest that higher concentration of neuroestrogen especially in the POA may inhibit male socio-sexual behavior. Dopamine may act as an alternative substrate for aromatase to compete with testosterone and prevent its transformation into neuroestrogen. Accordingly, dopamine may facilitate male socio-sexual behavior by decreasing aromatase activity in the cytosol after it enters the cell through dopamine transporter or receptor internalization. Glutamate was shown to decrease the activity of aromatase by phosphorylation of aromatase, whereas GnIH increases the activity of aromatase by its dephosphorylation. The effects of glutamate and GnIH on phosphorylation or dephosphorylation of aromatase are likely to be achieved by cell signaling processes triggered after binding to their receptors. Even if dopamine, glutamate, and GnIH can rapidly change the activity of aromatase and neuroestrogen concentration in the POA, we consider that neuroestrogen in the POA may not directly regulate the movement of the body to perform socio-sexual behaviors because synthesized neuroestrogen could not be degraded in milliseconds after constrictions and relaxations of related muscles, instead different concentrations of neuroestrogen is likely to facilitate or inhibit the action of neurotransmitters and neuromodulators, including dopamine, glutamate, and GnIH, which are released according to social or natural, favorable or unfavorable environment.

The key question arising from the above hypothesis is what is the possible mechanism of neuroestrogen action according to its concentration from facilitation to inhibition on male socio-sexual behavior? It was shown that ERαKO male mice display decreased aggression toward intruders in resident-intruder tests

(Ogawa et al., 1997). In contrast ERβKO male mice are more aggressive than wild type mice in resident-intruder tests (Ogawa et al., 1999). There are also studies showing different roles of ER subtypes on the behavior. ERα was shown to be essential for female-directed chemo-investigatory behavior of males (Wersinger and Rissman, 2000b) and ERβ was shown to regulate anxiety behavior (Choleris et al., 2003; Imwalle et al., 2005; Lund et al., 2005). It may be possible that neuroestrogen regulates different ER subtypes depending on its concentration in the brain. Further studies including detailed analyses of the localization of aromatase and ER subtypes and the time-course of their activations are required to answer this question.

ACKNOWLEDGMENTS

We thank Dr. Simone Meddle (The Roslin Institute, The University of Edinburgh, UK) for her valuable discussion on the manuscript. This work was supported by Grants-in-Aid for Scientific Research from the Ministry of Education, Science and Culture, Japan (23570091 to Takayoshi Ubuka; 22132004 and 22227002 to Kazuyoshi Tsutsui).

REFERENCES

Absil, P., Riters, L. V., and Balthazart, J. (2001). Preoptic aromatase cells project to the mesencephalic central gray in the male Japanese quail (*Coturnix japonica*). *Horm. Behav.* 40, 369–383. doi: 10.1006/hbeh.2001.1702

Adkins, E. K. (1977). Effects of diverse androgens on the sexual behavior and morphology of castrated male quail. *Horm. Behav.* 8, 201–207. doi: 10.1016/0018-506X(77)90037-X

Adkins, E. K., Boop, J. J., Koutnik, D. L., Morris, J. B., and Pniewski, E. E. (1980). Further evidence that androgen aromatization is essential for the activation of copulation in male quail. *Physiol. Behav.* 24, 441–446. doi: 10.1016/0031-9384(80)90233-4

Baillien, M., and Balthazart, J. (1997). A direct dopaminergic control of aromatase activity in the quail preoptic area. *J. Steroid Biochem. Mol. Biol.* 63, 99–113. doi: 10.1016/S0960-0760(97)00080-0

Bakker, J., Honda, S., Harada, N., and Balthazart, J. (2004). Restoration of male sexual behavior by adult exogenous estrogens in male aromatase knockout mice. *Horm. Behav.* 46, 1–10. doi: 10.1016/j.yhbeh.2004.02.003

Balthazart, J., Baillien, M., and Ball, G. F. (2001a). Rapid and reversible inhibition of brain aromatase activity. *J. Neuroendocrinol.* 13, 63–73. doi: 10.1046/j.1365-2826.2001.00598.x

Balthazart, J., Baillien, M., and Ball, G. F. (2001b). Phosphorylation processes mediate rapid changes of brain aromatase activity. *J. Steroid Biochem. Mol. Biol.* 79, 261–277. doi: 10.1016/S0960-0760(01)00143-1

Balthazart, J., Baillien, M., and Ball, G. F. (2002). Interactions between aromatase (estrogen synthase) and dopamine in the control of male sexual behavior in quail. *Comp. Biochem. Physiol. B Biochem. Mol. Biol.* 132, 37–55. doi: 10.1016/S1096-4959(01)00531-0

Balthazart, J., Baillien, M., and Ball, G. F. (2006). Rapid control of brain aromatase activity by glutamatergic inputs. *Endocrinology* 147, 359–366. doi: 10.1210/en.2005-0845

Balthazart, J., Baillien, M., Charlier, T. D., and Ball, G. F. (2003). Calcium-dependent phosphorylation processes control brain aromatase in quail. *Eur. J. Neurosci.* 17, 1591–1606. doi: 10.1046/j.1460-9568.2003.02598.x

Balthazart, J., Baillien, M., Cornil, C. A., and Ball, G. F. (2004). Preoptic aromatase modulates male sexual behavior: slow and fast mechanisms of action. *Physiol. Behav.* 83, 247–270. doi: 10.1016/j.physbeh.2004.08.025

Balthazart, J., Charlier, T. D., Cornil, C. A., Dickens, M. J., Harada, N., Konkle, A. T., et al. (2011). Sex differences in brain aromatase activity: genomic and non-genomic controls. *Front. Endocrinol. (Lausanne)* 2:34. doi: 10.3389/fendo.2011.00034

Balthazart, J., Cornil, C. A., Charlier, T. D., Taziaux, M., and Ball, G. F. (2009). Estradiol, a key endocrine signal in the sexual differentiation and activation of reproductive behavior in quail. *J. Exp. Zool. A Ecol. Genet. Physiol.* 311, 323–345. doi: 10.1002/jez.464

Balthazart, J., Evrard, L., and Surlemont, C. (1990). Effects of the nonsteroidal inhibitor R76713 on testosterone-induced sexual behavior in the Japanese quail (*Coturnix coturnix japonica*). *Horm. Behav.* 24, 510–531. doi: 10.1016/0018-506X(90)90039-Z

Balthazart, J., Foidart, A., Baillien, M., Harada, N., and Ball, G. F. (1998). Anatomical relationships between aromatase and tyrosine hydroxylase in the quail brain: double-label immunocytochemical studies. *J. Comp. Neurol.* 391, 214–226.

Balthazart, J., and Surlemont, C. (1990). Androgen and estrogen action in the preoptic area and activation of copulatory behavior in quail. *Physiol. Behav.* 48, 599–609. doi: 10.1016/0031-9384(90)90198-D

Beach, F. A. (1942). Copulatory behavior in prepubertally castrated male rats and its modification by estrogen administration. *Endocrinology* 31, 679–683. doi: 10.1210/endo-31-6-679

Beach, F. A. (1948). *Hormones and Behavior*. New York, NY: Paul B. Hoeber, Inc.

Beyer, C., Moralí, G., Naftolin, F., Larsson, K., and Pérez-palacios, G. (1976). Effect of some antiestrogens and aromatase inhibitors on androgen induced sexual behavior in castrated male rats. *Horm. Behav.* 7, 353–363. doi: 10.1016/0018-506X(76)90040-4

Beyer, C., and Vidal, N. (1971). Inhibitory action of MER-25 on adnrogen-induced oestrous behaviour in the ovariectomized rabbit. *J. Endocrinol.* 51, 401–402. doi: 10.1677/joe.0.0510401

Bitran, D., and Hull, E. M. (1987). Pharmacological analysis of male rat sexual behavior. *Neurosci. Biobehav. Rev.* 11, 365–389. doi: 10.1016/S0149-7634(87)80008-8

Black, M. P., Balthazart, J., Baillien, M., and Grober, M. S. (2005). Socially induced and rapid increases in aggression are inversely related to brain aromatase activity in a sex-changing fish, *Lythrypnus dalli*. *Proc. Biol. Sci.* 272, 2435–2440. doi: 10.1098/rspb.2005.3210

Blackburn, J. R., Pfaus, J. G., and Phillips, A. G. (1992). Dopamine functions in appetitive and defensive behaviours. *Prog. Neurobiol.* 39, 247–279. doi: 10.1016/0301-0082(92)90018-A

Charlier, T. D., Harada, N., Balthazart, J., and Cornil, C. A. (2011a). Human and quail aromatase activity is rapidly and reversibly inhibited by phosphorylating conditions. *Endocrinology* 152, 4199–4210. doi: 10.1210/en.2011-0119

Charlier, T. D., Newman, A. E., Heimovics, S. A., Po, K. W., Saldanha, C. J., and Soma, K. K. (2011b). Rapid effects of aggressive interactions on aromatase activity and oestradiol in discrete brain regions of wild male white-crowned sparrows. *J. Neuroendocrinol.* 23, 742–753. doi: 10.1111/j.1365-2826.2011.02170.x

Chevalier, G., and Deniau, J. M. (1990). Disinhibition as a basic process in the expression of striatal functions. *Trends Neurosci.* 13, 277–280. doi: 10.1016/0166-2236(90)90109-N

Choleris, E., Gustafsson, J. A., Korach, K. S., Muglia, L. J., Pfaff, D. W., and Ogawa, S. (2003). An estrogen-dependent four-gene micronet regulating social recognition: a study with oxytocin and estrogen receptor-alpha and -beta knockout mice. *Proc. Natl. Acad. Sci. U.S.A.* 100, 6192–6197. doi: 10.1073/pnas.0631699100

Christensen, L. W., and Clemens, L. G. (1975). Blockade of testosterone-induced mounting behavior in the male rat with intracranial application of the aromatization inhibitor, androst-1,4,6,-triene-3,17-dione. *Endocrinology* 97, 1545–1551. doi: 10.1210/endo-97-6-1545

Compaan, J. C., Wozniak, A., De Ruiter, A. J., Koolhaas, J. M., and Hutchison, J. B. (1994). Aromatase activity in the preoptic area differs between aggressive and nonaggressive male house mice. *Brain Res. Bull.* 35, 1–7. doi: 10.1016/0361-9230(94)90208-9

Corbin, C. J., Graham-Lorence, S., McPhaul, M., Mason, J. I., Mendelson, C. R., and Simpson, E. R. (1988). Isolation of a full-length cDNA insert encoding human aromatase system cytochrome P-450 and its expression in nonsteroidogenic cells. *Proc. Natl. Acad. Sci. U.S.A.* 85, 8948–8952. doi: 10.1073/pnas.85.23.8948

Cornil, C. A., Ball, G. F., and Balthazart, J. (2012). Rapid control of male typical behaviors by brain-derived estrogens. *Front. Neuroendocrinol.* 33, 425–446. doi: 10.1016/j.yfrne.2012.08.003

Cornil, C. A., Dalla, C., Papadopoulou-Daifoti, Z., Baillien, M., Dejace, C., Ball, G. F., et al. (2005). Rapid decreases in preoptic aromatase activity and brain monoamine concentrations after engaging in male sexual behavior. *Endocrinology* 146, 3809–3820. doi: 10.1210/en.2005-0441

Cornil, C., Foidart, A., Minet, A., and Balthazart, J. (2000). Immunocytochemical localization of ionotropic glutamate receptors subunits in the adult quail forebrain. *J. Comp. Neurol.* 428, 577–608. doi: 10.1002/1096-9861(20001225)428:4<577::AID-CNE1>3.0.CO;2-K

de Bournonville, C., Dickens, M. J., Ball, G. F., Balthazart, J., and Cornil, C. A. (2013). Dynamic changes in brain aromatase activity following sexual interactions in males: where, when and why? *Psychoneuroendocrinology* 38, 789–799. doi: 10.1016/j.psyneuen.2012.09.001

Dickens, M. J., Cornil, C. A., and Balthazart, J. (2011). Acute stress differentially affects aromatase activity in specific brain nuclei of adult male and female quail. *Endocrinology* 152, 4242–4251. doi: 10.1210/en.2011-1341

Dominguez, J. M., Gil, M., and Hull, E. M. (2006). Preoptic glutamate facilitates male sexual behavior. *J. Neurosci.* 26, 1699–1703. doi: 10.1523/JNEUROSCI.4176-05.2006

Fisher, C. R., Graves, K. H., Parlow, A. F., and Simpson, E. R. (1998). Characterization of mice deficient in aromatase (ArKO) because of targeted disruption of the cyp19 gene. *Proc. Natl. Acad. Sci. U.S.A.* 95, 6965–6970. doi: 10.1073/pnas.95.12.6965

Gooren, L. J. (1985). Human male sexual functions do not require aromatization of testosterone: a study using tamoxifen, testolactone, and dihydrotestosterone. *Arch. Sex. Behav.* 14, 539–548. doi: 10.1007/BF01541754

Harada, N. (1988). Cloning of a complete cDNA encoding human aromatase: immunochemical identification and sequence analysis. *Biochem. Biophys. Res. Commun.* 156, 725–732. doi: 10.1016/S0006-291X(88)80903-3

Harada, N., Wakatsuki, T., Aste, N., Yoshimura, N., and Honda, S. I. (2009). Functional analysis of neurosteroidal oestrogen using gene-disrupted and transgenic mice. *J. Neuroendocrinol.* 21, 365–369. doi: 10.1111/j.1365-2826.2009.01857.x

Harada, N., Yamada, K., Foidart, A., and Balthazart, J. (1992). Regulation of aromatase cytochrome P-450 (estrogen synthetase) transcripts in the quail brain by testosterone. *Brain Res. Mol. Brain Res.* 15, 19–26. doi: 10.1016/0169-328X(92)90146-3

Harding, C. F., Sheridan, K., and Walters, M. J. (1983). Hormonal specificity and activation of sexual behavior in male zebra finches. *Horm. Behav.* 17, 111–133. doi: 10.1016/0018-506X(83)90021-1

Hinuma, S., Shintani, Y., Fukusumi, S., Iijima, N., Matsumoto, Y., Hosoya, M., et al. (2000). New neuropeptides containing carboxy-terminal RFamide and their receptor in mammals. *Nat. Cell Biol.* 2, 703–708. doi: 10.1038/35036326

Honda, S., Harada, N., Ito, S., Takagi, Y., and Maeda, S. (1998). Disruption of sexual behavior in male aromatase-deficient mice lacking exons 1 and 2 of the cyp19 gene. *Biochem. Biophys. Res. Commun.* 252, 445–449. doi: 10.1006/bbrc.1998.9672

Huffman, L. S., O'Connell, L. A., and Hofmann, H. A. (2013). Aromatase regulates aggression in the African cichlid fish *Astatotilapia burtoni*. *Physiol. Behav.* 112–113, 77–83. doi: 10.1016/j.physbeh.2013.02.004

Hull, E. M., Bitran, D., Pehek, E. A., Warner, R. K., Band, L. C., and Holmes, G. M. (1986). Dopaminergic control of male sex behavior in rats: effects of an intracerebrally-infused agonist. *Brain Res.* 370, 73–81. doi: 10.1016/0006-8993(86)91106-6

Hull, E. M., Du, J., Lorrain, D. S., and Matuszewich, L. (1995). Extracellular dopamine in the medial preoptic area: implications for sexual motivation and hormonal control of copulation. *J. Neurosci.* 15, 7465–7471.

Hull, E. M., Lorrain, D. S., Du, J., Matuszewich, L., Lumley, L. A., Putnam, S. K., et al. (1999). Hormone-neurotransmitter interactions in the control of sexual behavior. *Behav. Brain Res.* 105, 105–116. doi: 10.1016/S0166-4328(99)00086-8

Imwalle, D. B., Gustafsson, J. A., and Rissman, E. F. (2005). Lack of functional estrogen receptor beta influences anxiety behavior and serotonin content in female mice. *Physiol. Behav.* 84, 157–163. doi: 10.1016/j.physbeh.2004.11.002

Kinoshita, E., Kinoshita-Kikuta, E., Takiyama, K., and Koike, T. (2006). Phosphate-binding tag, a new tool to visualize phosphorylated proteins. *Mol. Cell. Proteomics.* 5, 749–757. doi: 10.1074/mcp.T500024-MCP200

Kirby, E. D., Geraghty, A. C., Ubuka, T., Bentley, G. E., and Kaufer, D. (2009). Stress increases putative gonadotropin inhibitory hormone and decreases luteinizing hormone in male rats. *Proc. Natl. Acad. Sci. U.S.A.* 106, 11324–11329. doi: 10.1073/pnas.0901176106

Klaric, J. S., and Hendricks, S. E. (1986). Effects of two-stage lesions of the medial preoptic area on sexual behavior of male rats. *Physiol. Behav.* 37, 539–542. doi: 10.1016/0031-9384(86)90281-7

Kleitz-Nelson, H. K., Cornil, C. A., Balthazart, J., and Ball, G. F. (2010b). Differential effects of central injections of D1 and D2 receptor agonists and antagonists on male sexual behavior in Japanese quail. *Eur. J. Neurosci.* 32, 118–129. doi: 10.1111/j.1460-9568.2010.07257.x

Kleitz-Nelson, H. K., Dominguez, J. M., and Ball, G. F. (2010a). Dopamine release in the medial preoptic area is related to hormonal action and sexual motivation. *Behav. Neurosci.* 124, 773–779. doi: 10.1037/a0021490

Kriegsfeld, L. J., Mei, D. F., Bentley, G. E., Ubuka, T., Mason, A. O., Inoue, K., et al. (2006). Identification and characterization of a gonadotropin-inhibitory system in the brains of mammals. *Proc. Natl. Acad. Sci. U.S.A.* 103, 2410–2415. doi: 10.1073/pnas.0511003103

Kyomen, H. H., Satlin, A., Hennen, J., and Wei, J. Y. (1999). Estrogen therapy and aggressive behavior in elderly patients with moderate-to-severe dementia: results from a short-term, randomized, double-blind trial. *Am. J. Geriatr. Psychiatry.* 7, 339–348.

Liu, Y. C., Salamone, J. D., and Sachs, B. D. (1997). Lesions in medial preoptic area and bed nucleus of stria terminalis: differential effects on copulatory behavior and noncontact erection in male rats. *J. Neurosci.* 17, 5245–5253.

Lord, L. D., Bond, J., and Thompson, R. R. (2009). Rapid steroid influences on visually guided sexual behavior in male goldfish. *Horm. Behav.* 56, 519–526. doi: 10.1016/j.yhbeh.2009.09.002

Lund, T. D., Rovis, T., Chung, W. C., and Handa, R. J. (2005). Novel actions of estrogen receptor-beta on anxiety-related behaviors. *Endocrinology* 146, 797–807. doi: 10.1210/en.2004-1158

Malsbury, C. W. (1971). Facilitation of male rat copulatory behavior by electrical stimulation of the medial preoptic area. *Physiol. Behav.* 7, 797–805. doi: 10.1016/0031-9384(71)90042-4

Markowski, V. P., Eaton, R. C., Lumley, L. A., Moses, J., and Hull, E. M. (1994). A D1 agonist in the MPOA facilitates copulation in male rats. *Pharmacol. Biochem. Behav.* 47, 483–486. doi: 10.1016/0091-3057(94)90147-3

Matsumoto, T., Honda, S., and Harada, N. (2003). Alteration in sex-specific behaviors in male mice lacking the aromatase gene. *Neuroendocrinology* 77, 416–424. doi: 10.1159/000071313

McDonald, P., Beyer, C., Newton, F., Brien, B., Baker, R., Tan, H. S., et al. (1970). Failure of 5alpha-dihydrotestosterone to initiate sexual behaviour in the castrated male rat. *Nature* 227, 964–965. doi: 10.1038/227964a0

McPhaul, M. J., Noble, J. F., Simpson, E. R., Mendelson, C. R., and Wilson, J. D. (1988). The expression of a functional cDNA encoding the chicken cytochrome P-450arom (aromatase) that catalyzes the formation of estrogen from androgen. *J. Biol. Chem.* 263, 16358–16363.

Means, G. D., Mahendroo, M. S., Corbin, C. J., Mathis, J. M., Powell, F. E., Mendelson, C. R., et al. (1989). Structural analysis of the gene encoding human aromatase cytochrome P-450, the enzyme responsible for estrogen biosynthesis. *J. Biol. Chem.* 264, 19385–19391.

Melis, M. R., and Argiolas, A. (1995). Dopamine and sexual behavior. *Neurosci. Biobehav. Rev.* 19, 19–38. doi: 10.1016/0149-7634(94)00020-2

Mills, A. D., Crawford, L. L., Domjan, M., and Faure, J. M. (1997). The behavior of the Japanese or domestic quail *Coturnix japonica*. *Neurosci. Biobehav. Rev.* 21, 261–281. doi: 10.1016/S0149-7634(96)00028-0

Morali, G., Larsson, K., and Beyer, C. (1977). Inhibition of testosterone-induced sexual behavior in the castrated male rat by aromatase blockers. *Horm. Behav.* 9, 203–213. doi: 10.1016/0018-506X(77)90056-3

Naftolin, F., Ryan, K. J., Davies, I. J., Reddy, V. V., Flores, F., Petro, Z., et al. (1975). The formation of estrogens by central neuroendocrine tissues. *Recent. Prog. Horm. Res.* 31, 295–319.

Naftolin, F., Ryan, K. J., and Petro, Z. (1972). Aromatization of androstenedione by the anterior hypothalamus of adult male and female rats. *Endocrinology* 90, 295–298. doi: 10.1210/endo-90-1-295

Ogawa, S., Chan, J., Chester, A. E., Gustafsson, J. A., Korach, K. S., and Pfaff, D. W. (1999). Survival of reproductive behaviors in estrogen receptor beta gene-deficient (betaERKO) male and female mice. *Proc. Natl. Acad. Sci. U.S.A.* 96, 12887–12892. doi: 10.1073/pnas.96.22.12887

Ogawa, S., Lubahn, D. B., Korach, K. S., and Pfaff, D. W. (1997). Behavioral effects of estrogen receptor gene disruption in male mice. *Proc. Natl. Acad. Sci. U.S.A.* 94, 1476–1481. doi: 10.1073/pnas.94.4.1476

Orengo, C., Kunik, M. E., Molinari, V., Wristers, K., and Yudofsky, S. C. (2002). Do testosterone levels relate to aggression in elderly men with dementia? *J. Neuropsychiatry Clin. Neurosci.* 14, 161–166. doi: 10.1176/appi.neuropsych.14.2.161

Panzica, G. C., Viglietti-Panzica, C., and Balthazart, J. (1996). The sexually dimorphic medial preoptic nucleus of quail: a key brain area mediating steroid action on male sexual behavior. *Front. Neuroendocrinol.* 17, 51–125. doi: 10.1006/frne.1996.0002

Paredes, R. G., Tzschentke, T., and Nakach, N. (1998). Lesions of the medial preoptic area/anterior hypothalamus (MPOA/AH) modify partner preference in male rats. *Brain Res.* 813, 1–8. doi: 10.1016/S0006-8993(98)00914-7

Paredes, R., Haller, A. E., Manero, M. C., Alvarado, R., and Agmo, A. (1990). Medial preoptic area kindling induces sexual behavior in sexually inactive male rats. *Brain Res.* 515, 20–26. doi: 10.1016/0006-8993(90)90571-R

Pehek, E. A., Warner, R. K., Bazzett, T. J., Bitran, D., Band, L. C., Eaton, R. C., et al. (1988). Microinjection of cis-flupenthixol, a dopamine antagonist, into the medial preoptic area impairs sexual behavior of male rats. *Brain Res.* 443, 70–76. doi: 10.1016/0006-8993(88)91599-5

Phoenix, C. H. (1974). Effects of dihydrotestosterone on sexual behavior of castrated male rhesus monkeys. *Physiol. Behav.* 12, 1045–1055. doi: 10.1016/0031-9384(74)90153-X

Pineda, R., Garcia-Galiano, D., Sanchez-Garrido, M. A., Romero, M., Ruiz-Pino, F., Aguilar, E., et al. (2010). Characterization of the inhibitory roles of RFRP3, the mammalian ortholog of GnIH, in the control of gonadotropin secretion in the rat: *in vivo* and *in vitro* studies. *Am. J. Physiol. Endocrinol. Metab.* 299, E39-E46. doi: 10.1152/ajpendo.00108.2010

Rodríguez-Manzo, G., Pellicer, F., Larsson, K., and Fernández-Guasti, A. (2000). Stimulation of the medical preoptic area facilitates sexual behavior but does not reverse sexual satiation. *Behav. Neurosci.* 114, 553–560. doi: 10.1037/0735-7044.114.3.553

Roselli, C. E., Cross, E., Poonyagariyagorn, H. K., and Stadelman, H. L. (2003). Role of aromatization in anticipatory and consummatory aspects of sexual behavior in male rats. *Horm. Behav.* 44, 146–151. doi: 10.1016/S0018-506X(03)00123-5

Roselli, C. E., Liu, M., and Hurn, P. D. (2009). Brain aromatization: classic roles and new perspectives. *Semin. Reprod. Med.* 27, 207–217. doi: 10.1055/s-0029-1216274

Schlinger, B. A., and Callard, G. V. (1990). Aromatization mediates aggressive behavior in quail. *Gen. Comp. Endocrinol.* 79, 39–53. doi: 10.1016/0016-6480(90)90086-2

Schumacher, M., and Balthazart, J. (1987). Neuroanatomical distribution of testosterone-metabolizing enzymes in the Japanese quail. *Brain Res.* 422, 137–148. doi: 10.1016/0006-8993(87)90548-8

Selinger, H. E., and Bermant, G. (1967). Hormonal control of aggressive behavior in Japanese quail (*Coturnix coturnix japonica*). *Behaviour* 28, 255–268. doi: 10.1163/156853967X00037

Shen, P., Campagnoni, C. W., Kampf, K., Schlinger, B. A., Arnold, A. P., and Campagnoni, A. T. (1994). Isolation and characterization of a zebra finch aromatase cDNA: *in situ* hybridization reveals high aromatase expression in brain. *Brain Res. Mol. Brain Res.* 24, 227–237. doi: 10.1016/0169-328X(94)90136-8

Silverin, B., Baillien, M., and Balthazart, J. (2004). Territorial aggression, circulating levels of testosterone, and brain aromatase activity in free-living pied flycatchers. *Horm. Behav.* 45, 225–234. doi: 10.1016/j.yhbeh.2003.10.002

Simerly, R. B., Gorski, R. A., and Swanson, L. W. (1986). Neurotransmitter specificity of cells and fibers in the medial preoptic nucleus: an immunohistochemical study in the rat. *J. Comp. Neurol.* 246, 343–363. doi: 10.1002/cne.902460305

Simerly, R. B., and Swanson, L. W. (1988). Projections of the medial preoptic nucleus: a Phaseolus vulgaris leucoagglutinin anterograde tract-tracing study in the rat. *J. Comp. Neurol.* 270, 209–242. doi: 10.1002/cne.902700205

Simonin, F., Schmitt, M., Laulin, J. P., Laboureyras, E., Jhamandas, J. H., MacTavish, D., et al. (2006). RF9, a potent and selective neuropeptide FF receptor antagonist, prevents opioid-induced tolerance associated with hyperalgesia. *Proc. Natl. Acad. Sci. U.S.A.* 103, 466–471. doi: 10.1073/pnas.0502090103

Soma, K. K., Rendon, N. M., Boonstra, R., Albers, H. E., and Demas, G. E. (2014). DHEA effects on brain and behavior: insights from comparative studies of aggression. *J. Steroid Biochem. Mol. Biol.* doi: 10.1016/j.jsbmb.2014.05.011. [Epub ahead of print].

Soma, K. K., Sullivan, K., and Wingfield, J. (1999). Combined aromatase inhibitor and antiandrogen treatment decreases territorial aggression in a wild songbird during the nonbreeding season. *Gen. Comp. Endocrinol.* 115, 442–453. doi: 10.1006/gcen.1999.7334

Soma, K. K., Tramontin, A. D., and Wingfield, J. C. (2000). Oestrogen regulates male aggression in the non-breeding season. *Proc. Biol. Sci.* 267, 1089–1096. doi: 10.1098/rspb.2000.1113

Son, Y. L., Ubuka, T., Millar, R. P., Kanasaki, H., and Tsutsui, K. (2012). Gonadotropin-inhibitory hormone inhibits GnRH-induced gonadotropin subunit gene transcriptions by inhibiting AC/cAMP/PKA-dependent ERK pathway in LβT2 cells. *Endocrinology* 153, 2332–2343. doi: 10.1210/en.2011-1904

Son, Y. L., Ubuka, T., Narihiro, M., Fukuda, Y., Hasunuma, I., Yamamoto, K., et al. (2014). Molecular basis for the activation of gonadotropin-inhibitory hormone gene transcription by corticosterone. *Endocrinology* 155, 1817–1826. doi: 10.1210/en.2013-2076

Wersinger, S. R., and Rissman, E. F. (2000b). Oestrogen receptor alpha is essential for female-directed chemo-investigatory behaviour but is not required for the pheromone-induced luteinizing hormone surge in male mice. *J. Neuroendocrinol.* 12, 103–110. doi: 10.1046/j.1365–2826.2000.00418.x

Steele, R. E., Mellor, L. B., Sawyer, W. K., Wasvary, J. M., and Browne, L. J. (1987). *In vitro* and *in vivo* studies demonstrating potent and selective estrogen inhibition with the nonsteroidal aromatase inhibitor CGS 16949A. *Steroids* 50, 147–161. doi: 10.1016/0039-128X(83)90068-5

Szego, C. M., and Davis, J. S. (1967). Adenosine 3',5'-monophosphate in rat uterus: acute elevation by estrogen. *Proc. Natl. Acad. Sci. U.S.A.* 58, 1711–1718. doi: 10.1073/pnas.58.4.1711

Tobari, Y., Son, Y. L., Ubuka, T., Hasegawa, Y., and Tsutsui, K. (2014). A new pathway mediating social effects on the endocrine system: female presence acting via norepinephrine release stimulates gonadotropin-inhibitory hormone in the paraventricular nucleus and suppresses luteinizing hormone in quail. *J. Neurosci.* 34, 9803–9811. doi: 10.1523/JNEUROSCI.3706–13.2014

Toda, K., Okada, T., Takeda, K., Akira, S., Saibara, T., Shiraishi, M., et al. (2001a). Oestrogen at the neonatal stage is critical for the reproductive ability of male mice as revealed by supplementation with 17beta-oestradiol to aromatase gene (Cyp19) knockout mice. *J. Endocrinol.* 168, 455–463. doi: 10.1677/joe.0.1680455

Toda, K., Saibara, T., Okada, T., Onishi, S., and Shizuta, Y. (2001b). A loss of aggressive behaviour and its reinstatement by oestrogen in mice lacking the aromatase gene (Cyp19). *J. Endocrinol.* 168, 217–220. doi: 10.1677/joe.0.1680217

Tsai, M. J., and O'Malley, B. W. (1994). Molecular mechanisms of action of steroid/thyroid receptor superfamily members. *Annu. Rev. Biochem.* 63, 451–486. doi: 10.1146/annurev.bi.63.070194.002315

Tsutsui, K. (2009). A new key neurohormone controlling reproduction, gonadotropin-inhibitory hormone (GnIH): biosynthesis, mode of action and functional significance. *Prog. Neurobiol.* 88, 76–88. doi: 10.1016/j.pneurobio.2009.02.003

Tsutsui, K., Bentley, G. E., Bedecarrats, G., Osugi, T., Ubuka, T., and Kriegsfeld, L. J. (2010). Gonadotropin-inhibitory hormone (GnIH) and its control of central and peripheral reproductive function. *Front. Neuroendocrinol.* 31, 284–295. doi: 10.1016/j.yfrne.2010.03.001

Tsutsui, K., and Ishii, S. (1981). Effects of sex steroids on aggressive behavior of adult male Japanese quail. *Gen. Comp. Endocrinol.* 44, 480–486. doi: 10.1016/0016-6480(81)90336-1

Tsutsui, K., Saigoh, E., Ukena, K., Teranishi, H., Fujisawa, Y., Kikuchi, M., et al. (2000). A novel avian hypothalamic peptide inhibiting gonadotropin release. *Biochem. Biophys. Res. Commun.* 275, 661–667. doi: 10.1006/bbrc.2000.3350

Tsutsui, K., Saigoh, E., Yin, H., Ubuka, T., Chowdhury, V. S., Osugi, T., et al. (2009). A new key neurohormone controlling reproduction, gonadotrophin-inhibitory hormone in birds: discovery, progress and prospects. *J. Neuroendocrinol.* 21, 271–275. doi: 10.1111/j.1365–2826.2009.01829.x

Tsutsui, K., and Ubuka, T. (2013). "Gonadotropin-inhibitory hormone," in *Handbook of Biologically Active Peptides. Section on Brain Peptides,* eds A. J. Kastin and H. Vaudry (London: Academic Press), 802–811. doi: 10.1016/B978-0-12-385095-9.00107-X

Ubuka, T., and Bentley, G. E. (2011). "Neuroendocrine control of reproduction in birds," in *Hormones and Reproduction of Vertebrates. Birds,* Vol 4., eds D. O. Norris and K. H. Lopez (London: Academic Press), 1–25.

Ubuka, T., Bentley, G. E., Ukena, K., Wingfield, J. C., and Tsutsui, K. (2005). Melatonin induces the expression of gonadotropin-inhibitory hormone in the avian brain. *Proc. Natl. Acad. Sci. U.S.A.* 102, 3052–3057. doi: 10.1073/pnas.0403840102

Ubuka, T., Haraguchi, S., Tobari, Y., Narihiro, M., Ishikawa, K., Hayashi, T., et al. (2014). Hypothalamic inhibition of socio-sexual behaviour by increasing neuroestrogen synthesis. *Nat. Commun.* 4, 3061. doi: 10.1038/ncomms4061

Ubuka, T., Inoue, K., Fukuda, Y., Mizuno, T., Ukena, K., Kriegsfeld, L. J., et al. (2012a). Identification, expression, and physiological functions of Siberian hamster gonadotropin-inhibitory hormone. *Endocrinology* 153, 373–385. doi: 10.1210/en.2011-1110

Ubuka, T., Kim, S., Huang, Y. C., Reid, J., Jiang, J., Osugi, T., et al. (2008). Gonadotropin-inhibitory hormone neurons interact directly with gonadotropin-releasing hormone-I and -II neurons in European starling brain. *Endocrinology* 149, 268–278. Erratum in: *Endocrinology* 149, 4229. doi: 10.1210/en.2007-0983

Ubuka, T., Lai, H., Kitani, M., Suzuuchi, A., Pham, V., Cadigan, P. A., et al. (2009a). Gonadotropin-inhibitory hormone identification, cDNA cloning, and distribution in rhesus macaque brain. *J. Comp. Neurol.* 517, 841–855. doi: 10.1002/cne.22191

Ubuka, T., Mizuno, T., Fukuda, Y., Bentley, G. E., Wingfield, J. C., and Tsutsui, K. (2013b). RNA interference of gonadotropin-inhibitory hormone gene induces aggressive and sexual behaviors in birds. *Gen. Comp. Endocrinol.* 181, 179–186. doi: 10.1016/j.ygcen.2012.09.010

Ubuka, T., Morgan, K., Pawson, A. J., Osugi, T., Chowdhury, V. S., Minakata, H., et al. (2009b). Identification of human GnIH homologs, RFRP-1 and RFRP-3, and the cognate receptor, GPR147 in the human hypothalamic pituitary axis. *PLoS ONE* 4:e8400. doi: 10.1371/journal.pone.0008400

Ubuka, T., Mukai, M., Wolfe, J., Beverly, R., Clegg, S., Wang, A., et al. (2012b). RNA interference of gonadotropin-inhibitory hormone gene induces arousal in songbirds. *PLoS ONE* 7:e30202. doi: 10.1371/journal.pone.0030202

Ubuka, T., Son, Y. L., Bentley, G. E., Millar, R. P., and Tsutsui, K. (2013c). Gonadotropin-inhibitory hormone (GnIH), GnIH receptor and cell signaling. *Gen. Comp. Endocrinol.* 190, 10–17. doi: 10.1016/j.ygcen.2013.02.030

Ubuka, T., Son, Y. L., Tobari, Y., and Tsutsui, K. (2012c). Gonadotropin-inhibitory hormone action in the brain and pituitary. *Front. Endocrinol. (Lausanne)* 3:148. doi: 10.3389/fendo.2012.00148

Ubuka, T., and Tsutsui, K. (2014). Gonadotropin-inhibitory hormone inhibits aggressive behavior of male quail by increasing neuroestrogen synthesis in the brain beyond its optimum concentration. *Gen. Comp. Endocrinol.* 205, 49–54. doi: 10.1016/j.ygcen.2014.03.014

Ubuka, T., Ueno, M., Ukena, K., and Tsutsui, K. (2003). Developmental changes in gonadotropin-inhibitory hormone in the Japanese quail (*Coturnix japonica*) hypothalamo-hypophysial system. *J. Endocrinol.* 178, 311–318. doi: 10.1677/joe.0.1780311

Ubuka, T., Ukena, K., Sharp, P. J., Bentley, G. E., and Tsutsui, K. (2006). Gonadotropin-inhibitory hormone inhibits gonadal development and maintenance by decreasing gonadotropin synthesis and release in male quail. *Endocrinology* 147, 1187–1194. doi: 10.1210/en.2005-1178

Ukena, K., Ubuka, T., and Tsutsui, K. (2003). Distribution of a novel avian gonadotropin-inhibitory hormone in the quail brain. *Cell. Tissue. Res.* 312, 73–79.

Vasudevan, N., and Pfaff, D. W. (2008). Non-genomic actions of estrogens and their interaction with genomic actions in the brain. *Front. Neuroendocrinol.* 29, 238–257. doi: 10.1016/j.yfrne.2007.08.003

Voigt, C., Ball, G. F., and Balthazart, J. (2007). Neuroanatomical specificity of sex differences in expression of aromatase mRNA in the quail brain. *J. Chem. Neuroanat.* 33, 75–86. doi: 10.1016/j.jchemneu.2006.12.004

Wada, M. (1982). Effects of sex steroids on calling, locomotor activity, and sexual behavior in castrated male Japanese quail. *Horm. Behav.* 16, 147–157. doi: 10.1016/0018-506X(82)90015-0

Wade, J., Schlinger, B. A., Hodges, L., and Arnold, A. P. (1994). Fadrozole: a potent and specific inhibitor of aromatase in the zebra finch brain. *Gen. Comp. Endocrinol.* 94, 53–61. doi: 10.1006/gcen.1994.1059

Walters, M. J., and Harding, C. F. (1988). The effects of an aromatization inhibitor on the reproductive behavior of male zebra finches. *Horm. Behav.* 22, 207–218. doi: 10.1016/0018-506X(88)90067-0

Warner, R. K., Thompson, J. T., Markowski, V. P., Loucks, J. A., Bazzett, T. J., Eaton, R. C., et al. (1991). Microinjection of the dopamine antagonist cis-flupenthixol into the MPOA impairs copulation, penile reflexes and sexual motivation in male rats. *Brain Res.* 540, 177–182. doi: 10.1016/0006-8993(91)90505-P

Wersinger, S. R., and Rissman, E. F. (2000a). Dopamine activates masculine sexual behavior independent of the estrogen receptor alpha. *J. Neurosci.* 20, 4248–4254.

Wersinger, S. R., Sannen, K., Villalba, C., Lubahn, D. B., Rissman, E. F., and De Vries, G. J. (1997). Masculine sexual behavior is disrupted in male and female mice lacking a functional estrogen receptor alpha gene. *Horm. Behav.* 32, 176–183. doi: 10.1006/hbeh.1997.1419

Whalen, R. E., and Luttge, W. G. (1971). Testosterone, androstenedione and dihydrotestosterone effects on mating behaviour of male rats. *Horm. Behav.* 2, 117–125. doi: 10.1016/0018-506X(71)90027-4

Yahr, P. (1979). Data and hypotheses in tales of dihydrotestosterone. *Horm. Behav.* 13, 92–96. doi: 10.1016/0018-506X(79)90037-0

Yin, H., Ukena, K., Ubuka, T., and Tsutsui, K. (2005). A novel G protein-coupled receptor for gonadotropin-inhibitory hormone in the Japanese quail (*Coturnix japonica*): identification, expression and binding activity. *J. Endocrinol.* 184, 257–266. doi: 10.1677/joe.1.05926

Zumpe, D., Clancy, A. N., Bonsall, R. W., and Michael, R. P. (1996). Behavioral responses to Depo-Provera, Fadrozole, and estradiol in castrated, testosterone-treated cynomolgus monkeys (*Macaca fascicularis*): the involvement of progestin receptors. *Physiol. Behav.* 60, 531–540. doi: 10.1016/S0031-9384(96)80028-X

12

Contextual modulation of social and endocrine correlates of fitness: insights from the life history of a sex changing fish

Devaleena S. Pradhan[1*†], Tessa K. Solomon-Lane[2] and Matthew S. Grober[1,2]

[1] *Department of Biology, Georgia State University, Atlanta, GA, USA*
[2] *Neuroscience Institute, Georgia State University, Atlanta, GA, USA*

***Correspondence:**
Devaleena S. Pradhan, Department of Integrative Biology and Physiology, University of California, Los Angeles, 610 Charles E. Young Dr. East, CA 90095, USA.
e-mail: dspradhan@ucla.edu

†Present address:
Devaleena S. Pradhan, Department of Integrative Biology and Physiology, University of California, Los Angeles, CA, USA

Steroid hormones are critical regulators of reproductive life history, and the steroid sensitive traits (morphology, behavior, physiology) associated with particular life history stages can have substantial fitness consequences for an organism. Hormones, behavior and fitness are reciprocally associated and can be used in an integrative fashion to understand how the environment impacts organismal function. To address the fitness component, we highlight the importance of using reliable proxies of reproductive success when studying proximate regulation of reproductive phenotypes. To understand the mechanisms by which the endocrine system regulates phenotype, we discuss the use of particular endocrine proxies and the need for appropriate functional interpretation of each. Lastly, in any experimental paradigm, the responses of animals vary based on the subtle differences in environmental and social context and this must also be considered. We explore these different levels of analyses by focusing on the fascinating life history transitions exhibited by the bi-directionally hermaphroditic fish, *Lythrypnus dalli*. Sex changing fish are excellent models for providing a deeper understanding of the fitness consequences associated with behavioral and endocrine variation. We close by proposing that local regulation of steroids is one potential mechanism that allows for the expression of novel phenotypes that can be characteristic of specific life history stages. A comparative species approach will facilitate progress in understanding the diversity of mechanisms underlying the contextual regulation of phenotypes and their associated fitness correlates.

Keywords: androgen, cortisol, parenting, social status, reproduction

INTRODUCTION

Most organisms exhibit distinct developmental and reproductive stages during their life cycle. Physiological factors are critical orchestrators of life history transitions and coordinate dynamic, context-specific activities to increase fitness. In reproductively mature individuals, activities generally focus around nutrition and reproduction, and in turn, both of these activities are broadly dependent upon temporal patterns associated with circannual and seasonal rhythms (Ball et al., 2004; Prendergast et al., 2009). Within this realm, steroid hormones, the molecules of focus in this review, regulate phenotypes such as behavior and morphology in response to environmental change (Wingfield et al., 1990; Remage-Healey and Romero, 2001).

The environment can cause both predictable and unpredictable changes in endogenous hormones, either at the level of synthesis or signaling cascades to cause downstream consequences (Pradhan and Soma, 2012). Depending upon the particular environment, the behavior expressed by an individual (in isolation or toward conspecifics) can be modulated by steroid hormones, which has fitness consequences (**Figure 1**). The local environment can modulate the internal physiological state of an organism, with subsequent effects on both behavior and fitness, while the geographic location of the habitat can also serve as a selective pressure regulating physiological mechanisms (Nelson, 2011; Wingfield, 2012). For example, the patterns of genotype, phenotype, and plasticity of expression are rather different for animals living in the Tropics, Temperate, and Arctic regions (Wingfield et al., 1990; Borg, 1994; Wingfield and Hunt, 2002). In addition, whether data come from natural vs. laboratory environments has a major impact on their interpretation. For example, natural populations have high hormone levels, and natural predator stress can cause a greater glucocorticoid response than what can be simulated in a laboratory (e.g., via restraint) (Newman et al., 2013). It is imperative that sex steroids and glucocorticoids have differential responses to environmental stressors (Narayan et al., 2012) so that during a stressful event, the tradeoffs favor an instinct for survival, rather than reproduction. Given that fitness, hormones, and behavior are reciprocally associated, integrative studies that examine all three factors will provide critical insights into the evolution of life history strategies and regulation of processes that optimize fitness.

Sex changing fish are excellent models for understanding the fitness consequences associated with the behavioral and endocrine variation among individuals. In theory, an optimal life

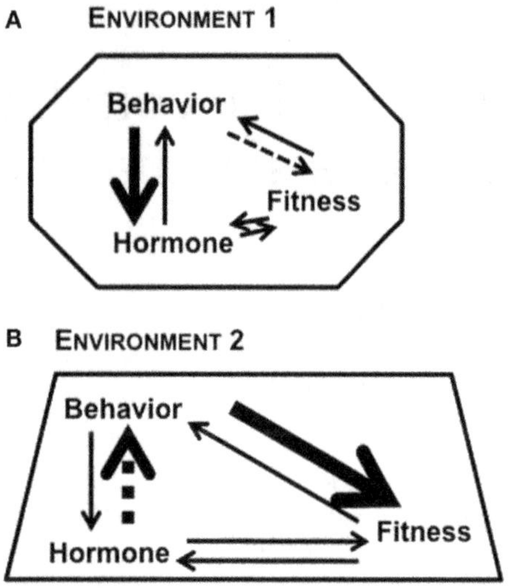

FIGURE 1 | Reciprocal relationships between hormone, behavior, and fitness of an individual. The strength of relationship between any two factors can be modulated based on context and the environment in which the organism lives. The different shapes in **(A)** Environment 1 and **(B)** Environment 2 represent the role of context in modulating the bi-directional links between any two factors. The varying thickness of arrows represents the complexity of links between factors.

history strategy for any species involves regulating behavior, physiology, and reproduction to match each context an individual finds itself in, as context changes over time, in order to maximize fitness (Horn and Rubenstein, 1984). Sex change allows individuals to reproduce as a different sex depending on the context or environmental conditions and can provide major increases to lifetime reproductive success (Warner et al., 1975). Generally, sex change should be favored in species for which male and female reproductive success differs over a lifetime and the reproductive success of one sex increases more rapidly than the other with time, age, or size. For example, in protogynous species, individuals reproduce as females when younger, smaller, and lower in social status and then as males when older, larger, and higher in social status (Ghiselin, 1969; Warner, 1975; Munday et al., 2006; Godwin, 2009). Functional sex change requires that an individual reproduce successfully as one sex and then as another. Integrative studies on sex change investigate multiple levels of analyses, including (1) behavior, such as establishing dominance initially and reproduction (courtship, mating, and parenting) at a later stage; (2) morphology, such as color change or gonadal and external genital rearrangement; (3) physiology, such as changes in profiles of sex hormones in the gonad, systemic circulation, and brain; and (4) reproduction, such as presence of fertilized eggs (Reavis and Grober, 1999; Black et al., 2005b; Rodgers, 2007).

The goal of this review is to bridge the gaps in understanding the links among fitness, hormones, and behavior when animals are working to adjust these factors in a variety of ethologically or ecologically relevant environmental/external contexts. First, we describe the fitness component of our model and propose how we can improve our understanding of behavioral endocrinology by incorporating fitness measures in our experiments. Second, we outline how to improve our understanding of endocrine regulation by considering different levels of analyses within the endocrinological context. The steroid hormones discussed herein [testosterone (T), 11-ketotestosterone (KT), 17β-estradiol (E_2), and cortisol (F)] are linked through steroidogenic conversion pathways (**Figure 2**) and can be produced and transduced at multiple sites across the body axis. Third, we discuss the integration of social and endocrine contexts, which allows us to better interpret the mechanisms that regulate transitions among phenotypes. Finally, we propose a model for how these factors interact to influence the expression of phenotype. Being cognizant of these different components and levels of analyses is especially important when designing experiments and interpreting results. Throughout this review, we present examples from several different vertebrate species but focus on data from the remarkable life history of the bi-directionally hermaphroditic, highly social marine fish, the bluebanded goby, *Lythrypnus dalli* (**Figure 3**).

FITNESS

To effectively incorporate a fitness component into our studies of hormones and behavior, it is critical to discuss how fitness is defined and measured. A variety of empirical measures of fitness have been utilized in field and laboratory experiments. Although the conceptual definition of fitness is widely agreed upon by scientists, a large number of operational definitions are presented in the literature. In fact, the significance and consequence of these different definitions has itself been the subject of study (Barker, 2009; Orr, 2009). In order to decide on the appropriate fitness component or proxy for a given experimental paradigm, a thorough analysis is necessary to identify constraints to measuring fitness. Through our synthesis, we aim to emphasize the value of integrating fitness measures into mechanistic studies of behavioral endocrinology.

BROAD DEFINITION

Generally, individual fitness is defined as passing genetic material to the next generation. However, fitness may also refer to a genotype, a population, or a species. Fitness is defined and measured differently at these levels of analyses and, as a result, requires the appropriate tools. For example, while the fitness of an individual may be reasonably estimated directly (i.e., by counting all the surviving offspring of an individual) or as its components, survival or reproductive success (e.g., offspring produced during an experimental time period), a population understanding of fitness might utilize genetic analyses of quantitative trait loci along with a variety mathematical fitness statistics (Barker, 2009; Orr, 2009). For the purposes of this article, which broadly concerns fitness, hormones, and behavior, we will focus on individual, i.e., phenotypic, fitness.

OPERATIONAL DEFINITION

Given the number of fitness definitions present in the scientific literature, it is critical for each study to provide a clear operational definition. From a survey of fitness definitions by Barker (2009), we would like to highlight three important considerations in defining fitness that are especially applicable to individual

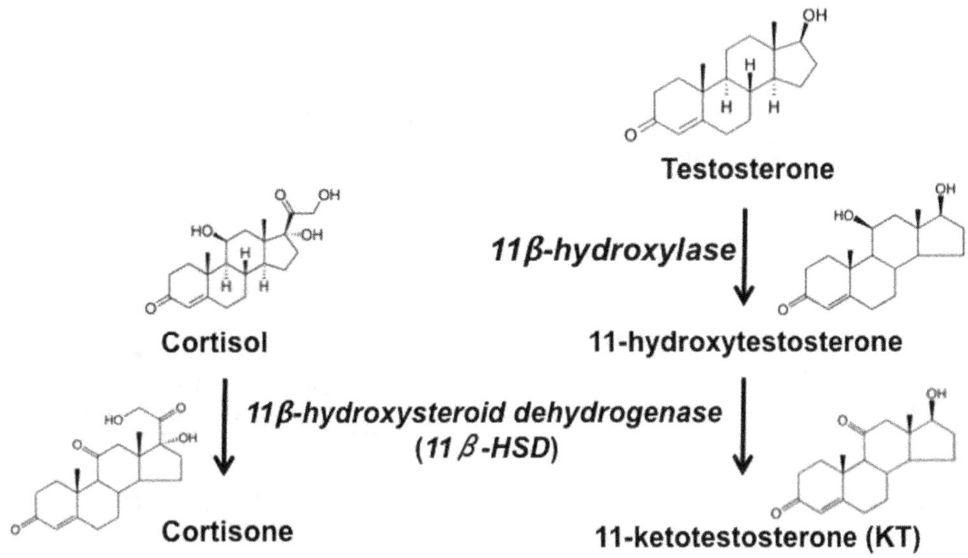

FIGURE 2 | Simplified pathway of steroidogenesis in fish. Testosterone is converted to 11-Ketotestosterone (KT) via the sequential action of 11β-hydroxylase, which converts KT to 11β-hydroxytestosterone (11β-OHT), and 11β-hydroxysteroid dehydrogenase, which converts 11β-OHT to KT and cortisol to cortisone. Adapted from Pradhan et al. (2014c).

fitness. First, experimental quantification of fitness and selection pressures should distinguish between two phases of selection. Within a generation, fitness differences among individuals can lead to change in the frequency distribution of phenotypes (e.g., via differential survival rates). If the fitness differences among individuals have a genetic basis and, therefore, are heritable, then these fitness differences will also lead to a change in the frequency distribution of phenotypes and genotypes in the next generation (Barker, 2009). Second, definitions frequently vary in the number of generations considered. Based on one definition, an individual might qualify as having high fitness if a large number of offspring are produced. By another definition, those offspring might also be required to produce a large number of offspring. An even more stringent definition might require that genetic material be passed down across multiple generations (Ellis, 1995; Barker, 2009). As discussed in more detail below, experimental limitations often affect how many generations can feasibly be quantified. Third, the importance of context in quantifying fitness is stated explicitly in some definitions, but not in others. The fitness of individuals must be compared within the same environmental context, for example, because gene by environment interactions can significantly affect the fitness of a given phenotype (Greenfield and Rodriguez, 2004; Barker, 2009). It is also critical to consider the life history stage of the individuals when fitness is quantified (Orr, 2009). For example, fish that undergo adult sex change, a primary focus of this paper, produce dramatically different numbers of offspring as females than as males (Warner, 1975; Munday et al., 2006). Estimates of reproductive success early in life, therefore, would fail to incorporate the increase in reproductive success following sex change. Similarly, when quantifying fitness proxies (discussed below), such as fighting ability, there may be age- and life history-dependent differences in the success of fighting using different methods (Lailvaux et al., 2004); therefore, accurate estimates of ability require assessment at multiple life history stages.

MEASURES OF FITNESS

In studies of hormones and behavior, individual fitness is measured most often as its components or via the use of proxies. The primary components of fitness are survival and reproductive success. Individuals must survive into reproductive maturity in order to have non-zero fitness, and for species in which individuals reproduce more the longer they live, age may be directly related to reproductive success. African elephants in musth, for example, experience an increase paternity success as they age (Hollister-Smith et al., 2007). The relationship between survival and reproductive success is not simple in all species. In *L. dalli*, territorial males are larger and likely to be older than subordinate females (Behrents, 1983), but the association between age (e.g., survival) and reproductive success is not likely to be causative. For species that experience reproductive senescence (e.g., Angelier et al., 2006; Aubry et al., 2009), increased survival beyond a certain age may or may not contribute significantly to reproductive success and, therefore, fitness. Finally, there may be a tradeoff for some species (e.g., elephant seals) between dominance/high reproductive success and life expectancy (Ellis, 1995).

Reproductive success refers to the number of offspring produced by an individual, usually within a time period shorter than a lifetime (to distinguish from a direct measure of fitness). As discussed above, definitions vary with respect to the number of generations genetic material must be passed down (Barker, 2009). Although an ideal measure would involve tracking genes across infinite generations, a strong definition of reproductive success is the number of offspring that survive until reproductive maturity (Ellis, 1995). Impressively, researchers studying chacma baboons (Silk et al., 2009), collared flycatchers (Brommer et al.,

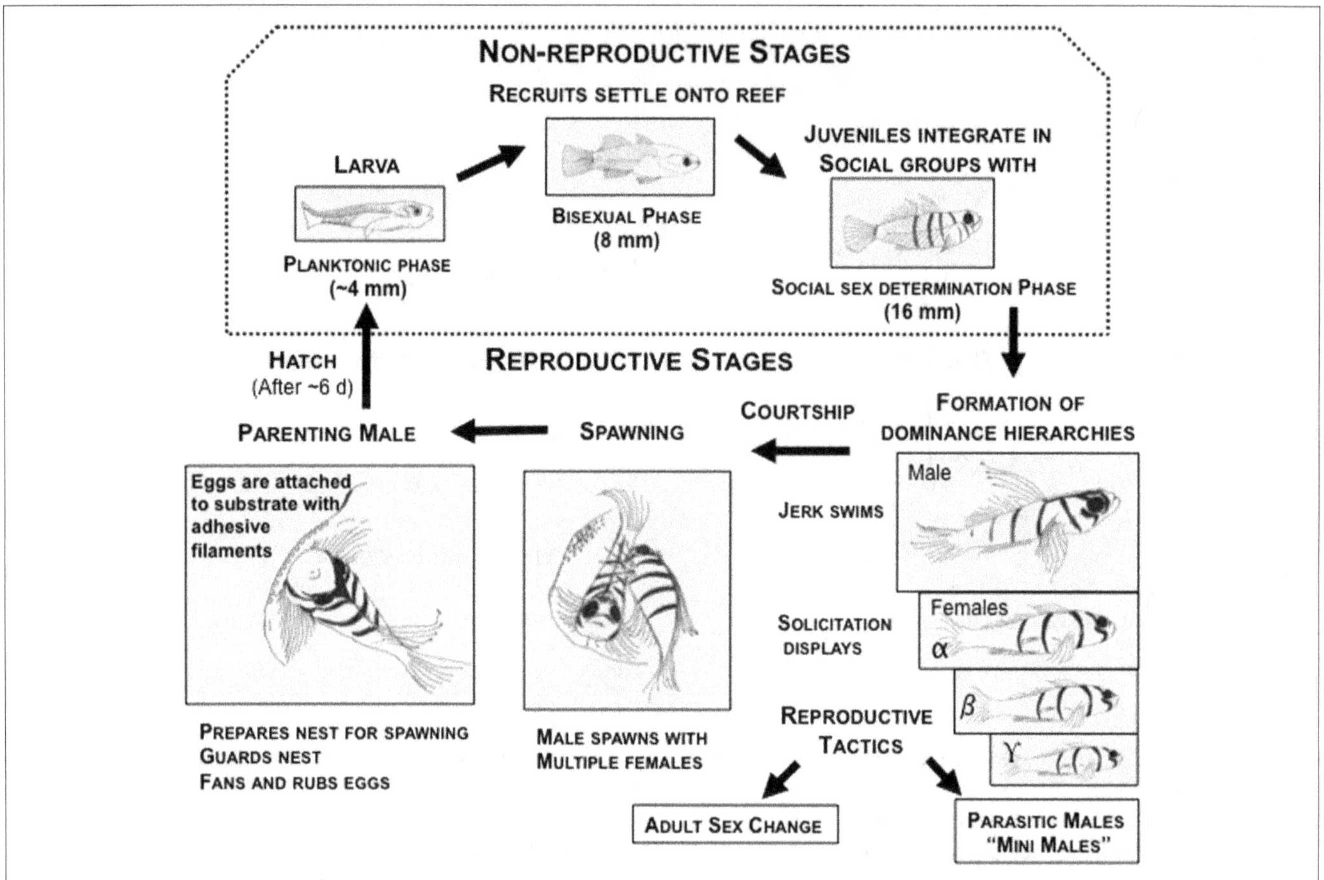

FIGURE 3 | Life cycle of bluebanded gobies, *Lythrypnus dalli*, depicting the life history stages during the breeding season in waters off the coast of Santa Catalina Island, California. The dotted box encompasses the non-reproductive stages, which are not discussed in this review. The remainder are parts of the reproductive stages, and each of these comprise sub-stages of territorial aggression, dominance hierarchies, courtship (male jerks and female solicitation), spawning, and parenting. In the laboratory, social groups are easily set up under conditions that are permissive for natural sex change and for spawning. These fish also show alternative reproductive strategies to increase lifetime reproductive success, such as socially controlled bi-directional adult sex change and parasitic male morphs.

2005), great reed warblers (Hasselquist, 1998), red-winged blackbirds (Forbes, 2011), feral horses (Cameron et al., 2009), dolphins (Frère et al., 2010), hyenas (Holekamp et al., 2012), meerkats (Hodge et al., 2008), and others (Ellis, 1995) all include reproductive success measures based on offspring survival and maturation. In practice, many reproductive proxies are used to estimate reproductive success, such as courtship (e.g., Shamble et al., 2009), mate choice (e.g., Clutton-Brock and McAuliffe, 2009), mating opportunities or attempts (e.g., Chen et al., 2011), successful copulations (e.g., White et al., 2010; Formica et al., 2011), the number of eggs laid (e.g., Ros et al., 2009), or the number of offspring born (e.g., Bell et al., 2011). While a number of reproductive proxies have been validated empirically by correlating the proxy with a more robust measure of reproductive success, others have not. In fact, some common proxies are not related at all to reproductive success in particular species, for example, male macaque copulation frequency (Ellis, 1995). Additionally, measuring different proxies within the same species can lead to different conclusions about the fitness consequences of a phenotype (Wong and Candolin, 2005). In the pygmy swordtail, although females prefer males with blue body coloration, gold-colored males outcompete blue males in agonistic interactions (Kingston et al., 2003). Dominance is itself a powerful predictor of status in many species (Ellis, 1995), and gold male dominance may constrain females' ability to act on their preference (Kingston et al., 2003).

Morphological and behavioral proxies are also common stand-ins for fitness and its components (survival, reproductive success). In some systems, the connection between morphological traits and fitness is well-documented. For example, male tail white in dark-eyed juncos has a genetic basis and is influenced by diet and age. Females prefer males with more tail white, males with more tail white tend to win male-male aggressive interactions, and larger males with more tail white produce offspring with more females (Hill et al., 1999; McGlothlin et al., 2005, 2007). Body parts of exaggerated size, such as weapons, horns, or claws, have also been linked to fighting ability, attractiveness, and reproductive success (Emlen, 2008). As with other proxies, however, rigorous tests of these associations are critical because, for example, empirical evidence linking ornamentation to body condition is generally lacking (Cotton et al., 2004), and the association between female ornamentation and offspring quality varies considerably (Nordeide et al., 2012). Perhaps the most common behavioral proxy for fitness is social dominance (Wilson, 1980; Ellis, 1995). Dominants may gain higher reproductive success by suppressing subordinate reproduction (Barrett et al., 1993; Clarke and Faulkes, 2001; White et al., 2002; Fitzpatrick et al., 2008), monopolizing mating opportunities, producing more offspring, and experiencing lower rates of abortion, egg loss, and offspring mortality (Smuts and Smuts, 1993; Trunzer et al., 1999; van Noordwijk and van Schaik, 1999; East and Hofer, 2001; Young et al., 2006; Robbins et al., 2007; Heg and Hamilton, 2008; Henry et al., 2013).

EXERCISE CAUTION WHEN INTERPRETING FITNESS DATA

Once a fitness proxy has been validated in the same or in a related species, morphological and behavioral traits are often used as stand-ins for fitness. Given that individual fitness is sensitive to context, however, it is important to differentiate between inferred and empirically quantified fitness consequences. While in many cases scientists have demonstrated consistent links, across species, between a given trait and fitness (Ellis, 1995; Emlen, 2008), it is critical not to assume fitness consequences or generalize without evidence across species and contexts. To demonstrate the importance of rigorously testing fitness hypotheses, we would like to highlight a few examples of unexpected fitness relationships. First, in the banded mongoose, there is a strong reproductive skew. Dominant females will evict pregnant subordinates from the social group, which causes abortion. Interestingly, dominant females that evict subordinates suffer reproductive costs, including lower offspring weight at birth and independence, as well as lower offspring survival (Bell et al., 2011). Second, in many hierarchical species, there is an association between status and glucocorticoid levels. Although subordinate status is often considered the more "stressful" social status, comparative data suggest that in approximately half of the species surveyed, dominant individuals were more stressed (Creel, 2001), which can itself be associated with negative fitness consequences (e.g., Sapolsky, 2005). Third, in many species, males adopt different reproductive strategies. In some species, there is evidence that alternative male morphs, long considered a less successful strategy than the more visible territorial or bourgeois male, may be equally reproductively successful (Taborsky, 1994). Finally, in a cooperatively breeding cichlid, subordinate females assist in caring for eggs produced by the dominant breeding pair. Neither kin selection nor the "pay-to-stay" hypothesis, which suggests group membership is the benefit to alloparenting, fully explains why subordinates help. Instead, subordinate females that alloparent are able to secure substrate on which to lay their own eggs (Heg et al., 2009). Ultimately, failing to rely on robust fitness measures to establish whether a trait, behavior, or phenotype is successful can lead to misleading or false statement about fitness consequences that may get repeated while remaining untested.

CONSTRAINTS OF INCORPORATING FITNESS MEASURES

In discussions about fitness, it is also important to acknowledge the practical constraints that make direct quantifications of fitness unfeasible, impossible, or arguably irrelevant to the specific research question. Although we have made clear the benefits of measuring fitness or fitness components directly in order to make strong statements about individual/phenotypic success and selection, we can recognize Dobzhansky's dictum about the importance of evolution for understanding biological phenomena (Dobzhansky, 1973) without calling for all experiments to be directly concerned with fitness measures. Some common constraints to experimentally measuring fitness include species that do not reproduce in the laboratory yet provide important insight into biological questions. For species that do reproduce in the laboratory, neither parents nor offspring are exposed to ethologically-relevant social and environmental pressures; therefore, extrapolations about fitness could be difficult to justify. The life history of some species makes it difficult to empirically quantify reproduction, such as species that are slow to mature and reproduce rarely. Similarly, life history transitions affect the ability to quantify offspring characteristics like condition, survival, and subsequent reproductive success if, for example, species undergo pelagic or dispersal periods. In field studies, species may cover too much area to track effectively, and courtship and mating events may be purposefully cryptic or difficult to observe due to crepuscular or nocturnal timing. Tracking fitness across generations typically requires long-term studies, which can be practically and monetarily difficult to conduct. Finally, in mechanistic studies, manipulations of hormones or neuropeptides alter physiology and behavior over relatively short periods of time, during which effects on reproduction or survival may not be feasible or generalizable to what might occur over a lifetime.

INTEGRATION OF BEHAVIORAL ENDOCRINOLOGY AND FITNESS

Hormones, behavior, and fitness are reciprocally related (**Figure 1**), and incorporating fitness measures may further elucidate the links between hormones and behavior, which are commonly measured together. In behavioral endocrinology, an important question to ask is whether hormones affect fitness indirectly via an affect on behavior or whether the fitness effect is direct. It must be clarified, however, that direct and indirect effects of hormones on fitness are not mutually exclusive. These effects can be important during different phases of life history of the same individual, and in many cases, it is challenging to tease apart direct and indirect effects. Direct effects of fitness on reproductive success could occur via effects on reproductive biology and behavior, while an indirect effect on reproductive success might affect a non-reproductive behavior that consequently affects reproductive success (e.g., social behavior).

Although the underlying mechanisms are far from simple, we will present some brief examples of direct and indirect fitness effects of two classes of hormones: glucocorticoids and androgens. Reproductive behavior can be energetically costly in terms of courtship displays (Fusani et al., 2014), spawning/mating (Watson et al., 1998), and parenting (Pradhan et al., 2014c, in press). For example, nesting male peacock blennies judge whether they can accept another clutch of eggs based on their energetic state (Olsson et al., 2009). Glucocorticoids are directly involved in the regulation of energy and behaviors related to acquiring energy, such as foraging (Schneider and Wade, 1999); therefore, glucocorticoids can directly affect the expression of reproductive behaviors. Glucocorticoids are also directly affect reproductive biology. The glucocorticoid cortisol, for example, is necessary for vitellogenesis (Brooks et al., 1997). Androgens also have direct effects on reproductive success, for example, via effects on spermatogenesis (Walker, 2011), expression of secondary sexual characteristics (Saraiva et al., 2010) and/or via androgen-dependent reproductive behaviors such as courtship displays (Vasconcelos et al., 2012; Schlinger et al., 2013) and parenting (Trainor and Marler, 2001; Foerster and Kempenaers, 2005). With respect to indirect effects, both glucocorticoids and androgens are associated with social status and agonistic behavior in a number of hierarchical species. High status individuals typically have a reproductive advantage over subordinates (Ellis, 1995), thus, behaviors such as territorial defense, dominance/submissive behavior, and aggression can all indirectly affect reproductive success (Foerster and Kempenaers, 2005). Both glucocorticoids and androgens are involved in numerous biological processes, and chronic exposure could impact fitness via more than one mechanism to incur reproductive costs (Wingfield et al., 2001; Breuner et al., 2008).

Sex changing fish are an excellent model for understanding how fitness can enhance our understanding of the causes and consequences of behavioral and endocrine state. Sex changing fish are useful because under a variety of contexts, hormones, behavior, and fitness can all be feasibly quantified. Furthermore, the foundational cannon of research on sex changing fish focused on fitness. As a life history strategy, sex change allows an individual to maximize reproductive success (Ghiselin, 1969; Warner, 1975). For example, for territorial species, young and small fish are not competitive territory holders. If males are the territory holders, an effective reproductive strategy would be to reproduce as female when young and small and then as a male when older, larger, and able to defend a territory. In the following section, we will discuss how the contextual regulation of fitness, hormones, and behavior has been measured in *L. dalli.*

INSIGHTS FROM *LYTHRYPNUS DALLI*

A number of fitness proxies have been utilized in research with *L. dalli*, most of which approximate reproductive success. These include estimates of gamete production, gonad morphology, social status, and various reproductive measures of eggs in the nest. Extensive work has been done classifying sexual allocation in males, females (St. Mary, 1993), and alternative male morphs, mini males (**Figure 3**) (Drilling and Grober, 2005). Mini males are considered to be a parasitic male morph in *L. dalli*, based on physiological and morphological traits, although their behavioral strategies remain to be described (Pradhan et al., 2014b). Adult male and female gonads contain both types of gametes, but the investment is heavily skewed toward the sex that the individual behaves and reproduces as St. Mary (1993). Mini males have an important allocation difference compared to nesting males. Mini males utilize the accessory gonadal structure to store sperm, while nesting males store mucus (Drilling and Grober, 2005).

Social groups of *L. dalli* are composed of a dominant male and multiple subordinate females. More than one female (and usually all females) lays eggs in the nest of the male, resulting in male reproductive success that is multiple times higher than any individual female in the group (Behrents, 1983). Female *L. dalli* routinely lay eggs and males readily parent in the laboratory (Pradhan et al., in press). Using sequential digital images of eggs in the nest, we can quantify the number of eggs laid, the number of clutches laid, average clutch size, inter-clutch interval, hatching success, and the number of eggs that hatch (**Figure 4**). Larval *L. dalli* are planktonic (**Figure 3**), making offspring survival and reproduction difficult to quantify in the laboratory and unfeasible in the field. Therefore, the number of eggs that hatch is our best estimate of reproductive success (Solomon-Lane et al., 2014).

In stable social groups, the quantity of eggs fertilized by the male is associated with the pattern of agonistic interaction in the group, especially among females (Solomon-Lane et al., 2014). More dominant females interrupt courtship solicitation displays by subordinate females and assume solicitation displays themselves (Pradhan et al., in press). Even though dominant and subordinate females display courtship at similar rates, number of eggs and number of eggs that advance to the "eyed" stage are positively associated with rates of dominant female courtship (Pradhan et al., in press). Therefore, agonistic interactions and social status could be used as one type of behavioral proxy. Once eggs are fertilized, males provide sole parental care, and they vary in their hatching success (Solomon-Lane et al., unpublished data), a quantitative measure of parenting efficacy, and in their rates of parenting (Pradhan et al., in press). In stable social groups, male reproductive success is negatively associated with the frequency of agonistic behavior, approaches and displacements, in the social group (**Figure 4C**) (Solomon-Lane et al., 2014). Males that fail to parent also suffer a reproductive cost because female *L. dalli* cannibalize eggs in an unguarded nest (**Figure 4D**) (Pradhan et al., 2014c). Following the removal of a male from the social group, the dominant female changes sex to male, and functional sex change is typically evaluated based on the ability of the new male to fertilize eggs (Reavis and Grober, 1999; Rodgers, 2007). Successful sex change is a life history transition that dramatically increases reproductive success (Behrents, 1983), and because this species functions as a sequential protogynous hermaphrodite, maleness itself (indicated by behavior, genital papilla morphology, and gonadal sex allocation) is a proxy for both survival and reproductive success.

ENDOCRINE CONTEXT

Steroid hormones respond to environmental signals in order to integrate environmental information into behavioral command decisions (Alcock, 2001). These signals can be detected only when the endogenous state of the organism is primed, via receptor expression, to respond. Signal transduction occurs via cellular and molecular mechanisms and must be considered within the context of response location (e.g., anatomical site). The end goal of the signal is to induce a phenotypic effect (Ball and Balthazart, 2008). Based on the organism studied, there are several different types of biological samples that could serve as proxies of steroid bioavailability. To understand the mechanisms by which steroids regulate structure and function, a variety of approaches to both quantifying steroids and manipulating steroid availability have been developed. This work has elucidated the multiple levels of endocrine context that should be considered when assessing the variation in behavior and fitness across life history transitions. We will now summarize the proxies of steroid function that are commonly used, how mechanisms of steroid function are

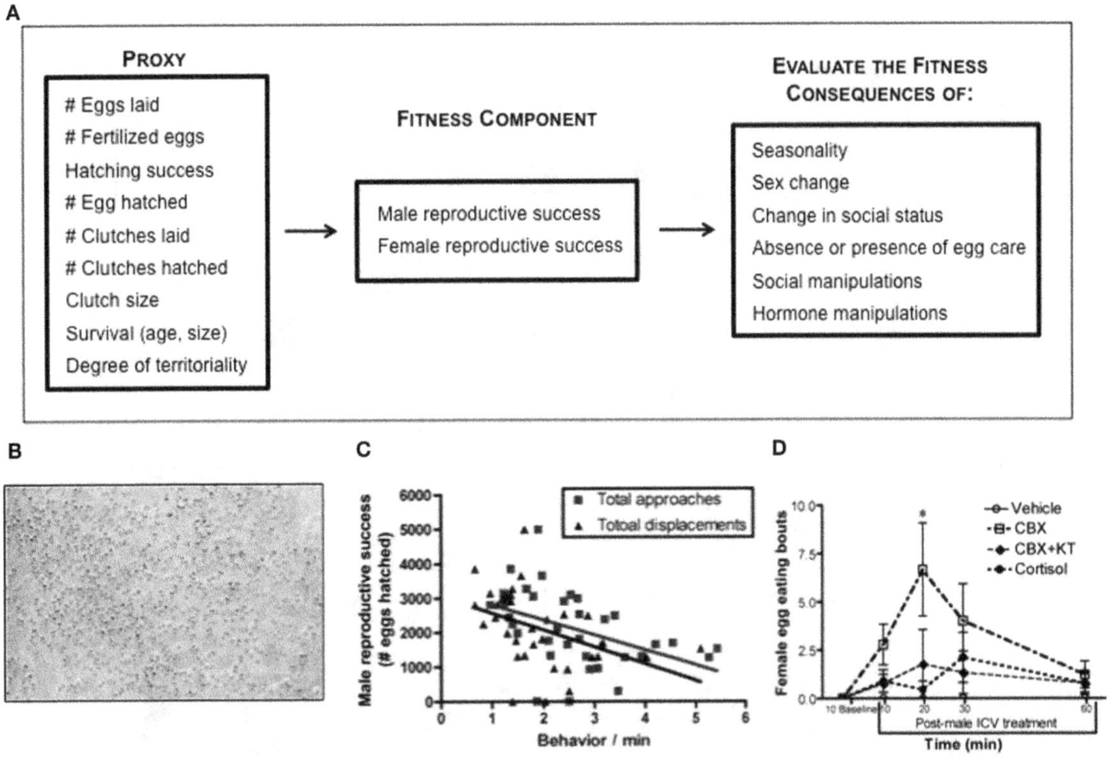

FIGURE 4 | Integration of fitness and behavioral neuroendocrinology in *Lythrypnus dalli*. (A) Examples of fitness proxies that are commonly used to estimate reproductive success. One or more of these measures can be evaluated during different life history stages and within a particular endocrinological or social context. **(B)** Eggs at different stages of development, such as newly laid and eyed. **(C)** In stable social groups male reproductive success is negatively associated with the frequency of approaches and displacements in the social group (total approaches is male, alpha, beta, gamma approaches). Adapted from Solomon-Lane et al. (2014). **(D)** Intracerebroventricular (ICV) treatment of males presented females with a new social opportunity, permitting them to enter the nest and eat eggs. CBX, Carbenoxolone; KT, 11-ketotestosterone, $*p < 0.05$. Adapted from Pradhan et al. (2014c).

investigated via endocrine manipulations, and the associated limitations.

PROXIES OF STEROID FUNCTION

Collectively, steroids affect many facets of phenotype, and specific steroids can have multiple effects (Nelson, 2011). These steroid functions include, but are not limited to, production of gametes, maintenance of homeostasis, activities related to survival and reproduction, development of secondary sexual morphological characteristics, and various aspects of social behavior (Wingfield et al., 1990; Borg, 1994; Cardwell et al., 1996; Trainor and Marler, 2001). At a fundamental level, the potent physiological impacts of steroid hormones occur primarily via steroid binding to membrane or nuclear associated receptors that up-regulate specific biochemical pathways via intracellular mechanisms, which then affect protein translation. As this level of experimental analysis is not possible for most behavioral investigations, proxies of steroid action are most often relied upon.

Which proxy is the most accurate representation of steroid levels that trigger and maintain activational effects in an organism? The answer to this question is anything but clear-cut because all proxies are indirect measures and have limitations (see below). There are many different levels of endocrine analyses, ranging from direct hormone measurements to receptor densities. Additionally, steroid receptor co-activators can modulate the downstream cellular response (Charlier et al., 2006). "Biomarkers" are naturally occurring molecules used to assess endogenous steroidal metabolites present in a biological sample of cells, tissues, and biofluids (Kotłowska, 2012). Often, the type of biological sample that is used as a proxy for steroid action is not based on accuracy, but rather on feasibility of collection and steroid detection (**Figure 5**). This results in many different levels of endocrine analyses, ranging from direct hormone measurements to receptor expression and binding kinetics. The site of steroid action—the cell—is probably the most appropriate location to measure levels of active steroids, but few techniques allow for the determination of cellular steroid levels associated with the production of specific behaviors. Microdialysis is a technique that allows for the determination of steroids in the extracellular fluid within specific regions of the forebrain of live, behaving animals (Ikeda et al., 2014; Rensel et al., 2014). While this may not be equivalent to steroid levels within specific cells, microdialysis is currently as close as we can get to measuring brain steroid levels in awake, behaving animals. In addition to sequestering steroids produced in the periphery, the brain

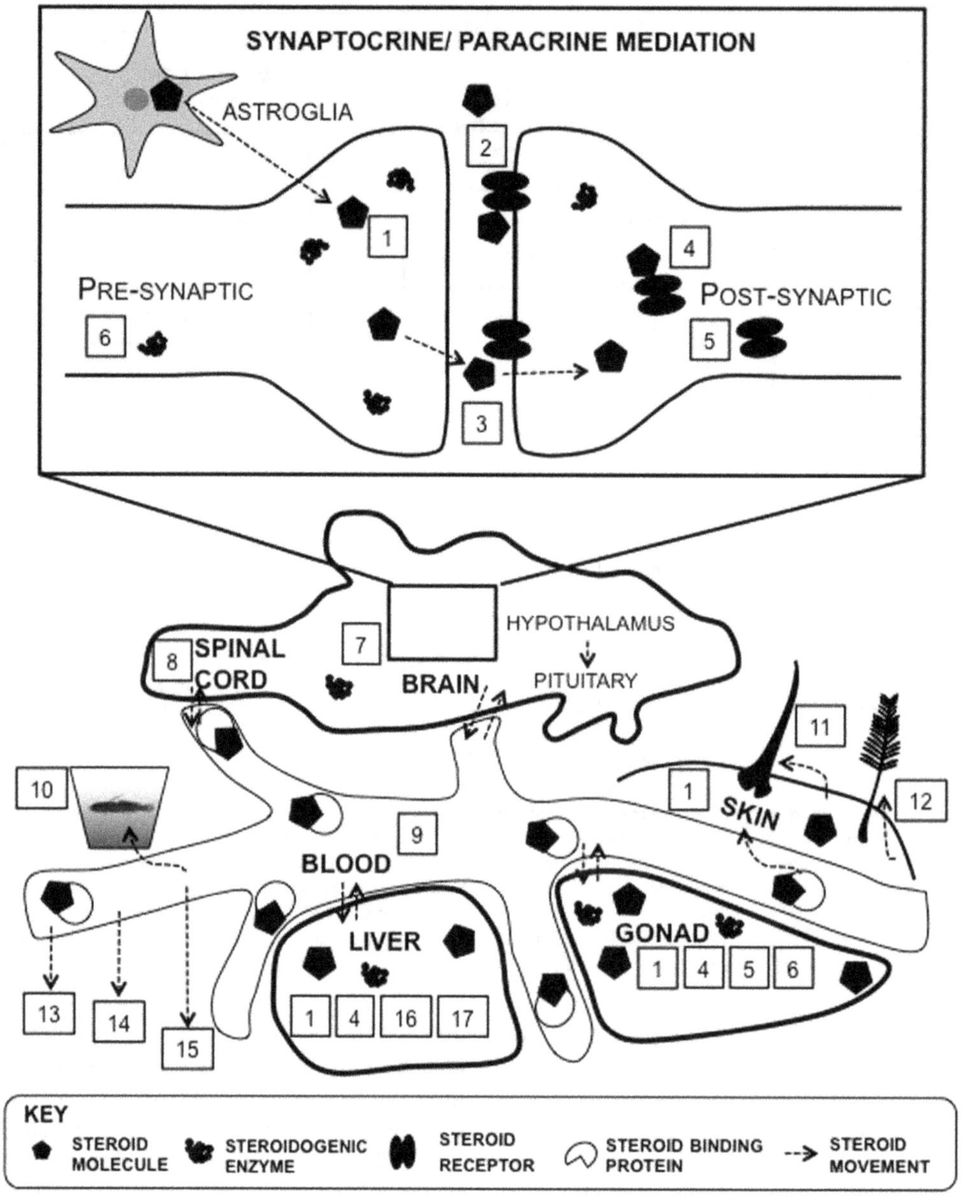

FIGURE 5 | Proxies of steroid function at multiple levels of analysis. There are many different approaches to determine steroid levels in organisms. Steroids can be measured within particular tissues such as the brain, and in systemic circulation, such as plasma. Direct proxies within brain tissue include steroid signaling molecules such as receptors and steroidogenic machinery, such as enzymes (#1–8): 1, tissue; 2, membrane receptor protein; 3, synapse; 4, intracellular receptor protein; 5, steroid receptor mRNA expression; 6, steroidogenic enzyme mRNA expression; 7, steroidogenesis; 8, cerebrospinal fluid. Steroids can be synthesized in astroglia and within the the synaptic bouton (Saldanha et al., 2011). There are many proxies of systemic measures (#9–17): 9, plasma; 10, water-borne; 11, hair/fur; 12, feather; 13, saliva; 14, urine; 15, feces; 16; steroid metabolism; 17, steroid conjugation.

is a remarkably heterogeneous organ that has specific sites of steroidogenic enzyme expression, steroidogenesis, and sex steroid receptor expression (Carere et al., 2007; Schmidt et al., 2008; Do Rego et al., 2009; Arterbery et al., 2010; Pradhan et al., 2010b) Another valid proxy is the steroidogenic potential of the brain, which can be measured at specific regions or subcellular compartments using *in vitro* assays (Black et al., 2005a; Pradhan et al., 2010a,b). The evidence for synaptocrine signaling, which encompasses steroid synthesis within the presynaptic bouton and release in the synaptic cleft for rapid neuromodulation, has spurred a re-evaluation of the most widely used proxies of hormone measurements (e.g., plasma) (Peterson et al., 2005; Saldanha et al., 2011). The primary advantage of local synthesis within a traditionally "target" organ is the speed and localization of steroid action due to temporal and spatial specificity (Schmidt and Soma, 2008; Saldanha et al., 2011). Another advantage is the reduction in costs of steroid synthesis: less hormone would need to be produced locally in the brain relative to the quantities needed to induce system-wide (including the brain) elevations in steroids (Wingfield et al., 2001).

Technological advancements have allowed for assay and equipment development that maximizes steroid extraction, separation, recovery, detection, and sensitivity from a wide array of sample types (Makin et al., 2010; Taves et al., 2011). At a very crude level, the weight of gland or the tissue that synthesizes the hormone can be measured to estimate the possible steroidogenic output (Buhimschi et al., 2008; Weathington et al., 2012). This is an indirect measure of steroid-releasing potential of that tissue. The most common estimate of steroid levels is also an indirect measure: plasma or serum is widely used because it is easily collected from most model organisms. This measure represents the systemic levels in circulation and is based on the view that steroids produced in specific organs are free to permeate the general circulation. Direct measures of steroids within specific tissues (both glands and targets) have been used successfully in fishes (Genova et al., 2012; Lorenzi et al., 2012) birds (Schmidt et al., 2009; Charlier et al., 2010), and rodents (Corpéchot et al., 1981) and provide an understanding of steroid function at the site of action. Steroid load can also be estimated by measuring specific proteins because steroids are generally bound to carrier proteins, such as sex hormone binding globulins (Heinlein and Chang, 2002), corticosteroid-binding globulin, or albumin (Huddleston et al., 2007), for transport to target organs.

A variety of non-invasive sampling methods are necessary for diagnostic testing of disease, detecting contamination, assessing responses to an environmental stressor or endogenous physiological factor, understanding the mechanism of steroid action, detecting steroids of abuse (Heitzman, 1976; De Jager et al., 2011; Divari et al., 2011), and assessing the reproductive status of wild and livestock populations. Fecal samples are used in wild or threatened populations (Borque et al., 2011). Urine samples can be easily collected from cattle (Doué et al., 2012) and amphibians (Narayan et al., 2012). For small fish, another non-invasive procedure involves measuring steroids exuded into water via gills, osmotic exchange through skin, and excretion (Sebire et al., 2007). For this procedure, the animal is temporarily kept in a beaker containing clean water for a long enough period of time for steroids to accumulate. As is the case with many non-invasive techniques, demonstrating correspondence between plasma hormone levels and water borne hormone is straightforward and necessary (Gabor and Contreras, 2012). It should not be assumed that multiple proxies of steroid function co-vary. For humans, salivary hormones are often measured because of the easy, non-invasive nature of sample collection (Hansen et al., 2008). Other non-invasive proxies of steroid measurement include feathers (Koren et al., 2012), hair [grizzly bears (Macbeth et al., 2010); humans (Dettenborn et al., 2012)], yolk [reptiles (Huang et al., 2013); fish (Feist et al., 1990), birds (Sockman et al., 2006)], and cerebrospinal fluid (Heidbrink et al., 2010). Taken together, other than direct measures of steroids at the site of action, all other measures should be regarded as proxies of steroid function and it is not clear if any one of those proxies (e.g., plasma/serum) is a "better" measure of steroid function than less traditionally employed measures. Our view is that each system has unique constraints on what can be sampled and each sampling method comes with specific limitations with regard to interpretation.

Limitations of endocrine proxies

In both field and laboratory settings, there are many constraints to measuring steroids from various species, including rodents. When studying free-living species, natural history, seasonality, type of sample availability, and ease of sample collection are all important considerations. The specific endocrine proxy used is also contingent upon other factors such as whether the species is dangerous to interact with, ease or ability to trap animals, lifespan, age, and population size. The degree of invasiveness of a procedure and how often samples are collected are also important considerations. By studying a species in a laboratory, some of these limitations can be circumvented and confounding factors can be controlled. Even under laboratory conditions, however, we need to be aware of the limitations and consequences of different sampling methods. The site from which a sample is collected should be reflective of the experimental question of interest, and carefully interpreted as such. This is especially critical when comparing steroid levels across a variety of sample types (e.g., plasma, tissue, waste). Due to the heterogeneity of steroid distribution in blood (Taves et al., 2010), one must exercise caution in interpreting plasma levels because it contains concentrated steroids compared to whole blood or red blood cells and might be an overestimation (Hiramatsu and Nisula, 1987; Taves et al., 2010). Environmental stressors can also have differential effects on steroids and their binding to proteins (Taves et al., 2010). In addition, the part of the body that blood is collected from must be considered. For example, cardiac, caudal, and brachial plasma represent systemic steroid levels. In comparison, the jugular vein represents blood that is exiting the brain, and is, therefore, an indirect measure of brain steroids (Schlinger and Arnold, 1993; Saldanha and Schlinger, 1997; Newman et al., 2008). Factors such as half-life (Cavaco et al., 1997), rate of elimination (Leshchenko et al., 2006), and rate of conversion to other active or inactive steroids can vary (Schlinger et al., 2008) depending on the site of blood collection, further complicating the interpretation of blood based steroid measures (Schmidt et al., 2008). Salivary samples are often collected from humans; however, context-specific variation limits its ability to be interpreted (Hansen et al., 2008; Kudielka et al., 2009).

ENDOCRINE MANIPULATIONS

Manipulative mechanistic studies have been integral to our understanding of the regulation of behavioral and morphological phenotypes. Steroids can be manipulated locally, in particular tissues of interest, or systemically. The context of the endocrine manipulation (e.g., anatomical location or form of manipulation) is critical to consider relative to the particular questions of interest. Classically, steroids have been administered chronically, founded on the theory that steroids take hours or days to exert their phenotypic effects via classical genomic mechanisms. However, some effects of steroid hormones occur on a much shorter time-scale, over seconds or minutes, via non-genomic mechanisms. Hence the appropriate type of manipulation and route of administration must be considered. Again, any steroidal manipulation should be performed within well-defined environmental contexts that are relevant to the life history of the animal being studied. We will now summarize some types of endocrine manipulations and discuss the associated limitations.

Systemic manipulations

Traditionally, studies on reproductive endocrinology focus separately on gonadally produced sex steroids and adrenally (or interrenally in fish) produced glucocorticoids. Early in the development of behavioral endocrinology, extirpation and replacement led to the discovery of blood borne "factors" that were released into circulation from the testes and controlled phenotype. In 1849, Arnold Berthold conducted a series of seminal experiments in which he either removed and/or transplanted testes in young male chickens (Quiring, 1944). He found, that removing the testes prevented the development of secondary sexual characteristics and the expression of male-typical sexual and aggressive behaviors, while transplanting testes from other birds rescued these traits (Quiring, 1944). Terminal examination of these animals in adulthood led him to conclude that substances released by the testes into blood are transported throughout the body, and largely to the nervous system (Quiring, 1944). Accordingly, systemic manipulations that investigate regulatory effects of hormones have largely focused on manipulating peripheral tissues by removal of source of the hormone (gonadectomy or adrenalectomy). There are several other methods by which peripheral hormones can be manipulated. Pharmacological manipulations that inhibit steroidogenic enzymes or serve as receptor antagonists can prevent the downstream effects of steroids (Nelson, 2011). After demonstrating the loss of phenotype in response to steroid removal, subsequent delivery of the hormone(s) under investigation can rescue or restore normal functioning. This step is critical for identifying the mechanism of specific steroid action. Intraperitoneal (IP) manipulations, such as injections and implants, are most often used to replace steroids after gland removal. Hormone implants (IP or subcutaneous, Fuenzalida, 1950) can be of several types and include incorporation into beeswax (Pradhan et al., 2014c), pure crystalline pellets (Pradhan et al., 2014a), controlled released pellets (Fuenzalida, 1950), *in situ* forming microparticle implants (Castillo-Briceno et al., 2013), and silastic tubing implants (Damassa et al., 1977). Additionally, steroids can also be ingested via mixing in food (Remage-Healey and Bass, 2006). Finally, on amphibians, non-invasive methods of steroid delivery have included patch-delivery (Knapp and Moore, 1997) or direct application on bare skin by dissolving in a vehicle (Belliure et al., 2004).

Local manipulations

Local steroid manipulations are often insightful because they occur at the site of hormone action. The effects of local manipulations are also less prone to interference from any indirect effects of the hormones acting on other target tissues (Friedman et al., 1964). This can be accomplished by performing implants directly within the tissue in question, for example, in thymus (Friedman et al., 1964) and brain (Ramirez et al., 1964; Hartmann et al., 1966). For central hormone manipulations, cannulae have been used for long-term experiments (Huddleston et al., 2006) and intracerebroventricular (ICV) injections have been used for short-term studies (Tehranipour and Moghimi, 2010; Solomon-Lane and Grober, 2012).

Limitations of endocrine manipulations

Any type of *in vivo* experimental manipulation has limitations. Both peripheral and local manipulation can affect an organism in unintended ways, based in part on the degree of invasiveness of the procedure. Administration of hormones can produce a high degree of individual variation in the amount of systemic and local hormone levels (Pradhan et al., 2014a). Steroid treatment can have effects at many different biological levels and differential rates of endogenous feedback loops or breakdown might be involved (Pradhan et al., 2014a). Some hormones are extremely potent with activating effects occurring at low levels. The effects of hormones do not tend to increase with added hormone, demonstrating that steroids do not generally exert effects in a dose-dependent manner (Nelson, 2011). If hormone is administered after gonadectomy, then timing becomes an important consideration because much higher does of hormones are required for restoring behavior relative to maintaining it (Damassa et al., 1977). High doses can also have costly physiological side-effects (Wingfield et al., 2001). In addition, frequent delivery, such as injections, might be too invasive and induce a variety of unwanted endocrine side affects (Wallis et al., 2014). Some drugs do not penetrate the blood brain barrier (Leshchenko et al., 2006) and cannot be used to investigate central effects on behavior (Pradhan et al., 2014c). We can also use different manipulations to consider endocrine vs. paracrine functions of hormones and discriminate between systemic vs. local effects. Different steroids also have differential rates of release, binding, breakdown, conversion, sequestration, and lipophilicity (Babuska and Pyaka, 2006). Hence, once introduced into the body, the timescale of effects and mechanisms of action may differ based on the particular steroid structure. Another consequence of hormone delivery is that the manipulation of one hormone, for example using an enzyme inhibitor, can cause unintended affects on other hormones in the steroidogenic pathway. Steroidogenic enzymes often act in more than one direction, and the same enzyme can participate in the conversion of multiple steroids. For example, administration of carbenoxolone (CBX), an 11β-hydroxysteroid dehydrogenase (11β-HSD) inhibitor, increases F while decreasing KT in fish (see **Figure 2**) (Pradhan et al., 2014c). Carbenoxolone, a glycyrrhetinic acid derivative, inhibits the gastric enzyme, pepsin. It has been used to treat ulcers since the 1960s (Henman, 1970). While at least two isoforms of 11β-HSD have been described (Payne and Hales, 2004), and both are inhibited by CBX (Jellinck et al., 1993; Ge et al., 1997; Ma et al., 2011), fish have only one isoform (Arterbery et al., 2010). The phenotypic effects of CBX treatment in fish could be due to the effects of either KT and/or F. Thus, presence of multiple isoforms of an enzyme and the ability of a chemical to affect more than one enzyme are important considerations for understanding the effects of any pharmacological manipulation, central or peripheral. Additionally, measures of systemic hormone levels following peripheral manipulations are not indicative of the degree to which exogenous steroids remain elevated in specific tissues and thus affect their subsequent biological effects. For example, systemic hormone manipulation differentially impacts the levels of that hormone found in different tissues (Pradhan et al., 2014a). It is likely that elevated peripheral hormones are transported to tissue via the blood supply; however, the vascular supply to the brain may not have a significant impact on total brain steroid levels (Taves et al., 2010). Some of these limitations of peripheral delivery can be circumvented via local steroid manipulations.

INSIGHTS FROM *LYTHRYPNUS DALLI*

Given the substantial independent data indicating the importance of both systemic and local steroidogenic regulation, we have utilized a variety of steroid measurements in our studies of hormonal regulation of reproductive life history in the bluebanded goby (**Figure 6A**), including tissue steroid levels (Lorenzi et al., 2012); steroids released in water (Lorenzi et al., 2008), distribution of steroid receptors and steroidogenic enzymes in tissue sections (Schuppe et al., unpublished results), and the potential for steroid synthesis in particular tissues (Pradhan et al., 2014c). The endocrine manipulations we have used in *L. dalli* include systemic treatment using IP implants (Pradhan et al., 2014a), addition of steroids or steroid inhibitors to the water (Schuppe et al., unpublished results) and local brain manipulations using ICV injections (Solomon-Lane and Grober, 2012) (**Figure 6B**). This combination of endocrine measures with endocrine manipulations at different levels of analysis has allowed us to empirically question the traditionally accepted phenomenon that sex steroids are synthesized in gonads and transported by the blood to target organs. This is particularly relevant when viewing the brain as a target organ because a behavioral change does not always correspond with changes in circulating steroid levels (Pradhan et al., 2010b) or gonad specific changes in steroid levels (Pradhan et al., 2014c). If the traditional dogma that the gonad being the primary site of sex steroid synthesis is true, then systemic levels should closely reflect gonadal steroid production or levels of hormone extracted from gonadal tissue. This relationship should hold true for other target tissues as well; however, this does not appear to be the case (Pradhan et al., 2014b).

In stable groups of *L. dalli*, there are no status or sex differences in water-borne steroid levels (Solomon-Lane et al., unpublished results; Lorenzi et al., 2008). However, three different tissues, brain, gonads, and muscle, show different patterns of steroid levels among males and females of different statuses (Pradhan et al., in review; Lorenzi et al., 2012). For example, the brain has 3× higher androgen levels than the gonad (Lorenzi et al., 2012), subordinate females have higher brain T, KT, and F compared to dominant females (Pradhan et al., in review), females have several fold higher ovarian E_2 compared to males (Lorenzi et al., 2012), and in mini males, brain and reproductive tissue levels of T, E_2, and KT are higher than in the muscle (Pradhan et al., 2014b). When the dominant male is removed from the social group, all the females in the hierarchy show tissue-specific changes in hormone levels (Lorenzi et al., 2012). This independent regulation is important because the brain modulates behavior and must respond to rapid changes in social context. Other tissues, such as the gonad, often have more delayed responses (Lorenzi et al., 2012). The speed of the response may not be as critical for non-behavioral traits. To evaluate the effect of exogenous steroid hormones on steroid load within tissue, we IP implanted females undergoing sex change with KT. We found that even though the KT load increases markedly in brain, gonads, and muscles within only 5 days of treatment, elevations in KT levels varries across the three tissues (Pradhan et al., 2014a). This indicates that there is differential penetration, sequestration, or breakdown of KT in tissue. In addition, there is a negative relationship between the amount of KT absorbed from the pellet and the level of KT measured from the gonads of KT implanted fish, but not control fish. Thus, a systemic steroid manipulation affects local steroid loads quite differently.

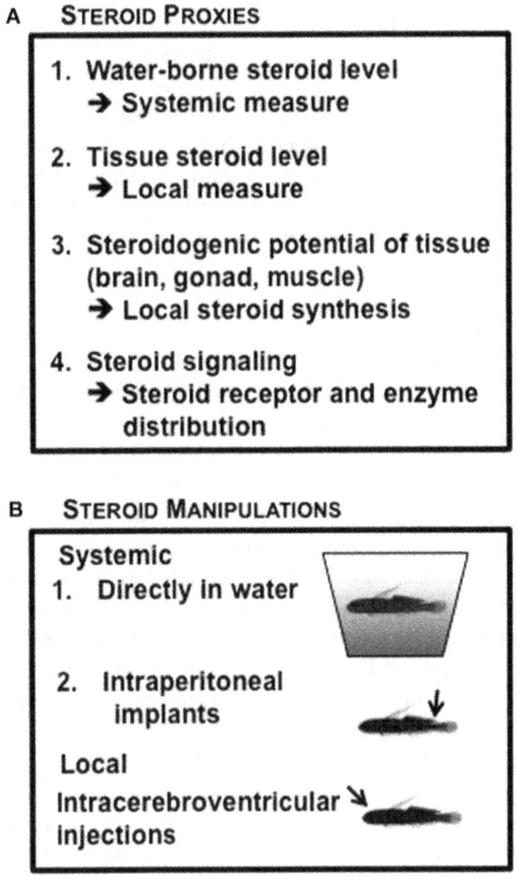

FIGURE 6 | Endocrine context of *Lythrypnus dalli*, commonly used in the laboratory. **(A)** Steroid measurement proxies **(B)** Steroid manipulation approaches.

When we consider the parenting stage of the life history, males that actively tend eggs have higher water-borne KT compared to experienced males not actively nesting, new males tending eggs, and females (Rodgers et al., 2006). To evaluate the role of KT in regulating male parenting, we performed two types of manipulations of 11β-HSD, an enzyme that synthesizes KT in both male gonad and brain (Pradhan et al., 2014c). First, using long-term IP implants of CBX, we found that KT synthesis is only transiently inhibited (Pradhan et al., 2014c). Second, using short-term ICV manipulation of parenting males, we show that the ratio of KT to F is rapidly (within 60 min) reduced in both brain and gonad (Pradhan et al., 2014c). Although water-borne KT is reduced by CBX in a dose dependent manner, F is not affected (Pradhan et al., unpublished results). Taken together, these results have important implications. First, local endocrine manipulations can have differential local and systemic effects. Second, endogenous steroids are linked through common enzymatic pathways, and manipulation of one enzyme can have differential and opposite effects on two active steroids.

SOCIAL CONTEXT

Interactions among conspecifics are frequent in social species and adaptive in particular environmental contexts (Wallen and Schneider, 1999). In the wild, an organism might experience variation in the type of social interaction with conspecifics and heteropecifics throughout its lifetime. For example, different types of interactions can emerge when dealing with parents, siblings, territorial or mate competitors, predators, prospective mates, and offspring. Two dramatic and highly escalated states of social interaction, sex and aggression, typically occur only under specific circumstances or contexts over the course of an organism's life history (Huber and Kravitz, 2010). Often, more than one type of interaction can overlap temporally, for example, warding off predators while providing brood care. Another change in social context can occur if a group member dies, and other individuals in a group compete to assume the open position in the hierarchy. For example, in *L dalli*, absence of the male from a social group creates a social context that is permissive for the highest ranking (alpha) female to establish dominance over the group, take over the nesting territory, and change sex to male (Pradhan et al., 2014a). Social context is also dynamic and is largely based on reciprocated interactions between or among individuals. For example, in a dyadic aggressive interaction, at least three components could be measured: (1) quality/intensity could range from threat displays to physical contact; (2) quantity could comprise the number of attacks and retaliations, and (3) duration of interaction would determine the timescale of interaction (Nilsen et al., 2004). In a status contest, individual variation in behavioral phenotype can lead to variation in the amount of time it takes for a resolution (Pradhan et al., 2014a). In addition, familiarity with a territory or residency status might also provide an advantage in social contests (e.g., "home advantage," Fuxjager et al., 2009). In any experimental paradigm, the response of animals might differ based on the particular social context; therefore, subtle changes in social context should be taken into consideration.

INTEGRATION OF BEHAVIORAL AND ENDOCRINE CONTEXT

Steroids can regulate social interactions in a context-dependent manner. To control for environmental variation and the logistical constraints of laboratory-based experiments, most studies use a very simplified and/or artificial social environment. However, in many group-living species, social complexity is integrated with endocrine function to regulate reproductive behavior. For example, in multi-female groups of rhesus monkeys, *Macaca mulatta*, males direct their reproductive behavior toward females only during the peri-ovulatory phase (Wallen and Winston, 1984). In pair-housing, however, males direct reproductive behavior toward females during both the follicular and peri-ovulatory phases (Wallen and Winston, 1984). Females are receptive to copulation only during particular reproductive stages in rhesus monkeys (Wallen and Winston, 1984), as well as in other vertebrates, such as rodents (Kow et al., 1978) and amphibians (Lynch et al., 2006). Thus, parameters of the mating system are shaped by cyclical ovarian patterns, which dictate the expression of specific reproductive behaviors in both males and females.

Social modulation of androgen levels is generally transient and occurs in animals during or right after an aggressive challenge. In song sparrows for example, winners of an aggressive encounter have high plasma T, while losers have low plasma T (Wingfield et al., 1990). These changes in plasma T are only seen during the breeding season, when the animals are already experiencing increased with marked increases in gonadal androgen synthesis (associated with spermatogenesis). Androgen synthesis is positively correlated with circulating androgens and sexual and territorial behavior (Borg, 1994). Song sparrows also maintain territorial aggression outside the breeding season despite low circulating androgen levels (Caldwell et al., 1984; Soma, 2006). One mechanism by which aggression during the non-breeding season can be maintained is through brain synthesis of androgens (Pradhan et al., 2010b). Thus, the behavioral output of an organism is affected by variation in both responses to social interactions and endocrine mechanisms of behavioral regulation.

Traditionally, hormone manipulations have been used to understand the role of steroids in the proximate regulation of behavior. The probability of increasing or decreasing the expression of behavior (e.g., aggressive, sexual) using a hormone manipulation is complicated because behaviors are often exhibited within tightly regulated windows that depend on the integration of ecological, social, and endogenous factors. For example, pharmacological treatment of spotted antbirds (*Hylophylax n. naevioides*) with androgen and estrogen inhibitors is during the breeding season is more effective in regulating aggressive behavior than during the non-breeding season. Effects also depend on the intensity of aggressive stimuli (Beebee, 2004). Experimentally elevated hormones often have impacts only during a short period after the manipulation and only specific components of aggression may be affected. In black redstarts (*Phoenicurus ochruros*), hormone manipulation causes short-term decreases in T and affects only specific components of song structure (Apfelbeck et al., 2013). Moreover, these effects also depend on whether the behavior occurs in a conspecific aggression or mating context (Apfelbeck et al., 2013). Thus, timing and social group dynamics are both important factors for determining the proximate hormonal mechanisms regulating behavior.

INSIGHTS FROM *LYTHRYPNUS DALLI*

In the laboratory, *L. dalli* social groups are easily set up under conditions permissive for natural sex change and spawning (**Figure 7**). The male, the most dominant member of the social group, is provided with a harem of 2–3 size-mismatched females and a piece of PVC tube that serves as his nest. These groups establish a robust linear hierarchy within 5 days (Reavis and Grober, 1999). The male regulates female entry into the nest

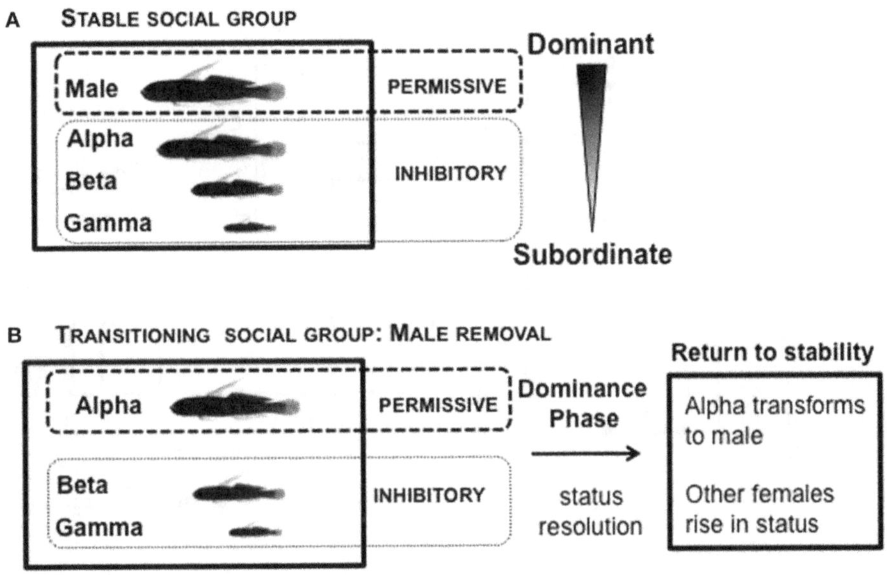

FIGURE 7 | Social context of *Lythrypnus dalli*. (A) Stable social groups form a linear social hierarchy in the laboratory within 5 days. In the presence of the male, all females are in an environment *inhibitory* to sex change. **(B)** Sex change can then be readily induced in the alpha female by removing the male, which changes the social context. The most dominant female is now in a transitioning social environment that is *permissive* for sex change, while the subordinate females are in an environment inhibitory for sex change. Depending upon the specific group, there is substantial variation in the time over which a stable social hierarchy is re-established ("Dominance Phase"), after which there is a decline in rates of agonistic interactions.

for spawning. The presence of eggs in the nest is important for understanding endocrine state: males only show high systemic KT levels when they are actively caring for eggs in their nest, but not when eggs are absent (Rodgers et al., 2006). In a stable social group, in the presence of the male, all females are in an environment inhibitory to sex change (**Figure 7A**). Immediately following male removal (first few minutes), the rates of agonistic interactions among the females increase while they re-establish social status relationships (Reavis and Grober, 1999). The highest-ranking female, usually the most aggressive, is not subordinated by any other female (Rodgers et al., 2007), and rapidly assumes the dominant/male position. The most dominant female is now in a transitioning social environment that is permissive for sex change, while the subordinate females are in an environment inhibitory for sex change (**Figure 7B**). There is substantial variation in the time required to re-established a stable social hierarchy ("Dominance Phase"), after which rates of agonistic interaction decline (Reavis and Grober, 1999).

Within 24 h of male removal, the dominant female undergoing sex change has transient increases in water-borne (Earley and Grober, unpublished results) and brain KT (Lorenzi et al., 2012). Water-borne F levels also transiently increase in the dominant female undergoing sex change and remain elevated up to 3 days, after which F declines to basal levels (Solomon-Lane et al., 2013). In pairs of size-mismatched females, implanting (IP) the subordinate (beta) female with KT causes her to transform morphologically into a male. However, because the social context predominates, betas retain their female-typical behavior and subordinate social status (Rodgers, 2007). In another experiment involving pairs of size-mismatched females, the dominant individual (alpha) undergoing sex change was implanted IP with KT or cholesterol (**Figure 8**). Aggressive behaviors increased transiently during the critical period of social instability but did not persist as a result of KT treatment (Pradhan et al., 2014a). Agonistic efficiency, a composite score of aggression (rate of displacements/rate of approaches) (Solomon-Lane et al., 2014), was only affected in cholesterol implanted individuals (**Figure 8A**). Alpha females implanted with cholesterol initially (Dominance Phase) exhibited a decline in agonistic efficiency but had dramatically higher agonistic efficiency the following day (Pradhan et al., 2014a). Overall, the data show that effects of the KT or cholesterol treatment cascade through the social group, such that in groups where alphas are less effective agonistically, betas have higher approach rates during the Dominance Phase (Pradhan et al., 2014a) (**Figures 8B,C**).

Transitioning *L. dalli* social groups also offer other opportunities to investigate the role of social and endocrine context on other types of behaviors. As mentioned above, in stable groups, males aggressively maintain their territory, control access to the nest, and exclusively exhibit parenting behavior. Through the use of ICV injections of CBX, we found that neural KT regulates male parenting behavior (Pradhan et al., 2014c). A new social context is created when specific ICV manipulations inhibits males from guarding their nests, allowing alpha females to enter the nesting site. Curiously, some alphas, in the absence of parenting males, demonstrate parenting behavior. After only 1 h, these parenting females that have significantly higher brain KT and lower gonadal KT compared to those alphas with males in the nest (Pradhan et al., 2014c). Levels of KT in betas are not affected, suggesting that behavioral and endocrine changes are specific to the expression of a particular behavior and not the sex of the individual. Additionally, there were no changes in T, E_2, or F levels (Pradhan et al., 2014c). Our results demonstrate that rapid changes in social

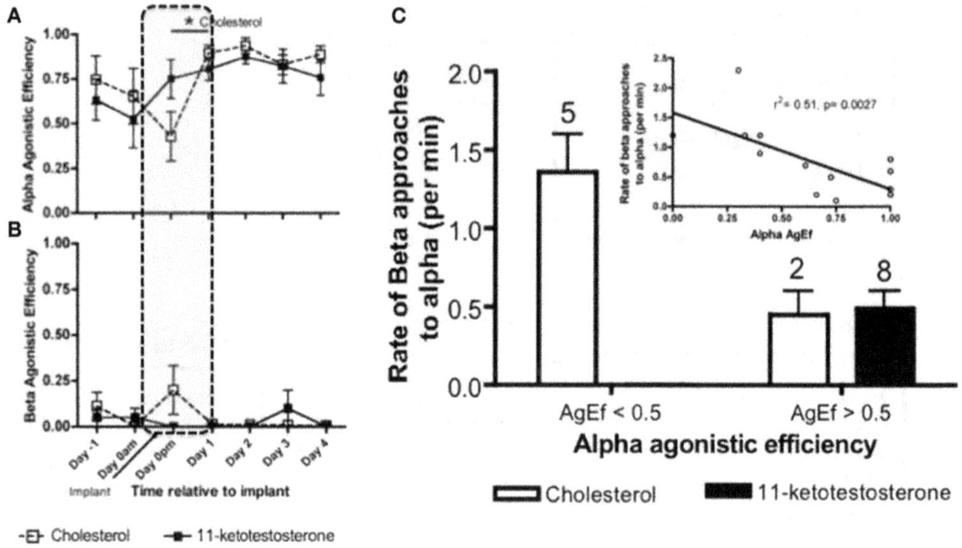

FIGURE 8 | Social context dependent effects of systemic (intraperitoneal) 11-ketotestosterone (KT) implants on agonistic interactions in *Lythrypnus dalli*. Alpha females were implanted with either KT or cholesterol and placed in a social environment that was permissive for sex change. **(A)** Alpha agonistic efficiency (AgEf) (displacements/approaches) toward betas relative to time after implant. Alpha females implanted with cholesterol had a decline in agonistic efficiency during the Dominance Phase (represented by dotted lines), but had dramatically higher agonistic efficiency the following day. **(B)** Beta Agonistic efficiency toward alphas relative to time after implant ($n = 8$ Chol and $n = 10$ KT). **(C)** Categorical representation of rates of beta approaches when alpha agonistic efficiecy was < or > 0.5. The numbers above bars represent the number of groups for each category. The inset is a regression of alpha agonistic efficiecy against rates of betas approaching alphas after alphas were treated with either KT or Cholesterol ($N = 15$). Note that some individuals were excluded from this analysis due to zero rates of interaction and overlap does not allow all data points to be seen clearly, $^{*}p < 0.05$.

context can have differential effects on local levels of specific steroids.

SYNTHESIS: FROM BROADCASTING FOR GENERAL EFFECT TO LOCAL SIGNALING FOR SPECIFIC EFFECT

We have presented a variety of endocrine and social factors that need to be integrated to elucidate how an animal expresses a phenotype. Proxies of endocrine function are based on the fact that centers in the hypothalamus and pituitary release regulatory hormones that stimulate the gonad or the adrenal gland to produce potent sex steroids or glucocorticoids, respectively. The traditional assumption follows that large quantities of steroids produced by endocrine organs, the "source," floods the circulatory system, and hormones are then transported to specific target organs to cause downstream effects on phenotype. A corollary to this conventional view is that gonadal steroids provide a system-wide signal that advertises or "screams" to the rest of the body that the gonad is ready to release gametes. Note that the scream is not directed. It is a systemic broadcast of remarkably high intensity and is a by-product of gonadal function. This "Screaming Gonad" hypothesis is generally applicable to species whose mating behavior is heavily regulated as a series of restricted reproductive cycles within and between mating seasons. In an evolutionary sense, the gonad does not know that it is screaming to the body; however, parts of the body express receptors to "hear" the signal. This has allowed for the coordination of reproductive function across many body tissues. For example, increased T in male rodents allows for the activation of sexual behavior, while gonadectomy gradually eliminates expression of sexual behavior (Damassa et al., 1977). These data indicate that most of the circulating T in rodents is likely to be gonadally produced. Testosterone acts as a signal to coordinate the expression of reproductive traits through affects on multiple organs that, together, enhance reproductive success. Gonadal T produced during the breeding season (when rats express reproductive behavior) is generally very high; however, the quantity of T required to maintain reproductive behavior is much lower (Damassa et al., 1977), suggesting that spermatogenesis drives T to circulating levels that are much higher than is needed to change physiology and behavior. Sexual selection results in direct fitness consequences and, as such, should co-opt the hormones that regulate gamete production to exert control over the expression of sexual behavior. Evolutionarily speaking, the rest of the organism is then entrained to reproductive signals from the gonad, so that all efforts of the organism work in a coordinated fashion toward increasing reproduction and thus fitness.

The mechanisms involved in the organization and activation of sexual behavior were proposed based primarily on work in rodents, starting with the classical study by Phoenix et al. (1959). Rodent models remain prevalent in laboratories investigating the function and mechanism of hormonal action, and the emergent principles derived from rodent models can have broad application. However, there are many species that express a level of sexual plasticity that cannot be explained by this existing model, primarily because many of the characteristics of adult sexual phenotype (Phoenix et al., 1959) are organized and therefore fixed during early development. In contrast to mammals that generally exhibit sexual canalization *in utero*, there are many species that have more flexibility and avoid the early fixation of sex. In these species, sex determination is environmental, not chromosomal (Devlin and Nagahama, 2002). For species in which the social environment determines sex, activating molecules, such as steroid hormones, play an important role in the reorganization of anatomy and behavior and maintaining sexually dimorphic phenotypes. For example, males generally have higher levels of circulating androgens than females. Males of species that show unidirectional sex change, such as wrasses, generally maintain dramatically higher circulating KT levels than females (Perry and Grober, 2003), and this might serve as a mechanism to canalize the terminal male phenotype. Species that have the capacity for bi-directional sex change, such as *L. dalli*, tend not to have dramatic sex differences in circulating androgen levels (Lorenzi et al., 2008, 2012), and this may allow them to avoid canalization. It is noteworthy that the absence of sexual dimorphism in KT levels in *L dalli* is a result of very low KT levels in males rather than elevated KT levels in females. While relatively low circulating KT levels in males may provide a mechanism that allows for male to female sex reversal, it does not preclude males from using KT to regulate sexually dimorphic behavior. One mechanism that allows for this behavioral plasticity is the local regulation of steroidogenesis and steroid signaling (e.g., brain KT is necessary for *L. dalli* parenting). Local regulation is the dissociation of specific endocrine glands as control centers, and allows specific target tissues, rather than endocrine glands, to control phenotypes.

The conventional view of the endocrine system that gonadal steroids regulate all aspects of reproductive behavior, allows for variation in environmental and social context to modulate the expression of behavior. Thus, in addition to circulating steroids entraining reproductive physiology, anatomy, and behavior, we should also expect to find local brain mechanisms that allow for contextual regulation of reproductive behavior. Local, tissue-specific regulatory systems provide checkpoints for the globally dispersed signal (Brenowitz and Lent, 2002). Gonadal function in some species can be regulated by social interactions, and rapid and fine-tuned control of behavior could only occur via local modulation. We propose that the activational phenotypic effects of hormones that are beneficial for attracting mates (e.g., the biochemical cascade of events involved in increasing muscle mass or change in coloration) could be triggered initially by a gonadally generated cue. If steroidogenic machinery (enzymes, cofactors, and substrates) is present in those initial steroid targets, then local synthesis of hormones (and receptors) could maintain those phenotypic effects. Gonadally produced sex steroids might be sequestered and used by those organs that do not have the capacity for local synthesis. For example, the supracarinalis muscle of *L. dalli* males expresses both, 11β-HSD and androgen receptor, while the external genetilia express androgen receptor but not 11β-HSD (Schuppe et al., unpublished results). These data suggest that while the muscle has local steroidogenic potential and could maintain its androgenic dimorphism via local regulation, the external genetilia only have the machinery for sensing androgen and is strictly a target organ.

Dissociating endocrine glands from their roles as control centers might serve as a mechanism to maintain reproductive plasticity by allowing more local control of target tissues phenotype. In those cases, the brain can regulate the expression of behavior regardless of signals from the gonad. The emancipation from strict gonadal control of reproductive behavior has occurred in a variety of species (humans, bonobos, sex changing fish) and seems to be associated with social systems where individuals can accrue non-procreative benefits from engaging in sexual behavior (e.g., resources, resolution of social conflict, manipulation of social hierarchy). In all of these cases, release from control by the "screaming gonad" requires the engagement of specific local mechanisms for regulating the expression of reproductive traits and, specifically, the control of courtship, mating, and parenting. To reduce the possible overstimulation produced by the sex hormones released from the "screaming gonad," and for reduction of unnecessary stimulation of target organs, specific receptors on either the cellular or nuclear membrane initiate the downstream intracellular events (Nelson, 2011). In order to maintain within-tissue control and be receptive to local steroid signals, tissues could filter out the high intensity gonadal "scream." Thus, binding globulins might be the proteins that bind with hormones in general circulation to regulate the unnecessary activation of target organs.

There are examples from a range of vertebrates, from fish to humans, that provide support for local brain regulation of reproductive behavior. First, female wrasses can behaviorally change sex to males when the social environment is permissive, even in the absence of gonads (Godwin et al., 1996). Second, when male *L. dalli* are ICV injected with CBX, a KT synthesis inhibitor, their parenting behavior is blocked (Pradhan et al., 2014c). However, upon delivery of KT along with CBX rescues those effects (Pradhan et al., 2014c). Thus, neurally produced KT can regulate male nest care behavior, and there is little evidence for gonadal involvement in the regulation of parenting. Finally, some primates, including human females, regularly display sexual activity outside of the fertile period of their reproductive cycle. These data demonstrate the presence of local control mechanisms, facilitated in some cases via local production of hormones. According to this view, hormones that originally were produced by the gonad, are now also being synthesized in the brain so as provide rapid regulation of behavior, allowing for a more adaptive matching to immediate context. Local synthesis of steroids allows for peripheral tissues to commandeer the ancestral pathway used for steroidogenic regulation, but under novel control processes that can be more carefully regulated in both time and space. Synaptocrine signaling (Saldanha et al., 2011) provides a cellular mechanisms within brain circuits that can exercise local control of behavior.

OVERALL SIGNIFICANCE AND FUTURE DIRECTIONS

The organization of the life cycle into distinct life history stages allows for specific adaptations to the unique environment experienced at each stage and the exploration of large and small scale mechanisms associated with the regulation of phenotypic traits. In an effort to increase fitness, individuals must respond to different social contexts in appropriate ways. The behavioral, physiological, and morphological components of these responses are closely regulated by the endocrine system. The use of validated fitness and endocrine proxies under different environmental (social and physical) contexts substantially add to our depth of knowledge regarding mechanisms that regulate the expression of context-dependent phenotypes. Caution should be exercised when interpreting results and drawing conclusions about the similarities and/or differences in mechanisms regulating phenotype based on proxies of measurement, because any two proxies may provide for widely different interpretations. Hypothesis testing should involve experimental designs that consider both the social and environmental context (**Figure 9**). According to our proposed model, the relative contribution of the particular social and/or endocrine context being investigated act together to affect phenotype. One or the other component may be more important in particular environments, but a balance is established, which allows for the expression of an adaptive phenotype in a variety of social and/or biotic environments. Finally, it is apparent that the comparative study of diverse species provides insights into unique mechanisms of behavioral regulation. While the establishment of small scale spatial (local steroid synthesis and action) and temporal (rapid time scale) effects of steroids have spurred a re-evaluation of the mechanisms by which hormones exert their effects, tremendous gaps in our knowledge remain. Given the diversity of mechanisms known to regulate steroid actions, a comparative species approach that integrates hormones and behavior in the service of fitness will greatly facilitate progress in this field.

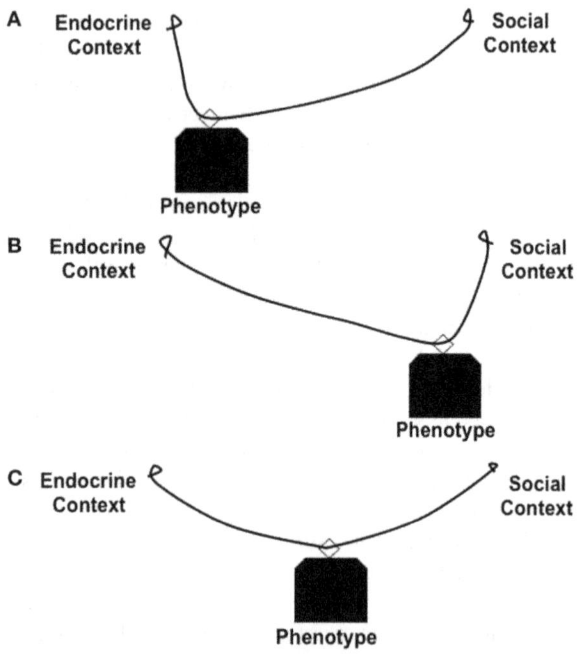

D

Factors to consider when designing experiments

Endocrine Context Factors	Social Context Factors
• Timing of endocrine measurements	• Ecology
• Route of endocrine measurements	• Interaction with conspecifics
• Route of endocrine measurements	• Life history (e.g. reproductive stage)
• Timing of endocrine changes	• Time scale of behavioral changes

FIGURE 9 | Functional interpretation of endocrine studies should be cognizant of the relevant proxy. Loose links exist, such that expression of phenotype is dependent upon both, **(A)** Endocrine and **(B)** Social factors. **(C)** Balance between these two factors is necessary for the regulation of function and increase lifetime reproductive success. **(D)** Several endocrine and social context factors must be considered when designing experiments.

ACKNOWLEDGMENTS

We thank Drs. Parhar, Ogawa, and Soga for the invitation to write this manuscript. We are also thankful to Drs. Bass and Somoza for comments on this manuscript. We thank staff at USC Wrigley Institute for Environmental Studies for assistance with the field studies. We are grateful for the grants from NSERC PGS D3, Sigma Xi, Brains and Behavior Program at Georgia State University and Georgia State University Dissertation Award to Devaleena S. Pradhan, NSF (IOB – 0548567) to Matthew S. Grober, and NSF Doctoral Dissertation Improvement Grant (1210382) to Matthew S. Grober and Devaleena S. Pradhan.

REFERENCES

Alcock, J. (2001). *Animal Behavior: An Evolutionary Approach, 7th Edn.* Sunderland, MA: Sinauer Associates Inc.

Angelier, F., Weimerskirch, H., Dano, S., and Chastel, O. (2006). Age, experience and reproductive performance in a long-lived bird: a hormonal perspective. *Behav. Ecol. Sociobiol.* 61, 611–621. doi: 10.1007/s00265-006-0290-1

Apfelbeck, B., Mortega, K. G., Kiefer, S., Kipper, S., and Goymann, W. (2013). Life-history and hormonal control of aggression in black redstarts: blocking testosterone does not decrease territorial aggression, but changes the emphasis of vocal behaviours during simulated territorial intrusions. *Front. Zool.* 10:8. doi: 10.1186/1742-9994-10-8

Arterbery, A. S., Deitcher, D. L., and Bass, A. H. (2010). Divergent expression of 11β-hydroxysteroid dehydrogenase and 11β-hydroxylase genes between male morphs in the central nervous system, sonic muscle and testis of a vocal fish. *Gen. Comp. Endocrinol.* 167, 44–50. doi: 10.1016/j.ygcen.2010.02.021

Aubry, L. M., Koons, D. N., Monnat, J.-Y., and Cam, E. (2009). Consequences of recruitment decisions and heterogeneity on age-specific breeding success in a long-lived seabird. *Ecology* 90, 2491–2502. doi: 10.1890/08-1475.1

Babuska, M., and Pyaka, A. (2006). Lipophilicity of selected steroid compounds. I. Investigations on RP18W stationary phase by RP–HPTLC. *J. Liq. Chromatogr. Relat. Technol.* 29, 1891–1903. doi: 10.1080/10826070600757748

Ball, G. F., Auger, C. J., Bernard, D. J., Charlier, T. D., Sartor, J. J., Riters, L. V., et al. (2004). Seasonal plasticity in the song control system: multiple brain sites of steroid hormone action and the importance of variation in song behavior. *Ann. N. Y. Acad. Sci.* 1016, 586–610. doi: 10.1196/annals.1298.043

Ball, G. F., and Balthazart, J. (2008). Individual variation and the endocrine regulation of behaviour and physiology in birds: a cellular/molecular perspective. *Philos. Trans. R. Soc. Lond. B. Biol. Sci.* 363, 1699–1710. doi: 10.1098/rstb.2007.0010

Barker, J. S. F. (2009). "Defining fitness in natural and domesticated populations," in *Adaptation and Fitness in Animal Populations: Evolutionary and Breeding Perspectives on Genetic Resource Management*, eds J. van der Werf, H.-U. Graser, R. Frankham, and C. Gondro (Heidelberg: Springer), 3–14. doi: 10.1007/978-1-4020-9005-9_1

Barrett, J., Abbott, D., and George, L. (1993). Sensory cues and the suppression of reproduction in subordinate female marmoset monkeys, *Callithrix jacchus*. *J. Reprod. Fertil.* 97, 301–310. doi: 10.1530/jrf.0.0970301

Beebee, M. (2004). The functions of multiple singing modes: experimental tests in yellow warblers, *Dendroica petechia*. *Anim. Behav.* 67, 1089–1097. doi: 10.1016/j.anbehav.2003.05.016

Behrents, K. (1983). *The Comparative Ecology and Interactions Between Two Sympatric Gobies (Lythrypnus dalli and Lythrypnus zebra), Biology*. University of Southern California, Los Angeles, 323.

Bell, M. B. V., Nichols, H. J., Gilchrist, J. S., Cant, M. A., and Hodge, S. J. (2011). The cost of dominance: suppressing subordinate reproduction affects the reproductive success of dominant female banded mongooses. *Proc. Biol. Sci.* 279, 619–624. doi: 10.1098/rspb.2011.1093

Belliure, J., Meylan, S., and Clobert, J. (2004). Prenatal and postnatal effects of corticosterone on behavior in juveniles of the common lizard, *Lacerta vivipara*. *J. Exp. Zool.* 301A, 401–410. doi: 10.1002/jez.a.20066

Black, M. P., Balthazart, J., Baillien, M., and Grober, M. S. (2005a). Socially induced and rapid increases in aggression are inversely related to brain aromatase activity in a sex-changing fish, *Lythrypnus dalli*. *Proc. Biol. Sci.* 272, 2435–2440. doi: 10.1098/rspb.2005.3210

Black, M. P., Moore, B., Canario, A. V. M., Ford, D., Reavis, R. H., and Grober, M. S. (2005b). Reproduction in context: field testing a laboratory model of socially controlled sex change in *Lythrypnus dalli* (Gilbert). *J. Exp. Mar. Biol. Ecol.* 318, 127–143. doi: 10.1016/j.jembe.2004.12.015

Borg, B. (1994). Androgens in teleost fishes. *Comp. Biochem. Physiol. C Comp. Pharmacol.* 109C, 219–245.

Borque, C., Perez-Garnelo, S. S., Delclaux, M., Martinez, E., and De la Fuente, J. (2011). Fecal steroid evaluation to monitor reproductive status in wild ungulate females using enzyme immunoassay commercial kits. *J. Zoo Wildl. Med.* 42, 537–551. doi: 10.1638/2009-0187.1

Brenowitz, E. A., and Lent, K. (2002). Act locally and think globally: intracerebral testosterone implants induce seasonal-like growth of adult avian song control circuits. *Proc. Natl. Acad. Sci. U.S.A.* 99, 12421–12426. doi: 10.1073/pnas.192308799

Breuner, C. W., Patterson, S. H., and Hahn, T. P. (2008). In search of relationships between the acute adrenocortical response and fitness. *Gen. Comp. Endocrinol.* 157, 288–295. doi: 10.1016/j.ygcen.2008.05.017

Brommer, J. E., Merila, J., Sheldon, B. C., and Gustafsson, L. (2005). Natural selection and genetic variation for reproductive reaction norms in a wild bird population. *Evolution* 59, 1362–1371. doi: 10.1111/j.0014-3820.2005.tb01785.x

Brooks, S., Tyler, C. R., and Sumpter, J. P. (1997). Egg quality in fish: what makes a good egg? *Rev. Fish Biol. Fisher* 7, 387–416. doi: 10.1023/A:1018400130692

Buhimschi, C. S., Turan, O. M., Funai, E. F., Azpurua, H., Bahtiyar, M. O., Turan, S., et al. (2008). Fetal adrenal gland volume and cortisol/dehydroepiandrosterone sulfate ratio in inflammation-associated preterm birth. *Obs. Gyn.* 111, 715–722. doi: 10.1097/AOG.0b013e3181610294

Caldwell, G. S., Glickman, S. E., and Smith, E. R. (1984). Seasonal aggression independent of seasonal testosterone in wood rats. *Proc. Natl. Acad. Sci. U.S.A.* 81, 5255–5257. doi: 10.1073/pnas.81.16.5255

Cameron, E. Z., Setsaas, T. H., and Linklater, W. L. (2009). Social bonds between unrelated females increase reproductive success in feral horses. *Proc. Natl. Acad. Sci. U.S.A.* 106, 13850–13853. doi: 10.1073/pnas.0900639106

Cardwell, J., Sorensen, P., Van der Kraak, G., and Liley, N. (1996). Effect of dominance status on sex hormone levels in laboratory and wild-spawning male trout. *Gen. Comp. Endocrinol.* 101, 333–341. doi: 10.1006/gcen.1996.0036

Carere, C., Ball, G. F., and Balthazart, J. (2007). Sex differences in projections from preoptic area aromatase cells to the periaqueductal gray in Japanese quail. *J. Comp. Neurol.* 500, 894–907. doi: 10.1002/cne.21210

Castillo-Briceno, P., Aguilla-Martinez, S., Liarte, S., Alcazar, A. G., Meseguer, J., Mulero, V., et al. (2013). *In situ* forming microparticle implants for delivery of sex steroids in fish: modulation of the immune response of gilthead seabream by testosterone. *Steroids* 78, 26–33. doi: 10.1016/j.steroids.2012.10.013

Cavaco, J., Vischer, H., Lambert, J., Goes, H., and Schulz, R. (1997). Mismatch between patterns of circulating and testicular androgens in African catfish, *Clarias gariepinus*. *Fish Physiol. Biochem.* 17, 155–162. doi: 10.1023/A:1007716514816

Charlier, T. D., Ball, G. F., and Balthazart, J. (2006). Plasticity in the expression of the steroid receptor coactivator 1 in the Japanese quail brain: effect of sex, testosterone, stress and time of the day. *Neuroscience* 140, 1381–1394. doi: 10.1016/j.neuroscience.2006.03.002

Charlier, T. D., Po, K. W. L., Newman, A. E. M., Shah, A. H., Saldanha, C. J., and Soma, K. K. (2010). 17β-estradiol levels in male zebra finch brain: combining Palkovits punch and an ultrasensitive radioimmunoassay. *Gen. Comp. Endocrinol.* 167, 18–26. doi: 10.1016/j.ygcen.2010.02.002

Chen, T., Beekman, M., and Ward, A. J. W. (2011). The role of female dominance hierarchies in the mating behaviour of mosquitofish. *Biol. Lett.* 7, 343–345. doi: 10.1098/rsbl.2010.1020

Clarke, F., and Faulkes, C. (2001). Intracolony aggression in the eusocial naked mole-rat, *Heterocephalus glaber*. *Anim. Behav.* 61, 311–324. doi: 10.1006/anbe.2000.1573

Clutton-Brock, T., and McAuliffe, K. (2009). Female mate choice in mammals. *Quart. Rev. Biol.* 84, 3–27. doi: 10.1086/596461

Corpéchot, C., Robel, P., Axelson, M., Sjövall, J., and Baulieu, E. E. (1981). Characterization and measurement of dehydroepiandrosterone sulfate in rat brain. *Proc. Natl. Acad. Sci. U.S.A.* 78, 4704–4707. doi: 10.1073/pnas.78.8.4704

Cotton, S., Fowler, K., and Pomiankowski, A. (2004). Do sexual ornaments demonstrate heightened condition-dependent expression as predicted by the handicap hypothesis? *Proc. Biol. Sci.* 271, 771–783. doi: 10.1098/rspb.2004.2688

Creel, S. (2001). Social dominance and stress hormones. *Trends Ecol. Evol.* 16, 491–497. doi: 10.1016/S0169-5347(01)02227-3

Damassa, D. A., Smith, E. R., Tennent, B., and Davidson, J. M. (1977). The relationship between circulating testosterone levels and male sexual behavior in rats. *Horm. Behav.* 8, 275–286. doi: 10.1016/0018-506X(77)90002-2

De Jager, N., Hudson, N. J., Reverter, A., Wang, Y.-H., Nagaraj, S. H., Cafe, L. M., et al. (2011). Chronic exposure to anabolic steroids induces the muscle expression of oxytocin and a more than fiftyfold increase in circulating oxytocin in cattle. *Physiol. Genomics* 43, 467–478. doi: 10.1152/physiolgenomics.00226.2010

Dettenborn, L., Muhtz, C., Skoluda, N., Stalder, T., Steudte, S., Hinkelmann, K., et al. (2012). Introducing a novel method to assess cumulative steroid concentrations: increased hair cortisol concentrations over 6 months in medicated patients with depression. *Stress* 15, 348–353. doi: 10.3109/10253890.2011.619239

Devlin, R. H., and Nagahama, Y. (2002). Sex determination and sex differentiation in fish: an overview of genetic, physiological, and environmental influences. *Aquaculture* 208, 191–364. doi: 10.1016/S0044-8486(02)00057-1

Divari, S., Mulasso, C., Uslenghi, F., Cannizzo, F. T., Spada, F., De Maria, R., et al. (2011). Progesterone receptor up-regulation: a diagnostic tool for the illicit use of oestrogens in adult beef cattle. *Food Addit. Contam.* 28, 1677–1686. doi: 10.1080/19440049.2011.609492

Dobzhansky, T. (1973). Nothing in biology makes sense except in the light of evolution. *Am. Biol. Teach.* 35, 125–129. doi: 10.2307/4444260

Do Rego, J. L., Seong, J. Y., Burel, D., Leprince, J., Luu-The, V., Tsutsui, K., et al. (2009). Neurosteroid biosynthesis: enzymatic pathways and neuroendocrine regulation by neurotransmitters and neuropeptides. *Front. Neuroendocrinol.* 30:259–301. doi: 10.1016/j.yfrne.2009.05.006

Doué, M., Bichon, E., Dervilly-Pinel, G., Pichon, V., Chapuis-Hugon, F., Lesellier, E., et al. (2012). Molecularly imprinted polymer applied to the selective isolation of urinary steroid hormones: an efficient tool in the control of natural steroid hormones abuse in cattle. *J. Chromatogr. A* 1270, 51–61. doi: 10.1016/j.chroma.2012.10.067

Drilling, C., and Grober, M. (2005). An initial description of alternative male reproductive phenotypes in the bluebanded goby, *Lythrypnus dalli* (Teleostei, Gobiidae). *Environ. Biol. Fish.* 72, 361–372. doi: 10.1007/s10641-004-2590-5

East, M., and Hofer, H. (2001). Male spotted hyenas (*Crocuta crocuta*) queue for status in social groups dominated by females. *Behav. Ecol.* 12, 558–568. doi: 10.1093/beheco/12.5.558

Ellis, L. (1995). Dominance and reproductive success among nonhuman animals: a cross-species comparison. *Ethol. Sociobiol.* 16, 257–333. doi: 10.1016/0162-3095(95)00050-U

Emlen, D. (2008). The evolution of animal weapons. *Ann. Rev. Ecol. Evol. Sys.* 39, 387–413. doi: 10.1146/annurev.ecolsys.39.110707.173502

Feist, G., Schreck, C. B., Fitzpatrick, M. S., and Redding, J. M. (1990). Sex steroid profiles of coho salmon (*Oncorhynchus kisutch*) during early development and sexual differentiation. *Gen. Comp. Endocrinol.* 80, 299–213. doi: 10.1016/0016-6480(90)90174-K

Fitzpatrick, J., Desjardins, J., Milligan, N., Stiver, K., Montgomerie, R., and Balshine, S. (2008). Female-mediated causes and consequences of status change in a social fish. *Proc. Biol. Sci.* 275, 929–936. doi: 10.1098/rspb.2007.1449

Foerster, K., and Kempenaers, B. (2005). Effects of testosterone on male-male competition and male-female interactions in blue tits. *Behav. Ecol. Sociobiol.* 57, 215–223. doi: 10.1007/s00265-004-0858-6

Forbes, S. (2011). Social rank governs the effective environment of siblings. *Biol. Lett.* 7, 346–348. doi: 10.1098/rsbl.2010.1064

Formica, V., Wood, C., Larsen, W., Butterfield, R., Augat, M., Hougen, H., et al. (2011). Fitness consequences of social network position in a wild population of forked fungus beetles (*Bolitotherus cornutus*). *J. Evol. Biol.* 25, 130–137. doi: 10.1111/j.1420-9101.2011.02411.x

Frère, C. H., Krützen, M., Mann, J., Connor, R. C., Bejder, L., and Sherwin, W. B. (2010). Social and genetic interactions drive fitness variation in a free-living dolphin population. *Proc. Natl. Acad. Sci. U.S.A.* 107, 19949–19954. doi: 10.1073/pnas.1007997107

Friedman, N. B., Bronze, E. J., and Drutz, R. E. (1964). The effects of local hormonal organ transplants and steroid hormone implants upon the thymus gland. *Ann. N. Y. Acad. Sci.* 113, 916–932. doi: 10.1111/j.1749-6632.1964.tb40712.x

Fuenzalida, F. (1950). Absorption of steroids from subcutaneously implanted tablets of the pure hormone and of the hormone mixed with cholesterol. *J. Clin. Endocrinol. Metab.* 10, 1511–1516. doi: 10.1210/jcem-10-11-1511

Fusani, L., Barske, J., Day, L. D., Fuxjager, M. J., and Schlinger, B. A. (2014). Physiological control of elaborate male courtship: female choice for neuromuscular systems. *Neurosci. Biobehav. Rev.* 46, 534–546. doi: 10.1016/j.neubiorev.2014.07.017

Fuxjager, M. J., Mast, G., Becker, E. A., and Marler, C. A. (2009). The 'home advantage' is necessary for a full winner effect and changes in post-encounter testosterone. *Horm. Behav.* 56, 214–219. doi: 10.1016/j.yhbeh.2009.04.009

Gabor, C. R., and Contreras, A. (2012). Measuring water-borne cortisol in *Poecilia latipinna*:is the process stressful, can stress be minimized and is cortisol correlated with sex steroid release rates? *J. Fish Biol.* 81, 1327–1339. doi: 10.1111/j.1095-8649.2012.03411.x

Ge, R. S., Gao, H. B., Nacharaju, V. L., Gunsalus, G. L., and Hardy, M. P. (1997). Identification of a kinetically distinct activity of 11β-hydroxysteroid dehydrogenase in rat Leydig cells. *Endocrinology* 138, 2435–2442.

Genova, R. M., Marchaterre, M. A., Knapp, R., Fergus, D., and Bass, A. H. (2012). Glucocorticoid and androgen signaling pathways diverge between advertisement calling and non-calling fish. *Horm. Behav.* 62, 426–432. doi: 10.1016/j.yhbeh.2012.07.010

Ghiselin, M. T. (1969). The evolution of hermaphroditism among animals. *Quart. Rev. Biol.* 44, 189–208. doi: 10.1086/406066

Godwin, J. (2009). Social determination of sex in reef fishes. *Semin. Cell Dev. Biol.* 20, 264–270. doi: 10.1016/j.semcdb.2008.12.003

Godwin, J., Crews, D., and Warner, R. R. (1996). Behavioural sex change in the absence of gonads in a coral reef fish. *Proc. Biol. Sci.* 263, 1683–1688. doi: 10.1098/rspb.1996.0246

Greenfield, M. D., and Rodriguez, R. L. (2004). Genotype–environment interaction and the reliability of mating signals. *Anim. Behav.* 68, 1461–1468. doi: 10.1016/j.anbehav.2004.01.014

Hansen, A. M., Garde, A. H., and Persson, R. (2008). Sources of biological and methodological variation in salivary cortisol and their impact on measurement among healthy adults: a review. *Scand. J. Clin. Lab. Invest.* 68, 448–458. doi: 10.1080/00365510701819127

Hartmann, G., Endröczi, E., and Lissák, K. (1966). The effect of hypothalamic implantation of 17β-oestradiol and systemic administration of prolactin (LTH) on sexual behaviour in male rabbits. *Acta Physiol. Acad. Sci. Hung.* 30, 53–59.

Hasselquist, D. (1998). Polygyny in great reed warblers: a long-term study of factors contributing to male fitness. *Ecology* 79, 2376–2390. doi: 10.1890/0012-9658(1998)079[2376:PIGRWA]2.0.CO;2

Heg, D., and Hamilton, I. M. (2008). Tug-of-war over reproduction in a cooperatively breeding cichlid. *Behav. Ecol. Soc.* 62, 1249–1257. doi: 10.1007/s00265-008-0553-0

Heg, D., Jutzeler, E., Mitchell, J. S., and Hamilton, I. M. (2009). Helpful female subordinate cichlids are more likely to reproduce. *PloS ONE* 4:e5458. doi: 10.1371/journal.pone.0005458

Heidbrink, C., Häusler, S. F., Buttmann, M., Ossadnik, M., Strik, H. M., Keller, A., et al. (2010). Reduced cortisol levels in cerebrospinal fluid and differential distribution of 11beta-hydroxysteroid dehydrogenases in multiple sclerosis: implications for lesion pathogenesis. *Brain Behav. Immun.* 24, 975–984. doi: 10.1016/j.bbi.2010.04.003

Heinlein, C. A., and Chang, C. (2002). The roles of androgen receptors and androgen-binding proteins in nongenomic androgen actions. *Mol. Endocrinol.* 16, 2181. doi: 10.1210/me.2002-0070

Heitzman, R. J. (1976). The effectiveness of anabolic agents in increasing rate of growth in farm animals; report on experiments in cattle. *Environ. Qual. Saf. Suppl.* 5, 89–98.

Henman, F. D. (1970). Inhibition of peptic activity by carbenoxolone and glycyrrhetinic acid. *Gut* 11, 344–351. doi: 10.1136/gut.11.4.344

Henry, M. D., Hankerson, S. J., Siani, J. M., French, J. A., and Dietz, J. M. (2013). High rates of pregnancy loss by subordinates leads to high reproductive skew in wild golden lion tamarins (*Leontopithecus rosalia*). *Horm. Behav.* 63, 675–683. doi: 10.1016/j.yhbeh.2013.02.009

Hill, J. A., Enstrom, D. A., Ketterson, E. D., Nolan, V., and Ziegenfus, C. (1999). Mate choice based on static versus dynamic secondary sexual traits in the dark-eyed junco. *Behav. Ecol.* 10, 91–96. doi: 10.1093/beheco/10.1.91

Hiramatsu, R., and Nisula, B. C. (1987). Erythrocyte-associated cortisol: measurement, kinetics of dissociation, potential physiological. *J. Clin. Endocrinol. Metabol.* 64, 1224–1232. doi: 10.1210/jcem-64-6-1224

Hodge, S. J., Manica, A., Flower, T. P., and Clutton-Brock, T. H. (2008). Determinants of reproductive success in dominant female meerkats. *J. Anim. Ecol.* 77, 92–102. doi: 10.1111/j.1365-2656.2007.01318.x

Holekamp, K. E., Smith, J. E., Strelioff, C. C., van Horn, R. C., and Watts, H. E. (2012). Society, demography and genetic structure in the spotted hyena. *Mol. Ecol.* 21, 613–632. doi: 10.1111/j.1365-294X.2011.05240.x

Hollister-Smith, J. A., Poole, J. H., Archie, E. A., Vance, E. A., Georgiadis, N. J., Moss, C. J., et al. (2007). Age, musth and paternity success in wild male African elephants, *Loxodonta africana*. *Anim. Behav.* 74, 287–296. doi: 10.1016/j.anbehav.2006.12.008

Horn, H., and Rubenstein, D. (1984). "Behavioural adaptations and life history," in *Behavioural Ecology: An Evolutionary Approach, 2nd Edn.*, eds J. Krebs, and N. Davies, (Sunderland, MA: Sinauer Associates Inc.), 279–298.

Huang, V., Bowden, R. M., and Crews, D. (2013). Yolk-albumen testosterone in a lizard with temperature-dependent sex determination: relation with development. *Gen. Comp. Endocrinol.* 186, 67–71. doi: 10.1016/j.ygcen.2013.02.019

Huber, R., and Kravitz, E. A. (2010). "Aggression: towards an integration of gene, brain and behaviour," in *Social Behaviour: Genes, Ecology and Evolution*, T. Székely, A. J. Moore, and J. Komdeur (New York, NY: S Cambridge University Press), 165–180.

Huddleston, G. G., Paisley, J. C., and Clancy, A. N. (2006). Effects of estrogen in the male rat medial amygdala: infusion of an aromatase inhibitor lowers mating and bovine serum albumin-conjugated estradiol implants do not promote mating. *Neuroendocrinology* 83, 106–116. doi: 10.1159/000094400

Huddleston, G. G., Paisley, J. C., Graham, S., Grober, M. S., and Clancy, A. N. (2007). Implants of estradiol conjugated to bovine serum albumin in the male rat medial preoptic area promote copulatory behavior. *Neuroendocrinology* 86, 249–259. doi: 10.1159/000107695

Ikeda, M., Rensel, M. A., Schlinger, B. A., and Remage-Healey, L. (2014). *In vivo* detection of fluctuating brain steroid levels in zebra finches. *Cold Spring Harb Protoc.* 12, 2367–1272. doi: 10.1101/pdb.prot084616

Jellinck, P. H., Monder, C., McEwen, B. S., and Sakai, R. R. (1993). Differential inhibition of 11β-hydroxysteroid dehydrogenase by carbenoxolone in rat brain regions and peripheral tissues. *J. Steroid Biochem. Mol. Biol.* 46, 209–213. doi: 10.1016/0960-0760(93)90296-9

Kingston, J. J., Rosenthal, G. G., and Ryan, M. J. (2003). The role of sexual selection in maintaining a colour polymorphism in the pygmy swordtail, *Xiphophorus pygmaeus*. *Anim. Behav.* 65, 735–743. doi: 10.1006/anbe.2003.2110

Knapp, R., and Moore, M. C. (1997). Male morphs in tree lizards have different testosterone responses to elevated levels of corticosterone. *Gen. Comp. Endocrinol.* 107, 273–279. doi: 10.1006/gcen.1997.6923

Koren, L., Nakagawa, S., Burke, T., Soma, K. K., Wynne-Edwards, K. E., and Geffen, E. (2012). Non-breeding feather concentrations of testosterone, corticosterone and cortisol are associated with subsequent survival in wild house sparrows. *Proc. R. Soc. Lond. B Biol. Sci.* 279, 1560–1566. doi: 10.1098/rspb.2011.2062

Kotłowska, A. (2012). Application of steroid hormone metabolomics in search of biomarkers in clinical research. *Drug Dev. Res.* 73, 381–389. doi: 10.1002/ddr.21028

Kow, L. M., Grill, H. J., and Pfaff, D. W. (1978). Elimination of lordosis in decerebrate female rats: observations from acute and chronic preparations. *Physiol. Behav.* 20, 171–174. doi: 10.1016/0031-9384(78)90069-0

Kudielka, B. M., Hellhammer, D. H., and Wüst, S. (2009). Why do we respond so differently? Reviewing determinants of human salivary cortisol responses to challenge. *Psychoneuroendocrinology* 34, 2–18. doi: 10.1016/j.psyneuen.2008.10.004

Lailvaux, S., Herrel, A., Vanhooydonck, B., Meyers, J., and Irschick, D. (2004). Performance capacity, fighting tactics and the evolution of life-stage male morphs in the green anole lizard (*Anolis carolinensis*). *Proc. R. Soc. Lond. B Biol. Sci.* 271, 2501–2508. doi: 10.1098/rspb.2004.2891

Leshchenko, Y., Likhodii, S., Yue, W., Burnham, W. M., and Perez Velazquez, J. L. (2006). Carbenoxolone does not cross the blood brain barrier: an HPLC study. *BMC Neurosci.* 7:3. doi: 10.1186/1471-2202-7-3

Lorenzi, V., Earley, R. L., and Grober, M. S. (2012). Differential responses of brain, gonad and muscle steroid levels to changes in social status and sex in a sequential and bidirectional hermaphroditic fish. *PLoS ONE* 7:e51158. doi: 10.1371/journal.pone.0051158

Lorenzi, V., Earley, R. L., Rodgers, E. W., Pepper, D. R., and Grober, M. S. (2008). Diurnal patterns and sex differences in cortisol, 11-ketotestosterone, testosterone, and 17β-estradiol in the bluebanded goby (*Lythrypnus dalli*). *Gen. Comp. Endocrinol.* 155, 438–446. doi: 10.1016/j.ygcen.2007.07.010

Lynch, K. S., Crews, D., Ryan, M. J., and Wilczynski, W. (2006). Hormonal state influences aspects of female mate choice in the Túngara frog (*Physalaemus pustulosus*). *Horm. Behav.* 49, 450–457. doi: 10.1016/j.yhbeh.2005.10.001

Ma, X., Lian, Q.-Q., Dong, Q., and Ge, R.-S. (2011). Environmental inhibitors of 11β-hydroxysteroid dehydrogenase type 2. *Toxicology* 285, 83–89. doi: 10.1016/j.tox.2011.04.007

Macbeth, B. J., Cattet, M. R. L., Stenhouse, G. B., Gibeau, M. L., and Janz, D. M. (2010). Hair cortisol concentration as a noninvasive measure of long-term stress in free-ranging grizzly bears (*Ursus arctos*): considerations with implications for other wildlife. *Can. J. Zool.* 88, 935–949. doi: 10.1139/Z10-057

Makin, H. L. J., Honour, J. W., and Shackleton, C. H. L. (2010). *Steroid Analysis.* Springer, New York.

St. Mary, C. (1993). Novel sexual patterns in two simultaneously hermaphroditic gobies, *Lythrypnus dalli* and *Lythrypnus zebra*. *Copeia* 4, 1062–1072. doi: 10.2307/1447085

McGlothlin, J. W., Duffy, D. L., Henry-Freeman, J. L., and Ketterson, E. D. (2007). Diet quality affects an attractive white plumage pattern in dark-eyed juncos (*Junco hyemalis*). *Behav. Ecol. Sociobiol.* 61, 1391–1399. doi: 10.1007/s00265-007-0370-x

McGlothlin, J. W., Parker, P. G., Nolan, V., and Ketterson, E. D. (2005). Correlational selection leads to genetic integration of body size and an attractive plumage trait in dark-eyed juncos. *Evolution* 59, 658–671. doi: 10.1111/j.0014-3820.2005.tb01024.x

Munday, P., Buston, P., and Warner, R. (2006). Diversity and flexibility of sex-change strategies in animals. *Trends Ecol. Evol.* 21, 89–95. doi: 10.1016/j.tree.2005.10.020

Narayan, E. J., Hero, J.-M., and Cockrem, J. F. (2012). Inverse urinary corticosterone and testosterone metabolite responses to different durations of restraint in the cane toad (*Rhinella marina*). *Gen. Comp. Endocrinol.* 179, 345–349. doi: 10.1016/j.ygcen.2012.09.017

Nelson, R. (2011). *An Introduction to Behavioral Endocrinology, 4th Edn.* Sunderland, MA: Sinauer Associates, Inc.

Newman, A. E. M., Pradhan, D. S., and Soma, K. K. (2008). Dehydroepiandrosterone and corticosterone are regulated by season and acute stress in a wild songbird: jugular versus brachial plasma. *Endocrinology* 149, 2537–2545. doi: 10.1210/en.2007-1363

Newman, A. E. M., Zanette, L. Y., Clinchy, M., Goodenough, N., and Soma, K. K. (2013). Stress in wild:chronic pressure acute restraint affect plasma DHEA and corticosterone levels in a songbird. *Stress* 16, 363–367. doi: 10.3109/10253890.2012.723076

Nilsen, S. P., Chan, Y., Huber, R., and Kravitz, E. A. (2004). Gender-selective patterns of aggressive behavior in *Drosophila melanogaster*. *Proc. Natl. Acad. Sci. U.S.A.* 101, 12342–12347. doi: 10.1073/pnas.0404693101

Nordeide, J. T., Kekäläinen, J., Janhunen, M., and Kortet, R. (2012). Female ornaments revisited – are they correlated with offspring quality? *J. Anim. Ecol.* 82, 26–38. doi: 10.1111/1365-2656.12021

Olsson, K. H., Kvarnemo, C., and Svensson, O. (2009). Relative costs of courtship behaviours in nest-building sand gobies. *Anim. Behav.* 77, 541–546. doi: 10.1016/j.anbehav.2008.10.021

Orr, H. A. (2009). Fitness and its role in evolutionary genetics. *Nat. Rev. Genet.* 10, 531–539. doi: 10.1038/nrg2603

Payne, A. H., and Hales, D. B. (2004). Overview of steroidogenic enzymes in the pathway from cholesterol to active steroid hormones. *Endocr. Rev.* 25, 947–970. doi: 10.1210/er.2003-0030

Perry, A. N., and Grober, M. S. (2003). A model for social control of sex change: interactions of behavior, neuropeptides, glucocorticoids, and sex steroids. *Horm. Behav.* 43, 31–38. doi: 10.1016/S0018-506X(02)00036-3

Peterson, R. S., Yarram, L., Schlinger, B. A., and Saldanha, C. J. (2005). Aromatase is pre-synaptic and sexually dimorphic in the adult zebra finch brain. *Proc. R. Soc. Lond. B Biol. Sci.* 272, 2089–2096. doi: 10.1098/rspb.2005.3181

Phoenix, C., Goy, R. W., Gerall, A. A., and Young, W. C. (1959). Organizing action of prenatally administered testosterone propionate on the tissues mediating mating behavior in the female guinea pig. *Endocrinology* 65, 369–382. doi: 10.1210/endo-65-3-369

Pradhan, D. S., Connor, K. R., Pritchett, E. M., and Grober, M. S. (2014a). Contextual modulation of androgen effects on agonistic interactions. *Horm. Behav.* 65, 47–56. doi: 10.1016/j.yhbeh.2013.11.006

Pradhan, D. S., Lau, L. Y. M., Schmidt, K. L., and Soma, K. K. (2010a). 3β-HSD in songbird brain: subcellular localization and rapid regulation by estradiol. *J. Neurochem.* 115, 667–675. doi: 10.1111/j.1471-4159.2010.06954.x

Pradhan, D. S., Newman, A. E. M., Wacker, D. W., Wingfield, J. C., Schlinger, B. A., and Soma, K. K. (2010b). Aggressive interactions rapidly increase androgen synthesis in the brain during the non-breeding season. *Horm. Behav.* 57, 381–389. doi: 10.1016/j.yhbeh.2010.01.008

Pradhan, D. S., Solomon-Lane, T. K., and Grober, M. S. (2014b). Water-borne and tissue endocrine profiles of an alternative male reproductive phenotype in the sex changing fish, *Lythrypnus dalli*. *Copeia* 4, 716–724. doi: 10.1643/CP-14-018

Pradhan, D. S., Solomon-Lane, T. K., Willis, M. C., and Grober, M. S. (2014c). A mechanism for rapid neurosteroidal regulation of parenting behaviour. *Proc. R. Soc. Lond. B Biol. Sci.* 281:20140239. doi: 10.1098/rspb.2014.0239

Pradhan, D. S., and Soma, K. K. (2012). Regulation of 3β-HSD activity in the songbird brain. *J. Ornithol.* 153, 227–234. doi: 10.1007/s10336-011-0808-9

Pradhan, D. S., Willis, M. C., Thonkulpitak, K., Solomon-Lane, T. K., and Grober, M. S. (in press). Simultaneous courtship and parenting in males and sex role reversal in females of the haremic bluebanded goby, *Lythrypnus dalli*. *Behaviour.* doi: 10.1163/1568539X-00003262

Prendergast, B. J., Nelson, R. J., and Zucker, I. (2009). *Mammalian Seasonal Rhythms: Behavior and Neuroendocrine Substrates, 2nd Edn.* San Diego: Elsevier.

Quiring, D. P. (1944). Transplantation of testes (by A.A. Berthold). *Bull. Hist. Med.* 16, 399–401.

Ramirez, V. D., Abrams, R. M., and McCann, S. M. (1964). Effect of estradiol implants in the hypothalamo-hypophysial region of the rat on the secretion of luteinizing hormone *Endocrinology* 75, 243–248. doi: 10.1210/endo-75-2-243

Reavis, R. H., and Grober, M. S. (1999). An integrative approach to sex change: social, behavioural and neurochemical changes in *Lythrypnus dalli* (Pisces). *Acta Ethol.* 2, 51–60. doi: 10.1007/PL00012232

Remage-Healey, L., and Bass, A. H. (2006). From social behavior to neural circuitry: steroid hormones rapidly modulate advertisement calling via a vocal pattern generator. *Horm. Behav.* 50, 432–441. doi: 10.1016/j.yhbeh.2006.05.007

Remage-Healey, L., and Romero, L. M. (2001). Corticosterone and insulin interact to regulate glucose and triglyceride levels during stress in a bird. *Am. J. Physiol.* 281, R994–R1003.

Rensel, M. A., Comito, D., Kosarussavadi, S., and Schlinger, B. A. (2014). Region-specific neural corticosterone patterns differ from plasma in a male songbird. *Endocrinology* 155, 3572–3581. doi: 10.1210/en.2014-1231

Robbins, M. M., Robbins, A. M., Gerald-Steklis, N., and Steklis, H. D. (2007). Socioecological influences on the reproductive success of female mountain gorillas (*Gorilla beringei beringei*). *Behav. Ecol. Sociobiol.* 61, 919–931. doi: 10.1007/s00265-006-0321-y

Rodgers, E. W. (2007). *Sexual Plasticity in a Marine Goby, Lythrypnus dalli: Social, Endocrine, and Genetic Influences on Functional sex.* Ph.D. thesis, Georgia State University, 1–107.

Rodgers, E. W., Earley, R. L., and Grober, M. S. (2006). Elevated 11-ketotestosterone during paternal behavior in the Bluebanded goby (*Lythrypnus dalli*). *Horm. Behav.* 49, 610–614. doi: 10.1016/j.yhbeh.2006.01.008

Rodgers, E. W., Earley, R. L., and Grober, M. S. (2007). Social status determines sexual phenotype in the bi-directional sex changing bluebanded goby *Lythrypnus dalli*. *J. Fish Biol.* 70, 1660–1668. doi: 10.1111/j.1095-8649.2007.01427.x

Ros, A. F. H., Fagundes, T., and Oliveira, R. F. (2009). Adjustment of brood size and androgen levels in a teleost species with exclusive male parental care. *Anim. Behav.* 78, 25–33. doi: 10.1016/j.anbehav.2009.03.006

Saldanha, C. J., Remage-Healey, L., and Schlinger, B. A. (2011). Synaptocrine signaling: steroid synthesis and action at the synapse. *Endocr. Rev.* 32, 532–549. doi: 10.1210/er.2011-0004

Saldanha, C. J., and Schlinger, B. A. (1997). Estrogen synthesis and secretion in the brown-headed cowbird (*Molothrus ater*). *Gen. Comp. Endocrinol.* 105, 390–401. doi: 10.1006/gcen.1996.6841

Sapolsky, R. (2005). The influence of social hierarchy on primate health. *Science* 308, 648–652. doi: 10.1126/science.1106477

Saraiva, J. L., Gonçalves, D. M., and Oliveira, R. F. (2010). Environmental modulation of androgen levels and secondary sex characters in two populations of the peacock blenny *Salaria pavo*. *Horm. Behav.* 57, 192–197. doi: 10.1016/j.yhbeh.2009.10.013

Schlinger, B. A., and Arnold, A. P. (1993). Estrogen synthesis *in vivo* in the adult zebra finch: additional evidence that circulating estrogens can originate in brain. *Endocrinology* 133, 2610–2616.

Schlinger, B. A., Barske, J., Day, L., Fusani, L., and Fuxjager, M. J. (2013). Hormones and the neuromuscular control of courtship in the golden-collared manakin (*Manacus vitellinus*). *Front. Neuroendocrinol.* 34, 143–156. doi: 10.1016/j.yfrne.2013.04.001

Schlinger, B. A., Pradhan, D. S., and Soma, K. K. (2008). 3β-HSD activates DHEA in the songbird brain. *Neurochem. Int.* 52, 611–620. doi: 10.1016/j.neuint.2007.05.003

Schmidt, K. L., Chin, E. H., Shah, A. H., and Soma, K. K. (2009). Cortisol and corticosterone in immune organs and brain of European starlings: developmental changes, effects of restraint stress, comparison with zebra finches. *Am. J. Physiol.* 297, R42–R51. doi: 10.1152/ajpregu.90964.2008

Schmidt, K. L., Pradhan, D. S., Shah, A. H., Charlier, T. D., Chin, E. H., and Soma, K. K. (2008). Neurosteroids, immunosteroids, and the Balkanization of endocrinology. *Gen. Comp. Endocrinol.* 157, 266–274. doi: 10.1016/j.ygcen.2008.03.025

Schmidt, K. L., and Soma, K. K. (2008). Cortisol and corticosterone in the songbird immune and nervous systems: local vs. systemic levels during development. *Am. J. Physiol.* 295, R103–R110. doi: 10.1152/ajpregu.00002.2008

Schneider, J. E., and Wade, G. N. (1999). "Inhibition of reproduction in service of energy balance," in *Reproduction in Context: Social and Environmental Influences on Reproduction,* eds K. Wallen and J. E. Schneider (Cambridge, MA: MIT Press), 35–84.

Sebire, M., Katsiadaki, I., and Scott, A. P. (2007). Non-invasive measurement of 11-ketotestosterone, cortisol and androstenedione in male three-spined stickleback (*Gasterosteus aculeatus*). *Gen. Comp. Endocr.* 152, 30–38. doi: 10.1016/j.ygcen.2007.02.009

Shamble, P. S., Wilgers, D. J., Swoboda, K. A., and Hebets, E. A. (2009). Courtship effort is a better predictor of mating success than ornamentation for male wolf spiders. *Behav. Ecol.* 20, 1242- 1251. doi: 10.1093/beheco/arp116

Silk, J. B., Beehner, J. C., Bergman, T. J., Crockford, C., Engh, A. L., Moscovice, L. R., et al. (2009). The benefits of social capital: close social bonds among female baboons enhance offspring survival. *Proc. R. Soc. Lond. B Biol. Sci.* 276, 3099–3104. doi: 10.1098/rspb.2009.0681

Smuts, B., and Smuts, R. (1993). Male aggression and sexual coercion of females in nonhuman primates and other mammals: evidence and theoretical implications. *Adv. Study Behav.* 22, 1–63. doi: 10.1016/S0065-3454(08)60404-0

Sockman, K. W., Sharp, P. J., and Schwabl, H. (2006). Orchestration of avian reproductive effort: an integration of the ultimate and proximate bases for flexibility in clutch size, incubation behaviour, and yolk androgen deposition. *Biol. Rev. Camb. Philos. Soc.* 81, 629. doi: 10.1017/S1464793106007147

Solomon-Lane, T. K., Crespi, E. J., and Grober, M. S. (2013). Stress and serial adult metamorphosis: multiple roles for the stress axis in socially regulated sex change. *Front. Neurosci.* 7:1–12. doi: 10.3389/fnins.2013.00210

Solomon-Lane, T. K., and Grober, M. S. (2012). Behavioral and physiological responses to central administration of corticotropin-releasing factor in the bluebanded goby (*Lythrypnus dalli*). *Physiol. Behav.* 106, 619–625. doi: 10.1016/j.physbeh.2012.04.017

Solomon-Lane, T. K., Pradhan, D. S., Willis, M. C., and Grober, M. S. (2014). Female, but not male, agonistic behaviour is associated with male reproductive success in stable bluebanded goby (*Lythrypnus dalli*) hierarchies. *Behaviour* 151, 1367–1387. doi: 10.1163/1568539X-00003188

Soma, K. K. (2006). Testosterone and aggression: berthold, birds and beyond. *J. Neuroendocrinol.* 18, 543–551. doi: 10.1111/j.1365-2826.2006.01440.x

Taborsky, M. (1994). Sneakers, satellites, and helpers – parasitic and cooperative behavior in fish reproduction. *Adv. Study Behav.* 23, 1–100. doi: 10.1016/S0065-3454(08)60351-4

Taves, M. D., Ma, C., Heimovics, S. A., Saldanha, C. J., and Soma, K. K. (2011). Measurement of steroid concentrations in brain tissue: methodological considerations. *Front. Endocrinol.* 2:39. doi: 10.3389/fendo.2011.00039

Taves, M., Schmidt, K., Ruhr, I., Kapusta, K., and Prior, N. H. (2010). Steroid concentrations in plasma, whole blood and brain: effects of saline perfusion to remove blood contamination from brain. *PLoS ONE* 5:e15727. doi: 10.1371/journal.pone.0015727

Tehranipour, M., and Moghimi, A. (2010). Neuroprotective effects of testosterone on regenerating spinal cord motoneurons in rats. *J. Mot. Behav.* 42, 151–155. doi: 10.1080/00222891003697921

Trainor, B. C., and Marler, C. A. (2001). Testosterone, paternal behavior, and aggression in the monogamous California mouse (*Peromyscus californicus*). *Horm. Behav.* 40, 32–42. doi: 10.1006/hbeh.2001.1652

Trunzer, B., Heinze, J., and Hölldobler, B. (1999). Social status and reproductive success in queenless ant colonies. *Behaviour* 136, 1093–1105. doi: 10.1163/156853999501775

van Noordwijk, M. A., and van Schaik, C. P. (1999). The effects of dominance rank and group size on female lifetime reproductive success in wild long-tailed macaques, *Macaca fascicularis*. *Primates* 40, 105–130. doi: 10.1007/BF02557705

Vasconcelos, R. O., Carrico, R., Ramos, A., Modesto, T., Fonseca, P. J., and Amorim, M. C. P. (2012). Vocal behavior predicts reproductive success in a teleost fish. *Behav. Ecol.* 23, 375–383. doi: 10.1093/beheco/arr199

Walker, W. H. (2011). Testosterone signaling and the regulation of spermatogenesis. *Spermatogenesis* 1, 116–120. doi: 10.4161/spmg.1.2.16956

Wallen, K., and Schneider, J. (1999). *Reproduction in Context: Social and Environmental Influences on Reproduction.* Cambridge, MA: MIT press.

Wallen, K., and Winston, L. A. (1984). Social complexity and hormonal influences on sexual behavior in rhesus monkeys (*Macaca mulatta*). *Physiol. Behav.* 32, 629–637. doi: 10.1016/0031-9384(84)90318-4

Wallis, L., Kleynhans, E., Toit, T. D., Gouws, C., Steyn, D., Steenekamp, J., et al. (2014). Novel non-invasive protein and peptide drug delivery approaches. *Protein Pept. Lett.* 2014, 1087–1101. doi: 10.2174/0929866521666140807112148

Warner, R. R. (1975). The adaptive significance of sequential hermaphroditism in animals. *Am. Nat.* 109, 61–82. doi: 10.1086/282974

Warner, R. R., Robertson, D. R., and Leigh, J. E. G. (1975). Sex change and sexual selection. *Science* 190, 633–638. doi: 10.1126/science.1188360

Watson, P. J., Arnqvist, G., and Stallmann, R. R. (1998). Sexual conflict and the energetic costs of mating and mate choice in water striders. *Am. Nat.* 151, 46–58. doi: 10.1086/286101

Weathington, J. M., Arnold, A. R., and Cooke, B. M. (2012). Juvenile social subjugation induces a sex-specific pattern of anxiety and depression-like behaviors in adult rats. *Horm. Behav.* 61, 91–99. doi: 10.1016/j.yhbeh.2011.10.008

White, D. J., Gersick, A. S., Freed-Brown, G., and Snyder-Mackler, N. (2010). The ontogeny of social skills: experimental increases in social complexity enhance reproductive success in adult cowbirds. *Anim. Behav.* 79, 385–390. doi: 10.1016/j.anbehav.2009.11.014

White, S., Nguyen, T., and Fernald, R. (2002). Social regulation of gonadotropin-releasing hormone. *J. Exp. Biol.* 205, 2567–2581.

Wilson, E., (1980). *Sociobiology: The Abridged Edn.* Cambridge, MA: The Belknap Press of Harvard University Press.

Wingfield, J. C. (2012). Regulatory mechanisms that underlie phenology, behavior, and coping with environmental perturbations: an alternative look at biodiversity. *Auk* 129, 1–7. doi: 10.1525/auk.2012.129.1.1

Wingfield, J. C., and Hunt, K. E. (2002). Arctic spring: hormone-behavior interactions in a severe environment. *Comp. Biochem. Physiol. B* 132, 275–286. doi: 10.1016/S1096-4959(01)00540-1

Wingfield, J. C., Lynn, S., and Soma, K. K. (2001). Avoiding the 'costs' of testosterone: ecological bases of hormone-behavior interactions. *Brain Behav. Evol.* 57, 239–251. doi: 10.1159/000047243

Wingfield, J., Hegner, R., Dufty, A. M., and Ball, G. F. (1990). The "Challenge hypothesis": theoretical implications for patterns of testosterone secretion. *Am. Nat.* 136, 829–846. doi: 10.1086/285134

Wong, B. B. M., and Candolin, U. (2005). How is female mate choice affected by male competition? *Biol. Rev.* 80, 559. doi: 10.1017/S1464793105006809

Young, A. J., Carlson, A. A., Monfort, S. L., Russell, A. F., Bennett, N. C., and Clutton-Brock, T. (2006). Stress and the suppression of subordinate reproduction in cooperatively breeding meerkats. *Proc. Natl. Acad. Sci. U.S.A.* 103, 12005–12010. doi: 10.1073/pnas.0510038103

13

Gender-typical olfactory regulation of sexual behavior in goldfish

Yutaro Kawaguchi, Akira Nagaoka, Asana Kitami, Tomomi Mitsuhashi, Youichi Hayakawa and Makito Kobayashi*

Department of Life Science, International Christian University, Mitaka, Tokyo, Japan

Correspondence:
Makito Kobayashi, Department of Life Science, International Christian University, 3-10-2 Osawa, Mitaka, Tokyo 181-8585, Japan
e-mail: makito@icu.ac.jp

It is known that olfaction is essential for the occurrence of sexual behavior in male goldfish. Sex pheromones from ovulatory females elicit male sexual behavior, chasing, and sperm releasing act. In female goldfish, ovarian prostaglandin F2α (PGF) elicits female sexual behavior, egg releasing act. It has been considered that olfaction does not affect sexual behavior in female goldfish. In the present study, we re-examined the involvement of olfaction in sexual behavior of female goldfish. Olfaction was blocked in male and female goldfish by two methods: nasal occlusion (NO) which blocks the reception of olfactants, and olfactory tract section (OTX) which blocks transmission of olfactory information from the olfactory bulb to the telencephalon. Sexual behavior of goldfish was induced by administration of PGF to females, an established method for inducing goldfish sexual behavior in both sexes. Sexual behavior in males was suppressed by NO and OTX as previously reported because of lack of pheromone stimulation. In females, NO suppressed sexual behavior but OTX did not affect the occurrence of sexual behavior. Females treated with both NO and OTX performed sexual behavior normally. These results indicate that olfaction is essential in female goldfish to perform sexual behavior as in males but in a different manner. The lack of olfaction in males causes lack of pheromonal stimulation, resulting in no behavior elicited. Whereas the results of female experiments suggest that lack of olfaction in females causes strong inhibition of sexual behavior mediated by the olfactory pathway. Olfactory tract section is considered to block the pathway and remove this inhibition, resulting in the resumption of the behavior. By subtract sectioning of the olfactory tract, it was found that this inhibition was mediated by the medial olfactory tracts, not the lateral olfactory tracts. Thus, it is concluded that goldfish has gender-typical olfactory regulation for sexual behavior.

Keywords: goldfish, sexual behavior, olfaction, olfactory tract, olfactory bulb, sex pheromone, prostaglandin

INTRODUCTION

In fishes, olfaction is one of the important senses for their life cycle activities such as feeding, avoiding predation, and reproduction (Hamdani et al., 2000, 2001; Weltzien et al., 2003; Zielinski and Hara, 2007). It has been known that many teleost fishes employ sex pheromones to coordinate their reproductive activity with successful fertilization of gametes (Stacey and Sorensen, 2006; Stacey, 2011). These sex pheromones released from a signaler transmit information on sex and sexual maturity of the signaler to a receiver. Since most of fish sex pheromones studied are from female to male, the involvement of olfaction in reproductive activity has been intensively studied in male fish, and few studies are conducted on the involvement of olfaction in female reproduction (Sorensen et al., 2005; Lastein et al., 2006; Appelt and Sorensen, 2007; Stacey, 2011; Hayakawa et al., 2012).

Goldfish *Carassius auratus* is a small cyprinid species and intensively used for environmental and physiological studies of behavior. As a result, hormonal, pheromonal, and neural regulation of sexual behavior in goldfish is probably the best understood among fish species (Stacey and Sorensen, 2006; Munakata and Kobayashi, 2010; Stacey, 2011; Kobayashi et al., 2013). Female sexual behavior (egg releasing act) is induced by prostaglandin F2α (PGF) produced in the ovary at the time of ovulation. PGF and its metabolites are released into the water as sex pheromones which stimulate male sexual behavior (chasing and sperm releasing act). For the occurrence of sexual behavior, estrogens are not required by females (Kobayashi and Stacey, 1993), but androgen is considered to be essential for males (Stacey and Kobayashi, 1996). When PGF is injected into non-ovulatory females, these fish are induced to perform female sexual behavior with normal males within several minutes after the PGF injection although no egg release is accompanied in this case (Stacey and Kyle, 1983). Thus, using PGF, sexual behavior can be induced easily in goldfish pairs.

Anatomy of olfactory system of goldfish and crucian carp *Carassius carassius*, closely related species of goldfish, is well studied (Von Bartheld et al., 1984; Hamdani et al., 2000, 2001; Weltzien et al., 2003; Stacey and Sorensen, 2006), which enables surgical block of olfaction in goldfish. In the present study, we examined involvement of olfaction in sexual behavior in male and female goldfish by two methods of olfactory blockage. The first method is occlusion of nasal cavity with glue which blocks reception of olfactants. The second method is olfactory tract section.

Since the olfactory bulbs of goldfish are the pedunculated type with elongated olfactory tracts, olfactory information from the olfactory bulbs to the telencephalon can be easily blocked by sectioning olfactory tracts (Stacey and Kyle, 1983; Von Bartheld et al., 1984; Kobayashi et al., 1986, 1994). Using these two methods, we compared the effects of olfactory blockage on sexual behavior between male and female goldfish.

MATERIALS AND METHODS

FISH

Goldfish *Carassius auratus* were obtained from a local dealer in Saitama Prefecture, Japan. Fish were kept in 800-L stock tanks maintained at 20°C under 16L/8D photoperiod. Fish were freely fed with commercial goldfish feed once a day. It is known that gonadal maturity of goldfish is generally maintained under these environmental conditions. Most of the stock males were spermiating and had tubercles on their pectoral fins (male secondary sexual characteristic), and females were found to have vitellogenic oocytes in the ovary when randomly sampled and dissected. Fish weighing 14–30 g were used for the experiments. The handling of fish in the present study was endorsed by Animal Experimentation Committee of International Christian University.

SEXUAL BEHAVIOR OF GOLDFISH

Natural and prostaglandin (PG)-induced spawning (sexual) behaviors are well documented in goldfish (Kobayashi et al., 2002; Munakata and Kobayashi, 2010). In brief, during natural spawning, ovulated females produce PGF in the ovary, and this PGF acts on the brain and triggers the female spawning act (egg releasing act) in the females. PGF and its metabolites are released into the water as sex pheromones which trigger male spawning behavior that are characterized as chasing and culminating in sperm release (i.e., male spawning act). Male chasing is persistent and interspersed with the spawning acts. Spawning acts (complete spawning act) are initiated by the entry of an ovulated female into the floating aquatic vegetation near the surface of the water and where the male follows the female. The female and the male turn on their sides and swim quickly through the vegetation, releasing eggs and sperm. The male always positions itself underneath and in contact with the female during this act. Then, they flip their tails to mix spawned eggs and sperm. Released eggs are characteristically sticky and quickly adhere to the vegetation. Female spawning will continue until most of her ovulated eggs are released, and this may involve hundreds or more spawning acts over several hours. Another type of spawning act of goldfish is called an incomplete spawning act. An incomplete (attempted) spawning act is similar to a complete spawning act except that the fish leave the vegetation without performing gamete release and tail flipping. In the present study, we considered both complete and incomplete spawning acts as normal behavior and were counted equally.

Female goldfish injected with PGF are induced to perform the female spawning act as do ovulated females with sexually mature males, although eggs are not released. Males do not distinguish between ovulated and PG-injected females. In the present paper, the female spawning act (egg releasing act) is referred to as female sexual behavior, and the male spawning act (sperm releasing act) is referred to as male sexual behavior in goldfish.

BEHAVIOR EXPERIMENTS

For the behavior experiments, fish were transferred from stock tanks to 60-L glass acclimating aquaria and kept at 20°C under 16L/8D photoperiod over the course of 1–10 days. Each behavior test was conducted in 60-L glass observation aquaria provided with artificial floating vegetation made of acrylic yarn, gravel, and an aerated box filter and water temperature maintained at 20°C and a 16L/8D photoperiod.

Prostaglandin F2α (PGF) (Panaseran Hi, Meiji Seika, Tokyo, Japan) was intramuscularly injected into females with a microsyringe for the induction of sexual behavior of goldfish just before each sexual behavior test. PGF was injected into experimental females at a dose of 0.1 μg/0.1 μL saline/g body weight for the female behavior experiments, and to partner females at a dose of 10 μg/2.0 μL saline/fish for the male behavior experiments (Stacey and Kyle, 1983; Saoshiro et al., 2013).

For male sexual behavior tests, experimental males and PG-injected partner females were paired in each observation aquarium and sexual behavior (total of complete and incomplete spawning acts) was counted for 60 or 90 min (Stacey and Kyle, 1983). For female behavior tests, PG-injected experimental females and partner males were paired in each observation aquarium and sexual behavior (total of complete and incomplete spawning acts) was counted for 60 or 90 min (Stacey and Kyle, 1983). Pre-treatment tests were conducted on Day 1 and Post-treatment tests were conducted on Day 3 (**Table 1**). Each experimental fish was paired with the same partner fish in pre- and post-treatment tests. Fish received no treatment or behavior test on Day 2 for the recovery from the treatment and behavior test. Experimental fish and partner fish were kept in 60-L glass acclimating aquaria between the tests.

Table 1 | Experimental design of sexual behavior in goldfish.

	Day 1	Day 3
Experiment 1	Sex behavior test	Nasal occlusion and sex behavior test
Experiment 2	Sex behavior test and OTX	Sex behavior test
Experiment 3	Sex behavior test	Nasal occlusion and sexual behavior test
Experiment 4	Sex behavior test and OTX	Sex behavior test
Experiment 5	Nasal occlusion, sex behavior test, and OTX	Nasal occlusion and sexual behavior test
Experiment 6	Sex behavior test and subtract section	Nasal occlusion and sexual behavior test
Experiment 7	Sex behavior test and subtract section	Nasal occlusion and sex behavior test

Fish received no treatment or behavior test on Day 2. OTX, olfactory tract section.

BLOCAKGE OF OLFACTION

For the blockage of olfaction, two methods were employed in this study: nasal occlusion which blocks reception of olfactants, and olfactory tract section (OTX) which blocks transmission of olfactory information from the olfactory bulb to the telencephalon where the neural center regulating sexual behavior is located (Kyle et al., 1982; Koyama et al., 1985).

Nasal occlusion was carried out according to the method previously reported (Partridge et al., 1976). Fish were anaesthetized by immersion in 0.02% tricaine methanesulfonate (Sigma-Aldrich, St. Louis, MO, USA) solution. The nasal cavities were occluded with denture fix (Shin-Poligrip-SA Mutenka, Earth Chemical, Tokyo, Japan). Then, fish were kept in dechlorinated water for 10–20 min for recovery from anesthesia before behavior tests.

For the complete blockage of olfaction, the nasal cavities of both sides were bilaterally occluded. As one of the controls, one side of nasal cavity was unilaterally occluded. As another control, fish were treated in the same manner without occlusion of the nasal cavities (intact). This method of occlusion was effective in blocking olfaction for 70–80 min since denture fix used in the present study is water-soluble and some bilaterally occluded males started male sexual behavior with PG-injected females around this time, probably due to the leakage of the water to the olfactory epithelium. Therefore, observation period of experiment using this method was set to 60 min.

It is well established that PG pheromone acts on the olfactory epithelium of sexually mature male goldfish and elicits chasing (courtship) of the males (Stacey and Sorensen, 2006). To assess the completeness of nasal occlusion, we examined the suppression of chasing of male goldfish in the presence of the PG-injected females. We tried other methods of olfactory blockage, such as cauterization of olfactory epithelium and application of silver nitrate solution on the epithelium, but these techniques were not successful (Kobayashi, unpublished data) and nasal occlusion was effective for 70–80 min. The methods that are effective for the olfactory blockage in males, nasal occlusion and olfactory tract section, were applied to the experiments of females in the present study.

Olfactory tract section was carried out according to the method previously reported (Stacey and Kyle, 1983; Kobayashi et al., 1986, 1994). Fish were anaesthetized with a 0.02% tricaine methanesulfonate solution. A four-sided flap was cut in the frontal bone using a disc saw in order to expose a pair of the olfactory tracts. After removal of a square flap of the frontal bone, the tracts were bilaterally or unilaterally sectioned at two places with Wecker's scissors, and the resultant sections were removed (OTX). Olfactory tracts were subdivided surgically into a lateral olfactory tract (LOT) and a medial olfactory tract (MOT) that can be further separated into lateral medial-olfactory tract (lMOT) and medial medial-olfactory tract (mMOT). Specific subtract section was also carried out. The cavity resulting from operation was filled with gelatin sponge (Spongel, Yamanouchi Pharamaceutical Co. Tokyo, Japan). Sham operations were performed in the same manner without cutting the olfactory tracts.

EFFECTS OF NASAL OCCLUSION ON MALE SEXUAL BEHAVIOR (EXPERIMENT 1)

In this experiment, involvement of olfaction in sexual behavior in male goldfish was examined by nasal occlusion which blocks the reception of sex pheromone from partner female. On Day 1, experimental males were paired with PG-injected partner females in observation aquaria, and male sexual behavior (sperm releasing act) was counted over a period of 60 min (pre-treatment test). On Day 3, experimental males were paired with PG-injected partner females after one of the following three treatments, bilateral nasal occlusion, unilateral nasal occlusion, and intact, and male sexual behavior was observed for 60 min (post-treatment test).

EFFECTS OF OLFACTORY TRACT SECTION ON MALE SEXUAL BEHAVIOR (EXPERIMENT 2)

In this experiment, involvement of olfaction in sexual behavior in male goldfish was examined by OTX which blocks the transmission of olfactory information from the olfactory bulb to the telencephalon. On Day 1, experimental males were paired with PG-injected partner females in observation aquaria, and male sexual behavior was counted over a period of 90 min (pre-treatment test). After the behavior tests, experimental males received either OTX or sham operation. On Day 3, experimental males were paired with PG-injected partner females, and male sexual behavior was observed for 90 min (post-treatment test).

EFFECTS OF NASAL OCCLUSION ON FEMALE SEXUAL BEHAVIOR (EXPERIMENT 3)

In this experiment, involvement of olfaction in sexual behavior in female goldfish was examined by nasal occlusion which blocks the reception of olfactants from the environment. On Day 1, experimental females were injected with PGF, paired with partner males in observation aquaria, and female sexual behavior (egg releasing act) was counted over a period of 60 min (pre-treatment test). On Day 3, experimental females were injected with PGF, paired with partner males after one of the following three treatments, bilateral nasal occlusion, unilateral nasal occlusion, and intact, and female sexual behavior was observed for 60 min (post-treatment test).

EFFECTS OF OLFACTORY TRACT SECTION ON FEMALE SEXUAL BEHAVIOR (EXPERIMENT 4)

In this experiment, involvement of olfaction in sexual behavior in female goldfish was examined by OTX. On Day 1, experimental females were injected with PGF, paired with partner males in observation aquaria, and female sexual behavior was counted over a period of 90 min (pre-treatment test). After the behavior tests, experimental females received either OTX or sham operation. On Day 3, experimental females were injected with PGF, paired with partner males, and female sexual behavior was observed for 90 min (post-treatment test).

EFFECTS OF NASAL OCCLUSION AND OLFACTORY TRACT SECTION ON FEMALE SEXUAL BEHAVIOR (EXPERIMENT 5)

In this experiment, effects of simultaneous treatments of nasal occlusion and OTX were examined in female goldfish. On Day 1, experimental females were injected with PGF, paired with partner males in observation aquaria after bilateral nasal occlusion, and female sexual behavior was counted over a period of

60 min (pre-treatment test). After the behavior tests, experimental females received either OTX or sham operation. On Day 3, experimental females were injected with PGF, paired with partner males after bilateral treatment of nasal occlusion, and female sexual behavior was observed for 60 min (post-treatment test).

EFFECTS OF LOT AND MOT SECTION ON FEMALE SEXUAL BEHAVIOR (EXPERIMENT 6)

In this experiment, effects of LOT and MOT section on sexual behavior were examined in female goldfish. On Day 1, experimental females were injected with PGF, paired with partner males in observation aquaria, and female sexual behavior was counted over a period of 60 min (pre-treatment test). After the behavior tests, experimental females received either LOT section or MOT section. On Day 3, experimental females were injected with PGF, paired with partner males after bilateral nasal occlusion, and female sexual behavior was observed for 60 min (post-treatment test).

EFFECTS OF LATERAL MOT AND MEDIAL MOT SECTION ON FEMALE SEXUAL BEHAVIOR (EXPERIMENT 7)

In this experiment, effects of lMOT and mMOT section on sexual behavior were examined in female goldfish. On Day 1, experimental females were injected with PGF, paired with partner males in observation aquaria, and female sexual behavior was counted over a period of 60 min (pre-treatment test). After the behavior tests, experimental females received either lMOT section or mMOT section. On Day 3, experimental females were injected with PGF, paired with partner males after bilateral nasal occlusion, and female sexual behavior was observed for 60 min (post-treatment test).

STATISTICS

Data among groups were statistically compared by ANOVA and Newman-Keuls test. Data between groups were statistically compared by Mann-Whitney U-test. Data within a group were statistically compared by paired t-test. Level of significance was 0.05 for all statistical tests. Statistical test could not be applied to some data of groups because mean values were zero or close to zero with very low deviation.

RESULTS

EFFECTS OF NASAL OCCLUSION ON MALE SEXUAL BEHAVIOR (EXPERIMENT 1)

Intact fish and unilaterally occluded fish actively performed male sexual behavior in pre- and post-treatment tests on Day 1 and Day 3, respectively (**Figure 1**). Levels of sexual behavior in these fish showed no change between Day 1 and Day 3 ($p > 0.05$). Level of sexual behavior in male goldfish significantly decreased after bilateral nasal occlusion ($p < 0.05$, compared to pre-treatment level and to levels of intact and unilaterally occluded fish of Day 3).

EFFECTS OF OLFACTORY TRACT SECTION ON MALE SEXUAL BEHAVIOR (EXPERIMENT 2)

Sham-operated fish actively performed male sexual behavior in pre- and post-treatment tests on Day 1 and Day 3, respectively (**Figure 2**). Levels of sexual behavior in sham-operated fish showed no change between Day 1 and Day 3 ($p > 0.05$). Level of sexual behavior in male goldfish significantly decreased after OTX ($p < 0.05$, compared to pre-treatment level and to level of sham operated fish of Day 3).

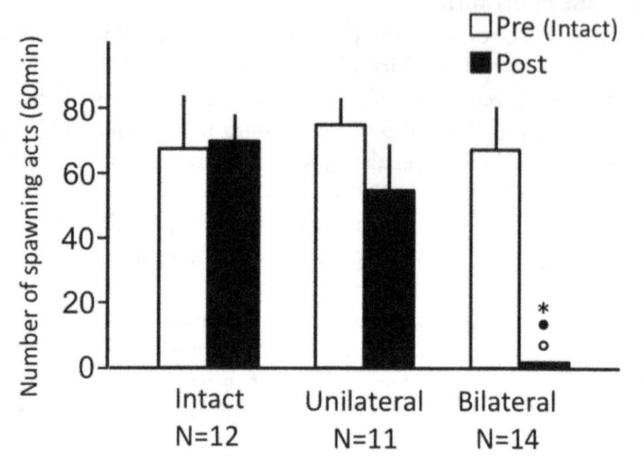

FIGURE 1 | Effects of nasal occlusion on male sexual behavior in male goldfish. Pre, Pre-treatment (open column). Post, post-treatment (solid column). Each column represents the mean and s.e.m. Difference compared to pre-treatment (asterisk), compared to intact fish (solid circle), and compared to unilaterally occluded fish (open circle). Level of significance, $p < 0.05$.

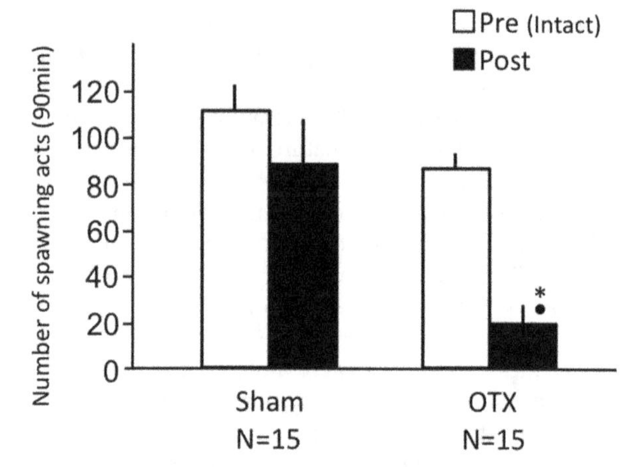

FIGURE 2 | Effects of olfactory tract section on male sexual behavior in male goldfish. Pre, Pre-treatment (open column). Post, post-treatment (solid column). Each column represents the mean and s.e.m. Difference compared to pre-treatment (asterisk), compared to sham-operated fish (solid circle). Level of significance, $p < 0.05$.

EFFECTS OF NASAL OCCLUSION ON FEMALE SEXUAL BEHAVIOR (EXPERIMENT 3)

Intact fish actively performed female sexual behavior in pre- and post-treatment tests on Day 1 and Day 3, respectively (**Figure 3**). Levels of sexual behavior in intact fish showed no change between Day 1 and Day 3 ($p > 0.05$). Level of sexual behavior in female goldfish significantly decreased after unilateral nasal occlusion ($p < 0.05$ compared to pre-treatment level). Female goldfish of bilateral occlusion showed no sexual behavior on Day 3.

EFFECTS OF OLFACTORY TRACT SECTION ON FEMALE SEXUAL BEHAVIOR (EXPERIMENT 4)

Both sham-operated fish and OTX fish actively performed female sexual behavior in pre- and post-treatment tests on Day 1 and Day 3, respectively (**Figure 4**). Levels of sexual behavior in these fish showed no change between Day 1 and Day 3 ($p > 0.05$).

EFFECTS OF NASAL OCCLUSION AND OLFACTORY TRACT SECTION ON FEMALE SEXUAL BEHAVIOR (EXPERIMENT 5)

Females with bilateral nasal occlusion showed almost no sexual behavior on Day 1 (**Figure 5**). Sham-operated fish with bilateral occlusion showed almost no sexual behavior on Day 3. OTX fish with bilateral occlusion actively performed sexual behavior on Day 3.

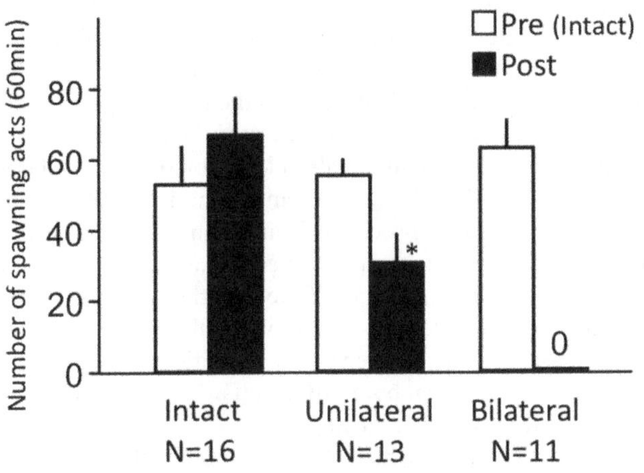

FIGURE 3 | Effects of nasal occlusion on female sexual behavior in female goldfish. Pre, Pre-treatment (open column). Post, post-treatment (solid column). Each column represents the mean and s.e.m. Difference compared to pre-treatment (asterisk), $p < 0.05$.

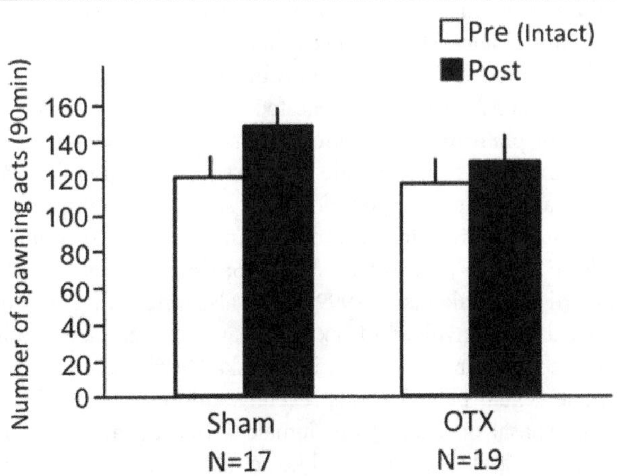

FIGURE 4 | Effects of olfactory tract section on female sexual behavior in female goldfish. Pre, Pre-treatment (open column). Post, post-treatment (solid column). Each column represents the mean and s.e.m.

EFFECTS OF LOT AND MOT SECTION ON FEMALE SEXUAL BEHAVIOR (EXPERIMENT 6)

Females before treatment actively performed sexual behavior on Day 1 (**Figure 6**). LOT-sectioned fish with bilateral nasal occlusion showed no sexual behavior on Day 3. MOT-sectioned fish with bilateral nasal occlusion actively performed sexual behavior on Day 3.

EFFECTS OF LATERAL MOT AND MEDIAL MOT SECTION ON FEMALE SEXUAL BEHAVIOR (EXPERIMENT 7)

Females before treatment actively performed sexual behavior on Day 1 (**Figure 7**). Levels of sexual behavior in lMOT-sectioned fish and mMOT-sectioned fish with bilateral nasal occlusion

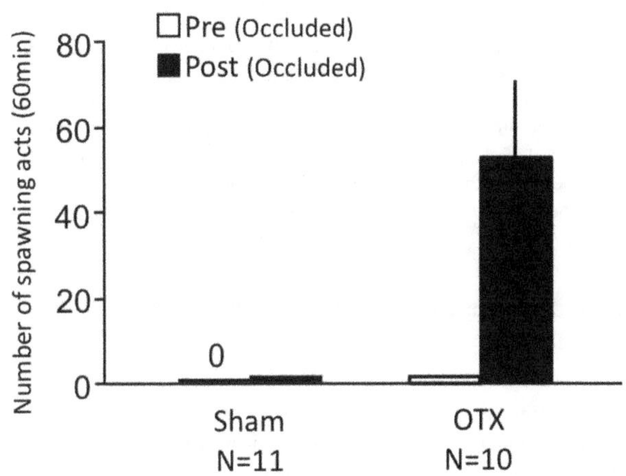

FIGURE 5 | Effects of nasal occlusion and olfactory tract section on female sexual behavior in female goldfish. Pre, Pre-treatment (bilaterally occluded). Post, post-treatment (bilaterally occluded and either sham-operated or olfactory-tract sectioned). Each column represents the mean and s.e.m.

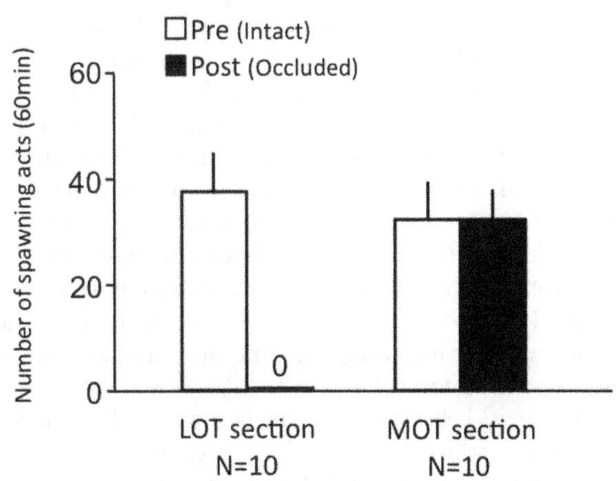

FIGURE 6 | Effects of olfactory subtract section on female sexual behavior in female goldfish. LOT section, Lateral olfactory tracts were sectioned. MOT, Medial olfactory tracts were sectioned. Pre-treatment (open column). Post, post-treatment (solid column). Each column represents the mean and s.e.m.

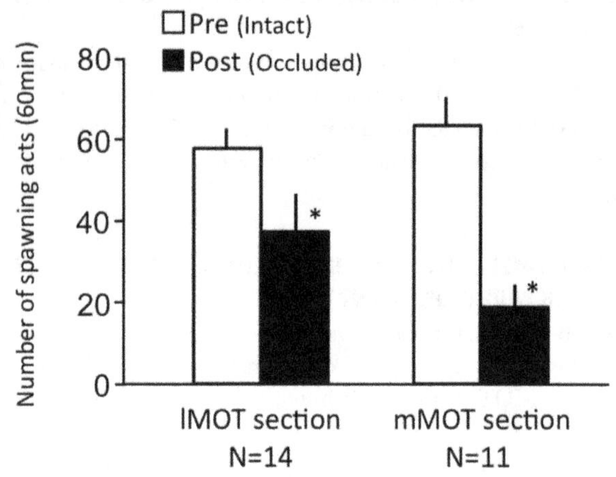

FIGURE 7 | Effects of section of medial olfactory tract components on female sexual behavior in female goldfish. lMOT section, lateral medial-olfactory tract section. mMOT section, medial medial-olfactory tract section. Pre-treatment (open column). Post, post-treatment (solid column, bilaterally occluded and either lMOT sectioned or mMOT sectioned). Each column represents the mean and s.e.m. Difference compared to pre-treatment (asterisk). Level of significance, $p < 0.05$.

significantly decreased on Day 3 ($p < 0.05$, compared to pretreatment level).

DISCUSSION

The present study indicates that olfaction is the key prerequisite for the occurrence of sexual behavior both in male and female goldfish, but its regulation for sexual behavior is different between male and female. In male goldfish, blockage of olfaction by nasal occlusion and OTX severely reduced activity of sexual behavior as previously reported (Partridge et al., 1976; Stacey and Kyle, 1983) because of lack of pheromonal stimulation. Since males with unilateral nasal occlusion actively performed sexual behavior as did intact males, chemical or physical damage of nasal occlusion on fish is considered to be negligible. Some males with bilateral nasal occlusion and OTX showed weak male sexual behavior. These males did not show vigorous chasing that intact males normally do to PG-injected partner females, and sexual behavior of these males occurred mostly when the partner females rose into the aquatic vegetation near these anosmic males. It is considered that anosmic males sometimes show sexual behavior by visual stimulus from females (Norm Stacey and Peter Sorensen, personal communication), and not due to incompleteness of nasal occlusion and OTX. Thus, we examined the involvement of olfaction in female sexual behavior using the same methods that were used for the experiments for males.

Female sexual behavior was strongly suppressed by bilateral nasal occlusion which blocks the reception of olfactants even under the stimulation of PGF. Level of sexual behavior was also reduced by unilateral nasal occlusion. The results of these experiments indicate that the olfaction is essential for the female sexual behavior to occur. However, OTX fish performed female sexual behavior after PG-injection as reported previously (Stacey and Kyle, 1983) although these females were unable to receive olfactory information from the olfactory bulbs. Since OTX did not affect the occurrence of female sexual behavior in PG-injected female goldfish in the previous study (Stacey and Kyle, 1983), it has been considered that olfaction is not essential for the female sexual behavior in goldfish. Nevertheless, nasal occlusion suppressed the female sexual behavior. Results of experiments of nasal occlusion and OTX look contradictory, but one of the possible interpretations we propose is as follows. Blockage of olfaction in females exerts strong inhibition of sexual behavior mediated by the olfactory pathway from the olfactory epithelium to the telencephalon via the olfactory bulb and the olfactory tract even in the presence of PGF stimulation. When females were treated with nasal occlusion and OTX simultaneously, the fish actively performed sexual behavior. Therefore, it is considered that OTX blocked the pathway and removed the inhibitory signaling for the behavior. Reduction of female sexual behavior in unilaterally occluded female may be caused by some inhibition from the occluded side of olfactory epithelium unlike the case of unilaterally occluded male goldfish. Sexual behavior of unilaterally occluded male can receive enough amount of pheromonal stimulation by one side of olfactory epithelium and perform full range of sexual behavior. We further examined the pathway of the inhibitory signaling in female goldfish by olfactory subtract section. Section of LOT did not remove the inhibition of sexual behavior in bilaterally occluded females, but by MOT section, bilaterally occluded females performed sexual behavior, indicating that the inhibition in the olfactory pathway is transmitted via MOT. When lMOT and mMOT was individually sectioned, bilateral nasal occlusion caused partial inhibition of female sexual behavior, suggesting that both lMOT and mMOT are involved in mediating the inhibitory signaling.

It is known that MOT mediates pheromonal information and that LOT mediates information of food odors in male and female goldfish and crucian carp (Stacey and Kyle, 1983; Hamdani et al., 2001; Weltzien et al., 2003). It is interesting that MOT is involved in regulation of sexual behavior both in male and female goldfish although its function is different, stimulatory in males and inhibitory in females. A clear functional difference of the olfactory bulb between male and female is reported in crucian carp. Electrophysiological study showed that the olfactory bulb of male carp discriminates sex pheromones but that of female does not (Lastein et al., 2006). It is suggested that these gender-typical function of pheromone detection and sexual behavior is developed by androgens since female fish start to perform male sexual behavior and male type gonadotropin secretion in response to sex pheromones in goldfish and crucian carp *Carassius auratus langsdorfii* (Stacey and Kobayashi, 1996; Kobayashi et al., 1997; Kobayashi and Nakanishi, 1999). It is also interesting to study how olfaction is involved in sexual behavior of females in other teleost species. Our recent study in medaka *Oryzias latipes* showed that male sexual behavior was severely suppressed by olfactory blockage (nasal occlusion) but female sexual behavior was not affected by nasal occlusion unlike female goldfish (Hayakawa et al., 2012).

The present study demonstrated the involvement of olfaction in female sexual behavior in goldfish. However, biological significance of olfactory regulation in female goldfish is not clarified.

There are some possible explanations of female olfactory system for the regulation of sexual behavior. One of the possible functions could be detection of special odorants, such as sex pheromone from males. There are some reports that female sexual activity is stimulated by sex pheromones from males (Stacey and Sorensen, 2006; Stacey, 2011). In the case of female goldfish, PGF triggers female sexual behavior and a male sex pheromone may not be a trigger but could facilitate the behavior. It is known that a large amount of androstenedione is released from sexually mature male goldfish into the water (Sorensen et al., 2005) and that PG-injected female goldfish show rise into vegetation (initial movement of female spawning act) more frequently in the presence of sexually mature males than in the absence of males (Appelt and Sorensen, 2007). It is possible that androstendione from males function as a sex pheromone which stimulates the initiation of female sexual behavior.

Another possible explanation is that female goldfish searches appropriate site and substrate for oviposition using sense of olfaction as well as vision and tactility. Normally females, not males, decide the site of oviposition in goldfish, and female goldfish need to select appropriate oviposition substrate which secures development of embryo and also appropriate site of water quality. Female goldfish may use olfaction for examining water quality of the spawning site. When olfaction is blocked in female goldfish which fails to examine the water quality of the spawning area, sexual behavior is inhibited even if the fish is stimulated by PGF. Such hypothesis can be applied in male tilapia *Oreochromis niloticus* which makes nest for spawning (Uchida et al., 2005). Olfactory blockage by removal of olfactory rosettes suppressed nest-buliding behavior in the male tilapia although activity of sexual behavior (courtship to female) was unchanged. Female salmonid fishes are known to stop nest-digging behavior and following spawning behavior when pH of the water is slightly lowered even when other environmental conditions are suitable for spawning (Ikuta et al., 2003). It is possible that these females sense the acidity by olfaction. It is of interest to examine whether water quality change may affect sexual behavior in intact and OTX female goldfish.

In conclusion, the present study demonstrated the involvement of olfaction in female sexual behavior in goldfish although it has been considered that olfaction does not affect the behavior. When reception of olfactants is blocked, female sexual behavior is severely suppressed. It is considered that lack of olfaction exerts inhibition of the behavior mediated by the olfactory pathway. Olfactory tract section removes this inhibition resulting in resumption of sexual behavior. Biological significance of this inhibitory system of female individual is unknown. Further behavioral and ecological studies are necessary for better understanding of the regulation of sexual behavior by olfaction in fishes. Also, it is interesting to study the gender typical-olfactory function could be induced heterotypically in goldfish since heterotypical sexual behavior and hormone secretion could be induced in goldfish (Stacey and Kobayashi, 1996; Kobayashi et al., 1997) and crucian carp *C. auratus langsdorfii* (Kobayashi and Nakanishi, 1999) which are considered to have sexually bipotential brain (Kobayashi et al., 2013).

ACKNOWLEDGMENTS

We are grateful to Prof. Naoyuki Yamamoto of Nagoya University for valuable comments and advices in conducting this study and for critical reading of the manuscript.

REFERENCES

Appelt, C. W., and Sorensen, P. W. (2007). Female goldfish signal spawning readiness by altering when and where they release a urinary pheromone. *Anim. Behav.* 74, 1329–1338. doi: 10.1016/j.anbehav.2007.02.032

Hamdani, E. H., Kasumyan, A., and Doving, K. B. (2001). Is feeding behavior in crucian carp mediated by the lateral olfactory tract? *Chem. Senses* 26, 1133–1138. doi: 10.1093/chemse/26.9.1133

Hamdani, E. H., Stabell, O. B., Alexander, G., and Doving, K. B. (2000). Alarm reaction in the crucian carp is mediated by the medial bundle of the medial olfactory tract. *Chem. Senses* 25, 103–109. doi: 10.1093/chemse/25.1.103

Hayakawa, Y., Takita, S., Kikuchi, K., Yoshida, A., and Kobayashi, M. (2012). Involvement of olfaction in spawning success of medaka *Oryzias latipes*. *Jpn. J. Ichthyol.* 59, 111–124.

Ikuta, K., Suzuki, Y., and Kitmura, S. (2003). Effects of low pH on the reproductive behavior of salmonid fishes. *Fish Physiol. Biochem.* 28, 407–410. doi: 10.1023/B:FISH.0000030607.75565.74

Kobayashi, M., Amano, M., Kim, M., Furukawa, K., Hasegawa, Y., and Aida, K. (1994). Gonadotropin-releasing hormones of terminal nerve origin are not essential to ovarian development and ovulation in goldfish. *Gen. Comp. Endocrinol.* 95, 192–200. doi: 10.1006/gcen.1994.1116

Kobayashi, M., Furukawa, K., Kim, M., and Aida, K. (1997). Induction of male-type gonadotropin secretion by 11-ketotestosterone in female goldfish. *Gen. Comp. Endocrinol.* 108, 434–445. doi: 10.1006/gcen.1997.6993

Kobayashi, M., Kobayashi, M., Aida, K., and Hanyu, I. (1986). Pheromone from ovulatory female goldfish induces gonadotropin surge in males. *Gen. Comp. Endocrinol.* 63, 451–455. doi: 10.1016/0016-6480(86)90145-0

Kobayashi, M., and Nakanishi, T. (1999). 11-Ketotestosterone induces male-type sexual behavior and gonadotropin secretion in gynogenetic crucian carp, *Carassius auratus langsdorfii*. *Gen. Comp. Endocrinol.* 115, 178–187. doi: 10.1006/gcen.1999.7314

Kobayashi, M., Saoshiro, S., Kawaguchi, Y., Hayakawa, Y., and Munakata, A. (2013). "Sexual plasticity of behavior in goldfish," in *Sexual Plasticity and Gametogenesis in Fishes*, ed B. Senthilkumaran (New York, NY: Nova Science Pub), 183–201.

Kobayashi, M., Sorensen, P. W., and Stacey, N. E. (2002). Hormonal and pheromonal control of spawning behavior in goldfish. *Fish Physiol. Biochem.* 26, 71–84. doi: 10.1023/A:1023375931734

Kobayashi, M., and Stacey, N. E. (1993). Prostaglandin-induced female spawning behavior in goldfish (*Carassius auratus*) appears independent of ovarien influence. *Horm. Behav.* 27, 38–55. doi: 10.1006/hbeh.1993.1004

Koyama, Y., Satou, M., and Ueda, K. (1985). Sexual behavior elicited by electrical stimulation of the telencephalic and preoptic areas in the goldfish, *Carassius auratus*. *Zool. Sci.* 2, 565–570.

Kyle, A. L., Stacey, N. E., and Peter, R. E. (1982). Ventral telencephalic lesions: effects on bisexual behavior, activity, and olfaction in the male goldfish. *Behav. Neural Biol.* 36, 229–221. doi: 10.1016/S0163-1047(82)90855-X

Lastein, S., Hamdani, E. H., and Doving, K. B. (2006). Gender distribution in neural discrimination of sex pheromones in the olfactory bulb of crucian carp, *Carassius carassius*. *Chem. Senses* 31, 69–77. doi: 10.1093/chemse/bjj007

Munakata, A., and Kobayashi, M. (2010). Endocrine control of sexual behavior in teleost fish. *Gen. Comp. Endocrinol.* 165, 456–468. doi: 10.1016/j.ygcen.2009.04.011

Partridge, B. L., Liley, N. R., and Stacey, N. E. (1976). The role of pheromones in the sexual behavior of the goldfish. *Anim. Behav.* 24, 291–299. doi: 10.1016/S0003-3472(76)80037-1

Saoshiro, S., Kawaguchi, Y., Hayakawa, Y., and Kobayashi, M. (2013). Sexual bipotentiality of behavior in male and female goldfish. *Gen. Comp. Endocrinol.* 181, 265–270. doi: 10.1016/j.ygcen.2012.08.022

Sorensen, P. W., Pinillos, M., and Scott, A. P. (2005). *Gen. Comp. Endocrinol.* 140, 164–175. doi: 10.1016/j.ygcen.2004.11.006

Stacey, N. E. (2011). "Hormonally derived sex pheromones in fishes," in *Hormones and Reproduction of Vertebrates, Vol.1*, eds D. O. Norris and K. H. Lopez (New York, NY: Academic Press, Elsevier), 169–192.

Stacey, N. E., and Kobayashi, M. (1996). Androgen induction of male sexual behaviors in female goldfish. *Horm. Behav.* 30,434–445. doi: 10.1006/hbeh.1996.0048

Stacey, N. E., and Kyle, A. L. (1983). Effects of olfactory tract lesions on sexual and feeding behavior in the goldfish. *Physiol. Behav.* 30, 621–628. doi: 10.1016/0031-9384(83)90231-7

Stacey, N. E., and Sorensen, P. W. (2006). "Reproductive pheromones," in *Behaviour and Physiology of Fish, Fish Physiology, Vol. 24*, eds K. A. Sloman, R. W. Wilson, and S. Balshine (New York, NY: Academic Press, Elsevier), 359–412.

Uchida, H., Ogawa, S., Harada, M., Matushita, M. Iwata, M., Sakuma, Y., and Parhar, I. S. (2005). The olfactory organ modulate gonadotropin-releasing hormone types and nest-building behavior in the tilapia *Oreochromis niloticus. J. Neurobiol.* 65, 1–11. doi: 10.1002/neu.20156

Von Bartheld, C. S., Meyer, D. L., Fiebig, E., and Ebbesson, S. O. E. (1984). Central connections of the olfactory bulb in the goldfish, *Carassius auratus. Cell Tissue Res.* 238, 475–487. doi: 10.1007/BF00219862

Weltzien, F. A., Hoglund, E. Hamdani, E. H., and Doving, K. B. (2003). Does the lateral bundle of the medial olfactory tract mediate reproductive behavior in male crucian carp? *Chem. Senses* 28, 293–300. doi: 10.1093/chemse/28.4.293

Zielinski, B. S., and Hara, T. J. (2007). "Olfaction," in *Sensory Systems Neuroscience, Fish Physiology, Vol. 25,* eds T. Hara and B. Zielinski (New York, NY: Academic Press, Elsevier), 1–43. doi: 10.1016/S1546-5098(06)25001-5

14

Fluorescent visualization of oxytocin in the hypothalamo-neurohypophysial system

Hirofumi Hashimoto, Takanori Matsuura and Yoichi Ueta*

Department of Physiology, School of Medicine, University of Occupational and Environmental Health, Kitakyushu, Japan

****Correspondence:***
Yoichi Ueta, Department of Physiology, School of Medicine, University of Occupational and Environmental Health, 1-1 Iseigaoka, Yahatanishi-ku, Kitakyushu 807-8555, Japan
e-mail: yoichi@med.uoeh-u.ac.jp

Oxytocin (OXT) is well known for its ability to the milk ejection reflex and uterine contraction. It is also involved in several other behaviors, such as anti-nociception, anxiety, feeding, social recognition, and stress responses. OXT is synthesized in the magnocellular neurosecretory cells (MNCs) in the hypothalamic paraventricular (PVN) and the supraoptic nuclei (SON) that terminate their axons in the posterior pituitary (PP). We generated transgenic rats that express the OXT and fluorescent protein fusion gene in order to visualize OXT in the hypothalamo-neurohypophysial system (HNS). In these transgenic rats, fluorescent proteins were observed in the MNCs and axon terminals in the PP. This transgenic rat is a new tool to study the physiological role of OXT in the HNS.

Keywords: CCK, c-fos, double transgenic rat, mRFP1, paraventricular nucleus, posterior pituitary, supraoptic nucleus

INTRODUCTION

Oxytocin (OXT), a nine amino acid neuropeptide, was discovered in 1906 as an extract with uterus-contracting effects from the pituitary (Dale, 1906). In 1953, OXT was the first peptide hormone to be sequenced and synthesized (du Vigneaud et al., 1953a,b, 1954). OXT is synthesized primarily in magnocellular neurosecretory cells (MNC) in the hypothalamic paraventricular (PVN) and the supraoptic nuclei (SON), which cells project their axon terminals into the posterior pituitary (PP), where it is released into the systemic circulation, in the same way as arginine vasopressin (AVP). OXT is well known for its roles in reproduction, especially during and after childbirth. Many previous studies have shown that OXT is involved in several physiological functions, such as antinociception, anxiety, feeding, social recognition, and stress responses (Carmichael et al., 1987, 1994; Stock and Uvnäs-Moberg, 1988; Uvnäs-Moberg et al., 1993; Leckman et al., 1994; Russell and Leng, 1998).

We recently have reported the generation and characterization of rats which faithfully express an AVP-enhanced green fluorescent protein (eGFP) fusion transgene (Ueta et al., 2005; Fujio et al., 2006; Shibata et al., 2007; Suzuki et al., 2009; Maruyama et al., 2010; Todoroki et al., 2010; Iwanaga et al., 2011; Ohno et al., 2012). Previous studies that used animals to examine OXT dynamics by fluorescent visualization reported about OXT-enhanced cyan fluorescent protein (eCFP) transgenic mice (Young et al., 1999; Zhang et al., 2002). Although we first generated an OXT-eCFP transgenic rat, the expression of the transgene was unstable for unknown reasons (Katoh et al., 2010). Monomeric red fluorescent protein (mRFP) was developed from DsRed, which is the red fluorescent protein from *Discosoma* (Campbell et al., 2002; Long et al., 2005), and we succeeded in generating transgenic rats bearing an OXT-mRFP1 fusion gene (Katoh et al., 2011).

In this review, we focus on (1) the distribution of OXT, (2) the regulation of synthesis and release of OXT, and (3) recent research about the visualization of OXT in OXT transgenic animals using a fluorescent protein, which is a new tool to study the physiological role of OXT in the hypothalamo-neurohypophysial system (HNS).

DISTRIBUTION OF OXYTOCIN AND OXYTOCIN RECEPTOR

In MNC in the PVN and the SON, OXT neurons project their axon terminals into the PP. In parvocellular neurosecretory cells (PNC) in the PVN, OXT neurons project their axon terminals to the spinal code, including the intermediolateral nucleus and gelatinous substance, where OXT have some role to modify pains and sympathetic nervous system (Sofroniew, 1980). OXT cells also project to the ambiguus nucleus, the nuclei of solitary tract (NTS), the dorsal motor nucleus of vagus, the Edinger–Westphal nucleus, circularis nucleus (CN), the parabrachial nucleus, the hippocampus, the amygdaloid nucleus, and the septulum (Reaves and Hayward, 1979; Nilaver et al., 1980; Sofroniew, 1980; Sofroniew et al., 1981; Hatton and Tweedle, 1982; Sawchenko and Swanson, 1982). Parvocellular OXT cells are found in the preoptic area and the lateral hypothalamus, whereas accessory magnocellular OXT cells are found scattered across the hypothalamus.

The central effects of OXT are mediated by OTRs distributed widely in the brain. OTR mRNAs are distributed in the ventromedial nucleus of the hypothalamus (VMH) and the PVN, which are involved in steroid-sensitive reproductive behaviors; in the substantia nigra and ventral tegmental area, which is involved in maternal behaviors; in the hippocampus, which is involved in learning and memory; and in the lateral septum, caudate putamen, amygdaloid nuclei, olfactory tubercle and cingulate, perirhinal, and frontal cortices, all of which are involved in reinforcement (Ostrowski, 1998).

REGULATION OF SYNTHESIS AND RELEASE OF OXYTOCIN

OXT is produced in the MNC of the PVN and the SON, and is released into the systemic circulation from axon terminals in the neurohypophysis, particularly during parturition, lactation and in response to osmotic challenges (Burbach et al., 2006). The structure of the OXT gene was elucidated in 1984 (Ivell and Richter, 1984). Expression of the OXT gene is stimulated during pregnancy and lactation (Van Tol et al., 1988; Zingg and Lefebvre, 1988). Interestingly, although estrogen or progesterone alone does not increase OXT synthesis expression of the OXT gene in the PVN and the SON was increased by the prolonged administration of estrogen and progesterone, followed by progesterone withdrawal (Thomas and Amico, 1996). By contrast, OXT gene expression in the uterine was highly stimulated by the combined application of estrogen and progesterone (Lefebvre et al., 1994).

OXT is well known for its roles in reproduction, especially during and after childbirth. The pulsatile OXT release into the circulation is stimulated by vaginocervical stimulation associated with labor and the stimulus of suckling on the nipple. The uterine muscle increases its OXT receptors (OTRs) and sensitivity to OXT during the latter few months of pregnancy. That level of OXT release from the neurohypophysis is considerably increased at the time of labor. In lactation, OXT causes milk to be expressed from the alveoli into the ducts of the breast so that the baby can obtain it by suckling. The suckling stimulus on the nipple of the breast causes signals to be transmitted through sensory nerves to the OXT, secreting neurons in the MNC in the PVN and the SON. OXT in plasma is carried to the breast, where it causes contraction of myoepithelial cells that lie outside of and form a latticework surrounding the alveoli of the mammary glands. In less than a minute after a baby starts suckling, milk begins to flow.

The sequence of the OTR was reported in 1992 (Kimura et al., 1992; Kubota et al., 1996). Gonadal steroids play an important role in mediating the regulation of OTR expression. Most peripheral OXT-binding sites, including the pituitary, renal, and uterine, are upregulated by estrogens (Fuchs et al., 1983; Soloff et al., 1983; Maggi et al., 1992). The upregulation is accompanied by OTR mRNA expression, suggesting that the upregulation is a consequence of a genomic estrogen effect on the OTR gene transcription (Breton et al., 1995; Larcher et al., 1995). Behavioral studies have clearly shown that a necessary potential of OXT to elicit maternal or sexual behavior is priming with estrogen alone or with both estrogen and progesterone (Pedersen et al., 1982; Fahrbach et al., 1985). This evidence suggests that OTRs are under the control of gonadal steroids in the central nervous system (CNS).

OTR gene expression increases during pregnancy and/or at parturition in the olfactory bulb, medial preoptic area, bed nucleus of the stria terminalis (BNST), the SON, and in the medial amygdala in rat (Young et al., 1997; Meddle et al., 2007). Studies have shown that OTR-binding sites increase in the medial preoptic area, the BNST, VMH, and the ventral tegmental area on postpartum day 1 (Insel, 1990; Pedersen et al., 1994; Young et al., 1997). These changes suggest that OXT and OTR receptors play a role in both lactation and the regulation of maternal behavior.

OXT is also recognized as having endocrine and paracrine roles in male reproduction. OXT is synthesized within the mammalian testis, epididymis and prostate, and OTRs in the reproductive tract support a local action for OXT (Ivell et al., 1990, 1997; Foo et al., 1991; Nicholson and Hardy, 1992; Frayne and Nicholson, 1995, 1998; Harris et al., 1996; Filippi et al., 2002; Whittington et al., 2004). In ejaculation, a burst of OXT is released from the neurohypophysis into the systemic circulation and stimulates contractions of the reproductive tract for sperm release (Ogawa et al., 1980; Carmichael et al., 1987; Murphy et al., 1987). OXT plays a paracrine role in stimulating contractility of the seminiferous tubules, epididymis and the prostate gland.

Interestingly, OXT is also released from soma and dendrites during parturition and lactation (Ludwig and Leng, 2006). Although OXT released from the soma and dendrites of the MNC in the SON and the PVN may act in a paracrine to activate distant receptors (Ludwig and Leng, 2006), OXT-like immunoreactivity (LI) fibers can be found throughout the brain, including the nucleus accumbens (NAcc), lateral septum, amygdala, and some areas in the hindbrain, brainstem, and spinal cord (Sofroniew, 1980; Castel and Morris, 1988). A notable reduction of OXT-LI fibers was observed throughout the brain by the lesioning of the PVN (De Vries and Buijs, 1983). Although little is known about the regulation of OXT release from these forebrain projections, they might contribute significantly to the regulation of behavior.

TRANSGENIC ANIMAL OF OXYTOCIN

OXT DEFICIENT MICE

Previous studies have generated mice carrying a deletion of the OXT-coding region using homologous recombination in embryonic stem cells (Nishimori et al., 1996; Young et al., 1996). Mice lacking OXT are both viable and fertile. Males do not have any reproduction behavioral or functional defects in the absence of OXT. Similarly, females have no obvious deficits in fertility or reproduction, including gestation and parturition. Although OXT-deficient females demonstrated normal maternal behavior, all their offspring died of starvation shortly after birth, because OXT-deficient mothers were unable to nurse. After injections of OXT to OXT-deficient mothers, milk ejection was induced and the offspring survived. OXT-deficient male mice fail to develop social memory (Ferguson et al., 2000). A measurement of both olfactory foraging and olfactory habituation tasks has indicated that olfactory detection of non-social stimuli is intact in OXT-deficient male mice, and treatment with OXT reinstates social memory in those mice. These data indicate that OXT is necessary for the normal development of social memory in mice and support the hypothesis that social memory has a neural basis distinct from other forms of memory.

OXTR DEFICIENT MICE

OXTR-deficient mice were viable and had no obvious deficits in fertility or reproductive behavior, the same as OXT-deficient mice (Takayanagi et al., 2005). OXTR-deficient dams mice exhibited normal parturition but demonstrated defects in lactation and maternal nurturing. Infant OXTR-deficient males emitted fewer ultrasonic vocalizations than their wild-type littermates in response to social isolation. Adult OXTR-deficient males also showed deficits in social discrimination, and demonstrated increased aggressive behavior. OXT-deficient males from

OXT-deficient but not from heterozygote dams showed high levels of aggression. These data suggest a developmental role for the OXT/OXTR system in shaping adult aggressive behavior.

ANIMALS BEARING FLUORESCENT FUSION TRANSGENES

Previous studies have shown the placement of the eGFP coding sequence (Young et al., 1999; Zhang et al., 2002) or chloramphenicol acetyltransferase (CAT) reporters at various locations within an OXT transgene (Jeong et al., 2001) (**Table 1**). We generated rats bearing an OXT-eCFP fusion transgene designed from a murine construct previously shown to be faithfully expressed in transgenic mice (Katoh et al., 2010) (**Table 1**). However, the expression of the transgene was unstable for unknown reasons.

The mRFP was developed from DsRed, which is the red fluorescent protein from *Discosoma* (Campbell et al., 2002; Long et al., 2005). We have succeeded in generating transgenic rats bearing an OXT-mRFP1 fusion gene (Katoh et al., 2011) (**Table 1**) (**Figure 1**). Interestingly, when the brains of these rats were mounted on a slide, the mRFP1 fluorescence was visible in the ventral part of the SON and in the PP without cutting. We could observe the mRFP1 fluorescence throughout the SON, especially in the dorsal parts. We could observe abundant mRFP1 fluorescence in the magnocellular division of the PVN and scattered mRFP1 fluorescence in the parvocellular division of the PVN. We also observed mRFP1 fluorescence in the internal layer of the median eminence (ME) and in the PP. *In situ* hybridization histochemistry showed mRFP1 mRNA localized in the SON and in the magnocellular and parvocellular divisions of the PVN. In comparing male and female transgenic rats under normal conditions, there were no differences in the expression of mRFP1 mRNA in the SON and the PVN. In comparing nontransgenic and transgenic rats under normal conditions, there were no differences between them in plasma osmorality, sodium, OXT, AVP, and the expression of the endogenous OXT gene and AVP gene in the SON and the PVN.

Previous studies have reported that OXT transcripts significantly increased in the rat hypothalamus after chronic osmotic stimuli, such as salt loading (Lightman and Young, 1987; McCabe et al., 1990; Yue et al., 2008). In our OXT-mRFP1 transgenic rats, the fluorescence of mRFP1 was remarkably increased by 5 to 7-fold throughout the SON and in the PVN, ME, and PP after salt loading for 5 days (Katoh et al., 2010) (**Figure 1**). *In situ* hybridization histochemistry showed dramatically increased the expression of the mRFP1 mRNA in the SON and the PVN after salt loading. Comparing nontransgenic and transgenic rats after salt loading, there were no differences in plasma osmorality, sodium, OXT, AVP, and the expression of the endogenous OXT gene and AVP gene in the SON and the PVN.

The peripheral administration of cholecystokinin (CCK) -8 stimulated secretion of OXT but not AVP (Verbalis et al., 1986; Ueta et al., 2000; Hashimoto et al., 2005), and excited OXT-secreting magnocellular neurons in the SON and the PVN in rats (Hamamura et al., 1991; Ueta et al., 1993, 2000; Hashimoto et al., 2005). CCK-8 stimulates gastric vagal afferents and activated noradrenergic neurons in the nucleus of the tractus solitarius (Luckman, 1992). It is postulated that these noradrenergic inputs activate OXT-secreting neurons in the SON and the PVN and cause the secretion of OXT into the systemic circulation in rats (Hamamura et al., 1991). Recently, we have developed a novel transgenic rat that enables the trivial visualization of c-*fos* expression using an eGFP tag (Katoh et al., 2014). These rats express a transgene consisting of c-*fos* gene regulatory sequences that drive the expression of a c-*fos*-eGFP fusion protein. Moreover, we generated a double transgenic rat that expresses both the c-*fos*-eGFP and an OXT-mRFP1 fusion gene. In these double transgenic rats, nuclear eGFP fluorescence appeared in OXT-mRFP1 neurons in the SON and the PVN 90 min after i.p. administration of CCK-8 (**Figure 2**). Three-dimensional reconstruction imaging enables the visualization of nuclear eGFP in the cytoplasm of OXT neurons illuminated and identified by virtue of their expression of mRFP1. In these neurons, abundant OXT granules in the cytoplasm are clearly visible by a plane image obtained from a higher magnification by confocal laser microscopy (Katoh et al., 2014).

CONCLUSIONS

We did not observe any fluorescence of mRFP1 in the ectopic area of OXT in the OXT-mRFP1 transgenic rats. The OXT neuron has the same proper response to physiological stimulation in the OXT-mRFP1 transgenic rats as in nontransgenic rats. Using OXT-mRFP1 rats, we can identify the OXT neuron

Table 1 | Oxytocin transgenes.

Transgenesis		Transgene	Reporter gene	Specificity expression in HNS	Ectopic expression	References
From	To					
Mouse	Mouse	AI-02	eGFP	None	None	Young et al., 1999
Mouse	Mouse	AI-01	eGFP	Few	None	Young et al., 1999
Mouse	Mouse	AI-03	eGFP	+	None	Young et al., 1999
Mouse	Mouse	JL-01	IRES-eGFP	+	None	Young et al., 1999
Mouse	Mouse	OT-3-CAT-3.5	CAT	+	None	Jeong et al., 2001
Mouse	Rat	AI-03	eCFP	+	None	Katoh et al., 2010
Rat	Rat	OXT-mRFP1	mRFP1	+	None	Katoh et al., 2011, 2014

HNS, hypothalamo-neurohypophysial system.

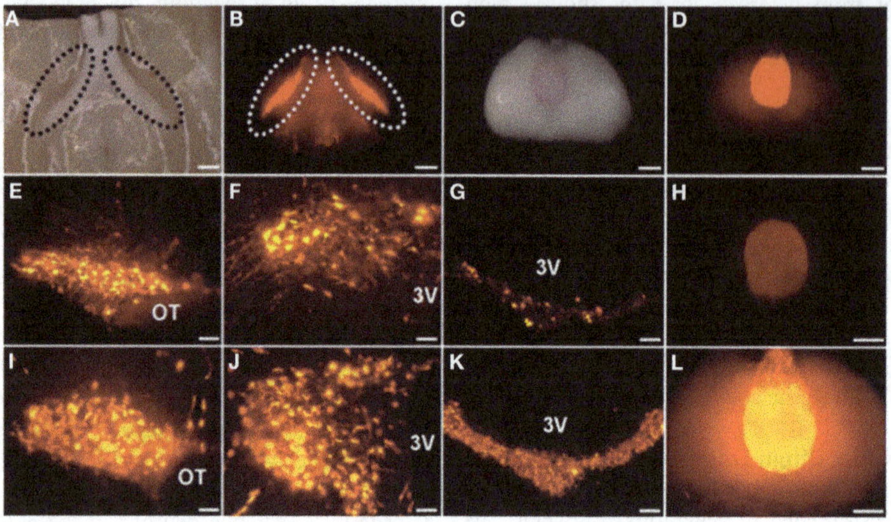

FIGURE 1 | The mRFP1 fluorescence was clearly observed in ventral parts of the supraoptic nucleus (SON) (A,B) and in the PP (C,D) without cutting. Endogenous florescence of mRFP1 in the SON **(E)**, the paraventricular nucleus (PVN) **(F)**, the median eminence (ME) **(G)**, and the posterior pituitary (PP) **(H)**. Effects of salt loading for 5 days on the mRFP1 fluorescence of the SON **(I)**, the PVN **(J)**, the ME **(K)**, and the PP **(L)**. Under light **(A,C)** and fluorescent **(B,D–L)**. *Scale bars*, 1 mm **(A–D,H,L)** and 0.1 mm **(E–G,I–K)**. OT, Optic tract; 3V, third ventricle. Modified with permission from Figure 1 in Katoh et al. (2011).

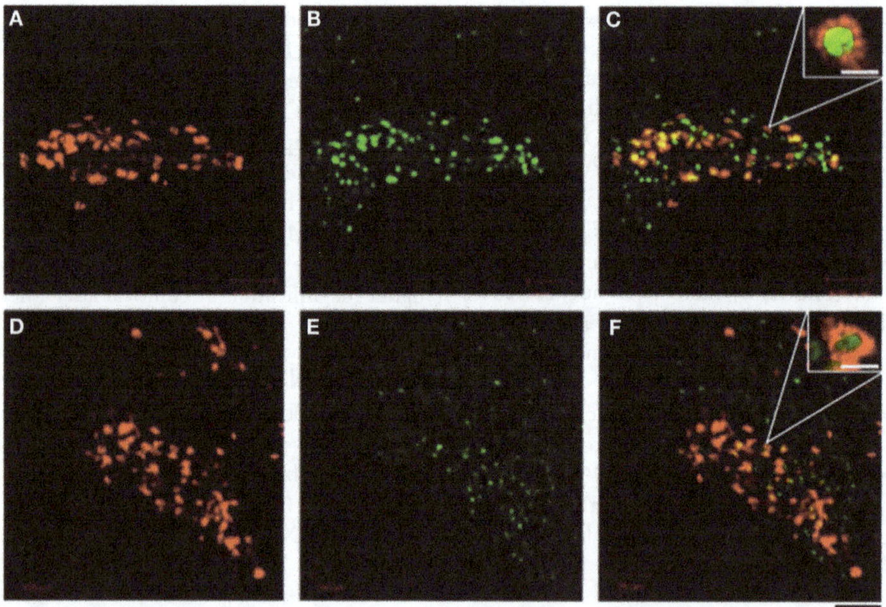

FIGURE 2 | Effects of i.p. administration of cholecystokinin-8 on the endogenous fluorescence of monomeric red fluorescent protein 1 (mRFP1) (A,D) and nuclear enhanced green fluorescent protein (eGFP) (B,E) in the supraoptic nucleus (A–C) and the paraventricular nucleus (D–F). The merged view of fluorescence of mRFP1 and eGFP was seen as a yellow color **(C,F)**. Scale bars shown in white represent 10 μm in **(C,F)**. The scale bar shown in black = 40 μm. Modified with permission from Figure 3 in Katoh et al. (2014).

easily and see changes in the neuron's activity and release of OXT in realtime. Moreover, we can see smaller changes that we had not been able to see before, because OXT-mRFP1 transcription is more sensitive than endogenous OXT transcription to the same stimulation. The OXT-mRFP1 transgenic rats are a useful animal model to study dynamic changes in OXT in the HNS.

ACKNOWLEDGMENTS

We thank to *Endocrine Society* and *British Society for Neuroendocrinology* for permission to use figures of journals, respectively, *Endocrinology* and *Journal of Neuroendocrinology*. This study was supported by Grant-in-Aid for Scientific Research (C) No. 25460324 (Hirofumi Hashimoto) and Grant-in-Aid for Scientific Research on Innovative Areas No. 25113721 (Yoichi

Ueta) from the Ministry of Education, Culture, Sports, Science and Technology (MEXT).

REFERENCES

Breton, C., Pechoux, C., Morel, G., and Zingg, H. H. (1995). Oxytocin receptor messenger ribonucleic acid: characterization, regulation, and cellular localization in the rat pituitary gland. *Endocrinology* 136, 2928–2936.

Burbach, P., Young, L. J., and Russell, J. (2006). "Oxytocin: synthesis, secretion and reproductive functions," in *Knobil and Neill's Physiology of Reproduction*, ed J. D. Neill (Amsterdam: Elsevier), 3055–3127.

Campbell, R. E., Tour, O., Palmer, A. E., Steinbach, P. A., Baird, G. S., Zacharias, D. A., et al. (2002). A monomeric red fluorescent protein. *Proc. Natl. Acad. Sci. U.S.A.* 99, 7877–7882. doi: 10.1073/pnas.082243699

Carmichael, M. S., Humbert, R., Dixen, J., Palmisano, G., Greenleaf, W., and Davidson, J. M. (1987). Plasma oxytocin increases in the human sexual response. *J. Clin. Endocrinol. Metab.* 64, 27–31. doi: 10.1210/jcem-64-1-27

Carmichael, M. S., Warburton, V. L., Dixen, J., and Davidson, J. M. (1994). Relationships among cardiovascular, muscular, and oxytocin responses during human sexual activity. *Arch. Sex. Behav.* 23, 59–79. doi: 10.1007/BF01541618

Castel, M., and Morris, J. (1988). The neurophysin-containing innervation of the forebrain of the mouse. *Neuroscience* 24, 937–966. doi: 10.1016/0306-4522(88)90078-4

Dale, H. H. (1906). On some physiological actions of ergot. *J. Physiol.* 34, 163–206.

De Vries, G. J., and Buijs, R. M. (1983). The origin of vasopressinergic and oxytocinergic innervation of the rat brain with special reference to the lateral septum. *Brain Res.* 273, 307–317. doi: 10.1016/0006-8993(83)90855-7

du Vigneaud, V., Ressler, C., Swan, J., and Roberts, C. (1954). The synthesis of oxytocin. *J. Am. Chem. Soc.* 76, 3115–3121. doi: 10.1021/ja01641a004

du Vigneaud, V., Ressler, C., Swan, J., Roberts, C., Katsoyannis, P., and Gordon, S. (1953b). The synthesis of an octapeptide amide with the hormonal activity of oxytocin. *J. Am. Chem. Soc.* 75, 4879–4880. doi: 10.1021/ja01115a553

du Vigneaud, V., Ressler, C., and Trippett, S. (1953a). The sequence of amino acids in oxytocin, with a proposal for the structure of oxytocin. *J. Biol. Chem.* 205, 949–957.

Fahrbach, S. E., Morrell, J. I., and Pfaff, D. W. (1985). Possible role for endogenous oxytocin in estrogen-facilitated maternal behavior in rats. *Neuroendocrinology* 40, 526–532. doi: 10.1159/000124125

Ferguson, J. N., Young, L. J., Hearn, E. F., Matzuk, M. M., Insel, T. R., and Winslow, J. T. (2000). Social amnesia in mice lacking the oxytocin gene. *Nat. Genet.* 25, 284–288. doi: 10.1038/77040

Filippi, S., Vannelli, G. B., Granchi, S., Luconi, M., Crescioli, C., Mancina, R., et al. (2002). Identification, localisation and functional activity of oxytocin receptors in epididymis. *Mol. Cell. Endocrinol.* 193, 89–100. doi: 10.1016/S0303-7207(02)00101-6

Foo, N. C., Carter, D., Murphy, D., and Ivell, R. (1991). Vasopressin and oxytocin gene expression in rat testis. *Endocrinology* 128, 2118–2128. doi: 10.1210/endo-128-4-2118

Frayne, J., and Nicholson, H. D. (1995). Effect of oxytocin on testosterone production by isolated rat Leydig cells is mediated via a specific oxytocin receptor. *Biol. Reprod.* 52, 1268–1273. doi: 10.1095/biolreprod52.6.1268

Frayne, J., and Nicholson, H. D. (1998). Localization of oxytocin receptors in the human and macaque monkey male reproductive tracts: evidence for a physiological role of oxytocin in the male. *Mol. Hum. Reprod.* 4, 527–532. doi: 10.1093/molehr/4.6.527

Fuchs, A. R., Periyasamy, S., Alexandrova, M., and Soloff, M. S. (1983). Correlation between oxytocin receptor concentration and responsiveness to oxytocin in pregnant rat myometrium: effects of ovarian steroids. *Endocrinology* 113, 742–749. doi: 10.1210/endo-113-2-742

Fujio, T., Fujihara, H., Shibata, M., Yamada, S., Onaka, T., Tanaka, K., et al. (2006). Exaggerated response of arginine vasopressin-enhanced green fluorescent protein fusion gene to salt loading without disturbance of body fluid homeostasis in rats. *J. Neuroendocrinol.* 18, 776–785. doi: 10.1111/j.1365-2826.2006.01476.x

Hamamura, M., Leng, G., Emson, P. C., and Kiyama, H. (1991). Electrical activation and c-fos mRNA expression in rat neurosecretory neurones after systemic administration of cholecystokinin. *J. Physiol.* 444, 51–63.

Harris, G. C., Frayne, J., and Nicholson, H. D. (1996). Epididymal oxytocin in the rat; its origin and regulation. *Int. J. Androl.* 19, 278–286. doi: 10.1111/j.1365-2605.1996.tb00476.x

Hashimoto, H., Onaka, T., Kawasaki, M., Chen, L., Mera, T., Soya, A., et al. (2005). Effects of cholecystokinin (CCK)-8 on hypothalamic oxytocin-secreting neurons in rats lacking CCK-A receptor. *Auton. Neurosci.* 121, 16–25. doi: 10.1016/j.autneu.2005.05.002

Hatton, G. I., and Tweedle, C. D. (1982). Magnocellular neuropeptidergic neurons in hypothalamus: increases in membrane apposition and number of specialized synapses from pregnancy to lactation. *Brain Res. Bull.* 8, 197–204. doi: 10.1016/0361-9230(82)90046-6

Insel, T. R. (1990). Regional changes in brain oxytocin receptors post-partum: time-course and relationship to maternal behaviour. *J. Neuroendocrinol.* 2, 539–545. doi: 10.1111/j.1365-2826.1990.tb00445.x

Ivell, R., Balvers, M., Rust, W., Bathgate, R., and Einspanier, A. (1997). Oxytocin and male reproductive function. *Adv. Exp. Med. Biol.* 424, 253–264. doi: 10.1007/978-1-4615-5913-9_47

Ivell, R., Furuya, K., Brackmann, B., Dawood, Y., and Khan-Dawood, F. (1990). Expression of the oxytocin and vasopressin genes in human and baboon gonadal tissues. *Endocrinology* 127, 2990–2996. doi: 10.1210/endo-127-6-2990

Ivell, R., and Richter, D. (1984). Structure and comparison of the oxytocin and vasopressin genes from rat. *Proc. Natl. Acad. Sci. U.S.A.* 81, 2006–2010. doi: 10.1073/pnas.81.7.2006

Iwanaga, M., Ohno, M., Katoh, A., Ohbuchi, T., Ishikura, T., Fujihara, H., et al. (2011). Upregulation of arginine vasopressin synthesis in the rat hypothalamus after kainic acid-induced seizures. *Brain Res.* 1424, 1–8. doi: 10.1016/j.brainres.2011.09.030

Jeong, S. W., Castel, M., Zhang, B. J., Fields, R. L., Paras, P., Arnheiter, H., et al. (2001). Cell-specific expression and subcellular localization of neurophysin-CAT-fusion proteins expressed from oxytocin and vasopressin gene promoter-driven constructs in transgenic mice. *Exp. Neurol.* 171, 255–271. doi: 10.1006/exnr.2001.7785

Katoh, A., Fujihara, H., Ohbuchi, T., Onaka, T., Hashimoto, T., Kawata, M., et al. (2011). Highly visible expression of an oxytocin-monomeric red fluorescent protein 1 fusion gene in the hypothalamus and posterior pituitary of transgenic rats. *Endocrinology* 152, 2768–2774. doi: 10.1210/en.2011-0006

Katoh, A., Fujihara, H., Ohbuchi, T., Onaka, T., Young, W. S. 3rd., Dayanithi, G., et al. (2010). Specific expression of an oxytocin-enhanced cyan fluorescent protein fusion transgene in the rat hypothalamus and posterior pituitary. *J. Endocrinol.* 204, 275–285. doi: 10.1677/JOE-09-0289

Katoh, A., Shoguchi, K., Matsuoka, H., Yoshimura, M., Ohkubo, J. I., Matsuura, T., et al. (2014). Fluorescent visualisation of the hypothalamic oxytocin neurones activated by cholecystokinin-8 in rats expressing c-fos-enhanced green fluorescent protein and oxytocin-monomeric red fluorescent protein 1 fusion transgenes. *J. Neuroendocrinol.* 26, 341–347. doi: 10.1111/jne.12150

Kimura, T., Tanizawa, O., Mori, K., Brownstein, M. J., and Okayama, H. (1992). Structure and expression of a human oxytocin receptor. *Nature* 356, 526–529. doi: 10.1038/356526a0

Kubota, Y., Kimura, T., Hashimoto, K., Tokugawa, Y., Nobunaga, K., Azuma, C., et al. (1996). Structure and expression of the mouse oxytocin receptor gene. *Mol. Cell. Endocrinol.* 124, 25–32. doi: 10.1016/S0303-7207(96)03923-8

Larcher, A., Neculcea, J., Breton, C., Arslan, A., Rozen, F., Russo, C., et al. (1995). Oxytocin receptor gene expression in the rat uterus during pregnancy and the estrous cycle and in response to gonadal steroid treatment. *Endocrinology* 136, 5350–5356.

Leckman, J. F., Goodman, W. K., North, W. G., Chappell, P. B., Price, L. H., Pauls, D. L., et al. (1994). The role of central oxytocin in obsessive compulsive disorder and related normal behavior. *Psychoneuroendocrinology* 19, 723–749. doi: 10.1016/0306-4530(94)90021-3

Lefebvre, D. L., Farookhi, R., Giaid, A., Neculcea, J., and Zingg, H. H. (1994). Uterine oxytocin gene expression. II. Induction by exogenous steroid administration. *Endocrinology* 134, 2562–2566.

Lightman, S. L., and Young, W. S. 3rd. (1987). Vasopressin, oxytocin, dynorphin, enkephalin and corticotrophin-releasing factor mRNA stimulation in the rat. *J. Physiol.* 394, 23–39.

Long, J. Z., Lackan, C. S., and Hadjantonakis, A. K. (2005). Genetic and spectrally distinct *in vivo* imaging: embryonic stem cells and mice with widespread expression of a monomeric red fluorescent protein. *BMC Biotechnol.* 5:20. doi: 10.1186/1472-6750-5-20

Luckman, S. M. (1992). Fos-like immunoreactivity in the brainstem of the rat following peripheral administration of cholecystokinin. *J. Neuroendocrinol.* 4, 149–152. doi: 10.1111/j.1365-2826.1992.tb00152.x

Ludwig, M., and Leng, G. (2006). Dendritic peptide release and peptide-dependent behaviours. *Nat. Rev. Neurosci.* 7, 126–136. doi: 10.1038/nrn1845

Maggi, M., Magini, A., Fiscella, A., Giannini, S., Fantoni, G., Toffoletti, F., et al. (1992). Sex steroid modulation of neurohypophysial hormone receptors in human nonpregnant myometrium. *J. Clin. Endocrinol. Metab.* 74, 385–392.

Maruyama, T., Ohbuchi, T., Fujihara, H., Shibata, M., Mori, K., Murphy, D., et al. (2010). Diurnal changes of arginine vasopressin-enhanced green fluorescent protein fusion transgene expression in the rat suprachiasmatic nucleus. *Peptides* 31, 2089–2093. doi: 10.1016/j.peptides.2010.08.010

McCabe, J. T., Kawata, M., Sano, Y., Pfaff, D. W., and Desharnais, R. A. (1990). Quantitative *in situ* hybridization to measure single-cell changes in vasopressin and oxytocin mRNA levels after osmotic stimulation. *Cell. Mol. Neurobiol.* 10, 59–71. doi: 10.1007/BF00733636

Meddle, S. L., Bishop, V. R., Gkoumassi, E., van Leeuwen, F. W., and Douglas, A. J. (2007). Dynamic changes in oxytocin receptor expression and activation at parturition in the rat brain. *Endocrinology* 148, 5095–5104. doi: 10.1210/en.2007-0615

Murphy, M. R., Seckl, J. R., Burton, S., Checkley, S. A., and Lightman, S. L. (1987). Changes in oxytocin and vasopressin secretion during sexual activity in men. *J. Clin. Endocrinol. Metab.* 65, 738–741. doi: 10.1210/jcem-65-4-738

Nicholson, H. D., and Hardy, M. P. (1992). Luteinising hormone differentially regulates the secretion of testicular oxytocin and testosterone by purified rat Leydig cells *in vitro*. *Endocrinology* 130, 671–677.

Nilaver, G., Zimmerman, E. A., Wilkins, J., Michaels, J., Hoffman, D., and Silverman, A. J. (1980). Magnocellular hypothalamic projections to the lower brain stem and spinal cord of the rat. Immunocytochemical evidence for predominance of the oxytocin-neurophysin system compared to the vasopressin-neurophysin system. *Neuroendocrinology* 30, 150–158. doi: 10.1159/000122991

Nishimori, K., Young, L. J., Guo, Q., Wang, Z., Insel, T. R., and Matzuk, M. M. (1996). Oxytocin is required for nursing but is not essential for parturition or reproductive behavior. *Proc. Natl. Acad. Sci. U.S.A.* 93, 11699–11704. doi: 10.1073/pnas.93.21.11699

Ogawa, S., Kudo, S., Kitsunai, Y., and Fukuchi, S. (1980). Increase in oxytocin secretion at ejaculation in male. *Clin. Endocrinol. (Oxf).* 13, 95–97. doi: 10.1111/j.1365-2265.1980.tb01027.x

Ohno, M., Fujihara, H., Iwanaga, M., Todoroki, M., Katoh, A., Ohbuchi, T., et al. (2012). Induction of arginine vasopressin-enhanced green fluorescent protein expression in the locus coeruleus following kainic acid-induced seizures in rats. *Stress* 15, 435–442. doi: 10.3109/10253890.2011.637185

Ostrowski, N. L. (1998). Oxytocin receptor mRNA expression in rat brain: implications for behavioral integration and reproductive success. *Psychoneuroendocrinology* 23, 989–1004. doi: 10.1016/S0306-4530(98)00070-5

Pedersen, C. A., Ascher, J. A., Monroe, Y. L., and Prange, A. J. Jr. (1982). Oxytocin induces maternal behavior in virgin female rats. *Science* 216, 648–650. doi: 10.1126/science.7071605

Pedersen, C. A., Caldwell, J. D., Walker, C., Ayers, G., and Mason, G. A. (1994). Oxytocin activates the postpartum onset of rat maternal behavior in the ventral tegmental and medial preoptic areas. *Behav. Neurosci.* 108, 1163–1171. doi: 10.1037/0735-7044.108.6.1163

Reaves, T. A. Jr., and Hayward, J. N. (1979). Immunocytochemical identification of vasopressinergic and oxytocinergic neurons in the hypothalamus of the cat. *Cell Tissue Res.* 196, 117–122. doi: 10.1007/BF00236352

Russell, J. A., and Leng, G. (1998). Sex, parturition and motherhood without oxytocin? *J. Endocrinol.* 157, 342–359. doi: 10.1677/joe.0.1570343

Sawchenko, P. E., and Swanson, L. W. (1982). Immunohistochemical identification of neurons in the paraventricular nucleus of the hypothalamus that project to the medulla or to the spinal cord in the rat. *J. Comp. Neurol.* 205, 260–272. doi: 10.1002/cne.902050306

Shibata, M., Fujihara, H., Suzuki, H., Ozawa, H., Kawata, M., Dayanithi, G., et al. (2007). Physiological studies of stress responses in the hypothalamus of vasopressin-enhanced green fluorescent protein transgenic rat. *J. Neuroendocrinol.* 19, 285–292. doi: 10.1111/j.1365-2826.2007.01532.x

Sofroniew, M. V. (1980). Projections from vasopressin, oxytocin, and neurophysin neurons to neural targets in the rat and human. *J. Histochem. Cytochem.* 28, 475–478. doi: 10.1177/28.5.7381192

Sofroniew, M. V., Weindl, A., Schrell, U., and Wetzstein, R. (1981). Immunohistochemistry of vasopressin, oxytocin and neurophysin in the hypothalamus and extrahypothalamic regions of the human and primate brain. *Acta Histochem. Suppl.* 24, 79–95.

Soloff, M. S., Fernstrom, M. A., Periyasamy, S., Soloff, S., Baldwin, S., and Wieder, M. (1983). Regulation of oxytocin receptor concentration in rat uterine explants by estrogen and progesterone. *Can. J. Biochem. Cell Biol.* 61, 625–630. doi: 10.1139/o83-078

Stock, S., and Uvnäs-Moberg, K. (1988). Increased plasma levels of oxytocin in response to afferent electrical stimulation of the sciatic and vagal nerves and in response to touch and pinch in anaesthetized rats. *Acta Physiol. Scand.* 132, 29–34. doi: 10.1111/j.1748-1716.1988.tb08294.x

Suzuki, H., Kawasaki, M., Ohnishi, H., Otsubo, H., Ohbuchi, T., Katoh, A., et al. (2009). Exaggerated response of a vasopressin-enhanced green fluorescent protein transgene to nociceptive stimulation in the rat. *J. Neurosci.* 29, 13182–13189. doi: 10.1523/JNEUROSCI.2624-09.2009

Takayanagi, Y., Yoshida, M., Bielsky, I. F., Ross, H. E., Kawamata, M., Onaka, T., et al. (2005). Pervasive social deficits, but normal parturition, in oxytocin receptor-deficient mice. *Proc. Natl. Acad. Sci. U.S.A.* 102, 16096–16101. doi: 10.1073/pnas.0505312102

Thomas, A., and Amico, J. A. (1996). Sequential estrogen and progesterone (P) followed by P withdrawal increases the level of oxytocin messenger ribonucleic acid in the hypothalamic paraventricular nucleus of the male rat. *Life Sci.* 58, 1615–1620. doi: 10.1016/0024-3205(96)00136-1

Todoroki, M., Ueta, Y., Fujihara, H., Otsubo, H., Shibata, M., Hashimoto, H., et al. (2010). Induction of the arginine vasopressin-enhanced green fluorescent protein fusion transgene in the rat locus coeruleus. *Stress* 13, 281–291. doi: 10.3109/10253890903383406

Ueta, Y., Fujihara, H., Serino, R., Dayanithi, G., Ozawa, H., Matsuda, K., et al. (2005). Transgenic expression of enhanced green fluorescent protein enables direct visualization for physiological studies of vasopressin neurons and isolated nerve terminals of the rat. *Endocrinology* 146, 406–413. doi: 10.1210/en.2004-0830

Ueta, Y., Kannan, H., Higuchi, T., Negoro, H., Yamaguchi, K., and Yamashita, H. (2000). Activation of gastric afferents increases noradrenaline release n the paraventricular nucleus and plasma oxytocin level. *J. Auton. Nerv. Syst.* 78, 69–76. doi: 10.1016/S0165-1838(99)00049-1

Ueta, Y., Kannan, H., Higuchi, T., Negoro, H., and Yamashita, H. (1993). CCK-8 excites oxytocin-secreting neurons in the paraventricular nucleus in rats—possible involvement of noradrenergic pathway. *Brain Res. Bull.* 32, 453–459. doi: 10.1016/0361-9230(93)90290-R

Uvnäs-Moberg, K., Bruzelius, G., Alster, P., and Lundeberg, T. (1993). The antinociceptive effect of non-noxious sensory stimulation is mediated partly through oxytocinergic mechanisms. *Acta Physiol. Scand.* 149, 199–204. doi: 10.1111/j.1748-1716.1993.tb09612.x

Van Tol, H. H., Bolwerk, E. L., Liu, B., and Burbach, J. P. (1988). Oxytocin and vasopressin gene expression in the hypothalamo–neurohypophyseal system of the rat during the estrous cycle, pregnancy, and lactation. *Endocrinology* 122, 945–951. doi: 10.1210/endo-122-3-945

Verbalis, J. G., McCann, M. J., McHale, C. M., and Stricker, E. M. (1986). Oxytocin secretion in response to cholecystokinin and food: differentiation of nausea from satiety. *Science* 232, 1417–1419. doi: 10.1126/science.3715453

Whittington, K., Assinder, S., Gould, M., and Nicholson, H. (2004). Oxytocin, oxytocin associated neurophysin and the oxytocin receptor in human prostate. *Cell Tissue Res.* 318, 375–382. doi: 10.1007/s00441-004-0968-5

Young, L. J., Winslow, J. T., Wang, Z., Gingrich, B., Guo, Q., Matzuk, M. M., et al. (1997). Gene targeting approaches to neuroendocrinology: oxytocin, maternal behavior, and affiliation. *Horm. Behav.* 31, 221–231. doi: 10.1006/hbeh.1997.1377

Young, W. S. 3rd., Iacangelo, A., Luo, X. Z., King, C., Duncan, K., and Ginns, E. I. (1999). Transgenic expression of green fluorescent protein in mouse oxytocin neurones. *J. Neuroendocrinol.* 11, 935–939. doi: 10.1046/j.1365-2826.1999.00410.x

Young, W. S. 3rd., Shepard, E., Amico, J., Hennighausen, L., Wagner, K. U., LaMarca, M. E., et al. (1996). Deficiency in mouse oxytocin prevents milk ejection, but not fertility or parturition. *J. Neuroendocrinol.* 8, 847–853. doi: 10.1046/j.1365-2826.1996.05266.x

Yue, C., Mutsuga, N., Sugimura, Y., Verbalis, J., and Gainer, H. (2008). Differential kinetics of oxytocin and vasopressin heteronuclear RNA expression in the rat supraoptic nucleus in response to chronic salt loading *in vivo*. *J. Neuroendocrinol.* 20, 227–232. doi: 10.1111/j.1365-2826.2007.01640.x

Zhang, B. J., Kusano, K., Zerfas, P., Iacangelo, A., Young, W. S. 3rd., and Gainer, H. (2002). Targeting of green fluorescent protein to secretory granules in oxytocin magnocellular neurons and its secretion from neurohypophysial nerve terminals in transgenic mice. *Endocrinology* 143, 1036–1046. doi: 10.1210/endo.143.3.8700

Zingg, H. H., and Lefebvre, D. L. (1988). Oxytocin and vasopressin gene expression during gestation and lactation. *Brain Res.* 464, 1–6. doi: 10.1016/0169-328X(88)90011-3

15

Social bonding: regulation by neuropeptides

Claudia Lieberwirth[1]* and Zuoxin Wang[2]

[1] *Department of Behavioral Science, Utah Valley University, Orem, UT, USA*
[2] *Department of Psychology and Program in Neuroscience, Florida State University, Tallahassee, FL, USA*

Correspondence:
Claudia Lieberwirth, Department of Behavioral Science, Utah Valley University, 800 West University Parkway, MS 115, Orem, UT 84058, USA
e-mail: clieberwirth@uvu.edu

Affiliative social relationships (e.g., among spouses, family members, and friends) play an essential role in human society. These relationships affect psychological, physiological, and behavioral functions. As positive and enduring bonds are critical for the overall well-being of humans, it is not surprising that considerable effort has been made to study the neurobiological mechanisms that underlie social bonding behaviors. The present review details the involvement of the nonapeptides, oxytocin (OT), and arginine vasopressin (AVP), in the regulation of social bonding in mammals including humans. In particular, we will discuss the role of OT and AVP in the formation of social bonds between partners of a mating pair as well as between parents and their offspring. Furthermore, the role of OT and AVP in the formation of interpersonal bonding involving trust is also discussed.

Keywords: pair bond, affiliation, social recognition, oxytocin, vasopressin

INTRODUCTION

Lasting, positive, and affiliative social relationships (e.g., among spouses, family members, and friends) play an essential role in human society (for review see Baumeister and Leary, 1995). These relationships affect psychological, physiological, and behavioral functions (for review see Baumeister and Leary, 1995). In particular, the enduring attachments between socio-sexual partners (e.g., marital relationships) seem to have profound impacts on the cognitive, social, emotional, and physical well-being. For example, social bonds that provide a sense of social belonging (social connectedness) seem to protect against feelings of loneliness, depression, and even anxiety (Lee and Robbins, 1998, 2000; Williams and Galliher, 2006). Furthermore, stable and positive marital relationships have been implicated to increase the life expectancy compared to that of non-attached singles (House et al., 1988; Lillard and Waite, 1995; Drefahl, 2012). There are also strong positive associations between high levels of marital satisfaction and immune function as well as cardiovascular health (Kiecolt-Glaser and Newton, 2001; Kiecolt-Glaser et al., 2010). Close parent relationships positively impact the psychological well-being of both parents and their children (Silverstein and Bengtson, 1991; Graziano et al., 2009). The presence of positive, secure attachments between parents and children provide protection against depression and anxiety in the child as well as lead to higher levels of child academic success (Bögels and Phares, 2008; Sarkadi et al., 2008; Graziano et al., 2009).

On the contrary, the disruption of social bonds (e.g., caused by marital problems, confrontations, isolation, or neglect) can have a negative impact on mental and physical health (Steptoe, 1991; Curtis, 1995). For example, low levels of intimacy between partners as well as perceived loneliness have been associated with negative psychological states, such as depression and depressive symptoms (Kiecolt-Glaser and Newton, 2001; Alpass and Neville, 2003; Adams et al., 2004). In addition, relationship conflict and interpersonal stress are associated with alterations in immune function (Kiecolt-Glaser and Newton, 2001; Kiecolt-Glaser et al., 2010; Jaremka et al., 2013). Similarly, adverse childhood experiences (such as parental separation or divorce, abuse, or neglect) have detrimental effects on the child's cognitive, physical, social, and emotional well-being. Early adverse childhood experiences are associated with poor child health at an early age (e.g., increased risk for asthma as well as cardio-respiratory and infectious diseases) as well as with the adoption of unhealthy lifestyles and medical problems (including but not limited to obesity, cancer, liver disease, chronic lung disease, and cardiovascular disease) in adulthood (Flaherty et al., 2006; Lanier et al., 2010; Leeb et al., 2011; Shonkoff et al., 2012). Adverse childhood experiences may also lead to reduced academic (i.e., failing in school) and post-academic (i.e., unemployment, poverty, and homelessness) success (Shonkoff et al., 2012). The experience of interpersonal distress during childhood is also correlated with depression, aggression, and drug misuse (e.g., cigarette smoking, alcohol consumption, and illegal drug use) later in life (DeFronzo and Pawlak, 1993; Anda et al., 1999; Nation and Heflinger, 2006; Leeb et al., 2011; Shonkoff et al., 2012).

It has been shown that abnormal social attachments and deficits in social interactions are core features of most psychopathologies, including autism spectrum disorder, social phobia, obsessive-compulsive disorder, post-traumatic stress disorder, and borderline personality disorder (reivewed by Bartz and Hollander, 2006). As social bonds play important roles in the psychological, physiological, and behavioral functioning and deficits in social bonding are core features of various psychopathologies, the research investigating the neural correlates of social bond formation is highly important. Research has provided ample evidence to suggest that social interactions (including the bond

Abbreviations: AAV, adeno-associated viral vector; AVP, arginine vasopressin; GABA, gamma-aminobutyric acid; OT, oxytocin; OTR, oxytocin receptor; V1aR, selective AVP receptor 1; SNP, single nucleotide polymorphism.

observed between socio-sexual partners and between parents and offspring, as well as trust in social interactions) seem to share similar neural mechanism (e.g., Curley and Keverne, 2005).

The structurally similar neuropeptides, oxytocin (OT), and arginine vasopressin (AVP), have repeatedly been implicated in the regulation of social cognition and behavior (including social recognition, affiliation, aggression, pair bonding, as well as parental behavior) (Lim and Young, 2006; Donaldson and Young, 2008; Heinrichs et al., 2009). OT and AVP may act as neurotransmitters, if released centrally via the hypothalamus (namely the paraventricular and supraoptic nuclei of the hypothalamus), or as neurohormones, if released peripherally via the pituitary gland (Ludwig and Leng, 2006; Debiec, 2007). It is believed that the behavioral effects of OT and AVP are primarily due to the central release from the parvocellular neurons of the paraventricular nucleus (Debiec, 2007). It should be noted that various other neurochemicals, including dopamine, endogenous opioids, adrenocorticotropic hormone (ACTH), gamma-aminobutyric acid (GABA), may also play a role in the regulation of social cognition and behavior (reviewed by Carter et al., 1995).

The following review will focus on the role of the neuropeptides OT and AVP in mediating social attachments between partners and between parents and their offspring. Such selective and enduring relationships are complex and likely depend on distinct processes, including approach behaviors, formation of social recognition memory, and subsequently the formation and maintenance of the bond. Therefore, we will discuss the role of OT and AVP in partner bonds and parent-offspring bonds focusing in particular on these aspects of social attachments. In addition, the influence of OT and AVP on relationships between close individuals, particularly trust between peers, will be discussed. We will focus exclusively on the mammalian literature, including evidence from studies in rodents, non-human primates, and humans. Finally, we will discuss how our current knowledge may shape future research to better understand the neural correlates of social bonding and its implications in pathologies.

SOCIAL BONDS BETWEEN PARTNERS IN A MATING PAIR

Romantic or passionate love, the intense attraction between mates, is an essential component of human social behavior and often precedes the formation of enduring preferential associations between two sexual partners. Such pair bonds are a type of social bond that occurs in nearly all human societies. While there are various definitions, a pair bond is commonly defined, across species, as an enduring preferential association between two sexually mature adults. The established social bond—a complex social behavior—is characterized by affiliative behaviors, copulation, and the selective preference toward the partner over a stranger (partner preference) (Gubernick, 1994). The bond is also often associated with mate guarding and bi-parental care of the offspring (Kleiman, 1977; Buss, 1988; Fraley et al., 2005). The significance of positive, enduring social bonds between human partners has been documented cross-culturally. For example, stable marital relationships are positively correlated with higher life expectancy compared to the life expectancy displayed by individuals who are single (House et al., 1988; Lillard and Waite, 1995; Drefahl, 2012). There are also strong positive associations between high levels of marital satisfaction and immune function as well as cardiovascular health (Kiecolt-Glaser and Newton, 2001; Kiecolt-Glaser et al., 2010). As enduring social bonds between partners are important to the psychological, physiological, and behavioral well-being (for review see Baumeister and Leary, 1995), considerable efforts have been made to identify the neurobiological mechanisms underlying pair bond formation. It should be mentioned that traditional laboratory rodents usually do not display pair bond formation, a behavioral characteristic that is displayed by less than 5% of mammalian species (Kleiman, 1977; Dewsbury, 1988). Therefore, various nontraditional animal models, which display pair bond formation—including marmosets (*Callithrix penicillata*), titi monkeys (*Callicebus cupreus*), California mice (*Peromyscus californicus*), and prairie voles (*Microtus ochrogaster*)—have emerged as better alternative animal models to study the neural correlates of pair bond formation (Carter et al., 1995; Bester-Meredith et al., 1999; Bales et al., 2007; de Jong et al., 2009; Smith et al., 2010). The nonapeptides, OT, and AVP, have been implicated in the regulation of social recognition and the display of prosocial/proximity-seeking behaviors—processes important for the formation of social bonds—as well as the formation of the bond itself (reviewed by Insel, 1992; Dluzen et al., 2001; Young, 2002; Bielsky and Young, 2004; Winslow and Insel, 2004; Wacker and Ludwig, 2012).

Using neuropharmacological manipulations, results suggest that OT and AVP play a role in pair bond formation across various mammalian species, including humans. Social recognition, an essential process to allow the formation of social bonds (Carter et al., 1995), allows members in a mating pair to distinguish between the familiar partner and an unfamiliar stranger. Several studies have implicated OT and AVP in mediating social recognition (reviewed by Engelmann et al., 1996; Dluzen et al., 2001; Bielsky and Young, 2004; Winslow and Insel, 2004; Wacker and Ludwig, 2012). In particular, the peripheral, central, and site-specific (e.g., into the lateral septum, main olfactory bulbs, and medial preoptic area) administration of OT facilitates social recognition in rats by increasing the retention time in a social discrimination test (Popik and van Ree, 1991; Popik et al., 1992a,b; Dluzen et al., 1998a,b, 2000), whereas the administration of a selective OT receptor, OTR, antagonist blocks short-term social recognition in rats and mice (Popik and van Ree, 1991; Engelmann et al., 1998; Dluzen et al., 2000; Ferguson et al., 2000). OT administration is also able to reverse the deficits in social memory observed in OT knockout mice (Ferguson et al., 2000, 2001). Similarly to OT, peripheral, central, and site-specific (e.g., into the lateral septum and main olfactory bulbs) AVP administration increases social recognition memory in rats (Dantzer et al., 1987, 1988; Le Moal et al., 1987; Popik et al., 1992b; Dluzen et al., 1998a,b) and rescues the social recognition impairment observed in Brattleboro rats, which carry a genetic mutation causing the lack of endogenous AVP (Engelmann and Landgraf, 1994). On the contrary, the peripheral, central, or site-specific (e.g., into the hippocampus, lateral septum, or main olfactory bulbs) administration of a non-selective AVP receptor antagonist, selective AVP receptor (V1aR) antagonist, or V1aR antisense oligodeoxynucleotide impairs social recognition memory in mice and rats (Dantzer et al., 1987, 1988; Bluthe et al., 1990; Popik et al., 1992b; Engelmann and Landgraf, 1994; Landgraf et al., 1995; van Wimersma Greidanus and Maigret, 1996; Everts and Koolhaas, 1997, 1999; Bielsky et al., 2005; Tobin et al., 2010). Rats treated site-specifically into the lateral septum with antisense oligodeoxynucleotides to the mRNA of V1aR investigate a familiar and a novel juvenile similarly, while rats treated with vehicle or scrambled-antisense oligodeoxynucleotide investigate the familiar significantly less than the novel juvenile—an indication of impaired social recognition (Landgraf et al., 1995). Similarly, the treatment with a V1aR antagonist, but not saline, into the lateral septum blocks the reduction in social investigation between a familiar and novel juveniles in rats (Dantzer et al., 1988; Popik et al., 1992b; Engelmann and Landgraf, 1994; Everts and Koolhaas, 1997, 1999; Bielsky et al., 2005). Site-specific treatment with anti-AVP serum into the ventral as well as dorsal hippocampus prevents the reduction of social investigation time between initial and second encounter of a juvenile as observed in control rats (van Wimersma Greidanus and Maigret, 1996). Treatment with an AVP antagonist into the main olfactory bulb inhibits the discrimination of a familiar vs. novel juvenile (Tobin et al., 2010). In extension to the memory-enhancing effects of OT in rats, intranasal OT administration also enhances the short- and long-term memory performance of both men and women in a face recognition test (Savaskan et al., 2008; Rimmele et al., 2009). However, it should be noted that additional research is necessary to interpret the effects of peripheral manipulations of the OT and AVP systems in affecting social recognition. In particular, research needs to systematically assess whether extrahypothalamic OT and AVP neurons are part of the neuronal circuit that is involved in social memory.

Further evidence for the involvement of OT and AVP in social bonds comes from neuropharmacological studies showing that OT and AVP play a role in the regulation of prosocial and affiliative behaviors. Such regulation is another essential component for the formation of a pair bond. For example, female prairie voles display higher levels of social behavior (including more side-by-side contact and less aggression) following a peripheral or central OT administration (Witt et al., 1990). Similarly, chronic OT administration increases social interactions of male rats with a female (as shown by an increase in the amount of side-by-side contact displayed and the duration of anogenital investigation) (Witt et al., 1992). The central OT administration increases approach, affiliative grooming (an important component of social interactions in various primate species) (Hinde and Berman, 1983), and huddle behavior toward a female in subordinate, but not dominant, male squirrel monkeys (*Saimiri sciureus*) (Winslow and Insel, 1991). In monogamous marmosets (*C. penicillata*), OT treatment increases the frequency of contact behavior, decreases the partner approach latency, and increases food sharing with the partner; whereas the treatment with a selective OTR antagonist reduces the frequency of contact behavior and decreased food sharing with the partner (Smith et al., 2010). Using adeno-viral vector-mediated (AAV) gene transfer, mice, rats, and meadow voles (*Microtus pennsylvanicus*, a promiscuous and nonsocial rodent species) can be engineered to express a similar V1aR pattern as the prairie vole. In turn, this receptor expression pattern in male mice, rats, and meadow voles significantly increases the affiliative behavior toward conspecific females (Young et al., 1999; Landgraf et al., 2003; Lim et al., 2004). Furthermore, intranasal AVP administration results in an increase in affiliative behavior (e.g., higher frequency of contact time) in male titi monkeys (*C. cupreus*) toward their female partner (Jarcho et al., 2011). Recent studies in humans have also provided evidence for the involvement of OT in the regulation of prosocial and affiliative behaviors. Using the Relationship Closeness Induction Task (a social psychology method used to introduce strangers to each other), intranasal OT administration increases conversational intimacy in women, but not men (Liu et al., 2012). Conversational intimacy is an index of human social approach behavior (Liu et al., 2012). Furthermore, intranasal OT treatment increases positive communication behavior in relation to negative behavior during a couple conflict discussion (Ditzen et al., 2009). In addition, researchers comparing plasma OT levels between new lovers (3 months after initiation of their romantic relationship) and non-attached singles, found that OT levels do not differ between men and women, are individually stable, and are higher in new lovers than singles (Schneiderman et al., 2012). Interestingly, the OT levels were positively correlated with the level of interactive reciprocity (i.e., affectionate touch) (Schneiderman et al., 2012). Similarly to plasma OT levels, plasma AVP levels also correlate positively with social functioning. In particular, higher levels of plasma AVP levels are associated with fewer negative marital interactions (Gouin et al., 2012).

Neuropharmacological manipulations of the OT and AVP systems, in particular using the socially monogamous prairie vole as an ideal model to study the neural correlates of pair bond formation between socio-sexual partners (Dewsbury, 1975; Williams et al., 1992b), provide further evidence that OT and AVP play an essential role in pair bond formation. Central or site-specific (e.g., into the nucleus accumbens) OT treatment, compared to artificial cerebrospinal fluid treatment, results in the formation of partner preference, an index of bond formation (Insel and Hulihan, 1995), in female prairie voles (Williams et al., 1992a; Insel and Hulihan, 1995; Cho et al., 1999; Liu and Wang, 2003). While mating (and/or cohabitation) is an essential component for pair bond formation (Getz et al., 1981; Williams et al., 1992b), OT-induced partner preference formation occurs even in the absence of mating. However, when females are pre-treated with a selective OTR antagonist, the OT treatment does not result in a partner preference (Williams et al., 1992a; Insel and Hulihan, 1995; Cho et al., 1999). In addition, a selective OTR antagonist given centrally before mating or in combination with OT also inhibits the formation of a partner preference in female prairie voles without affecting mating *per se* (Insel and Hulihan, 1995; Cho et al., 1999). The blockade of partner preference formation due to a selective OTR antagonist indicates that OT is working via an OTR-mediated mechanism. Interestingly, the effect of central OT seems to be gender-specific as OT administration does not result in partner preference formation and selective OTR antagonist administration does not block partner preference formation in males (Williams et al., 1992a; Winslow et al., 1993; Insel and Hulihan, 1995; but see Cho et al., 1999). Similarly to OT, AVP also plays a role in the formation of partner preference in prairie voles. In particular, central or site-specific (e.g., ventral pallidum) AVP treatment increases partner preference formation in male prairie voles in the absence of mating, while the treatment with a nonselective AVP receptor antagonist or a selective V1aR antagonist blocks the formation of partner preference formation (Winslow et al., 1993; Insel and Winslow, 1998; Cho et al., 1999; Lim and Young, 2004). It should be noted that such AVP-induced partner preference formation in female prairie voles is only observed when using a high dose of AVP (Insel, 1997; Cho et al., 1999).

Studies using genetic manipulations have also provided evidence indicating that social bonds (including the underlying components of social recognition, social affiliation, and, in turn, pair bond formation) are regulated in part by the neuropeptides, OT and AVP. For example, mice and Brattleboro rats that are null-mutants of the OT or AVP gene, respectively, show deficits in a social recognition task; but social recognition can be restored by OT and AVP administration (Ferguson et al., 2000, 2001; Winslow and Insel, 2002; Choleris et al., 2006; Crawley et al., 2007; Macbeth et al., 2009). In particular, OT treatment site-specifically into the medial amygdala is able to restore social recognition in OT knockout mice, indicating that amygdala OT plays an essential role in social recognition (Ferguson et al., 2001). Profound impairments in social recognition are also observed in OTR and V1aR knockout mouse species (Bielsky et al., 2004, 2005; Takayanagi et al., 2005; Macbeth et al., 2009). The re-expression of V1aR (using AAV) in the lateral septum of V1aR knockout mice can fully restore social recognition (Bielsky et al., 2005). In addition, the overexpression of the V1aR in the lateral septum of wild-type mice and rats can potentiate social recognition (Landgraf et al., 2003; Bielsky et al., 2005). Interestingly, CD38 knockout mice also show deficits in social recognition. CD38 knockout mice lack CD38, a type-II transmembrane protein. This protein is involved in the mobilization of intracellular Ca^{2+} via activation of cyclic ADP ribose (cADPR), a cellular messenger for calcium signaling (Jin et al., 2007). In turn, intracellular calcium signaling plays a key role in the central release of OT (Lopatina et al., 2013). Consequently, CD38 knockout mice have reduced levels of OT and display impairments in social recognition (Jin et al., 2007; Lopatina et al., 2013).

Genetic tools have also shown the involvement of OT and AVP in the display of prosocial and affiliative behaviors. Increasing the V1aR density via AAV-mediated gene transfer increases social affiliation and also shortens the length of cohabitation necessary for partner preference formation in male prairie voles (Pitkow et al., 2001). Interestingly, transgenic mice, expressing V1aR in a pattern resembling prairie vole V1aR expression, show an increase in affiliative behaviors toward females (including olfactory investigation and grooming) (Young et al., 1999). Prosocial behavior is also potentiated in male rats and prairie voles in response to the overexpression of V1aR in the lateral septum and ventral pallidum, respectively, (Pitkow et al., 2001; Landgraf et al., 2003). Furthermore, a recent study in humans indicates that single nucleotide polymorphisms (SNPs) of the OTR gene, namely the variants rs13316193, rs2254298, rs1042778, rs2268494, and rs226849, are associated with impairments in empathic communication (including less support-giving interactions and affective congruence) at the beginning of a romantic relationship. These impairments suggest that OT mediates human affiliative/prosocial behavior as an essential component of pair bond formation (Schneiderman et al., 2013).

Using genetic tools, researchers have also acquired evidence that OT and AVP play a role in the formation of the pair bond. For example, the overexpression of the V1aR in the ventral pallidum results in a strong partner preference formation in male prairie voles even in the absence of mating (Pitkow et al., 2001). Similarly, AAV-mediated V1aR gene transfer into the ventral forebrain of the promiscuous meadow vole (*M. pennsylvanicus*) enhances partner preference formation, a behavior that is not typically displayed by meadow voles (Lim et al., 2004). On the contrary, the knockdown of V1aR in the ventral pallidum of male prairie voles causes a deficit in partner preference formation (Barrett et al., 2013). Lastly, a number of recent findings suggest that OT and AVP may also play a role in the regulation of social bonding in humans. In particular, researchers assessed whether genetic variations in the OT and AVP receptor genes are associated with pair bonding and social behavior. The SNP in the OTR gene (rs7632287) seems to be associated with pair bonding in women. Women carrying one or two A-alleles score lower on the partner bonding scale and the relationship quality survey as well as are more likely to report martial problems than woman carrying two G alleles (Walum et al., 2012). The variation in the V1aR gene, *AVPR1A*, also seems to contribute to differences in human pair bonding. The allelic variant, RS3 334, is associated in men, but not women, with a lower bonding quality with the partner (characterized by lower scores on the partner bonding scale and a greater likelihood of reporting martial problems) (Walum et al., 2008). Interestingly, the association between the gene variants of the OTR and *AVPR1A* and the quality of pair bonding is also detected in the partner's perception of marital satisfaction (Walum et al., 2008, 2012).

PARENTAL BONDING

Most mammalian offspring, including human children, are dependent on parental care for survival (Bowlby, 1951; Ainsworth, 1979; Nowak et al., 2000). For the young, parental care is essential to their individual survival; for the parent, parental care—characterized by one or both parents providing offspring with nutrition, warmth, shelter, as well as predatory protection—is an essential component of mammalian fitness (de Jong et al., 2009). Positive, enduring bonds between parents and their children play a significant role for the psychological, physiological, and behavioral functions of both parents and children (Silverstein and Bengtson, 1991; Graziano et al., 2009). For example, the presence of positive, secure attachments between parents and children provide protection against depression and anxiety in the child as well as lead to higher levels of child academic success (Bögels and Phares, 2008; Sarkadi et al., 2008; Graziano et al., 2009). On the contrary, the lack of positive, enduring parental bonding is associated with poor child health at an early age (e.g., increased risk for asthma, as well as cardio-respiratory and infectious diseases) as well as with the adoption of unhealthy lifestyles and medical problems (including but not limited to obesity, cancer, liver disease, chronic lung disease, and cardiovascular disease) in adulthood (Flaherty et al., 2006; Lanier et al., 2010; Leeb et al., 2011; Shonkoff et al., 2012). In addition, the lack of positive parental bonds can also lead to reduced academic success, depression, aggression, and drug misuse (DeFronzo and Pawlak, 1993; Anda et al., 1999; Nation and Heflinger, 2006; Leeb et al., 2011; Shonkoff et al., 2012). As positive social bonds between parents and their children are essential for the psychological, physiological, and behavioral well-being of both parents and child, considerable efforts have been expanded to identify the neurobiological mechanisms underlying parental bond formation. Various animal models, primarily rats and sheep, have been used to study the neural correlates of maternal behavior (Kendrick, 2000). Very little is known about paternal behavior, which is relatively rare among mammals and is displayed by less than 5% of mammalian species that are monogamous, including humans (Kleiman, 1977). More recently, untraditional animal models including the male California mouse and the male prairie vole have emerged to study the neurobiological mechanism underlying paternal behavior (Kentner et al., 2010). Parental bonding depends on the approach (including the display of prosocial behavior), social recognition of the offspring, and subsequently the formation of a selective and enduring bond between parent and offspring. This complex social behavior seems to be regulated in part by OT and AVP (Kendrick, 2000; de Jong et al., 2009; Bosch and Neumann, 2012; Nagasawa et al., 2012).

Through neuropharmacological manipulations, evidence has accumulated suggesting that OT and AVP play a role in parental bond formation across various different mammalian species, including humans. The initiation of parental behavior depends on the approach and display of prosocial behavior, a process that seems to be facilitated in part by the neuropeptides, OT, and AVP. Central OT administration reduces the latency of female rats to show maternal behavior when exposed to pups (Pedersen and Prange, 1979; Pedersen et al., 1982; Fahrbach et al., 1984) and increases maternal behavior in mice (McCarthy, 1990). The central administration of the OTR agonist, Thr4, Fly7-OT, has a similar potency to OT in stimulating maternal behavior (Kendrick, 2000). In addition, central, but not peripheral, OT administration enhances the interest of nulliparous ewes toward newborns, increases the display of maternal behavior, and induces maternal responsiveness even without the experience of natural parturition (Kendrick et al., 1987; Keverne and Kendrick, 1992; Levy et al., 1992). Administration of an OTR antagonist site-specifically into the nucleus accumbens inhibits "spontaneous" maternal behavior in sexually naïve female prairie voles, which provides further evidence that OT may play a role in maternal behavior (Olazabal and Young, 2006). Furthermore, a correlational study in humans suggests the involvement of OT in maternal behavior. In particular, an increase in plasma OT level from the first to the third trimester is linked with maternal bonding to the fetus during the third trimester (Levine et al., 2007). Additionally, high levels of OT in the first trimester predict the amount of postpartum maternal behavior (including gaze, positive affect, and "motherese" vocalizations) (Feldman et al., 2007). Similarly to OT, central AVP administration also induces maternal behavior in rats (Pedersen et al., 1982). Chronic central AVP administration or overexpression of V1aR in the medial preoptic area (using AAV) increases arched back nursing behavior in female rats (Bosch and Neumann, 2008). On the contrary, antagonizing OT (via the administration of a selective OTR antagonist, antisera to OT, or an analog OT antagonist) centrally or site-specifically (e.g., into the medial preoptic area, olfactory bulb, or ventral tegmental area) can delay or block the onset of maternal behavior in rats (Fahrbach et al., 1985; Pedersen et al., 1985, 1994; van Leengoed et al., 1987; Yu et al., 1996) as well as reduce the display of arched back nursing behavior in rats (Bosch and Neumann, 2008). Similarly, the central or site-specific (e.g., into the medial preoptic area) administration of AVP antisera, V1aR antisense oligodeoxynucleotide, or V1aR antagonist decreases maternal behavior (Pedersen et al., 1985, 1994; Bosch and Neumann, 2008). Unfortunately due to the lack of an appropriate animal model to study the neural correlates of paternal behavior, only recently have researchers started to acquire knowledge about the underlying neural mechanisms. Congruent with the OT and AVP regulation of maternal affiliative behaviors toward pups (reviewed by Bosch and Neumann, 2012), these neuropeptides may also play a role in the onset of paternal affiliative behaviors toward pups. For example, parentally naïve male California mice show higher levels of OT when housed with a pregnant female than sexually naïve males or new fathers (Gubernick et al., 1995). There is also a transient increase of OT in male prairie voles that have been exposed to pups (Kenkel et al., 2012). Central treatment with OT, but not vehicle, in male common marmosets reduces the frequency of refusal of food transfer to the infant (Saito and Nakamura, 2011). As food transfer from mother or father to infant is considered caretaking behavior, the OT-induced reduction in food transfer refusal indicates an increase in parental behavior. There is evidence to suggest that AVP may also be involved. In early prairie vole studies, new fathers, compared to sexually naïve males, showed an increase in AVP mRNA expression in the bed nucleus of the stria terminalis (Wang et al., 1994b), but showed a decreased density of AVP-immunoreactive fibers in the lateral septum (Bamshad et al., 1993). These changes in the AVP system suggest an increased AVP release in the lateral septum, which is associated with the enhanced display of paternal behavior in the father voles (Wang et al., 1998). In a pharmacological experiment, the administration of AVP into the lateral septum of sexually naïve male prairie voles enhances paternal behavior (including grooming, crouching over, and contacting pups); whereas the administration of an AVP receptor antagonist inhibits paternal behavior (Wang et al., 1994a; Bales et al., 2004). These data demonstrate the functional role of central AVP in paternal behavior. Interestingly, central AVP treatment can also induce facultative paternal behavior in the typically non-paternal meadow vole, which can be blocked by the central treatment with a selective V1aR antagonist (Parker and Lee, 2001). In addition to the evidence that AVP plays a role in mediating paternal behavior in rodents, a study using male marmosets (*C. jacchus*) showed that fathers, both first time and experienced ones, have greater dendritic spine density on pyramidal neurons in the prefrontal cortex as compared to non-father marmosets (Kozorovitskiy et al., 2006). Most interestingly, the density of AVP V1aR and the proportion of V1aR-labeled dendritic spines increased significantly in fathers compared to non-fathers (Kozorovitskiy et al., 2006). These data indicate that AVP is involved in the neural reorganization associated with the experience of fatherhood in a bi-parental primate species. There is also evidence to suggest that OT and AVP interact in the regulation of paternal care. Bales et al. (2004) noted that only the combined treatment with OT and AVP antagonists fully reduces paternal care (i.e., inhibit kyphosis, pup approach, nonkyphotic contact, licking/grooming, and retrieving) in naïve male prairie voles. Furthermore, there is evidence indicating that OT and AVP may play a role in human parental behavior. In particular, the OT concentration in the mother's cerebrospinal fluid is significantly increased following birth (Takagi et al., 1985) and plasma OT levels after birth are correlated with maternal behavior (including gaze, vocalizations, positive affect, and affectionate touch) (Feldman et al., 2007). In addition, plasma OT levels show intra-individual stability across the first 6 months of parenthood and are positively correlated with maternal and paternal behavior (including "motherese" vocalizations, positive affect, and affectionate touch) (Feldman et al., 2010, 2011; Gordon et al., 2010a,c; Apter-Levi et al., 2013). Similarly, plasma AVP levels predict maternal and paternal behavior (particularly joint attention to inanimate objects and stimulatory contact) to their infant (Apter-Levi et al., 2013). Furthermore, triadic synchrony (defined as moments in which physical proximity and affectionate touch is displayed between parents and between parent and infant) is correlated with plasma OT (Gordon et al., 2010b).

Pharmacological manipulations suggest that the nonapeptides, OT and AVP, not only play a role in the initiation of maternal behavior, but also have an important role in mediating social recognition, another vital component for parental bonding. Indeed, social recognition between mothers and their offspring has been shown in various species including sheep (Ferreira et al., 2000), goats (Poindron et al., 2003), Southern pig-tailed macaques (*Macaca nemestrina*) (Jensen, 1965), Barbary macaques (*Macaca sylvanus*) (Hammerschmidt and Fischer, 1998), rhesus macaques (*Macaca mulatta*) (Jovanovic et al., 2000), and even rodents (Ostermeyer and Elwood, 1983). Using the sheep as a model to study the neural correlates for maternal bonding, OT has been shown to play a critical role in the olfactory recognition of the lamb (Kendrick et al., 1997). Once a ewe has formed such social recognition memory, it can distinguish its lamb from others and will reject all lambs other than their own—indicating the formation of a mother-offspring bond (Kendrick, 2000). Nephew and Bridges (2008) showed that the site-specific administration (into the medial amygdala, but not the lateral ventricles) of a V1aR antagonist blocks social recognition in female rats. While only very few studies have been performed to assess parent-offspring bonding in humans, it is still plausible to hypothesize that such parent-child bonding does occur in humans. In particular, human mothers are capable of recognizing their own infant within 30 min after birth (Porter et al., 1983).

Additional support of the involvement of OT and AVP in the initiation of parental behavior, comes from genetic studies. OTR and paternally expressed gene 3 (*peg3*) knockout mice display deficits in maternal behavior including nurturing of pups, nest building, pup retrieval, and crouching behavior (Li et al., 1999; Ragnauth et al., 2005; Pedersen et al., 2006; Champagne et al., 2009). The gene *peg3* codes for a large zinc finger protein, a transcription factor that has been implicated in p53-mediated apoptosis (Deng and Wu, 2000; Relaix et al., 2000), which may account for the reduction in hypothalamic OT neurons and OTR in *peg3* knockout mice (Relaix et al., 1998; Li et al., 1999). Further, Brattleboro rats, which are genetically incapable of producing AVP, also show deficits in maternal care evidenced by a lower survival rate of offspring (Wideman and Murphy, 1990). Female and male CD38 knockout mice, which exhibit low central OT levels in comparison to wild-type mice, as mentioned above, also display deficits in parental behavior (i.e., lower rate of pup retrieval and crouching over pups) (Jin et al., 2007; Akther et al., 2013). The re-expression of CD38 (using AAV) in the nucleus accumbens and OT administration in CD38 knockout mice can restore paternal behavior (including retrieval, pup grooming, crouching, and huddling) (Akther et al., 2013). In addition, the SNP of the prairie vole V1aR gene (*avpr1a*) is associated with parental behavior. Specifically, male prairie voles with the allele coding for a long *avpr1a* microsatellite display higher levels of licking/grooming behavior than male prairie voles with the short *avpr1a* microsatellite (Hammock and Young, 2005). Microsatellites, or short tandem repeats, consisting of one to six nucleotides, which are repeated several times and therefore contribute to genetic variation (Guichoux et al., 2011).

In humans, SNPs in the genes for the OTR and CD38 have been implicated in parental behavior. In particular, the OTR gene alleles rs2254298 and rs1042778 as well as the CD38 gene allele rs3796863 are associated with lower plasma OT levels, and in turn, lower rates of parental care (i.e., shorter duration of parent-infant gaze synchrony and less amount of touch toward the infant) (Feldman et al., 2012). Future studies are needed to address whether genetic manipulations can show the involvement of OT and AVP in the paternal recognition of offspring and the parental-offspring bond formation *per se*.

INTERPERSONAL BONDING

Similarly to the importance of attachment between partners of a mating pair and between parents and their offspring, mutually cooperative interactions involving the display of trust are an essential aspect of human society (Luhmann, 1979; Coleman, 1990). Trust is essential in love, families, and friendships. While a lot of effort has been expanded to investigate the neural correlates of social behavior, the neural mechanisms underlying trust are just beginning to be examined. Interestingly, it appears that the neuropeptide OT is not only involved in facilitating various social behaviors, such as pair bonding (Dluzen and Carter, 1979; Insel and Shapiro, 1992; Insel, 1997; Carter, 1998) and maternal attachment (Insel and Young, 2001; Bosch and Neumann, 2012), but has also been implicated in playing a role in trust (reviewed by De Dreu et al., 2010).

Research on the role of OT in regulating the display of trust revealed that OT levels increase in response to the display of intentional trust in a trust game with real monetary stakes. In particular, the level of peripheral OT (as assessed using blood) increases in subjects who received an intentional trust signal (Zak et al., 2004, 2005). However, it should be noted that currently the relationship between peripheral OT and central OT in humans is still unknown. Nevertheless, the findings of increased peripheral OT in response to intentional trust should be considered

Table 1 | Effects of pharmacological manipulations of OT and AVP on bonding behavior.

Type of bond	Treatment	Species	Effect	References
PAIR BOND				
Social recognition	Peripheral OT	Rat	↑	Popik et al., 1992a
	Central OT	OT KO mouse	↑	Ferguson et al., 2000
	Site-specific OT (e.g., AMY, LS, MPOA, OB)	OT KO mouse, rat	↑	Popik and van Ree, 1991; Popik et al., 1992b; Dluzen et al., 1998a,b, 2000; Ferguson et al., 2001; Winslow and Insel, 2002
	Intranasal OT	Human	↑	Savaskan et al., 2008; Rimmele et al., 2009
	Central OTR-A	Rat, mouse	↓	Engelmann et al., 1998; Ferguson et al., 2000
	Site-specific OTR-A (e.g., MPOA, OB)	Rat	↓	Popik and van Ree, 1991; Dluzen et al., 2000
	Peripheral AVP	Rat	↑	Dantzer et al., 1987
	Central AVP	Rat	↑	Le Moal et al., 1987
	Site-specific AVP (e.g., LS, OB)	Brattleboro rat, rat, V1aR KO mouse	↑	Dantzer et al., 1988; Popik et al., 1992b; Engelmann and Landgraf, 1994; Dluzen et al., 1998a,b; Landgraf et al., 2003; Bielsky et al., 2005
	Central AVP-A	Rat	↓	Bluthe et al., 1990; van Wimersma Greidanus and Maigret, 1996
	Site-specific AVP antisense, AVP-A, or V1aR-A (e.g., hippocampus, LS, OB)	Mouse, rat	↓	Dantzer et al., 1988; Popik et al., 1992b; Engelmann and Landgraf, 1994; Landgraf et al., 1995; van Wimersma Greidanus and Maigret, 1996; Everts and Koolhaas, 1997, 1999; Bielsky et al., 2005; Tobin et al., 2010
Prosocial behavior	Peripheral OT	Rat, prairie vole	↑	Witt et al., 1990
	Central OT	Prairie vole, rat, marmoset, squirrel monkey	↑	Witt et al., 1990, 1992; Winslow and Insel, 1991; Smith et al., 2010
	Intranasal OT	Human	↑	Liu et al., 2012
	Central OTR-A	Marmoset	↓	Smith et al., 2010
	Intranasal AVP	Titi monkey	↑	Jarcho et al., 2011
Bond	Central OT	Prairie vole	↑	Williams et al., 1992a; Insel and Hulihan, 1995; Cho et al., 1999
	Site-specifc OT (e.g., NAcc)	Prairie vole	↑	Liu and Wang, 2003
	Central OTR-A	Prairie vole	↓	Insel and Hulihan, 1995; Cho et al., 1999
	Central AVP	Prairie vole	↑	Winslow et al., 1993
	Central AVPR-A or V1aR-A	Prairie vole	↓	Winslow et al., 1993; Insel and Winslow, 1998; Cho et al., 1999
	Site-specific V1aR-A (e.g., VP)	Prairie vole	↓	Lim and Young, 2004
PARENTAL BOND				
Social recognition	OT or OTR-A	na	na	na
	AVP or AVPR-A	na	na	na
Prosocial behavior	Central OT	♂ common marmoset, ♀ mice, ♀ rat, ♀ sheep	↑	Pedersen and Prange, 1979; Pedersen et al., 1982; Fahrbach et al., 1984; Kendrick et al., 1987; McCarthy, 1990; Keverne and Kendrick, 1992; Levy et al., 1992; Saito and Nakamura, 2011
	Site-specific OT (e.g., NAcc)	♀♂ CD38KO mouse	↑	Akther et al., 2013
	Central OTR-A	♀ rats	↓	Fahrbach et al., 1985; Pedersen et al., 1985; van Leengoed et al., 1987
	Site-specific OTR-A (e.g., MPOA, NAcc, OB, and VTA)	♀ prairie voles, ♀ rats	↓	Pedersen et al., 1994; Yu et al., 1996; Olazabal and Young, 2006
	Central AVP	♂ meadow voles, ♀ rats	↑	Pedersen et al., 1982; Parker and Lee, 2001
	Site-specific AVP (e.g., LS)	♂ prairie vole	↑	Wang et al., 1994a
	Central AVPR-A	♂ meadow voles, ♀ rats	↓	Pedersen et al., 1985; Parker and Lee, 2001; Bosch and Neumann, 2008

(Continued)

Table 1 | Continued

Type of bond	Treatment	Species	Effect	References
	Site-specific AVPR-A or V1aR-A (e.g., MPOA and LS)	Rats, ♂ prairie vole	↓	Pedersen et al., 1994; Wang et al., 1994a
	Central AVP-A and OTR-A	♂ prairie vole	↓	Bales et al., 2004
Bond	OT or OTR-A	na	na	na
	AVP or AVPR-A	na	na	na
TRUST	Intranasal OT	Human	↑	Kosfeld et al., 2005; De Dreu et al., 2010; Mikolajczak et al., 2010a,b

Abbreviations used: AMY, amygdala; AVP, argenine vasopressin; AVP-A, non-selective AVP receptor antagonist; LS, lateral septum; MPOA, medial preoptic area; NAcc, nucleus accumbens; OB, olfacotry bulbs; OT, oxytocin, OTR-A, oxytocin receptor antagonist; VP, ventral pallidum; VTA, ventral tegmental area.

in the light of the hyperfunctional magnetic resonance imaging (hyperfMRI) study by Krueger et al. (2007). The authors report significant activity in the septal area when subjects display trust intentionally. Based on evidence from rodent studies, the septal area is involved in the regulation of social behavior (including pair bonding and paternal behavior) (Young et al., 2005; Skuse and Gallagher, 2009). In addition, the lateral septum via its connections to the nucleus accumbens may also represent a potential link between social behavior and reward circuitries (Young et al., 2005; Skuse and Gallagher, 2009). Furthermore, intranasal administration of OT increases interpersonal trust (see review by Van Ijzendoorn and Bakermans-Kranenburg, 2012), without affecting non-social risk-taking behaviors (Kosfeld et al., 2005). Specifically, 13 out of 29 subjects who received nasal spray containing OT showed the maximal trust level (i.e., sending all the money to another person in the "*trust game*" with real monetary stakes), whereas only 6 out of 29 subjects who received placebo showed maximal trust (Kosfeld et al., 2005). It should be noted that OT-induced trust only increases in the absence of cues that the partner is untrustworthy (Mikolajczak et al., 2010a). Exogenous administration of OT also increases the trust displayed toward one's own group (in-group trust). Using the intergroup prisoner's dilemma-maximizing difference game, it has been shown that intranasal OT increases in-group trust as displayed by an increase in the (monetary) contributions to the in-group, without affecting out-group distrust (De Dreu et al., 2010). In addition to the trust-increasing effects of OT in a monetary scenario, exogenous OT also increases trust in non-monetary scenarios. It has been observed that intranasal OT decreases the perceived risk of betrayal and increased trust in a scenario involving intimate and confidential information (Mikolajczak et al., 2010b). In particular, 60% of the participants who received OT, compared to only 3% of participants who received placebo, left a letter containing intimate and confidential information unsealed (Mikolajczak et al., 2010b). In addition, intranasal OT increases a person's willingness to share emotions, without affecting level of talkativeness (Lane et al., 2013).

Additional evidence for the involvement of OT in the regulation of trust comes from genetic studies (reviewed by Donaldson and Young, 2008). It should be noted that trust behavior appears to be heritable, indicating that a specific gene may be responsible for the variations in trust observed across individuals (Cesarini et al., 2008). In particular, using genetic screening for the OTR gene and the "*trust game*" showed that the rs53576, rs1042778, rs2268490, and rs237887 SNPs of the OTR gene is associated with greater trusting behavior (Israel et al., 2009; Krueger et al., 2012). Similarly to OT, AVP seems to play a role in mediating trust as well. In particular, the *AVPR1A* promoter region length (rs3 microsatellite polymorphism) is associated with greater money allocation, suggesting greater trusting behavior, in the "*trust game*" (Knafo et al., 2008).

CONCLUSION

Over the past decades, the understanding of the neurobiological mechanism underlying bonding behaviors has substantially increased. In particular, studies using various animal models have provided evidence of the involvement of the nonapeptides, OT and AVP, in the regulation of social bonding (including bonding between mates in a mating pair and bonding between parent and offspring) (see **Table 1**). In addition, experimental techniques (such as intranasal OT administration and gene sequencing) in humans have resulted in evidence suggesting that these nonapeptides may also play a role in the regulation of bonding in humans. However, it should be noted that other neurochemicals, such as prolactin, sex hormones, catecholamines, endogenous opiates, and GABA may also play a role in the regulation of social behaviors. Thus, future research is needed to determine the interplay of these various neurochemicals to regulate social bonding across various species. It is also of importance to mention that there are instances of sexual dimorphisms in the regulation of social bonding by OT and AVP (e.g., OT and AVP differently regulate social bonds in female and male prairie voles). Therefore, sex differences in the regulation of social bonding warrant further investigation.

ACKNOWLEDGMENTS

We are grateful to Hans Jorgensen for his critical reading of the manuscript. This manuscript was supported by NIH grant MHR01-058616.

REFERENCES

Adams, K. B., Sanders, S., and Auth, E. A. (2004). Loneliness and depression in independent living retirement communities: risk and resilience factors. *Aging Ment. Health* 8, 475–485. doi: 10.1080/13607860410001725054

Ainsworth, M. S. (1979). Infant–mother attachment. *Am. Psychol.* 34, 932–937. doi: 10.1037/0003-066X.34.10.932

Akther, S., Korshnova, N., Zhong, J., Liang, M., Cherepanov, S. M., Lopatina, O., et al. (2013). CD38 in the nucleus accumbens and oxytocin are related to paternal behavior in mice. *Mol. Brain* 6, 1–10. doi: 10.1186/1756-6606-6-41

Alpass, F. M., and Neville, S. (2003). Loneliness, health and depression in older males. *Aging Ment. Health* 7, 212–216. doi: 10.1080/1360786031000101193

Anda, R. F., Croft, J. B., Felitti, V. J., Nordenberg, D., Giles, W. H., Williamson, D. F., et al. (1999). Adverse childhood experiences and smoking during adolescence and adulthood. *JAMA* 282, 1652–1658. doi: 10.1001/jama.282.17.1652

Apter-Levi, Y., Zagoory-Sharon, O., and Feldman, R. (2013). Oxytocin and vasopressin support distinct configurations of social synchrony. *Brain Res.* doi: 10.1016/j.brainres.2013.1010.1052. [Epub ahead of print].

Bales, K. L., Kim, A. J., Lewis-Reese, A. D., and Sue Carter, C. (2004). Both oxytocin and vasopressin may influence alloparental behavior in male prairie voles. *Horm. Behav.* 45, 354–361. doi: 10.1016/j.yhbeh.2004.01.004

Bales, K. L., Mason, W. A., Catana, C., Cherry, S. R., and Mendoza, S. P. (2007). Neural correlates of pair-bonding in a monogamous primate. *Brain Res.* 1184, 245–253. doi: 10.1016/j.brainres.2007.09.087

Bamshad, M., Novak, M. A., and De Vries, G. J. (1993). Sex and species differences in the vasopressin innervation of sexually naive and parental prairie voles, *Microtus ochrogaster* and meadow voles, *Microtus pennsylvanicus*. *J. Neuroendocrinol.* 5, 247–255. doi: 10.1111/j.1365-2826.1993.tb00480.x

Barrett, C. E., Keebaugh, A. C., Ahern, T. H., Bass, C. E., Terwilliger, E. F., and Young, L. J. (2013). Variation in vasopressin receptor (*Avpr1a*) expression creates diversity in behaviors related to monogamy in prairie voles. *Horm. Behav.* 63, 518–526. doi: 10.1016/j.yhbeh.2013.01.005

Bartz, J. A., and Hollander, E. (2006). The neuroscience of affiliation: forging links between basic and clinical research on neuropeptides and social behavior. *Horm. Behav.* 50, 518–528. doi: 10.1016/j.yhbeh.2006.06.018

Baumeister, R. F., and Leary, M. R. (1995). The need to belong: desire for interpersonal attachments as a fundamental human motivation. *Psychol. Bull.* 117, 497–529. doi: 10.1037/0033-2909.117.3.497

Bester-Meredith, J. K., Young, L. J., and Marler, C. A. (1999). Species differences in paternal behavior and aggression in peromyscus and their associations with vasopressin immunoreactivity and receptors. *Horm. Behav.* 36, 25–38. doi: 10.1006/hbeh.1999.1522

Bielsky, I. F., Hu, S.-B., Ren, X., Terwilliger, E. F., and Young, L. J. (2005). The V1a vasopressin receptor is necessary and sufficient for normal social recognition: a gene replacement study. *Neuron* 47, 503–513. doi: 10.1016/j.neuron.2005.06.031

Bielsky, I. F., Hu, S. B., Szegda, K. L., Westphal, H., and Young, L. J. (2004). Profound impairment in social recognition and reduction in anxiety-like behavior in vasopressin V1a receptor knockout mice. *Neuropsychopharmacology* 29, 483–493. doi: 10.1038/sj.npp.1300360

Bielsky, I. F., and Young, L. J. (2004). Oxytocin, vasopressin, and social recognition in mammals. *Peptides* 25, 1565–1574. doi: 10.1016/j.peptides.2004.05.019

Bluthe, R.-M., Schoenen, J., and Dantzer, R. (1990). Androgen-dependent vasopressinergic neurons are involved in social recognition in rats. *Brain Res.* 519, 150–157. doi: 10.1016/0006-8993(90)90073-K

Bögels, S., and Phares, V. (2008). Fathers' role in the etiology, prevention and treatment of child anxiety: a review and new model. *Clin. Psychol. Rev.* 28, 539–558. doi: 10.1016/j.cpr.2007.07.011

Bosch, O. J., and Neumann, I. D. (2008). Brain vasopressin is an important regulator of maternal behavior independent of dams' trait anxiety. *Proc. Natl. Acad. Sci. U.S.A.* 105, 17139–17144. doi: 10.1073/pnas.0807412105

Bosch, O. J., and Neumann, I. D. (2012). Both oxytocin and vasopressin are mediators of maternal care and aggression in rodents: from central release to sites of action. *Horm. Behav.* 61, 293–303. doi: 10.1016/j.yhbeh.2011.11.002

Bowlby, J. (1951). *Maternal Care and Mental Health*. Geneva: World Health Organization.

Buss, D. M. (1988). From vigilance to violence: tactics of mate retention in American undergraduates. *Ethol. Sociobiol.* 9, 291–317. doi: 10.1016/0162-3095(88)90010-6

Carter, C. S. (1998). Neuroendocrine perspectives on social attachment and love. *Psychoneuroendocrinology* 23, 779–818. doi: 10.1016/S0306-4530(98)00055-9

Carter, C. S., DeVries, A. C., and Getz, L. L. (1995). Physiological substrates of mammalian monogamy: the prairie vole model. *Neurosci. Biobehav. Rev.* 19, 303–314. doi: 10.1016/0149-7634(94)00070-H

Cesarini, D., Dawes, C. T., Fowler, J. H., Johannesson, M., Lichtenstein, P., and Wallace, B. (2008). Heritability of cooperative behavior in the trust game. *Proc. Natl. Acad. Sci. U.S.A.* 105, 3721–3726. doi: 10.1073/pnas.0710069105

Champagne, F. A., Curley, J. P., Swaney, W. T., Hasen, N. S., and Keverne, E. B. (2009). Paternal influence on female behavior: the role of *Peg3* in exploration, olfaction, and neuroendocrine regulation of maternal behavior of female mice. *Behav. Neurosci.* 123, 469–480. doi: 10.1037/a0015060

Cho, M. M., DeVries, A. C., Williams, J. R., and Carter, C. S. (1999). The effects of oxytocin and vasopressin on partner preferences in male and female prairie voles (*Microtus ochrogaster*). *Behav. Neurosci.* 113, 1071–1079. doi: 10.1037/0735-7044.113.5.1071

Choleris, E., Ogawa, S., Kavaliers, M., Gustafsson, J. Å., Korach, K. S., Muglia, L. J., et al. (2006). Involvement of estrogen receptor α, β and oxytocin in social discrimination: a detailed behavioral analysis with knockout female mice. *Genes Brain Behav.* 5, 528–539. doi: 10.1111/j.1601-183X.2006.00203.x

Coleman, J. (1990). *Foundations of Social Theory*. Cambridge, MA: Belknap.

Crawley, J. N., Chen, T., Puri, A., Washburn, R., Sullivan, T. L., Hill, J. M., et al. (2007). Social approach behaviors in oxytocin knockout mice: comparison of two independent lines tested in different laboratory environments. *Neuropeptides* 41, 145–163. doi: 10.1016/j.npep.2007.02.002

Curley, J. P., and Keverne, E. B. (2005). Genes, brains and mammalian social bonds. *Trends Ecol. Evol.* 20, 561–567. doi: 10.1016/j.tree.2005.05.018

Curtis, R. (1995). Stress, personality and illness: the move from generality to specificity in current research trends. *Irish J. Psychol.* 16, 299–321. doi: 10.1080/03033910.1995.10558067

Dantzer, R., Bluthe, R. M., Koob, G. F., and Le Moal, M. (1987). Modulation of social memory in male rats by neurohypophyseal peptides. *Psychopharmacology(Berl)* 91, 363–368. doi: 10.1007/BF00518192

Dantzer, R., Koob, G. F., Bluthe', R.-M., and Le Moal, M. (1988). Septal vasopressin modulates social memory in male rats. *Brain Res.* 457, 143–147. doi: 10.1016/0006-8993(88)90066-2

Debiec, J. (2007). From affiliative behaviors to romantic feelings: a role of nanopeptides. *FEBS Lett.* 581, 2580–2586. doi: 10.1016/j.febslet.2007.03.095

De Dreu, C. K., Greer, L. L., Handgraaf, M. J., Shalvi, S., Van Kleef, G. A., Baas, M., et al. (2010). The neuropeptide oxytocin regulates parochial altruism in intergroup conflict among humans. *Science* 328, 1408–1411. doi: 10.1126/science.1189047

DeFronzo, J., and Pawlak, R. (1993). Effects of social bonds and childhood experiences on alcohol abuse and smoking. *J. Soc. Psychol.* 133, 635–642. doi: 10.1080/00224545.1993.9713918

de Jong, T. R., Chauke, M., Harris, B. N., and Saltzman, W. (2009). From here to paternity: neural correlates of the onset of paternal behavior in California mice (*Peromyscus californicus*). *Horm. Behav.* 56, 220–231. doi: 10.1016/j.yhbeh.2009.05.001

Deng, Y., and Wu, X. (2000). Peg3/Pw1 promotes p53-mediated apoptosis by inducing Bax translocation from cytosol to mitochondria. *Proc. Natl. Acad. Sci. U.S.A.* 97, 12050–12055. doi: 10.1073/pnas.97.22.12050

Dewsbury, D. A. (1975). Diversity and adaptation in rodent copulatory behavior. *Science* 190, 947–954. doi: 10.1126/science.1188377

Dewsbury, D. A. (1988). *The Comparative Psychology of Monogamy*. Lincoln: University of Nebraska Press.

Ditzen, B., Schaer, M., Gabriel, B., Bodenmann, G., Ehlert, U., and Heinrichs, M. (2009). Intranasal oxytocin increases positive communication and reduces cortisol levels during couple conflict. *Biol. Psychiatry* 65, 728–731. doi: 10.1016/j.biopsych.2008.10.011

Dluzen, D. E., and Carter, C. S. (1979). Ovarian hormones regulating sexual and social behaviors in female prairie voles, *Microtus ochrogaster*. *Physiol. Behav.* 23, 597–600. doi: 10.1016/0031-9384(79)90063-5

Dluzen, D. E., Muraoka, S., Engelmann, M., Ebner, K., and Landgraf, R. (2000). Oxytocin induces preservation of social recognition in male rats by activating alpha-adrenoceptors of the olfactory bulb. *Eur. J. Neurosci.* 12, 760–766. doi: 10.1046/j.1460-9568.2000.00952.x

Dluzen, D. E., Muraoka, S., Engelmann, M., and Landgraf, R. (1998a). The effects of infusion of arginine vasopressin, oxytocin, or their antagonists into the olfactory bulb upon social recognition responses in male rats. *Peptides* 19, 999–1005. doi: 10.1016/S0196-9781(98)00047-3

Dluzen, D. E., Muraoka, S., and Landgraf, R. (1998b). Olfactory bulb norepinephrine depletion abolishes vasopressin and oxytocin preservation of social recognition responses in rats. *Neurosci. Lett.* 254, 161–164. doi: 10.1016/S0304-3940(98)00691-0

Dluzen, D. E., Shang, Y., and Landgraf, R. (2001). "Oxytocin, norepinephrine and olfacotry bulb mediated recogntion," in *Chemical Signals in Vertebrates Nine*, eds A. Marchlewska-Koj, J. J. Lepri, and D. Müller-Schwarze (New York, NY: Springer US), 107–115. doi: 10.1007/978-1-4615-0671-3_14

Donaldson, Z. R., and Young, L. J. (2008). Oxytocin, vasopressin, and the neurogenetics of sociality. *Science* 322, 900–904. doi: 10.1126/science.1158668

Drefahl, S. (2012). Do the married really live longer? The role of cohabitation and socioeconomic status. *J. Marriage Fam.* 74, 462–475. doi: 10.1111/j.1741-3737.2012.00968.x

Engelmann, M., Ebner, K., Wotjak, C. T., and Landgraf, R. (1998). Endogenous oxytocin is involved in short-term olfactory memory in female rats. *Behav. Brain Res.* 90, 89–94. doi: 10.1016/S0166-4328(97)00084-3

Engelmann, M., and Landgraf, R. (1994). Microdialysis administration of vasopressin into the septum improves social recognition in Brattleboro rats. *Physiol. Behav.* 55, 145–149. doi: 10.1016/0031-9384(94)90022-1

Engelmann, M., Wotjak, C. T., Neumann, I., Ludwig, M., and Landgraf, R. (1996). Behavioral consequences of intracerebral vasopressin and oxytocin: focus on learning and memory. *Neurosci. Biobehav. Rev.* 20, 341–358. doi: 10.1016/0149-7634(95)00059-3

Everts, H. G., and Koolhaas, J. M. (1997). Lateral septal vasopressin in rats: role in social and object recognition? *Brain Res.* 760, 1–7. doi: 10.1016/S0006-8993(97)00269-2

Everts, H. G., and Koolhaas, J. M. (1999). Differential modulation of lateral septal vasopressin receptor blockade in spatial learning, social recognition, and anxiety-related behaviors in rats. *Behav. Brain Res.* 99, 7–16. doi: 10.1016/S0166-4328(98)00004-7

Fahrbach, S. E., Morrell, J. I., and Pfaff, D. W. (1984). Oxytocin induction of short-latency maternal behavior in nulliparous, estrogen-primed female rats. *Horm. Behav.* 18, 267–286. doi: 10.1016/0018-506X(84)90016-3

Fahrbach, S. E., Morrell, J. I., and Pfaff, D. W. (1985). Possible role for endogenous oxytocin in estrogen-facilitated maternal behavior in rats. *Neuroendocrinology* 40, 526–532. doi: 10.1159/000124125

Feldman, R., Gordon, I., Schneiderman, I., Weisman, O., and Zagoory-Sharon, O. (2010). Natural variations in maternal and paternal care are associated with systematic changes in oxytocin following parent–infant contact. *Psychoneuroendocrinology* 35, 1133–1141. doi: 10.1016/j.psyneuen.2010.01.013

Feldman, R., Gordon, I., and Zagoory–Sharon, O. (2011). Maternal and paternal plasma, salivary, and urinary oxytocin and parent–infant synchrony: considering stress and affiliation components of human bonding. *Dev. Sci.* 14, 752–761. doi: 10.1111/j.1467-7687.2010.01021.x

Feldman, R., Weller, A., Zagoory-Sharon, O., and Levine, A. (2007). Evidence for a neuroendocrinological foundation of human affiliation: plasma oxytocin levels across pregnancy and the postpartum period predict mother-infant bonding. *Psychol. Sci.* 18, 965. doi: 10.1111/j.1467-9280.2007.02010.x

Feldman, R., Zagoory-Sharon, O., Weisman, O., Schneiderman, I., Gordon, I., Maoz, R., et al. (2012). Sensitive parenting is associated with plasma oxytocin and polymorphisms in the *OXTR* and *CD38* genes. *Biol. Psychiatry* 72, 175–181. doi: 10.1016/j.biopsych.2011.12.025

Ferguson, J. N., Aldag, J. M., Insel, T. R., and Young, L. J. (2001). Oxytocin in the medial amygdala is essential for social recognition in the mouse. *J. Neurosci.* 21, 8278–8285.

Ferguson, J. N., Young, L. J., Hearn, E. F., Matzuk, M. M., Insel, T. R., and Winslow, J. T. (2000). Social amnesia in mice lacking the oxytocin gene. *Nat. Genet.* 25, 284–288. doi: 10.1038/77040

Ferreira, G., Terrazas, A., Poindron, P., Nowak, R., Orgeur, P., and Lévy, F. (2000). Learning of olfactory cues is not necessary for early lamb recognition by the mother. *Physiol. Behav.* 69, 405–412. doi: 10.1016/S0031-9384(00)00211-0

Flaherty, E. G., Thompson, R., Litrownik, A. J., Theodore, A., English, D. J., Black, M. M., et al. (2006). Effect of early childhood adversity on child health. *Arch. Pediatr. Adolesc. Med.* 160, 1232–1238. doi: 10.1001/archpedi.160.12.1232

Fraley, R. C., Brumbaugh, C. C., and Marks, M. J. (2005). The evolution and function of adult attachment: a comparative and phylogenetic analysis. *J. Pers. Soc. Psychol.* 89, 731–746. doi: 10.1037/0022-3514.89.5.751

Getz, L. L., Carter, C. S., and Gavish, L. (1981). The mating system of the prairie vole *Microtus ochrogaster*: field and laboratory evidence for pair-bonding. *Behav. Ecol. Sociobiol.* 8, 189–194. doi: 10.1007/BF00299829

Gordon, I., Zagoory-Sharon, O., Leckman, J. F., and Feldman, R. (2010a). Oxytocin and the development of parenting in humans. *Biol. Psychiatry* 68, 377–382. doi: 10.1016/j.biopsych.2010.02.005

Gordon, I., Zagoory-Sharon, O., Leckman, J. F., and Feldman, R. (2010b). Oxytocin, cortisol, and triadic family interactions. *Physiol. Behav.* 101, 679–684. doi: 10.1016/j.physbeh.2010.08.008

Gordon, I., Zagoory-Sharon, O., Leckman, J. F., and Feldman, R. (2010c). Prolactin, oxytocin, and the development of paternal behavior across the first six months of fatherhood. *Horm. Behav.* 58, 513–518. doi: 10.1016/j.yhbeh.2010.04.007

Gouin, J.-P., Carter, C. S., Pournajafi-Nazarloo, H., Malarkey, W. B., Loving, T. J., Stowell, J., et al. (2012). Plasma vasopressin and interpersonal functioning. *Biol. Psychol.* 91, 270–274. doi: 10.1016/j.biopsycho.2012.07.003

Graziano, F., Bonino, S., and Cattelino, E. (2009). Links between maternal and paternal support, depressive feelings and social and academic self-efficacy in adolescence. *Eur. J. Dev. Psychol.* 6, 241–257. doi: 10.1080/17405620701252066

Gubernick, D. J. (1994). *Biparental Care and Male-Female Relations in Mammals.* Chur: Harwood Academic Publishers.

Gubernick, D. J., Winslow, J. T., Jensen, P., Jeanotte, L., and Bowen, J. (1995). Oxytocin changes in males over the reproductive cycle in the monogamous, biparental California mouse, *Peromyscus californicus*. *Horm. Behav.* 29, 59–73. doi: 10.1006/hbeh.1995.1005

Guichoux, E., Lagache, L., Wagner, S., Chaumeil, P., Leger, P., Lepais, O., et al. (2011). Current trends in microsatellite genotyping. *Mol. Ecol. Res.* 11, 591–611. doi: 10.1111/j.1755-0998.2011.03014.x

Hammerschmidt, K., and Fischer, J. (1998). Maternal discrimination of offspring vocalizations in Barbary macaques (*Macaca sylvanus*). *Primates* 39, 231–236. doi: 10.1007/BF02557735

Hammock, E. A. D., and Young, L. J. (2005). Microsatellite instability generates diversity in brain and sociobehavioral traits. *Science* 308, 1630–1634. doi: 10.1126/science.1111427

Heinrichs, M., von Dawans, B., and Domes, G. (2009). Oxytocin, vasopressin, and human social behavior. *Front. Neuroendocrinol.* 30, 548–557. doi: 10.1016/j.yfrne.2009.05.005

Hinde, R. A., and Berman, C. M. (1983). *Primate Social Relationships: An Integrated Approach.* Oxford: Blackwell Scientific.

House, J. S., Landis, K. R., and Umberson, D. (1988). Social relationships and health. *Science* 241, 540–545. doi: 10.1126/science.3399889

Insel, T. R. (1992). Oxytocin–a neuropeptide for affiliation: evidence from behavioral, receptor autoradiographic, and comparative studies. *Psychoneuroendocrinology* 17, 3–35. doi: 10.1016/0306-4530(92)90073-G

Insel, T. R. (1997). A neurobiological basis of social attachment. *Am. J. Psychiatry* 154, 726–735.

Insel, T. R., and Hulihan, T. J. (1995). A gender-specific mechanism for pair bonding: oxytocin and partner preference formation in monogamous voles. *Behav. Neurosci.* 109, 782–789. doi: 10.1037/0735-7044.109.4.782

Insel, T. R., and Shapiro, L. E. (1992). Oxytocin receptor distribution reflects social organization in monogamous and polygamous voles. *Proc. Natl. Acad. Sci. U.S.A.* 89, 5981–5985. doi: 10.1073/pnas.89.13.5981

Insel, T. R., and Winslow, J. T. (1998). Serotonin and neuropeptides in affiliative behaviors. *Biol. Psychiatry* 44, 207–219. doi: 10.1016/S0006-3223(98)00094-8

Insel, T. R., and Young, L. J. (2001). The neurobiology of attachment. *Nat. Rev. Neurosci.* 2, 129–136. doi: 10.1038/35053579

Israel, S., Lerer, E., Shalev, I., Uzefovsky, F., Riebold, M., Laiba, E., et al. (2009). The oxytocin receptor (OXTR) contributes to prosocial fund allocations in the dictator game and the social value orientations task. *PLoS ONE* 4:e5535. doi: 10.1371/journal.pone.0005535

Jarcho, M. R., Mendoza, S. P., Mason, W. A., Yang, X., and Bales, K. L. (2011). Intranasal vasopressin affects pair bonding and peripheral gene expression in male Callicebus cupreus. *Gene Brain Behav.* 10, 375–383. doi: 10.1111/j.1601-183X.2010.00677.x

Jaremka, L. M., Fagundes, C. P., Peng, J., Bennett, J. M., Glaser, R., Malarkey, W. B., et al. (2013). Loneliness promotes inflammation during acute stress. *Psychol. Sci.* 24, 1089–1097. doi: 10.1177/0956797612464059

Jensen, G. D. (1965). Mother-infant relationship in the monkey *Macaca nemestrina*: development of specificity of maternal response to own infant. *J. Comp. Physiol. Psychol.* 59, 305–308. doi: 10.1037/h0021832

Jin, D., Liu, H.-X., Hirai, H., Torashima, T., Nagai, T., Lopatina, O., et al. (2007). CD38 is critical for social behaviour by regulating oxytocin secretion. *Nature* 446, 41–45. doi: 10.1038/nature05526

Jovanovic, T., Megna, N. L., and Maestripieri, D. (2000). Early maternal recognition of offspring vocalizations in rhesus macaques (*Macaca mulatta*). *Primates* 41, 421–428. doi: 10.1007/BF02557653

Kendrick, K. M. (2000). Oxytocin, motherhood and bonding. *Exp. Physiol.* 85, 111S–124S. doi: 10.1111/j.1469-445X.2000.tb00014.x

Kendrick, K. M., Da Costa, A. P. C., Broad, K. D., Ohkura, S., Guevara, R., Lévy, F., et al. (1997). Neural control of maternal behaviour and olfactory recognition of offspring. *Brain Res. Bull.* 44, 383–395. doi: 10.1016/S0361-9230(97)00218-9

Kendrick, K. M., Keverne, E. B., and Baldwin, B. A. (1987). Intracerebroventricular oxytocin stimulates maternal behaviour in the sheep. *Neuroendocrinology* 46, 56–61. doi: 10.1159/000124796

Kenkel, W. M., Paredes, J., Yee, J. R., Pournajafi-Nazarloo, H., Bales, K. L., and Carter, C. S. (2012). Neuroendocrine and behavioural responses to exposure to an infant in male prairie voles. *J. Neuroendocrinol.* 24, 874–886. doi: 10.1111/j.1365-2826.2012.02301.x

Kentner, A. C., Abizaid, A., and Bielajew, C. (2010). Modeling dad: animal models of paternal behavior. *Neurosci. Biobehav. Rev.* 34, 438–451. doi: 10.1016/j.neubiorev.2009.08.010

Keverne, E. B., and Kendrick, K. M. (1992). Oxytocin facilitation of maternal behavior in sheep. *Ann. N.Y. Acad. Sci.* 652, 83–101. doi: 10.1111/j.1749-6632.1992.tb34348.x

Kiecolt-Glaser, J. K., Gouin, J. P., and Hantsoo, L. (2010). Close relationships, inflammation, and health. *Neurosci. Biobehav. Rev.* 35, 33–38. doi: 10.1016/j.neubiorev.2009.09.003

Kiecolt-Glaser, J. K., and Newton, T. L. (2001). Marriage and health: his and hers. *Psychol. Bull.* 127, 472–503. doi: 10.1037/0033-2909.127.4.472

Kleiman, D. G. (1977). Monogamy in mammals. *Q. Rev. Biol.* 52, 39–69. doi: 10.1086/409721

Knafo, A., Israel, S., Darvasi, A., Bachner–Melman, R., Uzefovsky, F., Cohen, L., et al. (2008). Individual differences in allocation of funds in the dictator game associated with length of the arginine vasopressin 1a receptor RS3 promoter region and correlation between RS3 length and hippocampal mRNA. *Genes Brain Behav.* 7, 266–275. doi: 10.1111/j.1601-183X.2007.00341.x

Kosfeld, M., Heinrichs, M., Zak, P. J., Fischbacher, U., and Fehr, E. (2005). Oxytocin increases trust in humans. *Nature* 435, 673–676. doi: 10.1038/nature03701

Kozorovitskiy, Y., Hughes, M., Lee, K., and Gould, E. (2006). Fatherhood affects dendritic spines and vasopressin V1a receptors in the primate prefrontal cortex. *Nat. Neurosci.* 9, 1094–1095. doi: 10.1038/nn1753

Krueger, F., McCabe, K., Moll, J., Kriegeskorte, N., Zahn, R., Strenziok, M., et al. (2007). Neural correlates of trust. *Proc. Natl. Acad. Sci. U.S.A.* 104, 20084–20089. doi: 10.1073/pnas.0710103104

Krueger, F., Parasuraman, R., Iyengar, V., Thornburg, M., Weel, J., Lin, M., et al. (2012). Oxytocin receptor genetic variation promotes human trust behavior. *Front. Hum. Neurosci.* 6:4. doi: 10.3389/fnhum.2012.00004

Landgraf, R., Frank, E., Aldag, J. M., Neumann, I. D., Sharer, C. A., Ren, X., et al. (2003). Viral vector-mediated gene transfer of the vole V1a vasopressin receptor in the rat septum: improved social discrimination and active social behaviour. *Eur. J. Neurosci.* 18, 403–411. doi: 10.1046/j.1460-9568.2003.02750.x

Landgraf, R., Gerstberger, R., Montkowski, A., Probst, J. C., Wotjak, C. T., Holsboer, F., et al. (1995). V1 vasopressin receptor antisense oligodeoxynucleotide into septum reduces vasopressin binding, social discrimination abilities, and anxiety-related behavior in rats. *J. Neurosci.* 15, 4250–4258.

Lane, A., Luminet, O., Rimé, B., Gross, J. J., de Timary, P., and Mikolajczak, M. (2013). Oxytocin increases willingness to socially share one's emotions. *Int. J. Psychol.* 48, 676–681. doi: 10.1080/00207594.2012.677540

Lanier, P., Jonson-Reid, M., Stahlschmidt, M. J., Drake, B., and Constantino, J. (2010). Child maltreatment and pediatric health outcomes: a longitudinal study of low-income children. *J. Pediatr. Psychol.* 35, 511–522. doi: 10.1093/jpepsy/jsp086

Lee, R. M., and Robbins, S. B. (1998). The relationship between social connectedness and anxiety, self-esteem, and social identity. *J. Counsel. Psychol.* 45, 338–345. doi: 10.1037/0022-0167.45.3.338

Lee, R. M., and Robbins, S. B. (2000). Understanding social connectedness in college women and men. *J. Couns. Dev.* 78, 484–491. doi: 10.1002/j.1556-6676.2000.tb01932.x

Leeb, R. T., Lewis, T., and Zolotor, A. J. (2011). A review of physical and mental health consequences of child abuse and neglect and implications for practice. *Am. J. Lifestyle Med.* 5, 454–468. doi: 10.1177/1559827611410266

Le Moal, M., Dantzer, R., Michaud, B., and Koob, G. F. (1987). Centrally injected arginine vasopressin (AVP) facilitates social memory in rats. *Neurosci. Lett.* 77, 353–359. doi: 10.1016/0304-3940(87)90527-1

Levine, A., Zagoory-Sharon, O., Feldman, R., and Weller, A. (2007). Oxytocin during pregnancy and early postpartum: individual patterns and maternal–fetal attachment. *Peptides* 28, 1162–1169. doi: 10.1016/j.peptides.2007.04.016

Levy, F., Kendrick, K. M., Keverne, E. B., Piketty, V., and Poindron, P. (1992). Intracerebral oxytocin is important for the onset of maternal behavior in inexperienced ewes delivered under peridural anesthesia. *Behav. Neurosci.* 106, 427–432. doi: 10.1037/0735-7044.106.2.427

Li, L.-L., Keverne, E. B., Aparicio, S. A., Ishino, F., Barton, S. C., and Surani, M. A. (1999). Regulation of maternal rehavior and offspring growth by paternally expressed *peg3*. *Science* 284, 330–334. doi: 10.1126/science.284.5412.330

Lillard, L. A., and Waite, L. J. (1995). Til death do us part: marital disruption and mortality. *Am. J. Sociol.* 100, 1131–1156. doi: 10.1086/230634

Lim, M. M., Wang, Z., Olazabal, D. E., Ren, X., Terwilliger, E. F., and Young, L. J. (2004). Enhanced partner preference in a promiscuous species by manipulating the expression of a single gene. *Nature* 429, 754–757. doi: 10.1038/nature 02539

Lim, M. M., and Young, L. J. (2004). Vasopressin-dependent neural circuits underlying pair bond formation in the monogamous prairie vole. *Neuroscience* 125, 35–45. doi: 10.1016/j.neuroscience.2003.12.008

Lim, M. M., and Young, L. J. (2006). Neuropeptidergic regulation of affiliative behavior and social bonding in animals. *Horm. Behav.* 50, 506–517. doi: 10.1016/j.yhbeh.2006.06.028

Liu, J. C. J., Guastella, A. J., and Dadds, M. R. (2012). Effects of oxytocin on human social approach measured using intimacy equilibriums. *Horm. Behav.* 62, 585–591. doi: 10.1016/j.yhbeh.2012.09.002

Liu, Y., and Wang, Z. X. (2003). Nucleus accumbens oxytocin and dopamine interact to regulate pair bond formation in female prairie voles. *Neuroscience* 121, 537–544. doi: 10.1016/S0306-4522(03)00555-4

Lopatina, O., Inzhutova, A., Salmina, A. B., and Higashida, H. (2013). The roles of oxytocin and CD38 in social or parental behaviors. *Front. Neurosci.* 6:182. doi: 10.3389/fnins.2012.00182

Ludwig, M., and Leng, G. (2006). Dendritic peptide release and peptide-dependent behaviours. *Nat. Rev. Neurosci.* 7, 126–136. doi: 10.1038/nrn1845

Luhmann, N. (1979). *Trust and Power*. New York, NY: John Willey & Sons.

Macbeth, A. H., Lee, H. J., Edds, J., and Young, W. S. (2009). Oxytocin and the oxytocin receptor underlie intrastrain, but not interstrain, social recognition. *Genes Brain Behav.* 8, 558–567. doi: 10.1111/j.1601-183X.2009.00506.x

McCarthy, M. M. (1990). Oxytocin inhibits infanticide in female house mice (*Mus domesticus*). *Horm. Behav.* 24, 365–375. doi: 10.1016/0018-506X(90)90015-P

Mikolajczak, M., Gross, J. J., Lane, A., Corneille, O., de Timary, P., and Luminet, O. (2010a). Oxytocin makes people trusting, not gullible. *Psychol. Sci.* 21, 1072–1074. doi: 10.1177/0956797610377343

Mikolajczak, M., Pinon, N., Lane, A., de Timary, P., and Luminet, O. (2010b). Oxytocin not only increases trust when money is at stake, but also when confidential information is in the balance. *Biol. Psychol.* 85, 182–184. doi: 10.1016/j.biopsycho.2010.05.010

Nagasawa, M., Okabe, S., Mogi, K., and Kikusui, T. (2012). Oxytocin and mutual communication in mother-infant bonding. *Front. Hum. Neurosci.* 6:31. doi: 10.3389/fnhum.2012.00031

Nation, M., and Heflinger, C. A. (2006). Risk factors for serious alcohol and drug use: the role of psychosocial variables in predicting the frequency of substance use among adolescents. *Am. J. Drug Alcohol Abuse* 32, 415–433. doi: 10.1080/00952990600753867

Nephew, B. C., and Bridges, R. S. (2008). Arginine vasopressin V1a receptor antagonist impairs maternal memory in rats. *Physiol. Behav.* 95, 182–186. doi: 10.1016/j.physbeh.2008.05.016

Nowak, R., Porter, R. H., Levy, F., Orgeur, P., and Schaal, B. (2000). Role of mother-young interactions in the survival of offspring in domestic mammals. *Rev. Reprod.* 5, 153–163. doi: 10.1530/ror.0.0050153

Olazabal, D. E., and Young, L. J. (2006). Oxytocin receptors in the nucleus accumbens facilitate "spontaneous" maternal behavior in adult female prairie voles. *Neuroscience* 141, 559–568. doi: 10.1016/j.neuroscience.2006.04.017

Ostermeyer, M. C., and Elwood, R. W. (1983). Pup recognition in Mus musculus: parental discrimination between their own and alien young. *Dev. Psychobiol.* 16, 75–82. doi: 10.1002/dev.420160202

Parker, K. J., and Lee, T. M. (2001). Central vasopressin administration regulates the onset of facultative paternal behavior in *Microtus pennsylvanicus* (meadow voles). *Horm. Behav.* 39, 285–294. doi: 10.1006/hbeh.2001.1655

Pedersen, C. A., Ascher, J. A., Monroe, Y. L., and Prange, A. J. Jr. (1982). Oxytocin induces maternal behavior in virgin female rats. *Science* 216, 648–650. doi: 10.1126/science.7071605

Pedersen, C. A., Caldwell, J. D., Johnson, M. F., Fort, S. A., and Prange, A. J. Jr. (1985). Oxytocin antiserum delays onset of ovarian steroid-induced maternal behavior. *Neuropeptides* 6, 175–182. doi: 10.1016/0143-4179(85)90108-8

Pedersen, C. A., Caldwell, J. D., Walker, C., Ayers, G., and Mason, G. A. (1994). Oxytocin activates the postpartum onset of rat maternal behavior in the ventral tegmental and medial preoptic areas. *Behav. Neurosci.* 108, 1163–1171. doi: 10.1037/0735-7044.108.6.1163

Pedersen, C. A., and Prange, A. J. Jr. (1979). Induction of maternal behavior in virgin rats after intracerebroventricular administration of oxytocin. *Proc. Natl. Acad. Sci. U.S.A.* 76, 6661–6665. doi: 10.1073/pnas.76.12.6661

Pedersen, C. A., Vadlamudi, S. V., Boccia, M. L., and Amico, J. A. (2006). Maternal behavior deficits in nulliparous oxytocin knockout mice. *Genes Brain Behav.* 5, 274–281. doi: 10.1111/j.1601-183X.2005.00162.x

Pitkow, L. J., Sharer, C. A., Ren, X., Insel, T. R., Terwilliger, E. F., and Young, L. J. (2001). Facilitation of affiliation and pair-bond formation by vasopressin receptor gene transfer into the ventral forebrain of a monogamous vole. *J. Neurosci.* 21, 7392–7396.

Poindron, P., Gilling, G., Hernandez, H., Serafin, N., and Terrazas, A. (2003). Early recognition of newborn goat kids by their mother: I. Nonolfactory discrimination. *Dev. Psychobiol.* 43, 82–89. doi: 10.1002/dev.10123

Popik, P., and van Ree, J. M. (1991). Oxytocin but not vasopressin facilities social recognition following injection into the medial preoptic area of the rat brain. *Eur. Neuropsychopharmacol.* 1, 555–560. doi: 10.1016/0924-977X(91)90010-R

Popik, P., Vetulani, J., and van Ree, J. M. (1992a). Low doses of oxytocin facilitate social recognition in rats. *Psychopharmacology (Berl)* 106, 71–74. doi: 10.1007/BF02253591

Popik, P., Vos, P. E., and Van Ree, J. M. (1992b). Neurohypophyseal hormone receptors in the septum are implicated in social recognition in the rat. *Behav. Pharmacol.* 3, 351–358. doi: 10.1097/00008877-199208000-00011

Porter, R. H., Cernoch, J. M., and McLaughlin, F. J. (1983). Maternal recognition of neonates through olfactory cues. *Physiol. Behav.* 30, 151–154. doi: 10.1016/0031-9384(83)90051-3

Ragnauth, A. K., Devidze, N., Moy, V., Finley, K., Goodwillie, A., Kow, L. M., et al. (2005). Female oxytocin gene-knockout mice, in a semi-natural environment, display exaggerated aggressive behavior. *Genes Brain Behav.* 4, 229–239. doi: 10.1111/j.1601-183X.2005.00118.x

Relaix, F., Wei, X. J., Li, W., Pan, J., Lin, Y., Bowtell, D. D., et al. (2000). Pw1/Peg3 is a potential cell death mediator and cooperates with Siah1a in p53-mediated apoptosis. *Proc. Natl. Acad. Sci. U.S.A.* 97, 2105–2110. doi: 10.1073/pnas.040378897

Relaix, F., Wei, X. J., Wu, X., and Sassoon, D. A. (1998). Peg3/Pw1 is an imprinted gene involved in the TNF-NFkappaB signal transduction pathway. *Nat. Genet.* 18, 287–291. doi: 10.1038/ng0398-287

Rimmele, U., Hediger, K., Heinrichs, M., and Klaver, P. (2009). Oxytocin makes a face in memory familiar. *J. Neurosci.* 29, 38–42. doi: 10.1523/JNEUROSCI.4260-08.2009

Saito, A., and Nakamura, K. (2011). Oxytocin changes primate paternal tolerance to offspring in food transfer. *J. Comp. Physiol. A* 197, 329–337. doi: 10.1007/s00359-010-0617-2

Sarkadi, A., Kristiansson, R., Oberklaid, F., and Bremberg, S. (2008). Fathers' involvement and children's developmental outcomes: a systematic review of longitudinal studies. *Acta Paediatr.* 97, 153–158. doi: 10.1111/j.1651-2227.2007.00572.x

Savaskan, E., Ehrhardt, R., Schulz, A., Walter, M., and Schächinger, H. (2008). Post-learning intranasal oxytocin modulates human memory for facial identity. *Psychoneuroendocrinology* 33, 368–374. doi: 10.1016/j.psyneuen.2007.12.004

Schneiderman, I., Kanat-Maymon, Y., Ebstein, R. P., and Feldman, R. (2013). Cumulative risk on the oxytocin receptor gene (OXTR) underpins empathic communication difficulties at the first stages of romantic love. *Soc. Cogn. Affect. Neurosci.* doi: 10.1093/scan/nst142. [Epub ahead of print].

Schneiderman, I., Zagoory-Sharon, O., Leckman, J. F., and Feldman, R. (2012). Oxytocin during the initial stages of romantic attachment: relations to couples' interactive reciprocity. *Psychoneuroendocrinology* 37, 1277–1285. doi: 10.1016/j.psyneuen.2011.12.021

Shonkoff, J. P., Garner, A. S., Committee on Psychosocial Aspects of Child and Family Heath, Committee on Early Childhood, Adoption, and Dependent Care, and Section on Developmental and Behavioral Pediatrics. (2012). The lifelong effects of early childhood adversity and toxic stress. *Pediatrics* 129, e232–e246. doi: 10.1542/peds.2011-2663

Silverstein, M., and Bengtson, V. L. (1991). Do close parent-child relations reduce the mortality risk of older parents? *J. Health Soc. Behav.* 32, 382–395. doi: 10.2307/2137105

Skuse, D. H., and Gallagher, L. (2009). Dopaminergic-neuropeptide interactions in the social brain. *Trends Cogn. Sci.* 13, 27–35. doi: 10.1016/j.tics.2008.09.007

Smith, A. S., Agmo, A., Birnie, A. K., and French, J. A. (2010). Manipulation of the oxytocin system alters social behavior and attraction in pair-bonding primates, *Callithrix penicillata*. *Horm. Behav.* 57, 255–262. doi: 10.1016/j.yhbeh.2009.12.004

Steptoe, A. (1991). The links between stress and illness. *J. Psychosom. Res.* 35, 633–644. doi: 10.1016/0022-3999(91)90113-3

Takagi, T., Tanizawa, O., Otsuki, Y., Sugita, N., Haruta, M., and Yamaji, K. (1985). Oxytocin in the cerebrospinal fluid and plasma of pregnant and nonpregnant subjects. *Horm. Metab. Res.* 17, 308–310. doi: 10.1055/s-2007-1013526

Takayanagi, Y., Yoshida, M., Bielsky, I. F., Ross, H. E., Kawamata, M., Onaka, T., et al. (2005). Pervasive social deficits, but normal parturition, in oxytocin receptor-deficient mice. *Proc. Natl. Acad. Sci. U.S.A.* 102, 16096–16101. doi: 10.1073/pnas.0505312102

Tobin, V. A., Hashimoto, H., Wacker, D. W., Takayanagi, Y., Langnaese, K., Caquineau, C., et al. (2010). An intrinsic vasopressin system in the olfactory bulb is involved in social recognition. *Nature* 464, 413–417. doi: 10.1038/nature08826

Van Ijzendoorn, M. H., and Bakermans-Kranenburg, M. J. (2012). A sniff of trust: meta-analysis of the effects of intranasal oxytocin administration on face recognition, trust to in-group, and trust to out-group. *Psychoneuroendocrinology* 37, 438–443. doi: 10.1016/j.psyneuen.2011.07.008

van Leengoed, E., Kerker, E., and Swanson, H. H. (1987). Inhibition of post-partum maternal behaviour in the rat by injecting an oxytocin antagonist into the cerebral ventricles. *J. Endocrinol.* 112, 275–282. doi: 10.1677/joe.0.1120275

van Wimersma Greidanus, T. B., and Maigret, C. (1996). The role of limbic vasopressin and oxytocin in social recognition. *Brain Res.* 713, 153–159. doi: 10.1016/0006-8993(95)01505-1

Wacker, D. W., and Ludwig, M. (2012). Vasopressin, oxytocin, and social odor recognition. *Horm. Behav.* 61, 259–265. doi: 10.1016/j.yhbeh.2011.08.014

Walum, H., Lichtenstein, P., Neiderhiser, J. M., Reiss, D., Ganiban, J. M., Spotts, E. L., et al. (2012). Variation in the oxytocin receptor gene is associated with pair-bonding and social behavior. *Biol. Psychiatry* 71, 419–426. doi: 10.1016/j.biopsych.2011.09.002

Walum, H., Westberg, L., Henningsson, S., Neiderhiser, J. M., Reiss, D., Igl, W., et al. (2008). Genetic variation in the vasopressin receptor 1a gene (AVPR1A) associates with pair-bonding behavior in humans. *Proc. Natl. Acad. Sci. U.S.A.* 105, 14153–14156. doi: 10.1073/pnas.0803081105

Wang, Z., Ferris, C. F., and De Vries, G. J. (1994a). Role of septal vasopressin innervation in paternal behavior in prairie voles (*Microtus ochrogaster*). *Proc. Natl. Acad. Sci. U.S.A.* 91, 400–404. doi: 10.1073/pnas.91.1.400

Wang, Z., Smith, W., Major, D. E., and De Vries, G. J. (1994b). Sex and species differences in the effects of cohabitation on vasopressin messenger RNA expression in the bed nucleus of the stria terminalis in prairie voles (Microtus ochrogaster) and meadow voles (Microtus pennsylvanicus). *Brain Res.* 650, 212–218. doi: 10.1016/0006-8993(94)91784-1

Wang, Z., Young, L. J., De Vries, G. J., and Insel, T. R. (1998). Voles and vasopressin: a review of molecular, cellular, and behavioral studies of pair bonding and paternal behaviors. *Prog. Brain Res.* 119, 483–499. doi: 10.1016/S0079-6123(08)61589-7

Wideman, C. H., and Murphy, H. M. (1990). Vasopressin, maternal behavior, and pup well-being. *Curr. Psychol.* 9, 285–295. doi: 10.1007/BF02686866

Williams, J. R., Carter, C. S., and Insel, T. (1992a). Partner preference development in female prairie voles is facilitated by mating or the central infusion of oxytocin. *Ann. N.Y. Acad. Sci.* 652, 487–489. doi: 10.1111/j.1749-6632.1992.tb34393.x

Williams, J. R., Catania, K. C., and Carter, C. S. (1992b). Development of partner preferences in female prairie voles (*Microtus ochrogaster*): the role of social and sexual experience. *Horm. Behav.* 26, 339–349. doi: 10.1016/0018-506X(92)90004-F

Williams, K. L., and Galliher, R. V. (2006). Predicting depression and self-esteem from social connectedness, support, and competence. *J. Soc. Clin. Psychol.* 25, 855–874. doi: 10.1521/jscp.2006.25.8.855

Winslow, J. T., Hastings, N., Carter, C. S., Harbaugh, C. R., and Insel, T. R. (1993). A role for central vasopressin in pair bonding in monogamous prairie voles. *Nature* 365, 545–548. doi: 10.1038/365545a0

Winslow, J. T., and Insel, T. R. (1991). Social status in pairs of male squirrel monkeys determines the behavioral response to central oxytocin administration. *J. Neurosci.* 11, 2032–2038.

Winslow, J. T., and Insel, T. R. (2002). The social deficits of the oxytocin knockout mouse. *Neuropeptides* 36, 221–229. doi: 10.1054/npep.2002.0909

Winslow, J. T., and Insel, T. R. (2004). Neuroendocrine basis of social recognition. *Curr. Opin. Neurobiol.* 14, 248–253. doi: 10.1016/j.conb.2004.03.009

Witt, D. M., Carter, C. S., and Walton, D. M. (1990). Central and peripheral effects of oxytocin administration in prairie voles (*Microtus ochrogaster*). *Pharmacol. Biochem. Behav.* 37, 63–69. doi: 10.1016/0091-3057(90)90042-G

Witt, D. M., Winslow, J. T., and Insel, T. R. (1992). Enhanced social interactions in rats following chronic, centrally infused oxytocin. *Pharmacol. Biochem. Behav.* 43, 855–861. doi: 10.1016/0091-3057(92)90418-F

Young, L. J. (2002). The neurobiology of social recognition, approach, and avoidance. *Biol. Psychiatry* 51, 18–26. doi: 10.1016/S0006-3223(01)01268-9

Young, L. J., Murphy Young, A. Z., and Hammock, E. A. D. (2005). Anatomy and neurochemistry of the pair bond. *J. Comp. Neurol.* 493, 51–57. doi: 10.1002/cne.20771

Young, L. J., Nilsen, R., Waymire, K. G., MacGregor, G. R., and Insel, T. R. (1999). Increased affiliative response to vasopressin in mice expressing the V1a receptor from a monogamous vole. *Nature* 400, 766–768. doi: 10.1038/23650

Yu, G. Z., Kaba, H., Okutani, F., Takahashi, S., and Higuchi, T. (1996). The olfactory bulb: a critical site of action for oxytocin in the induction of maternal behaviour in the rat. *Neuroscience* 72, 1083–1088. doi: 10.1016/0306-4522(95)00600-1

Zak, P. J., Kurzban, R., and Matzner, W. T. (2004). "The neurobiology of trust," in *Biobehavioral Stress Response: Protective and Damaging Effects*, eds R. Yehuda and B. McEwen (New York, NY: New York Academy of Sciences), 224–227.

Zak, P. J., Kurzban, R., and Matzner, W. T. (2005). Oxytocin is associated with human trustworthiness. *Horm. Behav.* 48, 522–527. doi: 10.1016/j.yhbeh.2005.07.009

16

Effects of early life adverse experiences on the brain: implications from maternal separation models in rodents

Mayumi Nishi*, Noriko Horii-Hayashi and Takayo Sasagawa

Department of Anatomy and Cell Biology, Nara Medical University, Kashihara, Japan

****Correspondence:***
Mayumi Nishi, Department of Anatomy and Cell Biology, Faculty of Medicine, Nara Medical University, Kashihara, Nara 634-8521, Japan
e-mail: nmayumi@naramed-u.ac.jp

During postnatal development, adverse early life experiences affect the formation of neuronal networks and exert long-lasting effects on neural function. Many studies have shown that daily repeated maternal separation (MS), an animal model of early life stress, can regulate the hypothalamic-pituitary-adrenal axis (HPA axis) and affect subsequent brain function and behavior during adulthood. However, the molecular basis of the long-lasting effects of early life stress on brain function has not been fully elucidated. In this mini review, we present various cases of MS in rodents and illustrate the alterations in HPA axis activity by focusing on corticosterone (CORT). We then show a characterization of the brain regions affected by various patterns of MS, including repeated MS and single time MS at various stages before weaning, by investigating c-Fos expression. These CORT and c-Fos studies suggest that repeated early life stress may affect neuronal function in region- and temporal-specific manners, indicating a critical period for habituation to early life stress. Next, we introduce how early life stress can impact behavior, namely by inducing depression, anxiety or eating disorders, and alterations in gene expression in adult mice subjected to MS.

Keywords: maternal separation, HPA axis, depression, corticosteroid, gene expression, behavior, epigenetics

INTRODUCTION

As our contemporary society changes rapidly, changes in family structure can have a large influence on the mother–child relationship, as well as on other social environmental factors. In adult patients with various neuropsychiatric disorders, childhood abuse including sexual and/or physical abuse and neglect, is one of the most serious causes (Bremne and Vermetten, 2001; Heim and Nemeroff, 2001; Teicher et al., 2006). Adverse experiences occurring during critical periods of development, such as perinatal life, harmfully influence behavior, and physiological functions, including growth, metabolism, reproduction, and immune responses. Stressful environments in early life may induce permanent rather than transient consequences in animals. Previous studies have indicated that early unfavorable events augment the risk of behavioral disorders in adulthood, including neuropsychiatric disorders, such as depression (Kendler et al., 2002) and psychosis (Morgan et al., 2007). In rodent and primate models, adverse environments during the neonatal periods seem to play a critical role in developing the brain systems important to regulate behavior and stress responsiveness. In particular, the responsiveness of the hypothalamic-pituitary-adrenal (HPA) axis can be deteriorated by interrupting usual mother-pup interactions, which may induce persistent changes in the neurobiology, physiology, and emotional behavior in adult animals (Ellenbroek et al., 1998; Lyons et al., 1998; Pryce et al., 2005; Enthoven et al., 2008; Nishi et al., 2013).

In this mini review, we will focus on the response of corticosterone (CORT), an end product of the HPA axis in rodents, and c-Fos expression for examining the activated brain regions induced by maternal separation (MS), a model of rodent early life stress. Furthermore, we will also present alterations of behavioral aspects and alterations in gene expression.

EARLY MS

The inventive studies of Levine and colleagues, and consequently of Meaney, Plotsky, and their collaborators have demonstrated that changes in rodents' early postnatal experiences can induce profound long-lasting effects on emotionality and stress response (Levine, 1967; Meaney, 2001; Plotsky et al., 2005), which have spurred the employment of the rodent MS for investigating early life stress. This early life stress model is based on the evidence that unfavorable events in early life cause the vulnerability for developing various kinds of diseases in later life. In this type of study, MS should be carefully discussed in comparison to the appropriate control group, which may or may not be undisturbed from mother.

The procedure of MS showed a variety of the duration (e.g., 60 min–24 h) and the number of days (e.g., 1–14 days, 15–21 days) for the separation experiences among laboratories (Biagini et al., 1998; Caldji et al., 2000; Barreau et al., 2004; Arborelius and Eklund, 2007; Carrera et al., 2009; Tjong et al., 2010). In MS paradigm, many experiments, but certainly not all, have demonstrated that separation of pups from their mothers during the early postnatal period permanently increased anxiety-like behaviors in adulthood (Francis et al., 1999; Huot et al., 2001, 2004; Menard et al., 2004). As to the HPA axis activity, the response to stress is relatively low during early postnatal life (Walker et al., 1991; Levine, 2005), while MS could lead to life-long hyperactivity of the HPA axis (Holmes et al., 2005; Lippmann et al., 2007; Aisa et al., 2008; Marais et al., 2008). In contrast, short-term disturbance (e.g., 15 min), which has been called "handling," appeared to reduce anxiety-like behaviors, decrease HPA axis tone and reduce the response to stress in adulthood (Levine, 2005; Plotsky et al., 2005). The process of handling may imitate natural mice rearing, whereby the mother leaves her pups for short periods of time to collect foods. Thus, the short-term MS, handling, might be considered a more natural event.

The effect of MS also varies depending upon whether pups are separated in a group of littermates during MS or isolated singly. Miyazaki and colleagues recently reported that rat pups isolated singly from the mother during PND7 to PND11 presented disturbance of cortical function, whereas pups separated but gathered from PND7 to PND11 showed no cortical disruption (Miyazaki et al., 2012).

CHARACTERIZATION OF MATERNALLY SEPARATED ANIMALS

SERUM LEVEL OF CORT

In rodents, there is an unique period during which the HPA axis shows a rapid regression known as the stress hyporesponsive period (SHRP) (Levine, 2001). This period extends from PND4 to PND14 in rats and from PND2 to PND12 in mice. During the course of SHRP, ACTH in increased and baseline plasma glucocorticoid levels are lower than normal (Rosenfeld et al., 1991). Because, during ontogeny, the maintenance of low and stable levels of CORT is necessary for normal growth and development of the central nervous system (CNS), the SHRP is hypothesized to be neuroprotective against stress-induced excessive stimulation of glucocorticoid receptors (GRs) (Sapolsky and Meaney, 1986; Sapolsky, 1996). In rodents, the presence of the mother appears to suppress HPA axis activity, which primarily preserves the SHRP. Indeed, even during the SHRP, MS is a compelling inducer of a stress response. Meaney and his colleagues suggest that the quality of the mother-pup interactions, such as increased maternal licking, grooming, and arched-back nursing, is an important aspect for the preservation of this dampened HPA axis activity (Francis et al., 1999). The disturbance of SHRP induced by MS could cause an excessive exposure of the brain to high concentrations of glucocorticoids and activation of GRs, which may subsequently regulate brain and behavior in later life. Enhanced secretion of stress-induced CORT was observed in pups separated from their mothers for 1 h on PND2 to PND9 (McCormick et al., 1998). Nevertheless, a recent study indicated that repeated MS for 8 h daily from PND3 to PND5 rapidly desensitized the HPA axis activity of neonatal mice (Enthoven et al., 2008). We also reported that repeated MS for 3 h daily from PND1 to PND14 did not elevate a baseline level of CORT on PND14, whereas a single-time MS for 3 h at PND14 raised a baseline CORT level (**Figure 1**) (Horii-Hayashi et al., 2013). In contrast to the effects of MS on neonatal animals, repeated MS for 3 h daily from PND1 to PND14 significantly raises a CORT level in adulthood, as reported by many studies (Ryu et al., 2008; Jahng et al., 2010; Horii-Hayashi et al., 2013).

ACTIVATED BRAIN REGIONS ANALYZED BY c-FOS EXPRESSION

The expression of the immediate early gene product c-Fos is a reliable molecular marker to investigate neuronal activation. The examination of c-Fos expression has revealed that many brain regions are activated by MS, which differs depending on age and the type of stress. We recently analyzed the c-Fos expression induced by repeated MS and single-time MS during different developmental stages and time periods. Mice were exposed to 3 h repeated MS daily from PND1 to PND14 or from PND14 to PND21, or to single-time MS at PND14 or PND21 (Horii-Hayashi et al., 2013). We clarified that MS activated many brain regions and that c-Fos expression patterns

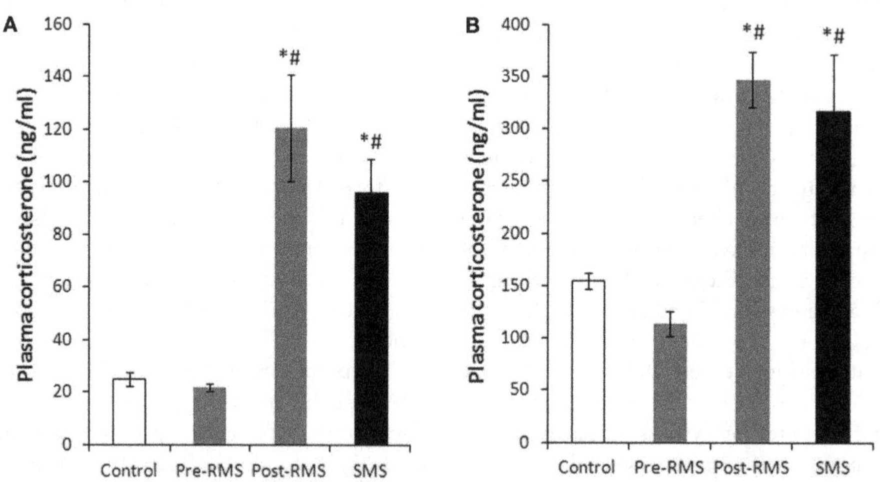

FIGURE 1 | Plasma CORT levels of repeated maternal separation (RMS) and single-time maternal separation (SMS) mice on PND14 and PND21 (Horii-Hayashi et al., 2013). The graphs show plasma CORT concentrations of PND14 **(A)** and PND21 **(B)** ($n = 5$–9 for each group). Blood samples were collected before (pre-RMS) and after (post-RMS) the final separation from RMS mice and after the separation from SMS mice. $^*P < 0.05$ vs. control, $^\#P < 0.05$ vs. Pre-MS.

changed developmentally (**Figure 2**). Single-time MS at both ages activated many regions of the hypothalamus and limbic forebrain, while the pattern of c-Fos expression in the repeated MS groups were significantly different on PND14 and PND21. In repeated MS of PND14 mice, the c-Fos expression levels in many regions were markedly increased compared with age-matched controls, excepting the VMH, Arc, BST, DG, Ce, MePV, and MePD. By contrast, in repeated MS on PND21 mice, c-Fos expression was reduced to control levels in all observed brain regions except for the LS and CA3. These findings suggest that repetition of a homotypic stimulus suppresses c-Fos expression by PND21, but that such suppression is barely observed on PND14. Moreover, in animals exposed to repeated homotypic stress during the postnatal period, increase in adrenal CORT secretion does not always associate with increased c-Fos expression in the PVN. Such developmental differences in c-Fos expression detected in the repeated MS groups may be associated with a developmental critical period for stress responses involving the HPA axis, during which animals are more susceptible to MS and other environments. In rodents, the critical period is the first two postnatal weeks. Thus, in early life, a repeated stress will be unlikely to suppress c-Fos expression. In turn, inappropriately activated c-Fos target genes may drastically alter how neurons function in critical neural circuits. Indeed, the suppression of increased c-Fos expression in repeated MS of PND14 mice was observed in specific regions (BST, Ce, MePD, and MePV) that form anatomical neural connections. These regions are referred to as an extended amygdala, which are closely associated with anxiety, fear, and psychiatric disorders (Davis et al., 2010). Therefore, even at PND14, repeated homotypic stress may reduce neural activity in the circuit of the extended amygdala. Moreover, in the SFO, where neurons are influenced by osmolality, calcium, and sodium concentrations in the systemic circulation (Smith and Ferguson, 2010), c-Fos expression was increased in both repeated and single-time MS mice, as compared to controls, on PND14. However, there were no changes in any of the groups

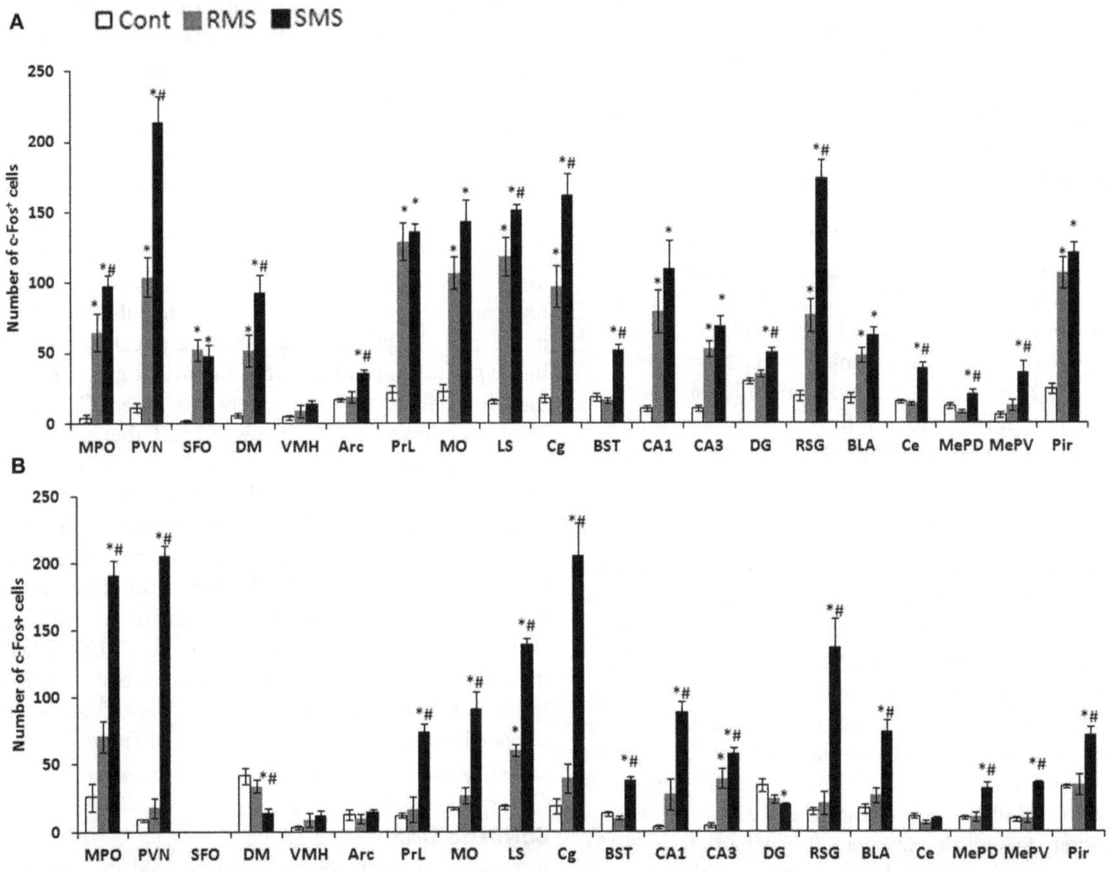

FIGURE 2 | c-Fos expression in the hypothalamus and limbic forebrain after MS (Horii-Hayashi et al., 2013). The graphs show the numbers of c-Fos-positive cells on PND14 **(A)** and PND21 **(B)** in non-separated control (white bar), RMS (gray bar), and SMS (black bar) mice ($n = 4$–5 for each group). In both RMS and SMS, the sampling point is just after MS procedure. $^{*}P < 0.05$ vs. control; $^{\#}P < 0.05$ vs. RMS. MPO, medial preoptic area; PVN, paraventricular nucleus; SFO, subfornical organ; DM, dorsomedial hypothalamic nucleus; VMH, ventromedial hypothalamic nucleus; PrL, prelimbic cortex; MO, medial orbital cortex; LS, lateral septum; Cg, cingulate cortex; BST, bed nucleus of stria terminalis; CA1, hippocampal area CA1; CA3, hippocampal area CA3; DG, dentate gyrus; RSG, retrosplenial granular cortex; La, lateral amygdaloid nucleus; BLA, anterior part of the basolateral amygdaloid nucleus; Ce, central amygdaloid nucleus; MePD, posterodorsal part of the medial amygdaloid nucleus; MePV, posteroventral part of the medial amygdaloid nucleus; Pir, piriform cortex.

on PND21. This difference may reflect the increased resistance of physical growth to the hyperosmolality induced by deprivation of lactation.

BEHAVIORAL CHANGES INDUCED BY MS IN RODENTS

Early life adverse experiences including MS is one of the greatest contributing factors for mental health problems across life stages (Levine, 2005), relating not only to risk for mental health disorders but also to transdiagnostic features common in many psychological disorders (Glaser et al., 2006). I will introduce some of the behavioral aspects observed in animal model of MS.

Depression- and anxiety-like behaviors

Numerous studies have demonstrated a strong relationship between traumatic events during early life and development of behavioral abnormalities later in life. Early life adversity, such as that induced by MS, child physical, sexual, and emotional abuse, and general neglect has been linked to serious psychiatric impairment in adulthood (MacMillan et al., 2001). Particularly, a stressful life event such as early parental loss is associated with unipolar and bipolar depression, as well as anxiety disorders, beyond familial or genetic factors (Kendler et al., 1992; Agid et al., 1999; Furukawa et al., 1999; Heim and Nemeroff, 2001). Many human studies have reported that major depression and anxiety disorders are frequent in adults with a history of childhood abuse (Stein et al., 1996; Felitti et al., 1998). There have been numerous reports of the behavioral changes induced by MS in animal studies. Neonatal MS induces permanent alterations in the characteristics of the HPA response to stress in the offspring later in life (Ladd et al., 1996; Vazquez et al., 2000). Many studies of repeated MS during the first 2 weeks of neonatal life showed depression- and anxiety-like behaviors in adulthood (Newport et al., 2002; Daniels et al., 2004; Lee et al., 2007; Ryu et al., 2009). In these studies, ambulation and rearing decreased, immobility during a forced swim test increased, and time spent in the closed arms of an elevated plus maze increased.

Fear response

Until recently, no one had investigated how early experiences affected fear retention and extinction development, although these forms of emotional learning could be critically involved in the pathogenesis and treatment of mental health problems. Recent several studies showed that the timing of the maturation of fear learning is not set in static, but can be dynamically regulated by early experiences. Although the exact mechanisms are still unknown, when rats are reared under stressful conditions then they exhibit adult-like fear retention and extinction behaviors at an earlier stage of development (Callaghan et al., 2013). Chocyk et al. reported that MS decreased freezing time in both contextual and auditory fear conditioning in adolescent and adult rats (Chocyk et al., 2014). These results suggest that early life stress may permanently affect fear learning and memory.

Food intake and response to food deprivation

Previous studies showed that repeated MS during the first 2 weeks after birth may not permanently affect food intake and body weight gain of the offspring as long as the pups are reared in a group (Iwasaki et al., 2000; Kalinichev et al., 2002; Ryu et al., 2008). In contrast, post-weaning social isolation promotes food intake and weight gain of adolescent MS pups, with impacts on anxiety-like behaviors (Ryu et al., 2008). Anhedonia to palatable food, one of the major symptoms of depression, was reported in adolescent MS pups with disruption of the mesolimbic dopaminergic activity in response to stress (Noh et al., 2008). Another study showed that sustained hyperphagia observed in the MS pups subjected to a fasting/re-feeding cycle repeated during adolescent period of MS pups induced a binge-like eating disorder, in which increased activity of the HPA axis responding to such metabolic challenges appeared to play a role, at least partly, in mediation with the hypothalamic neuro peptide Y (NPY) (Jahng, 2011).

GENE EXPRESSION

Many animal studies, including MS, have improved our knowledge of gene-environment interactions and elucidated the pathways that program an animal in response to its early life experiences (Meaney and Szyf, 2005). Epigenetic mechanisms involving DNA methylation, post-translational modification of histone proteins and non-coding RNAs (most notably micro-RNA) are major candidates for regulating gene expression and integrating intrinsic and environmental signals in the genome (Jaenisch and Bird, 2003). Murgatroyd and colleagues showed that in the parvocellular subdivision of the paraventricular nucleus of the hypothalamus, MS in mice persistently upregulates *Avp* gene expression associated with reduced DNA methylation of a region in the *Avp* enhancer. This early life stress-responsive region serves as a binding site for the methyl-CpG binding protein 2, which in turn is regulated through neuronal activity. They also found that the ability of methyl-CpG binding protein 2 to control transcription of the *Avp* gene and induce DNA methylation occurred by recruiting components of the epigenetic machinery (Murgatroyd et al., 2009; Murgatroyd and Nephew, 2013). Other groups investigated DNA methylation levels at a specific sequence motif upstream of the GR gene (Nr3c1) in the hippocampus of offspring, and found that subjecting pups to a single 24 h MS increases methylation levels (Kember et al., 2012). The epigenetic alterations of these genes suggest that the HPA axis could be dysregulated by MS. Importantly, however, the DNA methylation differences were also often strain specific (Kember et al., 2012). Taken together, these findings demonstrate the importance of investigating environmental effects on a range of genetic backgrounds, emphasizing the need for the further examination of environmental, genetic, and epigenetic interactions.

CONCLUSIONS

Adverse environments and experiences during the neonatal period can dramatically affect the development of the HPA axis that underlies adaptive behavioral responses. MS experiments, as a model of early life stress, demonstrate that CORT levels and c-Fos expression change depending upon the different experimental conditions of MS, e.g., age at testing and frequency of repetition. Furthermore, separation conditions (isolation with or without a littermate) could also influence the results of the MS experiments. MS can induce various behavioral changes manifested in later life, which could be caused, at least in part, by alterations in gene expression, particularly through epigenetic mechanisms.

ACKNOWLEDGMENTS

This work was supported by Grants-in-Aid for Scientific Research (23390040 to Mayumi Nishi and AstraZeneca Research Grant 2009). We thank Dr. Julian G. Mercer, a chief editor of J Neuroendocrinology, for permitting the reuse of our own figures published in J Neuroendocrinology.

REFERENCES

Agid, O., Shapira, B., Zislin, J., Ritsner, M., Hanin, B., Murad, H., et al. (1999). Environment and vulnerability to major psychiatric illness: a case control study of early parental loss in major depression, bipolar disorder and schizophrenia. *Mol. Psychiatry* 4, 163–172. doi: 10.1038/sj.mp.4000473

Aisa, B., Tordera, R., Lasheras, B., Del Rio, J., and Ramirez, M. J. (2008). Effects of maternal separation on hypothalamic-pituitary-adrenal responses, cognition and vulnerability to stress in adult female rats. *Neuroscience* 154, 1218–1226. doi: 10.1016/j.neuroscience.2008.05.011

Arborelius, L., and Eklund, M. B. (2007). Both long and brief maternal separation produces persistent changes in tissue levels of brain monoamines in middle-aged female rats. *Neuroscience* 145, 738–750. doi: 10.1016/j.neuroscience.2006.12.007

Barreau, F., Cartier, C., Ferrier, L., Fioramonti, J., and Bueno, L. (2004). Nerve growth factor mediates alterations of colonic sensitivity and mucosal barrier induced by neonatal stress in rats. *Gastroenterology* 127, 524–534. doi: 10.1053/j.gastro.2004.05.019

Biagini, G., Pich, E. M., Carani, C., Marrama, P., and Agnati, L. F. (1998). Postnatal maternal separation during the stress hyporesponsive period enhances the adrenocortical response to novelty in adult rats by affecting feedback regulation in the CA1 hippocampal field. *Int. J. Dev. Neurosci.* 16, 187–197. doi: 10.1016/S0736-5748(98)00019-7

Bremne, J. D., and Vermetten, E. (2001). Stress and development: behavioral and biological consequences. *Dev. Psychopathol.* 13, 473–489. doi: 10.1017/S0954579401003042

Caldji, C., Diorio, J., and Meaney, M. J. (2000). Variations in maternal care in infancy regulate the development of stress reactivity. *Biol. Psychiatry* 48, 1164–1174. doi: 10.1016/S0006-3223(00)01084-2

Callaghan, B. L., Graham, B. M., Li, S., and Richardson, R. (2013). From resilience to vulnerability: mechanistic insights into the effects of stress on transitions in critical period plasticity. *Front. Psychiatry* 4:90. doi: 10.3389/fpsyt.2013.00090

Carrera, O., Cerrato, M., Sanchez, A., and Gutierrez, E. (2009). Long maternal separation has protective effects in rats exposed to activity-based anorexia. *Dev. Psychobiol.* 51, 616–624. doi: 10.1002/dev.20396

Chocyk, A., Przyborowska, A., Makuch, W., Majcher-Maslanka, I., Dudys, D., and Wedzony, K. (2014). The effects of early-life adversity on fear memories in adolescent rats and their persistence into adulthood. *Behav. Brain Res.* 264, 161–172. doi: 10.1016/j.bbr.2014.01.040

Daniels, W. M., Pietersen, C. Y., Carstens, M. E., and Stein, D. J. (2004). Maternal separation in rats leads to anxiety-like behavior and a blunted ACTH response and altered neurotransmitter levels in response to a subsequent stressor. *Metab. Brain Dis.* 19, 3–14. doi: 10.1023/B:MEBR.0000027412.19664.b3

Davis, M., Walker, D. L., Miles, L., and Grillon, C. (2010). Phasic vs sustained fear in rats and humans: role of the extended amygdala in fear vs anxiety. *Neuropsychopharmacology* 35, 105–135. doi: 10.1038/npp.2009.109

Ellenbroek, B. A., Van Den Kroonenberg, P. T., and Cools, A. R. (1998). The effects of an early stressful life event on sensorimotor gating in adult rats. *Schizophr. Res.* 30, 251–260. doi: 10.1016/S0920-9964(97)00149-7

Enthoven, L., Oitzl, M. S., Koning, N., Van Der Mark, M., and De Kloet, E. R. (2008). Hypothalamic-pituitary-adrenal axis activity of newborn mice rapidly desensitizes to repeated maternal absence but becomes highly responsive to novelty. *Endocrinology* 149, 6366–6377. doi: 10.1210/en.2008-0238

Felitti, V. J., Anda, R. F., Nordenberg, D., Williamson, D. F., Spitz, A. M., Edwards, V., et al. (1998). Relationship of childhood abuse and household dysfunction to many of the leading causes of death in adults. The Adverse Childhood Experiences (ACE) study. *Am. J. Prev. Med.* 14, 245–258. doi: 10.1016/S0749-3797(98)00017-8

Francis, D. D., Champagne, F. A., Liu, D., and Meaney, M. J. (1999). Maternal care, gene expression, and the development of individual differences in stress reactivity. *Ann. N.Y. Acad. Sci.* 896, 66–84. doi: 10.1111/j.1749-6632.1999.tb08106.x

Furukawa, T. A., Ogura, A., Hirai, T., Fujihara, S., Kitamura, T., and Takahashi, K. (1999). Early parental separation experiences among patients with bipolar disorder and major depression: a case-control study. *J. Affect. Disord.* 52, 85–91. doi: 10.1016/S0165-0327(98)00054-8

Glaser, J. P., Van Os, J., Portegijs, P. J., and Myin-Germeys, I. (2006). Childhood trauma and emotional reactivity to daily life stress in adult frequent attenders of general practitioners. *J. Psychosom. Res.* 61, 229–236. doi: 10.1016/j.jpsychores.2006.04.014

Heim, C., and Nemeroff, C. B. (2001). The role of childhood trauma in the neurobiology of mood and anxiety disorders: preclinical and clinical studies. *Biol. Psychiatry* 49, 1023–1039. doi: 10.1016/S0006-3223(01)01157-X

Holmes, A., Le Guisquet, A. M., Vogel, E., Millstein, R. A., Leman, S., and Belzung, C. (2005). Early life genetic, epigenetic and environmental factors shaping emotionality in rodents. *Neurosci. Biobehav. Rev.* 29, 1335–1346. doi: 10.1016/j.neubiorev.2005.04.012

Horii-Hayashi, N., Sasagawa, T., Matsunaga, W., Matsusue, Y., Azuma, C., and Nishi, M. (2013). Developmental changes in desensitisation of c-Fos expression induced by repeated maternal separation in pre-weaned mice. *J. Neuroendocrinol.* 25, 158–167. doi: 10.1111/j.1365-2826.2012.02377.x

Huot, R. L., Gonzalez, M. E., Ladd, C. O., Thrivikraman, K. V., and Plotsky, P. M. (2004). Foster litters prevent hypothalamic-pituitary-adrenal axis sensitization mediated by neonatal maternal separation. *Psychoneuroendocrinology* 29, 279–289. doi: 10.1016/S0306-4530(03)00028-3

Huot, R. L., Thrivikraman, K. V., Meaney, M. J., and Plotsky, P. M. (2001). Development of adult ethanol preference and anxiety as a consequence of neonatal maternal separation in Long Evans rats and reversal with antidepressant treatment. *Psychopharmacology (Berl.)* 158, 366–373. doi: 10.1007/s002130100701

Iwasaki, S., Inoue, K., Kiriike, N., and Hikiji, K. (2000). Effect of maternal separation on feeding behavior of rats in later life. *Physiol. Behav.* 70, 551–556. doi: 10.1016/S0031-9384(00)00305-X

Jaenisch, R., and Bird, A. (2003). Epigenetic regulation of gene expression: how the genome integrates intrinsic and environmental signals. *Nat. Genet.* 33(Suppl.), 245–254. doi: 10.1038/ng1089

Jahng, J. W. (2011). An animal model of eating disorders associated with stressful experience in early life. *Horm. Behav.* 59, 213–220. doi: 10.1016/j.yhbeh.2010.11.010

Jahng, J. W., Ryu, V., Yoo, S. B., Noh, S. J., Kim, J. Y., and Lee, J. H. (2010). Mesolimbic dopaminergic activity responding to acute stress is blunted in adolescent rats that experienced neonatal maternal separation. *Neuroscience* 171, 144–152. doi: 10.1016/j.neuroscience.2010.08.063

Kalinichev, M., Easterling, K. W., Plotsky, P. M., and Holtzman, S. G. (2002). Long-lasting changes in stress-induced corticosterone response and anxiety-like behaviors as a consequence of neonatal maternal separation in Long-Evans rats. *Pharmacol. Biochem. Behav.* 73, 131–140. doi: 10.1016/S0091-3057(02)00781-5

Kember, R. L., Dempster, E. L., Lee, T. H., Schalkwyk, L. C., Mill, J., and Fernandes, C. (2012). Maternal separation is associated with strain-specific responses to stress and epigenetic alterations to Nr3c1, Avp, and Nr4a1 in mouse. *Brain Behav.* 2, 455–467. doi: 10.1002/brb3.69

Kendler, K. S., Neale, M. C., Kessler, R. C., Heath, A. C., and Eaves, L. J. (1992). Childhood parental loss and adult psychopathology in women. A twin study perspective. *Arch. Gen. Psychiatry* 49, 109–116. doi: 10.1001/archpsyc.1992.01820020029004

Kendler, K. S., Sheth, K., Gardner, C. O., and Prescott, C. A. (2002). Childhood parental loss and risk for first-onset of major depression and alcohol dependence: the time-decay of risk and sex differences. *Psychol. Med.* 32, 1187–1194. doi: 10.1017/S0033291702006219

Ladd, C. O., Owens, M. J., and Nemeroff, C. B. (1996). Persistent changes in corticotropin-releasing factor neuronal systems induced by maternal deprivation. *Endocrinology* 137, 1212–1218. doi: 10.1210/en.137.4.1212

Lee, J. H., Kim, H. J., Kim, J. G., Ryu, V., Kim, B. T., Kang, D. W., et al. (2007). Depressive behaviors and decreased expression of serotonin reuptake transporter in rats that experienced neonatal maternal separation. *Neurosci. Res.* 58, 32–39. doi: 10.1016/j.neures.2007.01.008

Levine, S. (1967). Maternal and environmental influences on the adrenocortical response to stress in weanling rats. *Science* 156, 258–260. doi: 10.1126/science.156.3772.258

Levine, S. (2001). Primary social relationships influence the development of the hypothalamic–pituitary–adrenal axis in the rat. *Physiol. Behav.* 73, 255–260. doi: 10.1016/S0031-9384(01)00496-6

Levine, S. (2005). Developmental determinants of sensitivity and resistance to stress. *Psychoneuroendocrinology* 30, 939–946. doi: 10.1016/j.psyneuen.2005.03.013

Lippmann, M., Bress, A., Nemeroff, C. B., Plotsky, P. M., and Monteggia, L. M. (2007). Long-term behavioural and molecular alterations associated with maternal separation in rats. *Eur. J. Neurosci.* 25, 3091–3098. doi: 10.1111/j.1460-9568.2007.05522.x

Lyons, D. M., Kim, S., Schatzberg, A. F., and Levine, S. (1998). Postnatal foraging demands alter adrenocortical activity and psychosocial development. *Dev. Psychobiol.* 32, 285–291. doi: 10.1002/(SICI)1098-2302(199805)32:4<285::AID-DEV3>3.0.CO;2-J

MacMillan, H. L., Fleming, J. E., Streiner, D. L., Lin, E., Boyle, M. H., Jamieson, E., et al. (2001). Childhood abuse and lifetime psychopathology in a community sample. *Am. J. Psychiatry* 158, 1878–1883. doi: 10.1176/appi.ajp.158.11.1878

Marais, L., Van Rensburg, S. J., Van Zyl, J. M., Stein, D. J., and Daniels, W. M. (2008). Maternal separation of rat pups increases the risk of developing depressive-like behavior after subsequent chronic stress by altering corticosterone and neurotrophin levels in the hippocampus. *Neurosci. Res.* 61, 106–112. doi: 10.1016/j.neures.2008.01.011

McCormick, C. M., Kehoe, P., and Kovacs, S. (1998). Corticosterone release in response to repeated, short episodes of neonatal isolation: evidence of sensitization. *Int. J. Dev. Neurosci.* 16, 175–185. doi: 10.1016/S0736-5748(98)00026-4

Meaney, M. J. (2001). Maternal care, gene expression, and the transmission of individual differences in stress reactivity across generations. *Annu. Rev. Neurosci.* 24, 1161–1192. doi: 10.1146/annurev.neuro.24.1.1161

Meaney, M. J., and Szyf, M. (2005). Maternal care as a model for experience-dependent chromatin plasticity? *Trends Neurosci.* 28, 456–463. doi: 10.1016/j.tins.2005.07.006

Menard, J. L., Champagne, D. L., and Meaney, M. J. (2004). Variations of maternal care differentially influence "fear" reactivity and regional patterns of cFos immunoreactivity in response to the shock-probe burying test. *Neuroscience* 129, 297–308. doi: 10.1016/j.neuroscience.2004.08.009

Miyazaki, T., Takase, K., Nakajima, W., Tada, H., Ohya, D., Sano, A., et al. (2012). Disrupted cortical function underlies behavior dysfunction due to social isolation. *J. Clin. Invest.* 122, 2690–2701. doi: 10.1172/JCI63060

Morgan, C., Kirkbride, J., Leff, J., Craig, T., Hutchinson, G., McKenzie, K., et al. (2007). Parental separation, loss and psychosis in different ethnic groups: a case-control study. *Psychol. Med.* 37, 495–503. doi: 10.1017/S0033291706009330

Murgatroyd, C., Patchev, A. V., Wu, Y., Micale, V., Bockmuhl, Y., Fischer, D., et al. (2009). Dynamic DNA methylation programs persistent adverse effects of early-life stress. *Nat. Neurosci.* 12, 1559–1566. doi: 10.1038/nn.2436

Murgatroyd, C. A., and Nephew, B. C. (2013). Effects of early life social stress on maternal behavior and neuroendocrinology. *Psychoneuroendocrinology* 38, 219–228. doi: 10.1016/j.psyneuen.2012.05.020

Newport, D. J., Stowe, Z. N., and Nemeroff, C. B. (2002). Parental depression: animal models of an adverse life event. *Am. J. Psychiatry* 159, 1265–1283. doi: 10.1176/appi.ajp.159.8.1265

Nishi, M., Horii-Hayashi, N., Sasagawa, T., and Matsunaga, W. (2013). Effects of early life stress on brain activity: implications from maternal separation model in rodents. *Gen. Comp. Endocrinol.* 181, 306–309. doi: 10.1016/j.ygcen.2012.09.024

Noh, S. J., Ryu, V., Yoo, S. B., Lee, J. H., Min, B. M., and Jahng, J. W. (2008). Suppressed intake of highly palatable food and dysfunctional of HPA axis response to restraint stress in adolescent rats that experienced neonatal maternal separation. *Appetite* 51:388. doi: 10.1016/j.appet.2008.04.174

Plotsky, P. M., Thrivikraman, K. V., Nemeroff, C. B., Caldji, C., Sharma, S., and Meaney, M. J. (2005). Long-term consequences of neonatal rearing on central corticotropin-releasing factor systems in adult male rat offspring. *Neuropsychopharmacology* 30, 2192–2204. doi: 10.1038/sj.npp.1300769

Pryce, C. R., Ruedi-Bettschen, D., Dettling, A. C., Weston, A., Russig, H., Ferger, B., et al. (2005). Long-term effects of early-life environmental manipulations in rodents and primates: potential animal models in depression research. *Neurosci. Biobehav. Rev.* 29, 649–674. doi: 10.1016/j.neubiorev.2005.03.011

Rosenfeld, P., Gutierrez, Y. A., Martin, A. M., Mallett, H. A., Alleva, E., and Levine, S. (1991). Maternal regulation of the adrenocortical response in preweanling rats. *Physiol. Behav.* 50, 661–671. doi: 10.1016/0031-9384(91)90001-5

Ryu, V., Lee, J. H., Yoo, S. B., Gu, X. F., Moon, Y. W., and Jahng, J. W. (2008). Sustained hyperphagia in adolescent rats that experienced neonatal maternal separation. *Int. J. Obes. (Lond.)* 32, 1355–1362. doi: 10.1038/ijo.2008.108

Ryu, V., Yoo, S. B., Kang, D. W., Lee, J. H., and Jahng, J. W. (2009). Post-weaning isolation promotes food intake and body weight gain in rats that experienced neonatal maternal separation. *Brain Res.* 1295, 127–134. doi: 10.1016/j.brainres.2009.08.006

Sapolsky, R. M. (1996). Stress, glucocorticoids, and damage to the nervous System: the current state of confusion. *Stress* 1, 1–19. doi: 10.3109/10253899609001092

Sapolsky, R. M., and Meaney, M. J. (1986). Maturation of the adrenocortical stress response: neuroendocrine control mechanisms and the stress hyporesponsive period. *Brain Res.* 396, 64–76. doi: 10.1016/0165-0173(86)90010-X

Smith, P. M., and Ferguson, A. V. (2010). Circulating signals as critical regulators of autonomic state–central roles for the subfornical organ. *Am. J. Physiol. Regul. Integr. Comp. Physiol.* 299, R405–R415. doi: 10.1152/ajpregu.00103.2010

Stein, M. B., Walker, J. R., Anderson, G., Hazen, A. L., Ross, C. A., Eldridge, G., et al. (1996). Childhood physical and sexual abuse in patients with anxiety disorders and in a community sample. *Am. J. Psychiatry* 153, 275–277.

Teicher, M. H., Tomoda, A., and Andersen, S. L. (2006). Neurobiological consequences of early stress and childhood maltreatment: are results from human and animal studies comparable? *Ann. N.Y. Acad. Sci.* 1071, 313–323. doi: 10.1196/annals.1364.024

Tjong, Y. W., Ip, S. P., Lao, L., Wu, J., Fong, H. H., Sung, J. J., et al. (2010). Neonatal maternal separation elevates thalamic corticotrophin releasing factor type 1 receptor expression response to colonic distension in rat. *Neuro Endocrinol. Lett.* 31, 215–220.

Vazquez, D. M., Lopez, J. F., Van Hoers, H., Watson, S. J., and Levine, S. (2000). Maternal deprivation regulates serotonin 1A and 2A receptors in the infant rat. *Brain Res.* 855, 76–82. doi: 10.1016/S0006-8993(99)02307-0

Walker, C. D., Scribner, K. A., Cascio, C. S., and Dallman, M. F. (1991). The pituitary-adrenocortical system of neonatal rats is responsive to stress throughout development in a time-dependent and stressor-specific fashion. *Endocrinology* 128, 1385–1395. doi: 10.1210/endo-128-3-1385

17

Urinary oxytocin positively correlates with performance in facial visual search in unmarried males, without specific reaction to infant face

Atsuko Saito[1]*, Hiroki Hamada[2], Takefumi Kikusui[3], Kazutaka Mogi[3], Miho Nagasawa[3], Shohei Mitsui[3], Takashi Higuchi[4], Toshikazu Hasegawa[1] and Kazuo Hiraki[2,5]*

[1] Department of Cognitive and Behavioral Science, Graduate School of Arts and Sciences, The University of Tokyo, Tokyo, Japan
[2] Department of General Systems Studies, Graduate School of Arts and Sciences, The University of Tokyo, Tokyo, Japan
[3] Department of Animal Science and Biotechnology, Azabu University, Kanagawa, Japan
[4] Faculty of Medical Sciences, University of Fukui, Fukui, Japan
[5] JST, CREST, Tokyo, Japan

***Correspondence:**
Atsuko Saito, Department of Cognitive and Behavioral Science, Graduate School of Arts and Sciences, The University of Tokyo, 3-8-1 Komaba, Meguro-ku, Tokyo 153-8902, Japan
e-mail: casaito@mail.ecc.u-tokyo.ac.jp;
Kazuo Hiraki, Department of General Systems Studies, Graduate School of Arts and Sciences, The University of Tokyo, 3-8-1 Komaba, Meguro-ku, Tokyo 153-8902, Japan
e-mail: khiraki@idea.c.u-tokyo.ac.jp

The neuropeptide oxytocin plays a central role in prosocial and parental behavior in non-human mammals as well as humans. It has been suggested that oxytocin may affect visual processing of infant faces and emotional reaction to infants. Healthy male volunteers ($N = 13$) were tested for their ability to detect infant or adult faces among adult or infant faces (facial visual search task). Urine samples were collected from all participants before the study to measure the concentration of oxytocin. Urinary oxytocin positively correlated with performance in the facial visual search task. However, task performance and its correlation with oxytocin concentration did not differ between infant faces and adult faces. Our data suggests that endogenous oxytocin is related to facial visual cognition, but does not promote infant-specific responses in unmarried men who are not fathers.

Keywords: oxytocin, social cognition, infant, visual search, cognitive task

INTRODUCTION

Oxytocin is a 9-amino-acid peptide that is produced in the hypothalamus and is released into the brain and bloodstream (Donaldson and Young, 2008). It was originally known as a hormone that increases uterus contractions during labor and stimulates the ejection of milk. In the past few decades, although controversial, current evidence suggest that oxytocin has a role to play in social and maternal behavior. Rats treated with oxytocin receptor antagonists and oxytocin knockout mice are unable to recognize previously encountered conspecifics (Engelmann et al., 1998; Ferguson et al., 2000). In prairie voles, infusion of oxytocin in the ventricle promotes pair bond formation in virgin females (Williams et al., 1994; Insel and Hulihan, 1995). Infusion of oxytocin into the ventricle can also initiate maternal behaviors in virgin female rats, such as nest building as well as licking and retrieving pups (Pedersen and Prange, 1979; Pedersen et al., 1982).

In humans, the role of oxytocin in maternal behavior and mother–infant relations, as well as in paternal behavior and father–infant relations, has been investigated. Plasma oxytocin levels in mothers positively correlated to the amount of maternal bonding behaviors, such as gaze, vocalizations, affectionate touch, mother–infant behavioral synchrony, and attachment style (Feldman et al., 2007, 2011; Strathearn et al., 2009; Gordon et al., 2010a,b). Paternal behavior and father–infant affect synchrony have also been associated with oxytocin levels in plasma and saliva (Gordon et al., 2010a,b,c; Feldman et al., 2011). Both fathers and mothers who provide high levels of contact toward their infants show increased salivary oxytocin following parent–infant interactions, and such an increase is not observed among parents displaying low levels of contact (Feldman et al., 2010). These results suggest that peripheral oxytocin levels are positively related to maternal and paternal behavior, and to parental attachment to infants in mothers and fathers.

Evidence indicating that intranasal oxytocin administration affects social perception, cognition, and behavior in a non-parental context is accumulating (Bos et al., 2012; Churchland and Winkielman, 2012; Guastella and Macleod, 2012; Van Ijzendoorn and Bakermans-Kranenburg, 2012; Zink and Meyer-Lindenberg, 2012). However, it is still not clear whether exogenously administered oxytocin, which increases oxytocin level temporally, has the same effects on social cognition or behavior as basal oxytocin levels. In fact, in the context of a trust game, administered oxytocin causes a substantial increase in trust (Kosfeld et al., 2005), but baseline plasma oxytocin levels do not associate with trust (Zak et al., 2005). In parental contexts, although some research investigated the relationship between oxytocin and perception for infants stimuli or paternal behavior by using intranasal oxytocin administration (Riem et al., 2011; Rupp et al., 2012; Weisman et al., 2012, 2014), the role of oxytocin in infant stimuli perception remains to be evaluated (Van Ijzendoorn and Bakermans-Kranenburg, 2012).

The cognitive processes associated with the perception of infant stimuli that relate to parental behavior are unknown. As mentioned above, many previous studies investigating the relationship between parental behavior and endocrinology focused on observed, direct behavior toward infants, or subjective evaluation of emotion against infants in parents (Fleming et al., 1987; Feldman et al., 2007; Gordon et al., 2010a). In addition, some neuroimaging studies have examined brain activation in response to infant stimuli (Swain, 2008), and a few researchers have reported the cognitive effects of infant stimuli (Brosch et al., 2007, 2008; Nittono et al., 2012). However, the question of how infant stimuli are processed, cognitively, remains open. Given the response to infant stimuli can be related to maltreatment of infants, it is important for researchers to understand these cognitive processes.

In rodents, the role of endocrinological factors, including oxytocin, in parental behavior has been investigated in both parental and non-parental individuals. However, in humans, it is mainly investigated in parents. Currently, we do not know whether oxytocin has the same role in non-parental humans as observed in parental individuals because parents have a different physiological status from those of non-parents. For example, fathers and mothers who have young children have lower testosterone levels than non-fathers and non-mothers (Kuzawa et al., 2010; Gettler et al., 2011). Compared to non-fathers, primate fathers that help mothers raise their young like humans have an increased density of dendritic spines on pyramidal neurons and increased vasopressin receptors in the prefrontal cortex (Kozorovitskiy et al., 2006). Therefore, the effect of oxytocin on parental behavior or response to infant stimuli in non-parents may differ from that in parents.

The purpose of this study was to investigate the role of oxytocin in non-parents in response to infant faces with comparison to adult faces. We measured urinary oxytocin levels just before the cognitive test in non-married, non-father men. We adopted the baseline peripheral oxytocin levels because nearly all previous research about oxytocin's role in parental behavior has treated them as mentioned above. We measured urinary oxytocin because it is related to social interactions (Fries et al., 2005; Nagasawa et al., 2009; Seltzer et al., 2010; Snowdon et al., 2010; Crockford et al., 2013; Wittig et al., 2014) and its sampling is non-invasive. Urinary oxytocin has a linear association with plasma oxytocin level (Amico et al., 1987; Romero et al., 2014). Women were excluded from our study to rule out possible interactions with circulating gonadal steroids (Salonia et al., 2005). Because infant faces attract human attention in the dot-probe task (Brosch et al., 2007, 2008), we measured non-parents' reaction to infants by using the attention task. The task was visual search of infant and adult faces. This task is important, requiring attention during an active scan of the visual environment, as participants search for a particular object or feature (the target) among other objects or features (distracters); it is considered a key paradigm in attention research for the investigation of selective attention (Muller and Krummenacher, 2006). If oxytocin is positively related to the responsiveness to infants, the performance for infant faces, or the performance difference between the reaction time for infant faces and that for adult faces, will negatively correlate with urinary oxytocin levels.

MATERIALS AND METHODS

PARTICIPANTS

Thirteen healthy young men aged 21–33 years ($M = 26.08$, $SD = 3.43$) were recruited from the student population of the University of Tokyo. All had normal or corrected-to-normal vision according to self-report. All were non-married and had no offspring. All protocols were approved by the Research Ethics Committee of the University of Tokyo (subject No. 229-2). Written informed consent was obtained from the participants and participants gave permission to use their data in the analyses.

STIMULI AND APPARATUS

The stimuli consisted of adult stimuli and infant stimuli. Twenty chromatic infant face photographs consisting of 10 male and 10 female Japanese infants aged from 6 to 9 months old ($M = 6.5$, $SD = 0.81$) were prepared to make infant stimuli. Ten chromatic adult face photographs consisting of 6 male and 4 female Japanese adults aged 19–34 years ($M = 23.7$, $SD = 4.43$) and 10 photographs from the Ekman and Friesen (1976) database consisting of 4 male and 6 female Asian neutral faces were prepared to make adult stimuli. These 40 photographs were morphed using Sqirlz Morph software (Xiberpix, Solihull, UK; http://www.xiberpix.net/SqirlzMorph.html). First, 4 morphed faces were made from the following categories: adult males, adult females, infant males, and infant females. These 4 morphed faces were mixed with each original face of the same category with a mixture ratio of 1:2. All photographs were presented in gray scale, matched in brightness and contrast, and pasted onto a black background.

A 16-inch color CRT monitor attached to a PC was used to display the experimental tasks. The experimental control software was written with E-Prime 2.0 (Psychological Software Tools).

PROCEDURE

Performances were tested using a within-subjects design with 3 factors: target (present vs. absent), distracter's age category (adult vs. infant), and set size—the number of elements in the presentation. We used a variety of set sizes: 3, 4, and 6. Each trial started with the presentation of a white fixation cross (1.2×1.2 cm) for 500 ms. Next, the stimulus faces were presented. The faces were 5.7 cm high × 4.5 cm wide on the screen, and were presented at a distance of 5.8 cm between the fixation cross and the center of the image. Participants were placed 60 cm from the screen using a chin-rest. This resulted in a visual angle of 5.5° between the fixation cross and the center of the image. Participants were instructed to press the "same" button (a numeric key 1 or 2) if all faces were the same age category and the "different" button (a numeric key 2 or 1) if one of the faces differed in the age category from the rest. The combinations of numeric keys were assigned randomly to each participant. Participants were also asked to respond as quickly and accurately as possible. The stimulus faces remained on the screen for 6000 ms or until the participant responded (**Figure 1**).

For each set size, there were 160 trials composed of 4 blocks of 40. There were 12 blocks in total, which were preceded by a block of 8 practice trials. The order of the blocks differed across participants.

MEASUREMENT OF URINARY OXYTOCIN

Urine was collected from participants just before the visual search task between 1400 and 1800. Participants were instructed to abstain from food and drink for 2 h before urine sampling. An hour before this urine sampling, participants urinated and were instructed to abstain from exercise, stressful activity (e.g., seeing exciting movies), and sleeping. Immediately after collection, urine samples were centrifuged at 4°C in a refrigerated centrifuge, and frozen at −80°C until assayed. Urinary oxytocin concentrations were measured using radioimmunoassays (Mitsui et al., 2011). Creatinine concentrations were measured using the Jaffe reaction using 96-well microplates (3881-096, Asahi Glass Co., Japan). The plate was read at an optical density of 450 nm by using a microplate reader. Urinary oxytocin levels are expressed as the oxytocin to creatinine ratio. The intra-assay coefficient of variation was 4.26%.

RESULTS

BEHAVIORAL DATA

Data from all participants were analyzed because error rates were lower than 10%. The average error rate was 5.0%. Only reaction times (RTs) to correctly identified targets and correctly rejected non-targets were included in the analyses. Before the analysis, RTs were filtered for outliers. All RTs lying more than 2 standard deviations above or below the individual mean were excluded from the analyses. Average RTs and differences between the reaction time for infant faces and for adult faces (RTs for Infant target or distracters - RTs for Adult target or distracters) are summarized in **Table 1**.

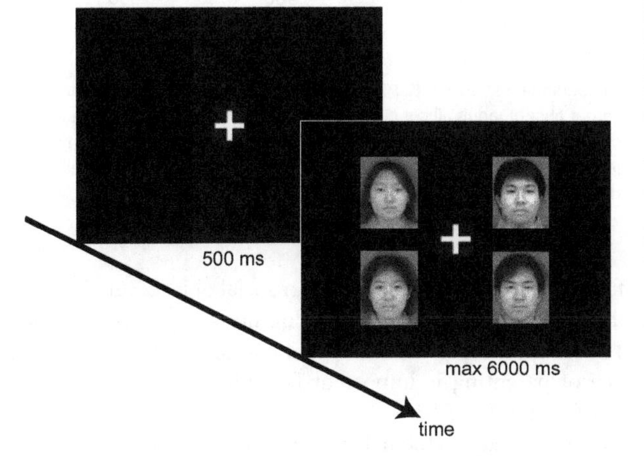

FIGURE 1 | Experimental sequence of the visual search task.

ASSOCIATION BETWEEN OXYTOCIN LEVELS AND PERFORMANCE IN VISUAL SEARCH

As one participant's oxytocin concentration was extremely high (2031.79 pg/mg), we analyzed other 12 participants' data. The average oxytocin concentrations was 344.38 pg/mg (range: 117.38–753.36, $SD = 196.18$). We calculated Speaman's correlation coefficients between RTs in the visual search task and urinary oxytocin levels (**Figure 2**). As shown in **Figures 2A–L**, the reaction time for the visual search task negatively correlated with urinary oxytocin levels; that is, the performance positively correlated with oxytocin levels. The correlation coefficients (Speamans rho) were significant for the adult target conditions of set size 3 ($rho = -0.587$, $p = 0.045$, **Figure 2A**), and the adult condition of set size 6 and the infant condition of set size 3 in target absent condition ($rho = -0.706$, $p = 0.010$; $rho = -0.587$, $p = 0.045$, respectively, **Figures 2I,J**). We also calculated the statistical power of our experiments. This analysis revealed that correlations that were statistically significant had sufficient statistical power (~0.5, **Figure 2**). In contrast, there were no consistent tendencies in the differences between the reaction time for infant faces and adult faces (**Figures 3A–F**).

DISCUSSION

Our results show that performance of the visual search task positively correlated with urinary oxytocin levels. This is the first presentation of the relationship between peripheral oxytocin levels and the performance of cognitive tasks. The response for social stimuli, both of infant and adult faces, was accelerated by high oxytocin levels. This result is consistent with many previous studies in which intranasal oxytocin administration promoted positive responses in social contexts (Kosfeld et al., 2005; Zak et al., 2007; Baumgartner et al., 2008; Petrovic et al., 2008; Theodoridou et al., 2009). However, arginine vasopressin, a neuropeptide that has a similar amino acid sequence and function as oxytocin, enhanced performance in a simple reaction time task when it was delivered by intranasal spray (Beckwith et al., 1983; Jennings

Table 1 | Average RTs (ms) and standard deviations for target-present and target-absent trials and differences between the reaction time for infant faces and that for adult faces.

Set size	3		4		6	
	M	*SD*	*M*	*SD*	*M*	*SD*
TARGET PRESENT						
Adult target	855.259	155.215	873.335	117.583	972.834	123.608
Infant target	843.201	135.803	875.097	137.499	963.807	90.290
Difference	−12.059	50.304	1.762	70.636	−9.027	65.710
TARGET ABSENT						
Adult all	856.670	149.689	860.864	120.309	1046.755	138.065
Infant all	742.284	102.438	752.219	101.178	937.447	105.662
Difference	−114.386	68.782	−108.645	64.621	−109.308	86.976

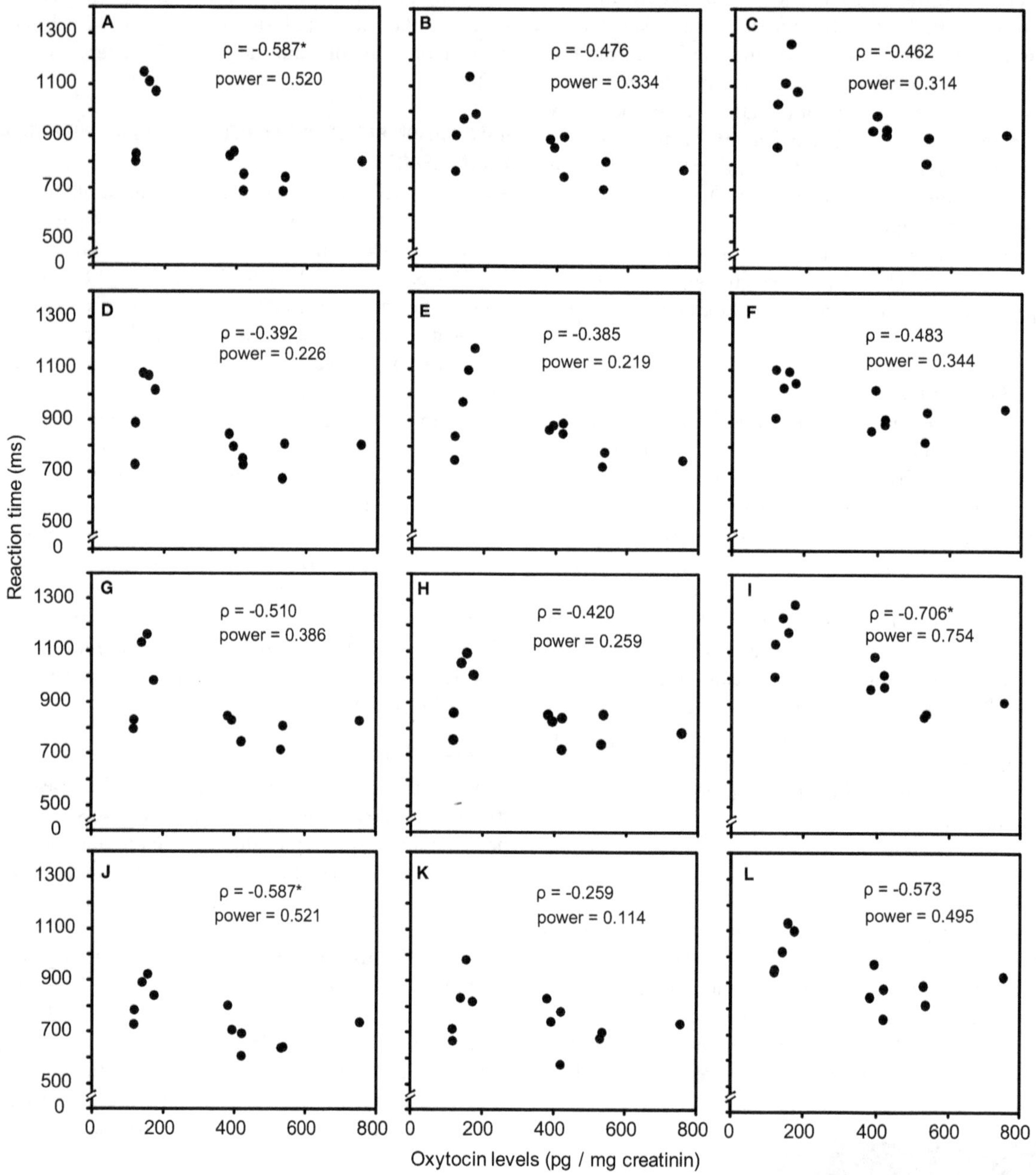

FIGURE 2 | Correlation between urinary oxytocin levels and reaction times (A–L). (A) Target present, adult target condition, set size 3; **(B)** Target present, adult target condition, set size 4; **(C)** Target present, adult target condition, set size 6; **(D)** Target present, infant target condition, set size 3; **(E)** Target present, infant target condition, set size 4; **(F)** Target present, infant target condition, set size 6; **(G)** Target absent, adult all condition, set size 3; **(H)** Target absent, adult all condition, set size 4; **(I)** Target absent, adult all condition, set size 6; **(J)** Target absent, infant all condition, set size 3; **(K)** Target absent, infant all condition, set size 4; **(L)** Target absent, infant all condition, set size 6. *indicates $p < 0.05$.

et al., 1986). Oxytocin may also have a similar effect. In this case, the current results can easily be explained by the enhancement effect of oxytocin on the simple reaction time task. To clarify this issue, it is necessary to perform experiments using non-social stimuli. Collectively, although the results are preliminary due to the relatively small sample size, this is the first presentation of the relationship between endogenous oxytocin levels and the performance of cognitive tasks, which can explain the individual differences in visual search ability for social object. But we cannot find any relationship between endogenous oxytocin and visual search for infant faces in unmarried males, indicating that experience of parenting is important for enhance the visual search ability for infants.

We measured oxytocin levels in urine. There is some controversy surrounding the relationship between oxytocin levels in urine and plasma (Amico et al., 1987; Feldman et al., 2011).

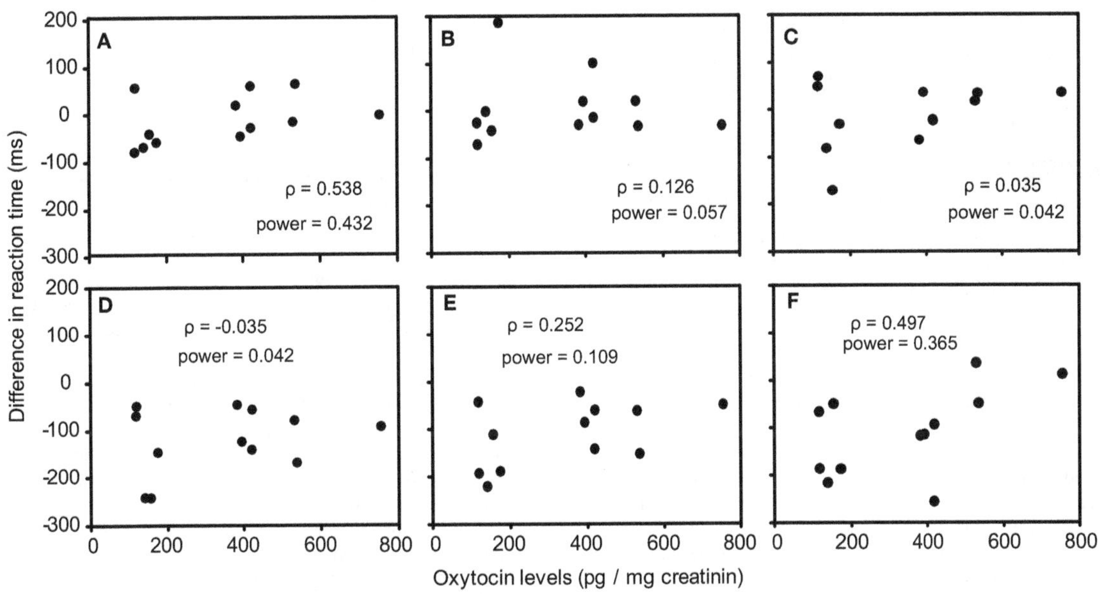

FIGURE 3 | Correlation between urinary oxytocin levels and differences between the reaction times for infant faces and adult faces (A–F). (A) Target present, set size 3; **(B)** Target present, set size 4; **(C)** Target present, set size 6; **(D)** Target absent, set size 3; **(E)** Target present, set size 4; **(F)** Target present, set size 6.

However, it is understandable that Feldman et al. (2011) described no correlation between urinary oxytocin and plasma oxytocin, as they measured urine and plasma at a single time point. Urinary oxytocin reflects oxytocin that has accumulated in the kidney over a period of approximately an hour. In our study, participants urinated an hour before urine sampling, and were then instructed to abstain from exercise, stressful activities (e.g., watching exciting movies), and sleeping. Therefore, our samples reflect accumulated oxytocin, excreted from the kidney over the course of an hour. In addition, we recently demonstrated a significant positive correlation between plasma oxytocin and urinary oxytocin levels in dogs (Romero et al., 2014). These results indicate that urinary oxytocin is a non-invasive biomarker that can be used to assess oxytocin activity. There is still debate over whether peripheral measures of oxytocin are related to central measures of oxytocin. However, non-invasive measures, such as urinary oxytocin, hold research and therapeutic advantages (Crockford et al., 2014). Our results improve the understanding of effects of peripheral oxytocin.

The results were somewhat different from the expected ones. The oxytocin levels positively correlated to the detected speed of infant faces as well as to that for adult faces. In addition, oxytocin levels did not relate to differences between the reaction time for infant faces and that for adult faces. A positive relationship between peripheral oxytocin and specific reaction to infants was not observed. These results seem inconsistent with the previous results showing that peripheral oxytocin levels positively correlated with paternal behavior (Gordon et al., 2010a,b,c; Feldman et al., 2011). The reason for this inconsistency may be caused by the difference in features of the participants. Almost all of the previous studies investigating the effect of oxytocin on parental behavior targeted actual parents. In contrast, the participants in our studies were non-married and non-father males. Although fathers do not have different peripheral oxytocin levels from non-fathers (Gray et al., 2007), the physical conditions of fathers, including testosterone levels, differ from those of non-fathers (Kuzawa et al., 2010; Gettler et al., 2011). These differences may explain the inconsistency between the previous studies and our study. There is the possibility that other hormonal levels interact with oxytocin and affect parent-like behavior. For example, testosterone affects expression of the oxytocin receptor in central nervous system (Arsenijevic and Tribollet, 1998) and oxytocin interacts with testosterone level and parental behavior (Weisman et al., 2014). That is, people who have different attributions, including marital status or parenthood, have different effects of oxytocin on parental behavior. Becoming fathers may change the response to infants: the effect of oxytocin on responses specialized for infants will be shown in fathers.

Our results reveal that high oxytocin levels do not always facilitate the specific reaction to infants. As Bartz et al. (2011) pointed out, the effects of oxytocin are constrained by situations and/or individualities. Therefore, it is necessary to study them by considering the features of the participants as discussed above. In addition to the different effects of oxytocin depending on the individual traits, a couple of recent studies demonstrated that oxytocin's social effects are context-dependent (Cardoso et al., 2013; Scheele et al., 2014). We should also take the difference in context into consideration when we investigate the effects of oxytocin.

AUTHOR CONTRIBUTIONS

Conceived and designed the experiments: Atsuko Saito, Hiroki Hamada, and Kazuo Hiraki. Performed the experiments: Hiroki Hamada Analyzed the data: Hiroki Hamada, Atsuko Saito, and Kazuo Hiraki. Hormonal measurement: Hiroki Hamada, Takefumi Kikusui, Kazutaka Mogi, Miho Nagasawa, and Shohei Mitsui and Takashi Higuchi. Prepared the manuscript: Atsuko Saito and Hiroki Hamada. Organized the research project: Kazuo Hiraki and Toshikazu Hasegawa.

ACKNOWLEDGMENTS

This work was supported by JSPS KAKENHI Grant Number 23700307 (to Atsuko Saito), 25118007 (to Takefumi Kikusui), 25118003 (to Toshikazu Hasegawa), 22240026 (to Kazuo Hiraki) and Crest JST (to Kazuo Hiraki).

REFERENCES

Amico, J. A., Ulbrecht, J. S., and Robinson, A. G. (1987). Clearance studies of oxytocin in humans using radioimmunoassay measurements of the hormone in plasma and urine. *J. Clin. Endocrinol. Metab.* 64, 340–345. doi: 10.1210/jcem-64-2-340

Arsenijevic, Y., and Tribollet, E. (1998). Region-specific effect of testosterone on oxytocin receptor binding in the brain of the aged rat. *Brain Res.* 785, 167–170. doi: 10.1016/S0006-8993(97)01429-7

Bartz, J. A., Zaki, J., Bolger, N., and Ochsner, K. N. (2011). Social effects of oxytocin in humans: context and person matter. *Trends Cogn. Sci.* 15, 301–309. doi: 10.1016/j.tics.2011.05.002

Baumgartner, T., Heinrichs, M., Vonlanthen, A., Fischbacher, U., and Fehr, E. (2008). Oxytocin shapes the neural circuitry of trust and trust adaptation in humans. *Neuron* 58, 639–650. doi: 10.1016/j.neuron.2008.04.009

Beckwith, B. E., Couk, D. I., and Till, T. S. (1983). Vasopressin analog influences the performance of males on a reaction time task. *Peptides* 4, 707–709. doi: 10.1016/0196-9781(83)90022-0

Bos, P. A., Panksepp, J., Bluthe, R. M., and Van Honk, J. (2012). Acute effects of steroid hormones and neuropeptides on human social-emotional behavior: a review of single administration studies. *Front. Neuroendocrinol.* 33, 17–35. doi: 10.1016/j.yfrne.2011.01.002

Brosch, T., Sander, D., Pourtois, G., and Scherer, K. R. (2008). Beyond fear: rapid spatial orienting toward positive emotional stimuli. *Psychol. Sci.* 19, 362–370. doi: 10.1111/j.1467-9280.2008.02094.x

Brosch, T., Sander, D., and Scherer, K. R. (2007). That baby caught my eye attention capture by infant faces. *Emotion* 7, 685–689. doi: 10.1037/1528-3542.7.3.685

Cardoso, C., Ellenbogen, M. A., Serravalle, L., and Linnen, A.-M. (2013). Stress-induced negative mood moderates the relation between oxytocin administration and trust: evidence for the *tend-and-befriend* response to stress? *Psychoneuroendocrinology* 38, 2800–2804. doi: 10.1016/j.psyneuen.2013.05.006

Churchland, P. S., and Winkielman, P. (2012). Modulating social behavior with oxytocin: how does it work? What does it mean? *Horm. Behav.* 61, 392–3099. doi: 10.1016/j.yhbeh.2011.12.003

Crockford, C., Deschner, T., Ziegler, T. E., and Wittig, R. M. (2014). Endogenous peripheral oxytocin measures can give insight into the dynamics of social relationships: a review. *Front. Behav. Neurosci.* 8:68. doi: 10.3389/fnbeh.2014.00068

Crockford, C., Wittig, R. M., Langergraber, K., Ziegler, T. E., Zuberbuhler, K., and Deschner, T. (2013). Urinary oxytocin and social bonding in related and unrelated wild chimpanzees. *Proc. R. Soc. B Biol. Sci.* 280, 1471–2954. doi: 10.1098/rspb.2012.2765

Donaldson, Z. R., and Young, L. J. (2008). Oxytocin, vasopressin, and the neurogenetics of sociality. *Science* 322, 900–904. doi: 10.1126/science.1158668

Ekman, P., and Friesen, W. V. (1976). *Pictures of Facial Affect*. Palo Alto, CA: Consulting Psychologists Press.

Engelmann, M., Ebner, K., Wotjak, C. T., and Landgraf, R. (1998). Endogenous oxytocin is involved in short-term olfactory memory in female rats. *Behav. Brain Res.* 90, 89–94. doi: 10.1016/S0166-4328(97)00084-3

Feldman, R., Gordon, I., Schneiderman, I., Weisman, O., and Zagoory-Sharon, O. (2010). Natural variations in maternal and paternal care are associated with systematic changes in oxytocin following parent-infant contact. *Psychoneuroendocrinology* 35, 1133–1141. doi: 10.1016/j.psyneuen.2010.01.013

Feldman, R., Gordon, I., and Zagoory-Sharon, O. (2011). Maternal and paternal plasma, salivary, and urinary oxytocin and parent-infant synchrony: considering stress and affiliation components of human bonding. *Dev. Sci.* 14, 752–761. doi: 10.1111/j.1467-7687.2010.01021.x

Feldman, R., Weller, A., Zagoory-Sharon, O., and Levine, A. (2007). Evidence for a neuroendocrinological foundation of human affiliation: plasma oxytocin levels across pregnancy and the postpartum period predict mother-infant bonding. *Psychol. Sci.* 18, 965–970. doi: 10.1111/j.1467-9280.2007.02010.x

Ferguson, J. N., Young, L. J., Hearn, E. F., Matzuk, M. M., Insel, T. R., and Winslow, J. T. (2000). Social amnesia in mice lacking the oxytocin gene. *Nat. Genet.* 25, 284–288. doi: 10.1038/77040

Fleming, A. S., Steiner, M., and Anderson, V. (1987). Hormonal and attitudinal correlates of maternal behavior during the early postpartum period in first-time mothers. *J. Reprod. Infant Psyc.* 5, 193–205. doi: 10.1080/02646838708403495

Fries, A. B., Ziegler, T. E., Kurian, J. R., Jacoris, S., and Pollak, S. D. (2005). Early experience in humans is associated with changes in neuropeptides critical for regulating social behavior. *Proc. Natl. Acad. Sci. U.S.A.* 102, 17237–17240. doi: 10.1073/pnas.0504767102

Gettler, L. T., McDade, T. W., Feranil, A. B., and Kuzawa, C. W. (2011). Longitudinal evidence that fatherhood decreases testosterone in human males. *Proc. Natl. Acad. Sci. U.S.A.* 108, 16194–16199. doi: 10.1073/pnas.1105403108

Gordon, I., Zagoory-Sharon, O., Leckman, J. F., and Feldman, R. (2010a). Oxytocin and the development of parenting in humans. *Biol. Psychiatry* 68, 377–382. doi: 10.1016/j.biopsych.2010.02.005

Gordon, I., Zagoory-Sharon, O., Leckman, J. F., and Feldman, R. (2010b). Oxytocin, cortisol, and triadic family interactions. *Physiol. Behav.* 101, 679–684. doi: 10.1016/j.physbeh.2010.08.008

Gordon, I., Zagoory-Sharon, O., Leckman, J. F., and Feldman, R. (2010c). Prolactin, Oxytocin, and the development of paternal behavior across the first six months of fatherhood. *Horm. Behav.* 58, 513–518. doi: 10.1016/j.yhbeh.2010.04.007

Gray, P. B., Parkin, J. C., and Samms-Vaughan, M. E. (2007). Hormonal correlates of human paternal interactions: a hospital-based investigation in urban Jamaica. *Horm. Behav.* 52, 499–507. doi: 10.1016/j.yhbeh.2007.07.005

Guastella, A. J., and Macleod, C. (2012). A critical review of the influence of oxytocin nasal spray on social cognition in humans: evidence and future directions. *Horm. Behav.* 61, 410–418. doi: 10.1016/j.yhbeh.2012.01.002

Insel, T. R., and Hulihan, T. J. (1995). A gender-specific mechanism for pair bonding: oxytocin and partner preference formation in monogamous voles. *Behav. Neurosci.* 109, 782–789. doi: 10.1037/0735-7044.109.4.782

Jennings, J. R., Nebes, R. D., and Reynolds, C. F. 3rd. (1986). Vasopressin peptide (DDAVP) may narrow the focus of attention in normal elderly. *Psychiatry Res.* 17, 31–39. doi: 10.1016/0165-1781(86)90039-9

Kosfeld, M., Heinrichs, M., Zak, P. J., Fischbacher, U., and Fehr, E. (2005). Oxytocin increases trust in humans. *Nature* 435, 673–676. doi: 10.1038/nature03701

Kozorovitskiy, Y., Hughes, M., Lee, K., and Gould, E. (2006). Fatherhood affects dendritic spines and vasopressin V1a receptors in the primate prefrontal cortex. *Nat. Neurosci.* 9, 1094–1095. doi: 10.1038/nn1753

Kuzawa, C. W., Gettler, L. T., Huang, Y. Y., and McDade, T. W. (2010). Mothers have lower testosterone than non-mothers: evidence from the Philippines. *Horm. Behav.* 57, 441–447. doi: 10.1016/j.yhbeh.2010.01.014

Mitsui, S., Yamamoto, M., Nagasawa, M., Mogi, K., Kikusui, T., Ohtani, N., et al. (2011). Urinary oxytocin as a noninvasive biomarker of positive emotion in dogs. *Horm. Behav.* 60, 239–243. doi: 10.1016/j.yhbeh.2011.05.012

Muller, H. J., and Krummenacher, J. (2006). Visual search and selective attention. *Vis. Cogn.* 14, 389–410. doi: 10.1080/13506280500527676

Nagasawa, M., Kikusui, T., Onaka, T., and Ohta, M. (2009). Dog's gaze at its owner increases owner's urinary oxytocin during social interaction. *Horm. Behav.* 55, 434–441. doi: 10.1016/j.yhbeh.2008.12.002

Nittono, H., Fukushima, M., Yano, A., and Moriya, H. (2012). The power of kawaii: viewing cute images promotes a careful behavior and narrows attentional focus. *PLoS ONE* 7:e46362. doi: 10.1371/journal.pone.0046362

Pedersen, C. A., Ascher, J. A., Monroe, Y. L., and Prange, A. J. Jr. (1982). Oxytocin induces maternal behavior in virgin female rats. *Science* 216, 648–650. doi: 10.1126/science.7071605

Pedersen, C. A., and Prange, A. J. Jr. (1979). Induction of maternal behavior in virgin rats after intracerebroventricular administration of oxytocin. *Proc. Natl. Acad. Sci. U.S.A.* 76, 6661–6665. doi: 10.1073/pnas.76.12.6661

Petrovic, P., Kalisch, R., Singer, T., and Dolan, R. J. (2008). Oxytocin attenuates affective evaluations of conditioned faces and amygdala activity. *J. Neurosci.* 28, 6607–6615. doi: 10.1523/JNEUROSCI.4572-07.2008

Riem, M. M., Bakermans-Kranenburg, M. J., Pieper, S., Tops, M., Boksem, M. A., Vermeiren, R. R., et al. (2011). Oxytocin modulates amygdala, insula, and inferior frontal gyrus responses to infant crying: a randomized controlled trial. *Biol. Psychiatry.* 70, 291–297. doi: 10.1016/j.biopsych.2011.02.006

Romero, T., Nagasawa, M., Mogi, K., Hasegawa, T., and Kikusui, T. (2014). Oxytocin promotes social bonding in dogs. *Proc. Natl. Acad. Sci. U.S.A.* 111, 9085–9090. doi: 10.1073/pnas.1322868111

Rupp, H. A., James, T. W., Ketterson, E. D., Sengelaub, D. R., Ditzen, B., and Heiman, J. R. (2012). Amygdala response to negative images in postpartum vs nulliparous women and intranasal oxytocin. *Soc. Cogn. Affect. Neurosci.* 9, 48–54. doi: 10.1093/scan/nss100

Salonia, A., Nappi, R. E., Pontillo, M., Daverio, R., Smeraldi, A., Briganti, A., et al. (2005). Menstrual cycle-related changes in plasma oxytocin are relevant to normal sexual function in healthy women. *Horm. Behav.* 47, 164–169. doi: 10.1016/j.yhbeh.2004.10.002

Scheele, D., Kendrick, K. M., Khouri, C., Kretzer, E., Schläpfer, T. E., Stoffel-Wagner, B., et al. (2014). An oxytocin-induced facilitation of neural and emotional responses to social touch correlates inversely with autism traits. *Neuropsychopharmacology* 39, 2078–2085. doi: 10.1038/npp.2014.78

Seltzer, L. J., Ziegler, T. E., and Pollak, S. D. (2010). Social vocalizations can release oxytocin in humans. *Proc. R. Soc. B Biol. Sci.* 277, 2661–2666. doi: 10.1098/rspb.2010.0567

Snowdon, C. T., Pieper, B. A., Boe, C. Y., Cronin, K. A., Kurian, A. V., and Ziegler, T. E. (2010). Variation in oxytocin is related to variation in affiliative behavior in monogamous, pairbonded tamarins. *Horm. Behav.* 58, 614–618. doi: 10.1016/j.yhbeh.2010.06.014

Swain, J. E. (2008). Baby stimuli and the parent brain: functional neuroimaging of the neural substrates of parent-infant attachment. *Psychiatry* 5, 28–36.

Strathearn, L., Fonagy, P., Amico, J., and Montague, P. R. (2009). Adult attachment predicts maternal brain and oxytocin response to infant cues. *Neuropsychopharmacology* 34, 2655–2666. doi: 10.1038/npp.2009.103

Theodoridou, A., Rowe, A. C., Penton-Voak, I. S., and Rogers, P. J. (2009). Oxytocin and social perception: oxytocin increases perceived facial trustworthiness and attractiveness. *Horm. Behav.* 56, 128–132. doi: 10.1016/j.yhbeh.2009.03.019

Van Ijzendoorn, M. H., and Bakermans-Kranenburg, M. J. (2012). A sniff of trust: meta-analysis of the effects of intranasal oxytocin administration on face recognition, trust to in-group, and trust to out-group. *Psychoneuroendocrinology* 37, 438–443. doi: 10.1016/j.psyneuen.2011.07.008

Weisman, O., Zagoory-Sharon, O., and Feldman, R. (2012). Oxytocin administration to parent enhances infant physiological and behavioral readiness for social engagement. *Biol. Psychiatry* 72, 982–989. doi: 10.1016/j.biopsych.2012.06.011

Weisman, O., Zagoory-Sharon, O., and Feldman, R. (2014). Oxytocin administration, salivary testosterone, and father-infant social behavior. *Prog. Neuropsychopharmacol. Biol. Psychiatry* 49, 47–52. doi: 10.1016/j.pnpbp.2013.11.006

Williams, J. R., Insel, T. R., Harbaugh, C. R., and Carter, C. S. (1994). Oxytocin administered centrally facilitates formation of a partner preference in female prairie voles (Microtus ochrogaster). *J. Neuroendocrinol.* 6, 247–250. doi: 10.1111/j.1365-2826.1994.tb00579.x

Wittig, R. M., Crockford, C., Deschner, T., Langergraber, K. E., Ziegler, T. E., and Zuberbuhler, K. (2014). Food sharing is linked to urinary oxytocin levels and bonding in related and unrelated wild chimpanzees. *Proc. R. Soc. B Biol. Sci.* 281:20133096. doi: 10.1098/rspb.2013.3096

Zak, P. J., Kurzban, R., and Matzner, W. T. (2005). Oxytocin is associated with human trustworthiness. *Horm. Behav.* 48, 522–527. doi: 10.1016/j.yhbeh.2005.07.009

Zak, P. J., Stanton, A. A., and Ahmadi, S. (2007). Oxytocin increases generosity in humans. *PLoS ONE* 2:e1128. doi: 10.1371/journal.pone.0001128

Zink, C. F., and Meyer-Lindenberg, A. (2012). Human neuroimaging of oxytocin and vasopressin in social cognition. *Horm. Behav.* 61, 400–409. doi: 10.1016/j.yhbeh.2012.01.016

18

Pairmate-dependent pup retrieval as parental behavior in male mice

Mingkun Liang[1,2], Jing Zhong[1,2], Hong-Xiang Liu[1], Olga Lopatina[1], Ryusuke Nakada[2], Agnes-Mikiko Yamauchi[2] and Haruhiro Higashida[1]*

[1] *Department of Basic Research on Social Recognition and Memory, Research Center for Child Mental Development, Kanazawa University, Kanazawa, Japan*
[2] *Department of Biophysical Genetics, Graduate School of Medical Sciences, Kanazawa University, Kanazawa, Japan*

***Correspondence:**
*Haruhiro Higashida, Department of Basic Research on Social Recognition and Memory, Research Center for Child Mental Development, Kanazawa University, 13-1 Takara-machi, Kanazawa 920-8640, Japan
e-mail: haruhiro@med.kanazawa-u.ac.jp*

Appropriate parental care by fathers can greatly facilitate healthy human family life. However, much less is known about paternal behavior in animals compared to those regarding maternal behavior. Previously, we reported that male ICR strain laboratory mice, although not spontaneously parental, can be induced to display maternal-like parental care (pup retrieval) when separated from their pups by signals from the pairmate dam (Liu et al., 2013). This parental behavior by the ICR sires, which are not genetically biparental, is novel and has been designated as pairmate-dependent paternal behavior. However, the factors critical for this paternal behavior are unclear. Here, we report that the pairmate-dependent paternal retrieval behavior is observed especially in the ICR strain and not in C57BL/6 or BALB/c mice. An ICR sire displays retrieval behavior only toward his biological pups. A sire co-housed with an unrelated non-pairing dam in a new environment, under which 38-kHz ultrasonic vocalizations are not detected, does not show parenting behavior. It is important for sires to establish their own home territory (cage) by continuous housing and testing to display retrieval behavior. These results indicated that the ICR sires display distinct paternity, including father-child social interaction, and shed light on parental behavior, although further analyses of paternal care at the neuroendocrinological and neurocircuitry levels are required.

Keywords: parental behavior, paternal care, pup retrieval behavior, paternity, mouse

INTRODUCTION

According to Schor and others, "a stable, well-functioning family that consists of two parents and children is potentially the most secure, supportive, and nurturing environment in which children may be raised" (Schor and American Academy of Pediatrics Task Force on the Family, 2003; Fortunato and Archetti, 2010; Benbassat and Priel, 2012). Thus, the role of a father in the home is highly significant, and currently, the physical absence of the father in the home is seen as a major problem facing families worldwide (Feinberg, 2002; Fleming et al., 2002; Amato, 2005; Benbassat and Priel, 2012; Morrongiello et al., 2013; Bornovalova et al., 2014). This raises questions regarding which factors determine paternal care and how they are maintained. This may be addressed by behavioral studies and neuroendocrinological analysis of oxytocin, stress hormones, sex hormones, or epigenetic mechanisms (Ogawa et al., 1998; Pfaff et al., 1999; Nunes et al., 2001; Gammie, 2005; Jin et al., 2007; Bridges, 2008; Nishimori et al., 2008; Lee et al., 2009; Neumann, 2009; Chourbaji et al., 2011; Douglas, 2011; Morgan and Bale, 2011; Hashimoto et al., 2012; Higashida et al., 2012a,b; Parhar et al., 2012; Soga et al., 2012; Bambico et al., 2013; Salmina et al., 2013; Morrison et al., 2014).

Although a number of animal models have been used in experimental studies of parental care (Reburn and Wynne-Edwards, 1999; Carter et al., 2009; de Jong et al., 2009; McGraw and Young, 2010; Ozawa et al., 2010; Kuroda et al., 2011; Mogi et al., 2011; Saltzman and Maestripieri, 2011; Lambert et al., 2013; Tachikawa et al., 2013; Yoshida et al., 2013), given its value for genetic studies, a mouse model of paternal behavior may be especially useful (Hager and Johnstone, 2003; Jin et al., 2007; Liu et al., 2013). While some strains of the laboratory mouse *Mus musculus* become biparental (Wright and Brown, 2000; Chourbaji et al., 2011), a phenomenon called sensitization (Rosenblatt, 1967; Rosenblatt et al., 1996), little information is available regarding the factors that specifically induce male parental behavior (Gubernick and Alberts, 1987, 1989; Lonstein and De Vries, 2000; Kentner et al., 2010; Leuner et al., 2010).

Previously, we reported that the outbred ICR strain is uniparental and is a good model for studies of parental behavior (Jin et al., 2007; Liu et al., 2008, 2013; Higashida et al., 2012a), because these mice actively reproduce offspring and exhibit easily monitored pup retrieval after separation (Fujimoto et al., 2013; Liu et al., 2013), which is a reliable indicator of parental behavior (Gammie, 2005; Wynne-Edwards and Timonin, 2007; Yoshida et al., 2013). We demonstrated that male ICR mice display robust parental care, which is induced by signaling from the pairmate dam, after separation from the pups (Liu et al., 2013). We demonstrated that this signaling is mediated through as yet unidentified olfactory pheromonal cues and auditory 38-kHz ultrasonic vocalization (USV) cues (Liu et al., 2013), that the male response can be modified hormonally via oxytocin (Akther et al., 2013), that CD38 in the nucleus accumbens is critical (Akther et al., 2013), and that the central cholinergic system is involved (Fujimoto et al., 2013). However, the factors influencing singly isolated sires in which there is no direct communicative interaction between dams and sires remain unclear.

In the present study, to simplify fatherhood evaluation, we used an all-or-nothing type of pup retrieval behavior by calculating the percentage of sires that displayed retrieval behavior (Liu et al., 2013). We investigated paternal behavior in terms of the types of conditions that can induce or maintain paternal retrieval behavior by sires when the males are isolated before the offspring are delivered by pregnant mates, and the males are held separately to prevent them being sires by physically separating them from other family members for 3 days. Then, family ties are formed with or without mate information. In other experiments, we examined isolation from pups under different housing conditions in which either pairmate dam and pup olfactory information is present or excluded.

MATERIALS AND METHODS

ANIMALS

Male and female Slc:ICR, C57BL/6, and BALB/c mice were obtained from Japan SLC, Inc. (Hamamatsu, Japan) via a local distributor (Sankyo Laboratory Service Corporation, Toyama, Japan). The ICR mice were originally obtained from Charles River Laboratories in 1965 and since then bred in Japan with the alternative name Swiss CD1. The offspring of these mice were born in our laboratory colony, weaned at 21–28 days of age, and housed in same-sex groups of 3–5 animals until pairing (Liu et al., 2013). The animals were paired and kept in our laboratory under standard conditions (24°C; 12-h light/dark cycle, lights on at 08:00) with food and water *ad libitum*. The mice were housed together continuously in standard mouse maternity cages. The experiments were performed in accordance with the Guidelines for the Care and Use of Laboratory Animals of Kanazawa University.

BEHAVIORAL TESTING

Virgin males and females were paired at 45–55 d. A single male and a single female were continuously housed together in a standard mouse maternity cage from the mating period until the delivery of pups. In some experiments, the males were separated in new cages 1 day before parturition to prevent formation of family relationships and kept in the new cages for 3 days. Then, the males were allowed to meet their pups with or without pairmates from day 3 to day 5. All family units composed of a new sire (first-time father), dam, and their first litter were experimentally naïve.

One male parent was placed for 10 min in the original cage or new cage alone or with his pairmate (separation environment). Five pups were randomly selected from the litter and placed individually at a site remote from the nest in the original cage. The sires were returned to the original home cage or a new cage in the presence of their five biological or foster pups to assess parental behavior. Parental retrieval behavior (percentage of sires exhibiting retrieval) was examined for 10 min following reunion. The behavioral tests were performed in a randomly mixed sequence of experimental groups. Experiments were usually performed at 10:00–15:00. We defined retrieval as positive if the sires carried all 5 pups to the original nesting place or within two thirds of the distance between the nest and the place at which the pups had been placed (Liu et al., 2013). We also observed other parental behaviors (grooming, crouching, and huddling) as defined by Gubernick and Alberts (1987, 1989). The animals in this and subsequent experiments were tested only once.

MEASUREMENT OF USVs

Experiments were carried out in a soundproof chamber measuring 600 × 500 × 500 mm (model MC-050/VA; Muromachi Kikai, Tokyo, Japan). USVs were detected with a condenser microphone (Type 7016; Aco, Tokyo, Japan) and a preamplifier (type 4116; Aco) designed for sound pressure level (SPL) measurements between 20 Hz and 90 kHz. A 4-kHz band-pass filter was used to minimize background noise during recordings; however, most WAV files still contained a considerable amount of "non-USV" signal. Extraneous noise was identified and removed from the sonograms as far as possible. When a rater found an ultrasound signal that was difficult to interpret, the call was evaluated by a minimum of one additional trained observer and identification required a consensus by all raters. Each sonogram was then evaluated with a series of automated parameters. The microphone was placed 50 cm above the cage in a soundproof chamber and connected to an amplifier (model UMA-2; Muromachi Kikai). Acoustic signals were transmitted to a vocalization analyzer system (model MK-1500; Muromachi Kikai) with functions such as an analog-to-digital converter (192 kHz), frequency filters, a digital fast-Fourier-transform analyzer, and signal input—output terminals. Input signals were visualized on SpectraLAB (Sound Technology Inc., State College, PA) in the analyzer system on a personal computer. USVs were recorded as WAVE files and analyzed; the number of calls, frequency, and wave width (>40 ms) were measured using a USV monitor (Muromachi Kikai).

STATISTICAL ANALYSIS

The data were calculated as the means or the means ± s.e.m. Two-tailed Fisher's exact probability test was used for single comparisons of retrieval behaviors. The remaining data were analyzed by two-tailed Student *t*-test.

RESULTS

It has been reported that parental behavior in mice is dependent on the strain (Wright and Brown, 2000). Therefore, we first examined and compared parent–pup family units in three strains, i.e., ICR, C57BL/6, and BALB/c mice, under various experimental settings. The data are summarized in **Table 1**. Maternal nurturing behavior was observed in dams of all three strains, in a strain-nonspecific fashion, except for the low rate of retrieval by the BALB/c dams. In contrast, paternal behavior was variable between the strains. No retrieval behavior was observed by BALB/c sires ($n = 15$). C57BL/6 sires displayed retrieval during reunion after single-separation in new cages (approximately 40%, $n = 15$). However, isolation together with the partner in new cages did not potentiate but rather decreased this rate to 13.3% ($n = 15$). This parental behavior suggests that C57BL/6 males display mate-independent paternal behavior. Interestingly, 38-kHz USVs were

Table 1 | Parental behaviors in three strains of mice.

Behavior		Mouse strain		
		ICR ($n = 15$)	**C57BL/6 ($n = 15$)**	**BALB/c ($n = 15$)**
Dam	Retrieval	100% fast, rhythmic	100% fast, rhythmic	60% slow, interrupted
	Crouching	Over all pups	Over not all pups	Over all pups
	Grooming	Rare	Rare	Rare
	Nest building	Sometimes	Sometimes	Sometimes
Sire	Retrieval by separation	10%	40%	0%
	After co-housing pairmates	60%	10%	0%
		Fast (<4 min)	Very slow	–
		Smooth	Intermittent	–
	Crouching	Over not all pups	Not often	–
	Grooming	Rare	Rare	–
	Nest building	Not often	Rare	–
Pup	Number of pups per litter	~15	~5	~7
	Survival ratio	~100%	60–70%	~100%
	USVs	>70 calls/2 min	<20 calls/2 min	>80 calls/2 min
Communication from dams to sires with 38 kHz USVs		Detected	Not detected	Not detected
Pattern of paternal care		Mate-dependent	Mate-independent	None

not recorded from any dam–sire pairs of C57BL/6 and BALB/c strains separated in new cages for 10 min. These results indicated that pairmate-dependent care is specific to the ICR strain. Therefore, in the following experiments, we examined various critical conditions under which ICR strain males did or did not show paternal behavior.

RETRIEVAL BEHAVIOR BY SIRES SEPARATED ALONE IN HOME CAGES

The experimental paradigms for each experiment are shown schematically in each figure. In **Figure 1**, we first reproduced our previous results (Liu et al., 2013). Male and female ICR strain mice were paired and housed together continuously in a standard mouse maternity cage (**Figure 1A**). The mice were left undisturbed during the first 3 days after the birth of their pups (**Figure 1B**), during which they displayed distinct paternal and maternal behaviors as described previously (Liu et al., 2013). The sire and dam nursed the pups. This involved nest-building, pup retrieval, licking, and huddling over the pups and lactating. However, as described in the Methods section, we mainly analyzed the male's retrieval behavior, as a parental role, in the following experiments.

The sire in the first family was left alone in the vacated cage during the period of separation (**Figure 1C**), whereas the pups and dam were removed and placed in a new cage (**Figure 1D**) separated from the family cage. After 10 min, the five selected pups of the sire (biological offspring) were returned to the nursing cage in a remote area away from the nest, where the sire was present (**Figure 1E**). The sire retrieved the offspring over 10 min (86% of the sires, $n = 15$; **Figures 1F,S**).

If the non-biological (foster) pups (**Figure 1N**) of the third family (**Figures 1M,N**) were introduced into the vacated home cage with the second sire (**Figures 1I,K**) in the second family (**Figures 1G,H**), instead of the biological pups (**Figures 1H,J**), 33% of the 15 sires displayed pup retrieval (**Figures 1L,S**; two-tailed Fisher's exact probability test between sires toward biological (F) and non-biological (L) pups, $P < 0.01$).

When a sire from the third family (**Figure 1N**) was placed and isolated for 10 min in the home cage of the second family (**Figure 1O**), the third sire did not retrieve any of the foster (second family's) pups (**Figures 1R,S**; $n = 15$, two-tailed Fisher's exact probability test between unrelated sires (R) and sires with non-biological (L) or biological (F) pups, $P < 0.05$ and $P < 0.0001$, respectively). These results suggested that paternal pup retrieval behavior in the home cage is maintained by biological family cues of their mate dams and remaining pups.

RETRIEVAL BEHAVIOR BY SIRES AFTER SEPARATION IN NEW CAGES

Male parental care in **Figure 1** may have been induced by the fact that the males were left in the nursing environment during parent–pup separation. To select out pup information during isolation, we used the co-housing paradigm presented in **Figure 2**. We examined whether sires developed paternal behavior following time spent with the family. Pup retrieval increased on a daily basis after parturition, while dams displayed a higher retrieval ratio from the first day of parturition than the sires (**Table 2**).

The sires alone (**Figure 2D**) or together with the mate dams (**Figure 2H**) were placed in a new cage for 10 min, whereas the pups alone (**Figure 2G**) or together with dams (**Figure 2C**)

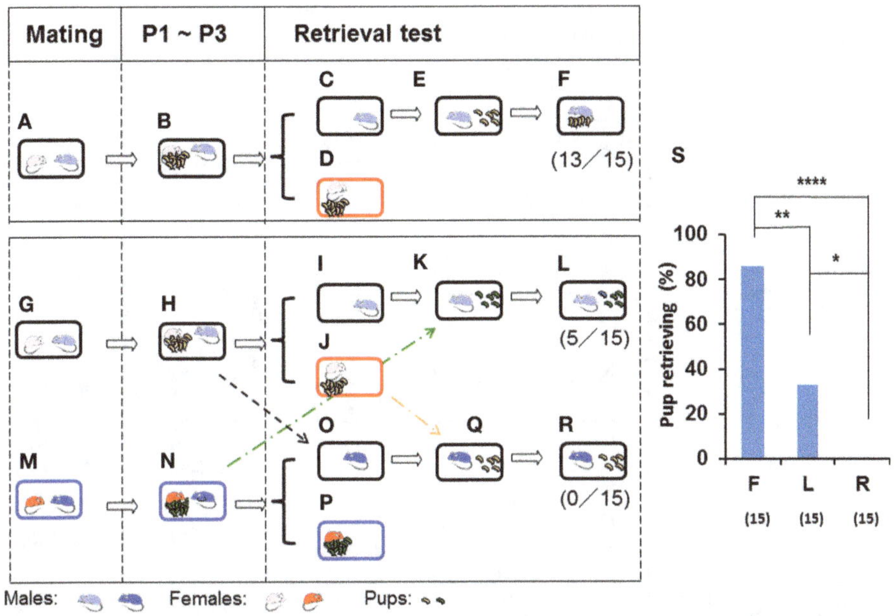

FIGURE 1 | Parental retrieval test in ICR mice for biological and non-biological pups. Schematic representations of the parental care test in three mated pairs **(A,G,M)**. After cohabiting with their pups as a family for 3 days from postnatal day 1 (P1) until postnatal day 3 (P3) **(B,H,N)**, the sires were separated in the home cage **(C,I,O)** from the pups and pairmates **(D,J,P)** for 10 min. The sires were then reunited with five biological **(E)** or non-biological **(K)** pups. Subsequent pup retrieval behavior over a 10-min period was then observed **(F,L)**. The third sire **(M,N)** was placed in the home cage **(O)** of another family **(H)**, and retrieval was tested for non-biological (another family's) pups in an unrelated cage **(Q,R)**. The numbers of positive mice/number of mice tested are shown in parentheses. The number of sires displaying retrieval behavior out of sires tested was expressed as a percentage **(S)**. $N = 15$ for each experiment. Two-tailed Fisher's exact probability test: between sires toward biological **(F)** and non-biological **(L)** pups or unrelated sires **(R)**, $^{**}P < 0.01$ and $^{****}P < 0.0001$, respectively; and between sires tested toward non-biological pups **(L)** and unrelated sires **(R)**, $^{*}P < 0.05$.

were left in the home cage. Then, the sires were returned to the home cages in which five pups remained (**Figures 2E,I**). The male's retrieval behavior was undiminished when housed with the pairmate (66%, $n = 30$; **Figures 2J,U**) but was strongly reduced when housed alone (24%, $n = 41$; **Figures 2F,U**). As expected, a high level of sire care was displayed after isolation in the new environment together with mate dams and pups (as the whole family (**Figures 2K,L**) (66%, $n = 15$; **Figure 2U**): two-tailed Fisher's exact probability test between sires separated alone (F) and together (J) or as a whole family (N), $P < 0.001$, equally.

The latter was specifically associated with co-habitation with the pairmate dam during the separation period (**Figure 2H**), because negligible retrieval behavior was apparent if the sire was housed with the dam of another brood (**Figures 2O–T**; 20%, $n = 15$); two-tailed Fisher's exact probability test shows no significant difference between sires separated together with unrelated dams (T) and alone (F); and separated together (J), $P < 0.01$; and separated as a whole family (N), $P < 0.05$, **Figure 2U**). Thus, it appears that the mate dam provides some signal(s) during the separation period to induce parental behavior in the sire, in agreement with the results reported previously (Liu et al., 2013). Whereas parental care by the dam is independent of the presence of the male or the housing environment, that by the male is strongly dependent on cues from the pairmate dam and/or home cage.

We recorded USVs (with >40 ms in wave width) to determine their role as one form of critical interactive information in this paradigm. We detected 38-kHz USVs identical to those reported previously (Liu et al., 2013) under isolation conditions in new cages for 10 min between sires and mate dams at a frequency of 25.9 ± 4.8 calls/10 min ($n = 8$, **Table 3**; $P < 0.01$ from other values, two-tailed Student t-test). No identical 38-kHz USVs were recorded between sires and unrelated dams. Instead, 30–80-kHz USVs were recorded infrequently at 40.7 ± 26.7 calls/10 min ($n = 11$) between unfamiliar couples. These 30–80-kHz USVs were emitted when a sire was co-housed with a virgin female at 313.6 ± 64.9 calls/10 min ($n = 11$, $P < 0.001$ from two other values, two-tailed Student t-test). These data clearly support the suggestion that paternal retrieval is essentially triggered by the pairmate's 38-kHz USVs.

RETRIEVAL BY ISOLATED BEFORE PAIRMATE PARTURITION

The retrieval behavior displayed by males may have been induced by family formation in the nursing cage environment. To assess this possibility, data were obtained from parting males (**Figures 3, 4**) that remained with the paired pregnant females 1 day before parturition of their first litter and were then separated into a new cage (**Figures 3A–C**). The males were then isolated alone for 3 days (**Figure 3E**). When sire paternal retrieval was examined immediately on day 3 in the sire home cage (**Figure 3K**), 21.4% of sires with no prior contact with their biological pups and pairmate dam, i.e., the paternity unformed state (**Figure 3E**), displayed retrieval behavior ($n = 42$; **Figure 3N**). Next, when the isolated males were relocated in the home cage

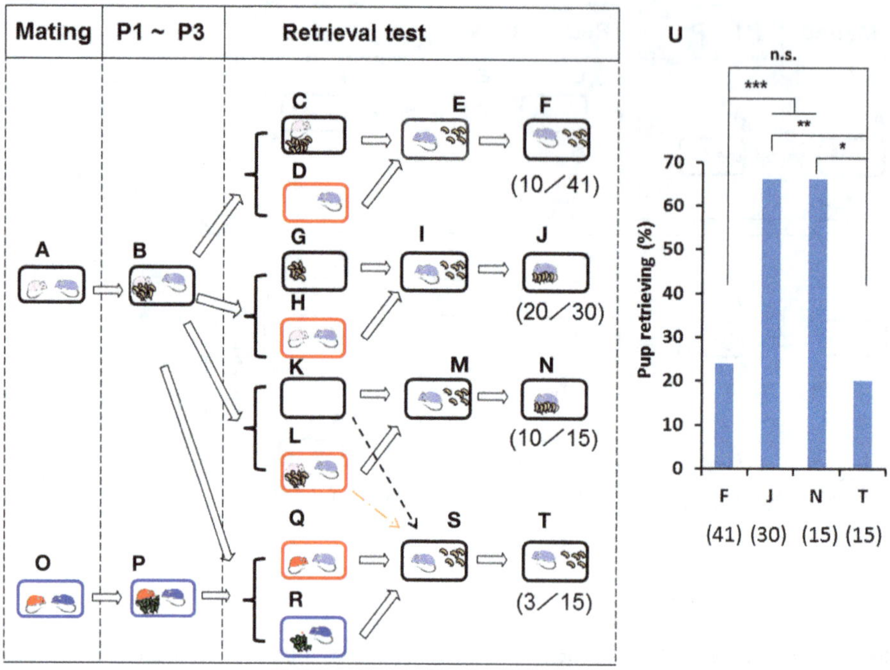

FIGURE 2 | Paternal retrieval test in ICR mice isolated in new cages. Paired couples were kept in rearing cages from mating to postnatal day 3 (P3) **(A,B,O,P)**. In **(C,D)**, the pups and the mating dam were left in their home cages **(C)**, and the sire alone was placed in a new holding cage **(D)**. In **(G,H)**, the pups were kept in the original cage, and the parents were placed in a new cage **(H)**. In **(K,L)**, the whole family was moved to a new cage **(L)**. In **(Q,R)**, the sire was kept during the separation period **(Q)** with a non-mating dam of another family **(O,P)**. After isolation for 10 min in each cage, pup retrieval behavior over a 10-min period was observed in each case **(E,I,M,S)**. The number of sires displaying retrieval behavior was scored **(F,J,N,T)**. The numbers of positive mice/number of mice tested are shown in parentheses and expressed as percentages **(U)**. Two-tailed Fisher's exact probability test: between sires separated alone **(F)** and together **(J)** or as a whole family **(N)**, $^{***}P < 0.001$ equally; between sires separated together **(J)** and as a whole family **(N)**, $^{**}P < 0.01$; between sires separated alone **(F)** and co-housed with unrelated dams **(T)**, not significant (n.s.); sires separated as a whole family **(N)** and co-housed with unrelated dams **(T)**, $^{*}P < 0.05$.

Table 2 | Percentages of sire's or dam's exhibiting retrieval behavior during the postpartum period.

Postnatal day of pups	Percentage of exhibiting retrieval behavior	
	By sires	By dams
1	14 (15)	55 (20)
2	40 (20)	90* (20)
3	65** (20)	90* (20)
4	70** (17)	85 (20)
5	65** (20)	75 (16)

*Number of mice tested are shown in parentheses. *, **Significantly different from day 1, $^{*}P < 0.05$ and $^{**}P < 0.01$, respectively, two-tailed Fisher's exact probability test.*

Table 3 | Number of USVs recorded from cages of sires co-housed with different types of females for 10 min.

	Type*	Number of USVs (calls/10 min)	(*n*)
	38-kHz	30–80-kHz	
With pairmate dam	25.9 ± 4.8**	0	(8)
With unrelated dam	0	40.7 ± 26.7	(11)
With virgin female	0	313.6 ± 64.9***	(11)

USVs (with >40 ms in duration) were recorded in n pairs.

**Judging from the previous results (Liu et al., 2013), 38-kHz USVs appear to be emitted from pairmate dams and 30–80-kHz USVs from sires.*

$^{**}P < 0.01$ or $^{***}P = 0.001$, from pairmate dams, unrelated dams or virgin females, respectively, two-tailed Student's t-test.

and stayed with the family (pups and pairmate dam) for 3 days (**Figure 3F**), the rate of retrieval in their home cage was only 4% ($n = 25$; **Figures 3G–J**). Although the sire lived together with the family for 3 days, such treatment made no contribution to the formation of paternity (two values in **Figure 3O** were equally very low; no significance, two-tailed Fisher's exact probability test).

To further analyze the relevance of family interaction during the stay as a whole family on postnatal days 3–5 (P3–P5) (**Figure 3**), we used the short-term pup exposure method (twice for 3 h for a total 6 h a day; **Figure 4**) to acquire or learn the process of paternity for the family. Males were isolated in new cages prior to parturition (**Figures 4B,C**) and kept in the cages for 2 days (**Figures 4D,E**). Then, pairmate dams and pups were relocated to the male's cage, and the whole family was kept there for 3 days (**Figure 4F**). Retrieval behavior was displayed by 8 (62%) of 13 sires (**Figures 4G–J**). The high level of retrieval appears to

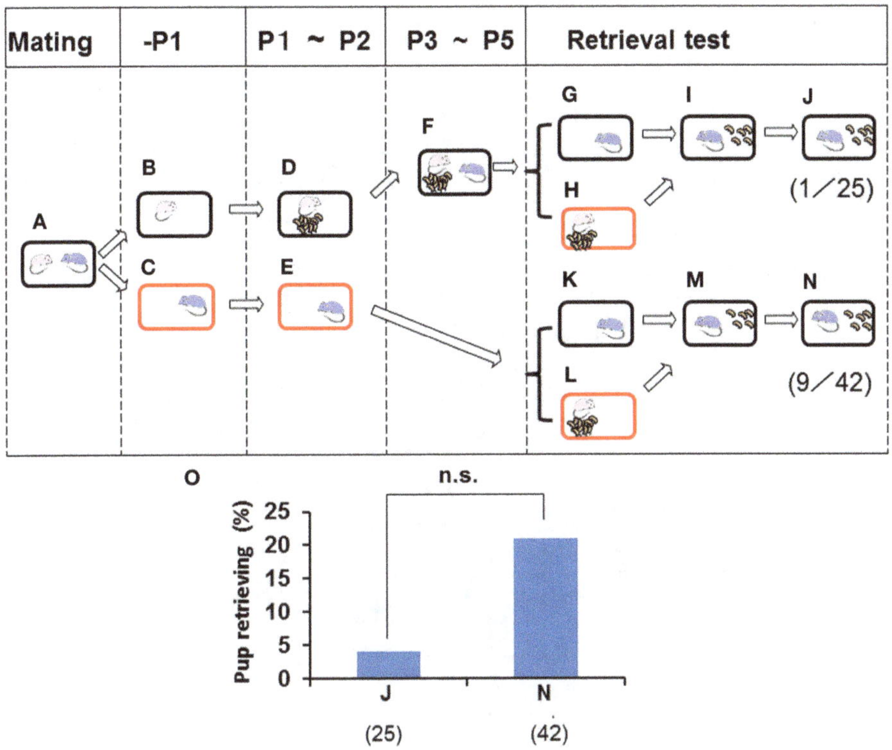

FIGURE 3 | Paternal retrieval test in ICR mice isolated prior parturition from the mating pair and then united as a whole family. A paired couple was kept in a rearing cage from mating **(A)** to 1 day before parturition, and the female and male were then kept in a home cage **(B)** or in a new cage **(C)**. The next day, the female delivered her pups **(D)** and remained until postnatal day 2 (P2). The male was kept continuously in the new cage until P2 **(E)**. From P3 to P5, the sire was introduced to the family cage with the dam and pups **(F)**. In another experiment, pup retrieval behavior over a 10-min period was examined for sires at P2 **(K–N)** or at P5 **(G–J)**. The number of sires displaying retrieval behavior was scored **(J,N)**. The numbers of positive mice/number of mice tested are shown in parentheses and expressed as percentages **(O)**. Note that two values in O are equally very low: no significance (n.s.) between **(J)** and **(N)**, two-tailed Fisher's exact probability test.

have been caused by continuously living in new cages that had been established as the male's territory.

In this suitable condition, we examined whether the presence of the dam was necessary for parental behavior by the isolated males. From P3 to P5, the pups and dam were kept together in their original home cages (**Figure 4K**), but the pups were temporarily transferred to the sire's cage twice for 3 h (a total of 6 h) per day (**Figure 4L**), and the males were otherwise alone for the rest of the day (18 h; **Figure 4M**). These sires showed retrieval behavior at a very high rate (17 (85%) of 20 sires tested; **Figures 4O–Q**). In both cases, the sires displayed a very high frequency of retrieval after living as the whole family or only with pups shortly in new cages that had, nevertheless, been established as the territory and established nest of the male, although no significant differences were observed between two types of sire (J and Q in **Figure 4R**; not significant, two-tailed Fisher's exact probability test). Furthermore, these results indicated that direct interaction with the mate dam is not necessary if the home territory is established by the sires.

Finally, we further examined the impact of territorial information on male retrieval behavior. Family cues were learned by individual sires in a manner identical to that shown in **Figure 4** (**Figures 5A–F**) during P3–P5, but in this case, via short exposure by transferring of their biological pups with their dams in new cages to the nursing cage with the sires. Then, retrieval behavior was examined under two housing conditions: in the sire's home cage in which the sire had stayed continuously (**Figures 5F,G,I–L**), or in a new cage (to the sires) in which the mate dams and pups had been staying (**Figures 5G,H,M–P**). In the home cages, 10 (50%) of 20 sires showed retrieval (**Figure 5L**), whereas only 3 (15%) of 20 sires in new cages displayed retrieval behavior ($P < 0.05$ between testing in old (L) and new (P) cages shown in **Figure 5Q**, two-tailed Fisher's exact probability test). In both cages, nests were established by the sire and dam. However, the new cages established by the sires' mate dams were quite new to the sires, even if the cages were fully filled with the mate dam's olfactory information.

DISCUSSION

The studies described here were performed to test several hypotheses that had not been explored previously (Akther et al., 2013; Fujimoto et al., 2013; Liu et al., 2013), pertaining to the various conditions responsible for parental behaviors other than the communicative interaction between sires and dams. Four findings are of particular interest: (1) among the mouse strains tested, the mate-dependent paternal retrieval behavior was observed only in

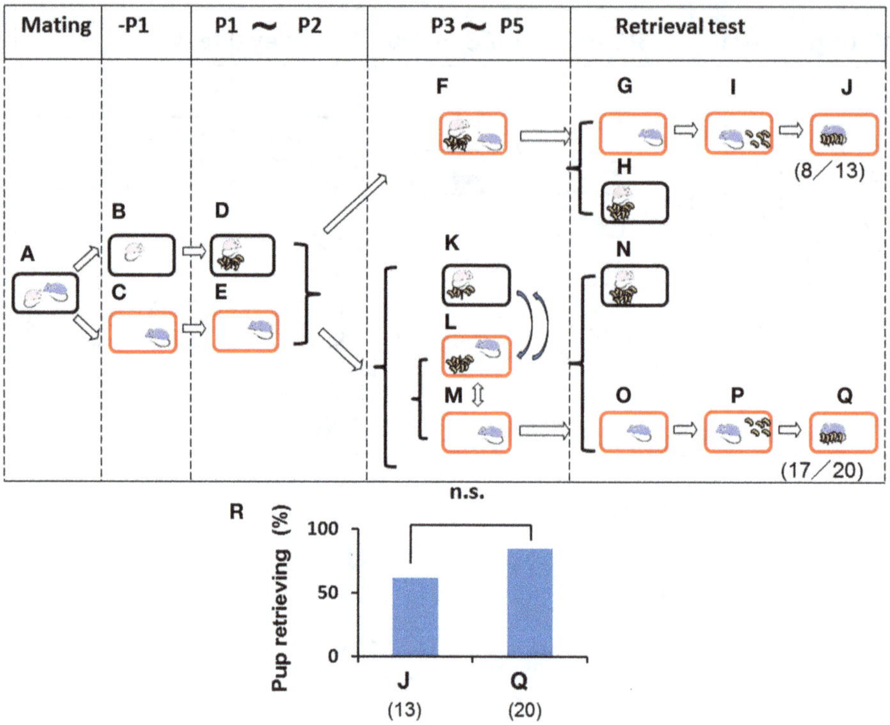

FIGURE 4 | Paternal retrieval test in mice isolated prior parturition from the mating pair and then united as a whole family or with pups only. A paired couple was kept in a rearing cage from mating **(A)** to 1 day before parturition. The female was kept in a home cage **(B)** and delivered her pups **(D)** and remained until postnatal day 2 (P2) **(D)**. The male was kept in a new cage before meeting the pups **(C)** and kept until P2 **(E)**. The dam and pups were introduced in the sire's own (new) cage and stayed as a whole family until P5 **(F)**. Instead of the whole family, in another experiment, only pups in home cages with their dams **(K)** were transferred twice for 3 h (total 6 h) a day to the sire's cage **(L)**. During the rest of the time from P3 to P5, the sire stayed alone **(M)**, and pups were located with the dam **(K)**. Pup retrieval behavior over a period of 10 min was examined (**G–J** and **N–Q**, respectively). The number of sires displaying retrieval behavior was scored **(J,Q)**. The numbers of positive mice/number of mice tested are shown in parentheses, and the numbers of sires displaying retrieval were expressed as percentages **(R)**. Note that the retrieval rate in two cases **(J,Q)** was high enough to have no significance (n.s.), two-tailed Fisher's exact probability test.

the ICR strain (**Table 1**), and acquisition of such paternal behavior increased slowly following parturition of the dam (**Table 2**); (2) the ICR sires displayed parental retrieval behavior only for their own biological pups (**Figure 1**); (3) interaction between the sires and unrelated non-mating dams is not effective (**Figure 2**) and does not involve 38-kHz USVs (**Table 3**); (4) it is important for the sire to establish its home cage (territory) by continuous housing to display parental retrieval behavior (**Figures 3–5**).

After separation from pups in the home or new cages with the sires alone or together with the pairmate dam, the sires displayed retrieval behavior, as shown in **Figures 2J,N**, in agreement with previous reports (Liu et al., 2013). We designated this behavior of the sire as mate-dependent parental behavior. In the present study, this particular behavior was specific to the ICR strain and was not observed in two other laboratory strains, i.e., C57BL/6 and BALB/c mice. Therefore, the ICR strain's mate-dependent retrieval is not a general behavior observed equally in all mice but is strain-specific. However, this does not reduce the value of our findings because the observed paternal behavior is unique. Furthermore, when considering human society, human males are not completely and genetically predisposed to display parental behavior. In this context, the behavior of the ICR strain may be a more suitable and novel model for investigating paternal behavior, comparing the genetically determined paternity, observed in animals such as voles or California mice (de Jong et al., 2009; Ahern et al., 2011).

The ICR sires displayed parental retrieval behavior only for their biological pups, indicating that they can discriminate between their biological and non-biological offspring. This discrimination likely depends on odor or USV (Kuroda et al., 2007, 2011). The characteristic 38-kHz USVs were not recorded during co-housing of ICR sires with non-mate dams, suggesting that the sires can distinguish the mate from non-mate dams or that the dams can distinguish the mate from non-mate sires. These results strongly support our suggestion that 38-kHz USVs are critical and have context for sires to induce retrieval behavior.

In these experiments, we examined the olfactory information of pups and cages (homes) for the sires prior to separation from the mate dam and their offspring. In habituation as a family, the presence of the mate was not completely essential. Interestingly, we estimated that the territory information is much more important to sires than the pheromones in the cages once they had established their home cage. Surprisingly, when the sires were continuously housed in their newly established home

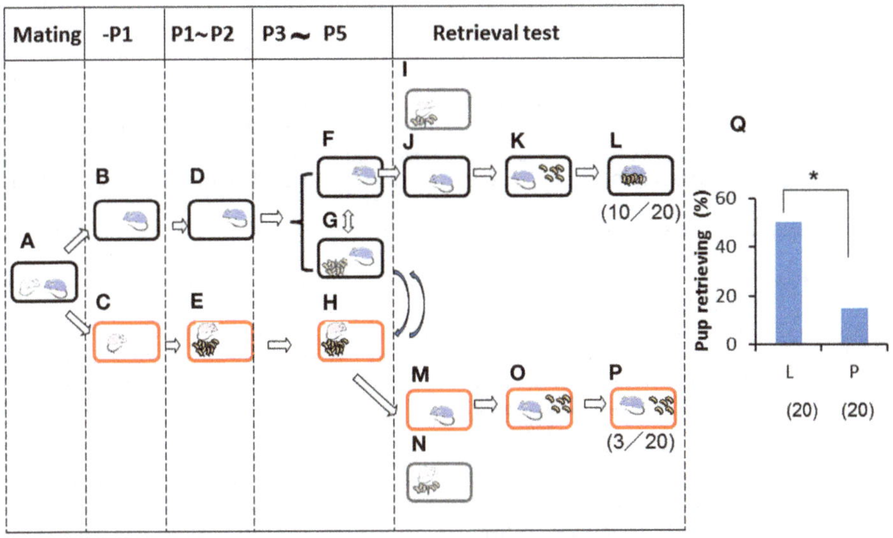

FIGURE 5 | Paternal retrieval test in ICR mice isolated prior parturition from the mating pair and then united with pups only. A paired couple was kept in a rearing cage from mating to 1 day before parturition **(A)**. The male was kept in the old cage **(B)** before meeting the pups and kept until P2 **(D)**. The female was kept in a new cage **(C)**, delivered her pups, and remained until postnatal day 2 **(E)**. The pups were transferred twice for 3 h (total 6 h) a day **(G)** from the dam's (new) cage **(H)** during P3 to P5. During the rest of the time, the sires stayed alone in the home cages **(F)** and the dams were with the pups **(H)**. Pup retrieval behavior over a period of 10 min was examined at P5 **(I–L** and **M–P**, respectively). The number of sires displaying retrieval behavior was scored **(L,P)**, and the numbers of positive mice/number of mice tested are shown in parentheses. Pup retrieval was expressed as percentages (**Q**; $*P < 0.05$ between old **(L)** and new **(P)** cages, two-tailed Fisher's exact probability test).

cages, they displayed paternal retrieval. In sharp contrast, if the cage was new to the sire, even though the dam's and sire's olfactory information was there, the sire failed to display retrieval behavior. These observations suggested that territory establishment is critical to maintaining paternity (Wright and Brown, 2000).

Pup retrieval as a parental behavior is rare among laboratory mice that are not genetically monogamous (Wright and Brown, 2000; Kalueff et al., 2007). We found conditions in which the ICR sires retrieved their pups related to their family structure. This unique ability of the ICR sires will contribute to the increased survival rate after reproduction and to the high level of social attachment and interaction. We have recently reported that central cholinergic cellular signaling (Fujimoto et al., 2013) and CD38 and oxytocin signaling in the nucleus accumbens (NAcc) (Akther et al., 2013) are critical for the expression of paternal care of the ICR mice. We also demonstrated the modulatory roles of the mPOA and VP on parental behavior in rodents (Akther et al., 2014). These published findings suggest that the neural circuitry mediating paternal behavior includes the mPOA, VTA, NAcc, and VP, and may be similar to those that mediate maternal behavior as proposed by Numan and others (Numan et al., 2005; Lee and Brown, 2007; Wynne-Edwards and Timonin, 2007; Numan and Stolzenberg, 2009). In addition, it is particularly interesting to test if mPOA galanin neurons regulate mate-dependent parental behavior in the ICR strain (Wu et al., 2014). Further neuroendocrinological and neurocircuitry analyses in ICR mice will be useful for understanding disorders with social impairment, such as autism spectrum disorders and schizophrenia (Insel, 2010; Munesue et al., 2010; Riebold et al., 2011; Feldman et al., 2012; Salmina et al., 2013).

AUTHOR CONTRIBUTIONS

Haruhiro Higashida designed experiments. Mingkun Liang, Jing Zhong, Hong-Xiang Liu, Olga Lopatina, Ryusuke Nakada, Agnes-Mikiko Yamauchi, and Haruhiro Higashida performed animal experiments. Haruhiro Higashida and Mingkun Liang wrote the manuscript.

ACKNOWLEDGMENTS

This work was supported in part by the Core Research for Evolutional Science and Technology (CREST) from the Japan Science and Technology Agency and by the Strategic Research Program for Brain Sciences from Ministry of Education, Culture, Sports, Science, and Technology, Japan.

REFERENCES

Ahern, T. H., Hammock, E. A., and Young, L. J. (2011). Parental division of labor, coordination, and the effects of family structure on parenting in monogamous prairie voles (Microtus ochrogaster). *Dev. Psychobiol.* 53, 118–131. doi: 10.1002/dev.20498

Akther, S., Fakhrul, A. A., and Higashida, H. (2014). Effects of electrical lesions of the medial preoptic area and the ventral pallidum on mate-dependent paternal behavior in mice. *Neurosci. Lett.* 570, 21–25. doi: 10.1016/j.neulet.2014.03.078

Akther, S., Korshnova, N., Zhong, J., Liang, M., Cherepanov, S. M., Lopatina, O., et al. (2013). CD38 in the nucleus accumbens and oxytocin are related to paternal behavior in mice. *Mol. Brain* 6:41. doi: 10.1186/1756-6606-6-41

Amato, P. R. (2005). The impact of family formation change on the cognitive, social, and emotional well-being of the next generation. *Future Child* 15, 75–96. doi: 10.1353/foc.2005.0012

Bambico, F. R., Lacoste, B., Hattan, P. R., and Gobbi, G. (2013). Father absence in the monogamous california mouse impairs social behavior and modifies dopamine and glutamate synapses in the medial prefrontal cortex. *Cereb. Cortex*. doi: 10.1093/cercor/bht310. [Epub ahead of print].

Benbassat, N., and Priel, B. (2012). Parenting and adolescent adjustment: the role of parental reflective function. *J. Adolesc.* 35, 163–174. doi: 10.1016/j.adolescence.2011.03.004

Bornovalova, M. A., Cummings, J. R., Hunt, E., Blazei, R., Malone, S., and Iacono, W. G. (2014). Understanding the relative contributions of direct environmental effects and passive genotype-environment correlations in the association between familial risk factors and child disruptive behavior disorders. *Psychol. Med.* 44, 831–844. doi: 10.1017/S0033291713001086

Bridges, R. (2008). "Parenting and the brain: an overview," in *Neurobiology of The Parental Brain*, ed R. S. Bridges (Elsevier, MA: Academic Press), 1–550. doi: 10.1016/B978-012374285-8.00037-8

Carter, C. S., Boone, E. M., Pournajafi-Nazarloo, H., and Bales, K. L. (2009). Consequences of early experiences and exposure to oxytocin and vasopressin are sexually dimorphic. *Dev. Neurosci.* 31, 332–341. doi: 10.1159/000216544

Chourbaji, S., Hoyer, C., Richter, S. H., Brandwein, C., Pfeiffer, N., Vogt, M. A., et al. (2011). Differences in mouse maternal care behavior - is there a genetic impact of the glucocorticoid receptor? *PLoS ONE* 6:e19218. doi: 10.1371/journal.pone.0019218

de Jong, T. R., Chauke, M., Harris, B. N., and Saltzman, W. (2009). From here to paternity: neural correlates of the onset of paternal behavior in California mice (*Peromyscus californicus*). *Horm. Behav.* 56, 220–231. doi: 10.1016/j.yhbeh.2009.05.001

Douglas, A. J. (2011). Mother-offspring dialogue in early pregnancy: impact of adverse environment on pregnancy maintenance and neurobiology. *Prog. Neuropsychopharmacol. Biol. Psychiatry* 35, 1167–1177. doi: 10.1016/j.pnpbp.2010.07.024

Feinberg, M. E. (2002). Coparenting and the transition to parenthood: a framework for prevention. *Clin. Child Fam. Psychol. Rev.* 5, 173–195. doi: 10.1023/A:1019695015110

Feldman, R., Zagoory-Sharon, O., Weisman, O., Schneiderman, I., Gordon, I., Maoz, R., et al. (2012). Sensitive parenting is associated with plasma oxytocin and polymorphisms in the OXTR and CD38 genes. *Biol. Psychiatry* 72, 175–181. doi: 10.1016/j.biopsych.2011.12.025

Fleming, A. S., Kraemer, G. W., Gonzalez, A., Lovic, V., Rees, S., and Melo, A. (2002). Mothering begets mothering: the transmission of behaviour and its neurobiology across generation. *Pharmacol. Biochem. Behav.* 73, 61–75. doi: 10.1016/S0091-3057(02)00793-1

Fortunato, L., and Archetti, M. (2010). Evolution of monogamous marriage by maximization of inclusive fitness. *J. Evol. Biol.* 23, 149–156. doi: 10.1111/j.1420-9101.2009.01884.x

Fujimoto, H., Liu, H. X., Lopatina, O., Brown, D. A., and Higashida, H. (2013). Scopolamine modulates paternal parental retrieval behavior in mice induced by the maternal mate. *Neurosci. Lett.* 546, 63–66. doi: 10.1016/j.neulet.2013.04.059

Gammie, S. C. (2005). Current models and future directions for understanding the neural circuitries of maternal behaviors in rodents. *Behav. Cogn. Neurosci. Rev.* 4, 119–135. doi: 10.1177/1534582305281086

Gubernick, D. J., and Alberts, J. R. (1987). The biparental care system of the California mouse, *Peromyscus californicus*. *J. Comp. Psychol.* 101, 169–177. doi: 10.1037/0735-7036.101.2.169

Gubernick, D. J., and Alberts, J. R. (1989). Postpartum maintenance of paternal behaviour in the biparental California mouse, *Peromyscus californicus*. *Anim. Behav.* 37, 656–664. doi: 10.1016/0003-3472(89)90044-4

Hager, R., and Johnstone, R. A. (2003). The genetic basis of family conflict resolution in mice. *Nature* 421, 533–535. doi: 10.1038/nature01239

Hashimoto, H., Uezono, Y., and Ueta, Y. (2012). Pathophysiological function of oxytocin secreted by neuropeptides: a mini review. *Pathophysiology* 19, 283–298. doi: 10.1016/j.pathophys.2012.07.005

Higashida, H., Yokoyama, S., Huang, J. J., Liu, L., Ma, W. J., Akther, S., et al. (2012a). Social memory, amnesia, and autism: brain oxytocin secretion is regulated by NAD+ metabolites and single nucleotide polymorphisms of CD38. *Neurochem. Int.* 61, 828–838. doi: 10.1016/j.neuint.2012.01.030

Higashida, H., Yokoyama, S., Kikuchi, M., and Munesue, T. (2012b). CD38 and its role in oxytocin secretion and social behavior. *Horm. Behav.* 61, 351–358. doi: 10.1016/j.yhbeh.2011.12.011

Insel, T. R. (2010). The challenge of translation in social neuroscience: a review of oxytocin, vasopressin, and affiliative behavior. *Neuron* 65, 768–779. doi: 10.1016/j.neuron.2010.03.005

Jin, D., Liu, H. X., Hirai, H., Torashima, T., Nagai, T., Lopatina, O., et al. (2007). CD38 is critical for social behaviour by regulating oxytocin secretion. *Nature* 446, 41–45. doi: 10.1038/nature05526

Kalueff, A. V., Keisala, T., Minasyan, A., and Tuohimaa, P. (2007). Influence of paternal genotypes on F1 behaviors: lessons from several mouse strains. *Behav. Brain Res.* 177, 45–50. doi: 10.1016/j.bbr.2006.11.005

Kentner, A. C., Abizaid, A., and Bielajew, C. (2010). Modeling dad: animal models of paternal behavior. *Neurosci. Biobehav. Rev.* 34, 438–451. doi: 10.1016/j.neubiorev.2009.08.010

Kuroda, K. O., Meaney, M. J., Uetani, N., Fortin, Y., Ponton, A., and Kato, T. (2007). ERK-FosB signaling in dorsal MPOA neurons plays a major role in the initiation of parental behavior in mice. *Mol. Cell Neurosci.* 36, 121–131. doi: 10.1016/j.mcn.2007.05.010

Kuroda, K. O., Tachikawa, K., Yoshida, S., Tsuneoka, Y., and Numan, M. (2011). Neuromolecular basis of parental behavior in laboratory mice and rats: with special emphasis on technical issues of using mouse genetics. *Prog. Neuropsychopharmacol. Biol. Psychiatry* 35, 1205–1231. doi: 10.1016/j.pnpbp.2011.02.008

Lambert, K. G., Franssen, C. L., Hampton, J. E., Rzucidlo, A. M., Hyer, M. M., True, M., et al. (2013). Modeling paternal attentiveness: distressed pups evoke differential neurobiological and behavioral responses in paternal and nonpaternal mice. *Neuroscience* 234, 1–12. doi: 10.1016/j.neuroscience.2012.12.023

Lee, A. W., and Brown, R. E. (2007). Comparison of medial preoptic, amygdala, and nucleus accumbens lesions on parental behavior in California mice (*Peromyscus californicus*). *Physiol. Behav.* 92, 617–628. doi: 10.1016/j.physbeh.2007.05.008

Lee, H. J., Macbeth, A. H., Pagani, J. H., and Young, W. S. 3rd. (2009). Oxytocin: the great facilitator of life. *Prog. Neurobiol.* 88, 127–151. doi: 10.1016/j.pneurobio.2009.04.001

Leuner, B., Glasper, E. R., and Gould, E. (2010). Parenting and plasticity. *Trends Neurosci.* 33, 465–473. doi: 10.1016/j.tins.2010.07.003

Liu, H. X., Lopatina, O., Higashida, C., Fujimoto, H., Akther, S., Inzhutova, A., et al. (2013). Displays of paternal mouse pup retrieval following communicative interaction with maternal mates. *Nat. Commun.* 4, 1346. doi: 10.1038/ncomms2336

Liu, H. X., Lopatina, O., Higashida, C., Tsuji, T., Kato, I., Takasawa, S., et al. (2008). Locomotor activity, ultrasonic vocalization and oxytocin levels in infant CD38 knockout mice. *Neurosci. Lett.* 448, 67–70. doi: 10.1016/j.neulet.2008.09.084

Lonstein, J. S., and De Vries, G. J. (2000). Sex differences in the parental behavior of rodents. *Neurosci. Biobehav. Rev.* 24, 669–686. doi: 10.1016/S0149-7634(00)00036-1

McGraw, L. A., and Young, L. J. (2010). The prairie vole: an emerging model organism for understanding the social brain. *Trends Neurosci.* 33, 103–109. doi: 10.1016/j.tins.2009.11.006

Mogi, K., Nagasawa, M., and Kikusui, T. (2011). Developmental consequences and biological significance of mother-infant bonding. *Prog. Neuropsychopharmacol. Biol. Psychiatry* 35, 1232–1241. doi: 10.1016/j.pnpbp.2010.08.024

Morgan, C. P., and Bale, T. L. (2011). Early prenatal stress epigenetically programs dysmasculinization in second-generation offspring via the paternal lineage. *J. Neurosci.* 31, 11748–11755. doi: 10.1523/JNEUROSCI.1887-11.2011

Morrison, K. E., Rodgers, A. B., Morgan, C. P., and Bale, T. L. (2014). Epigenetic mechanisms in pubertal brain maturation. *Neuroscience* 264C, 17–24. doi: 10.1016/j.neuroscience.2013.11.014

Morrongiello, B. A., Schwebel, D. C., Stewart, J., Bell, M., Davis, A. L., and Corbett, M. R. (2013). Examining parents' behaviors and supervision of their children in the presence of an unfamiliar dog: does the blue dog intervention improve parent practices? *Accid. Anal. Prev.* 54, 108–113. doi: 10.1016/j.aap.2013.02.005

Munesue, T., Yokoyama, S., Nakamura, K., Anitha, A., Yamada, K., Hayashi, K., et al. (2010). Two genetic variants of CD38 in subjects with autism spectrum disorder and controls. *Neurosci. Res.* 67, 181–191. doi: 10.1016/j.neures.2010.03.004

Neumann, I. D. (2009). The advantage of social living: brain neuropeptides mediate the beneficial consequences of sex and motherhood. *Front. Neuroendocrinol.* 30, 483–496. doi: 10.1016/j.yfrne.2009.04.012

Nishimori, K., Takayanagi, Y., Yoshida, M., Kasahara, Y., Young, L. J., and Kawamata, M. (2008). New aspects of oxytocin receptor function revealed by knockout mice: sociosexual behaviour and control of energy balance. *Prog. Brain Res.* 170, 79–90. doi: 10.1016/S0079-6123(08)00408-1

Numan, M., Numan, M. J., Schwarz, J. M., Neuner, C. M., Flood, T. F., and Smith, C. D. (2005). Medial preoptic area interactions with the nucleus accumbens–ventral pallidum circuit and maternal behavior in rats, *Behav. Brain Res.* 158, 53–68. doi: 10.1016/j.bbr.2004.08.008

Numan, M., and Stolzenberg, D. S. (2009). Medial preoptic area interactions with dopamine neural systems in the control of the onset and maintenance of maternal behavior in rats. *Front. Neuroendocrinol.* 30, 46–64. doi: 10.1016/j.yfrne.2008.10.002

Nunes, S., Fite, J. E., Patera, K. J., and French, J. A. (2001). Interactions among paternal behavior, steroid hormones, and parental experience in male marmosets (*Callithrix kuhlii*). *Horm. Behav.* 39, 70–82. doi: 10.1006/hbeh.2000.1631

Ogawa, S., Washburn, T. F., Taylor, J., Lubahn, D. B., Korach, K. S., and Pfaff, D. W. (1998). Modifications of testosterone-dependent behaviors by estrogen receptor-alpha gene disruption in male mice. *Endocrinology* 139, 5058–5069.

Ozawa, M., Kikusui, T., Takeuchi, Y., and Mori, Y. (2010). Comparison of parental behavior and offspring's anxiety behavior using a reciprocal F1 hybrid model. *J. Vet. Med. Sci.* 72, 1589–1596. doi: 10.1292/jvms.10-0173

Parhar, I., Ogawa, S., and Kitahashi, T. (2012). RFamide peptides as mediators in environmental control of GnRH neurons. *Prog. Neurobiol.* 98, 176–196. doi: 10.1016/j.pneurobio.2012.05.011

Pfaff, D. W., Ogawa, S., and Kow, L. M. (1999). Neural oxytocinergic systems as genomic targets for hormones and as modulators of hormone-dependent behaviors. *Results Probl. Cell Differ.* 26, 91–105. doi: 10.1007/978-3-540-49 421-8_5

Reburn, C. J., and Wynne-Edwards, K. E. (1999). Hormonal changes in males of a naturally biparental and a uniparental mammal. *Horm. Behav.* 35, 163–176. doi: 10.1006/hbeh.1998.1509

Riebold, M., Mankuta, D., Lerer, E., Israel, S., Zhong, S., Nemanov, L., et al. (2011). All-trans retinoic acid upregulates reduced CD38 transcription in lymphoblastoid cell lines from Autism spectrum disorder. *Mol. Med.* 17, 799–806. doi: 10.2119/molmed.2011.00080

Rosenblatt, J. S. (1967). Nonhormonal basis of maternal behavior in the rat. *Science* 156, 1512–1514. doi: 10.1126/science.156.3781.1512

Rosenblatt, J. S., Hazelwood, S., and Poole, J. (1996). Maternal behavior in male rats: effects of medial preoptic area lesions and presence of maternal aggression. *Horm. Behav.* 30, 201–215. doi: 10.1006/hbeh.1996.0025

Salmina, A. B., Lopatina, O., Kuvacheva, N. V., and Higashida, H. (2013). Integrative neurochemistry and neurobiology of social recognition and behavior analyzed with respect to CD38-dependent brain oxytocin secretion. *Curr. Top. Med. Chem.* 13, 2965–2977.

Saltzman, W., and Maestripieri, D. (2011). The neuroendocrinology of primate maternal behavior. *Prog. Neuropsychopharmacol. Biol. Psychiatry* 35, 1192–1204. doi: 10.1016/j.pnpbp.2010.09.017

Schor, E. L., and American Academy of Pediatrics Task Force on the Family. (2003). Family pediatrics: report of the task force on the family. *Pediatrics* 111, 1541–1571.

Soga, T., Dalpatadu, S. L., Wong, D. W., and Parhar, I. S. (2012). Neonatal dexamethasone exposure down-regulates GnRH expression through the GnIH pathway in female mice. *Neuroscience* 218, 56–64. doi: 10.1016/j.neuroscience.2012.05.023

Tachikawa, K. S., Yoshihara, Y., and Kuroda, K. O. (2013). Behavioral transition from attack to parenting in male mice: a crucial role of the vomeronasal system. *J. Neurosci.* 33, 5120–5126. doi: 10.1523/JNEUROSCI.2364-12.2013

Wright, S. L., and Brown, R. E. (2000). Maternal behavior, paternal behavior, and pup survival in CD-1 albino mice (*Mus musculus*) in three different housing conditions. *J. Comp. Psychol.* 114, 183–192. doi: 10.1037/0735-7036.114.2.183

Wu, Z., Autry, A. E., Bergan, J. F., Watabe-Uchida, M., and Dulac, C. G. (2014). Galanin neurons in the medial preoptic area govern parental behaviour. *Nature* 509, 325–330. doi: 10.1038/nature13307

Wynne-Edwards, K. E., and Timonin, M. E. (2007). Paternal care in rodents: weakening support for hormonal regulation of the transition to behavioral fatherhood in rodent animal models of biparental care. *Horm. Behav.* 52, 114–121. doi: 10.1016/j.yhbeh.2007.03.018

Yoshida, S., Esposito, G., Ohnishi, R., Tsuneoka, Y., Okabe, S., Kikusui, T., et al. (2013). Transport Response is a filial-specific behavioral response to maternal carrying in C57BL/6 mice. *Front. Zool.* 10:50. doi: 10.1186/1742-9994-10-50

19

Identification of neural cells activated by mating stimulus in the periaqueductal gray in female rats

Shunji Yamada and Mitsuhiro Kawata *

Department of Anatomy and Neurobiology, Kyoto Prefectural University of Medicine, Kyoto, Japan

***Correspondence:**
*Mitsuhiro Kawata, Department of Anatomy and Neurobiology, Kyoto Prefectural University of Medicine, Kawaramachi-Hirokoji, Kamigyo-ku, Kyoto 602-8566, Japan
e-mail: mkawata@koto.kpu-m.ac.jp*

Induction of lordosis as typical female sexual behavior in rodents is dependent on a mount stimulus from males and blood levels of estrogen. Periaqueductal gray (PAG) efferent neurons have been suggested to be important for lordosis behavior; however, the neurochemical basis remains to be understood. In this study, we neuroanatomically examined (1) whether PAG neurons activated by mating stimulus project to the medullary reticular formation (MRF), which is also a required area for lordosis; and (2) whether these neurons are glutamatergic. Mating stimulus significantly increased the number of cFos-immunoreactive (ir) neurons in the PAG, particularly in its lateral region. Half of cFos-ir neurons in the lateral PAG were positive for a retrograde tracer (FluoroGold; FG) injected into the MRF. cFos-ir neurons also colocalized with mRNA of *vesicular glutamate transporter 2 (vGLUT2)*, a molecular marker for glutamatergic neurons. Using retrograde tracing and *in situ* hybridization in conjunction with fluorescent microscopy, we also found FG and *vGLUT2* mRNA double-positive neurons in the lateral PAG. These results suggest that glutamatergic neurons in the lateral PAG project to the MRF and are involved in lordosis behavior in female rats.

Keywords: periaqueductal gray, cFos, mating stimulus, vesicular glutamate transporter 2, FluoroGold, lordosis

INTRODUCTION

Lordosis is a typical sexual behavior of a female rodent and is induced by a male mount stimulus under proestrus levels of estrogen. The mount stimulus passes through the anterolateral column of the spinal cord and then inputs into the medullary reticular formation (MRF) and periaqueductal gray (PAG) (Pfaff, 1980). Daniels et al. demonstrated an efferent pathway for lordosis behavior using a pseudorabies virus (PRV) as a transneuronal retrograde tracer (Daniels et al., 1999). When PRV was injected into the lumbar epaxial muscles, which produce a lordosis posture in female rats, the PRV was sequentially labeled in the MRF, PAG, and ventromedial nucleus of the hypothalamus (VMH). The VMH is the main site of action of estrogen for inducing lordosis (Rubin and Barfield, 1983) and estrogen receptor-expressing neurons in this nucleus project to the PAG (Calizo and Flanagan-Cato, 2003). Thus, the PAG and MRF are important relay areas that reflexively change a male mount stimulus into an output for lordosis posture (Pfaff, 1980).

Electrical stimulation of the PAG induces lordosis behavior (Sakuma and Pfaff, 1979a). Conversely, lesions of the PAG (Sakuma and Pfaff, 1979b) or local lesions in the caudal ventrolateral PAG (Lonstein and Stern, 1998) reduce lordosis in female rats. Manual vaginocervical stimulation (VCS), which induces lordosis, is increased cFos expression in the PAG (Pfaus et al., 1996). Neural connections of the PAG to the MRF are involved in induction of an electromyogram (EMG) response in muscles regulating lordosis in female rats (Robbins et al., 1990). These results suggest that PAG efferent neurons activated by a mating stimulus may be related to induction of lordosis, but the neurotransmitter in PAG neurons projecting to the MRF remains to be understood.

Many reports have shown involvement of glutamate and its receptor in lordosis. Intracerebroventricular (icv) administration of N-methyl-D-aspartic-acid (NMDA), an agonist of the glutamate NMDA receptor, facilitated lordosis in ovariectomized (OVX) rats treated with low-dose estrogen (Gargiulo and Donoso, 1995), and activation of lordosis induced by progesterone in estrogen-treated OVX rats was blocked by icv injection of a NMDA antagonist (Gargiulo et al., 1992). A mRNA for *vesicular glutamate transporter 2 (vGLUT2)*, a molecular marker for glutamatergic neurons (Ziegler et al., 2002, 2012), is expressed in the lateral part of the PAG (Oka et al., 2008). Therefore, we hypothesized that the lateral PAG neurons projecting to the MRF are glutamatergic neurons and that these neurons are involved in lordosis. To investigate this hypothesis, we used neuroanatomical methods to examine (1) whether lateral PAG neurons activated by a mating stimulus directly project to the MRF, and (2) whether these neurons are glutamatergic in estrogen-treated OVX rats.

MATERIALS AND METHODS

ANIMALS AND TREATMENTS

Wistar female rats aged 8 weeks were purchased from Shimizu Laboratory Supplies Co. (Kyoto, Japan) and housed under a 12-h reverse light/dark cycle with free access to food and water. After two consecutive estrus cycles, rats were bilaterally ovariectomized and silastic tubing (1.5 mm i.d.; 3.0 mm o.d.; 25 mm length; Dow Corning, Midland, MI) containing crystalline 17 β-estradiol (E2,

Nachalai, Osaka, Japan) was implanted subcutaneously under anesthesia with 2–3% isoflurane. We confirmed that the E2 treatment caused hypertrophy of the uterus and induced a high lordosis quotient (>90) against male mount behavior. All experimental procedures were authorized by the Committee for Animal Research, Kyoto Prefectural University of Medicine.

SEXUAL STIMULATION AND TISSUE PREPARATION

One week after OVX and E2 treatment, the rats were assigned randomly to a sexual stimulus condition. Some female rats were placed into a test arena (60 cm long × 30 cm wide × 30 cm high) with a sexually vigorous male (age > 12 weeks) for 1 h for mating stimulus at 17:00, and others were placed into the same arena without a male to serve as non-mating stimulated controls. Mating-stimulated female rats received >10 mating stimuli within 15 min. At the conclusion of sexual stimulation, all animals were anesthetized with pentobarbital (Somnopentyl; Kyouritsu Seiyaku, Tokyo, Japan) and perfused with physiological saline followed by 4% paraformaldehyde in 0.05 M PB. The brain was immediately removed, postfixed with the same fixative overnight at 4°C, and then kept in 30% sucrose in 0.05 M PB at 4°C. Serial coronal sections (30 μm) containing the PAG were obtained using a cryostat (CM 3050 S; Leica, Wetzlar, Germany).

cFos IMMUNOHISTOCHEMISTRY (IHC)

Every fourth section through the PAG (8 sections, from 7.0 to 8.2 mm posterior to the bregma in the brain atlas (Paxinos and Watson, 2006)) from mating-stimulated ($n = 5$) and control ($n = 5$) rats was sequentially incubated with 0.3% H_2O_2 in PBS with 0.3% Triton X-100 for 30 min and 2% normal goat serum (NGS) in PBS for 1 h at room temperature (RT). Sections were then incubated with primary rabbit antiserum against cFos (1:15,000; Ab-5, Calbiochem, Merck, Tokyo, Japan) for 24 h at RT. Immunoreactive (ir) neurons were visualized with a streptavidin-biotin kit (Nichirei, Tokyo, Japan), followed by 3,3′-diaminobenzidine (DAB) with 2.5% nickel chloride, as described our previous method (Takanami et al., 2010).

FLUOROGOLD (FG) INJECTION INTO THE MRF AND FG AND cFos DOUBLE-IHC

Five days after OVX and E2 treatment, rats ($n = 9$) were stereotaxically implanted with a stainless-steel guide cannula (23-gage; Plastics One, Roanoke, VA) in the MRF with the tip end at 11.4 mm posterior and 9.0 mm ventral to the bregma and 0.7 lateral to the midline, according to the brain atlas (Paxinos and Watson, 2006). FluoroGold (FG; Invitrogen, Carlsbad, CA) was dissolved in saline at 2% and unilaterally injected into the MRF at a rate of 0.25 μl/min for 2 min using a microsyringe pump through an internal cannula (26 gage). This procedure was performed under anesthesia with pentobarbital (13 mg/ml Somnopentyl, 0.15 ml/100 g body weight). Two days after FG injection, some rats ($n = 6$) received sexual stimulation and others ($n = 3$) were used as non-stimulated controls. Brains were processed for FG and cFos double-IHC. After cFos-ir was detected as described above, free-floating sections were sequentially incubated with 0.3% H_2O_2 in PBS for 15 min, 2% NGS in PBS for 1 h, and primary rabbit antiserum against FG (1:20,000; Invitrogen) for 24 h at RT. FG-ir neurons were visualized with a streptavidin-biotin kit, followed by DAB as a chromogen.

vGLUT2 mRNA IN SITU HYBRIDIZATION (ISH) AND cFos IHC

To detect *vGLUT2* mRNA, cDNA for vGLUT2 (734 bp) was generated by RT-PCR from total RNA of rat hypothalamus. Primers were based on the sequence of rat vGLUT2 (accession number AF271235). The upstream and downstream primers were 5′-CTT CTT GGT GCT TGC AGT GG and 5′-GGA CGA ATG GCC TGA ATG GA, respectively (Ziegler et al., 2002). Non-radioactive free-floating ISH was performed as described previously (Yamada et al., 2007, 2012). Briefly, every fourth section containing the PAG (8 sections, $n = 6$) was acetylated and then hybridized with 2 mg/ml DIG-labeled *vGLUT2* antisense cRNA probes synthesized from cDNA of vGLUT2 using a DIG-labeling kit (Boehringer Mannheim GmbH, Mannheim, Germany) overnight at 55°C. After elimination of excess cRNA probes, the sections were incubated with 1.5% blocking reagent (Boehringer Mannheim) and then with an alkaline phosphatase (AP)-conjugated anti-DIG antibody (1:1000, Roche Diagnostics Corp., Indianapolis, IN) for 2 h at 37°C. *vGLUT2*-positive neurons were visualized with a BCIP/NBT solution (1:50, Roche Diagnostics Corp.). After *vGLUT2* ISH, cFos IHC was performed as described above.

FLUORESCENT *vGLUT2 mRNA* ISH AND FG IHC

Preparation of PAG sections ($n = 3$) after FG injection into the MRF and the procedure until blocking with 1.5% blocking solution is described in the section on ISH for *vGLUT2* mRNA. After blocking, the sections were incubated with a mixture of sheep horseradish peroxidase-conjugated anti-DIG antibody (1:20, Roche Diagnostics Corp.) and rabbit anti-FG antibody (1:1000, Invitrogen) overnight at RT. Then the sections were incubated for 30 min in biotin-conjugated tyramide (1:50 in amplification diluent, PerkinElmer, Waltham, MA). Following several washings, the sections were incubated with a mixture of Alexa 488-conjugated streptavidin and Alexa 546-conjugated anti-rabbit IgG (1:500, Molecular Probes, Eugene, OR) for 2 h at RT.

ANALYSIS AND STATISTICS

After staining, the sections were mounted on APS-coated glass slides and covered with a glass micro-cover slip. Non-fluorescent staining was observed under a light microscope (BX 50; Olympus) and photographs of ipsilateral PAG were captured using a CCD camera (DP 21; Olympus). A frame of size of 0.5 × 0.5 mm (region of interest, ROI) was made in the captured lateral PAG and the numbers of cFos-ir, FG-ir, *vGLUT2* mRNA-positive, FG-ir and cFos-ir, and *vGLUT2* mRNA-positive and cFos-ir neurons in the ROI were counted. Immunofluorescent staining was viewed and captured using a LSM510META confocal laser-scanning microscope (Carl Zeiss, Jena, Germany). All values are expressed as means ± SEM. The significance of a difference between mating-stimulated and non-stimulated control rats was evaluated by Student *t*-test.

RESULTS

ACTIVATION OF LATERAL PAG NEURONS BY MATING STIMULUS

In non-mating stimulated control rats, which were placed in the test arena without male rats, there were few cFos-ir neurons in the PAG (**Figure 1A**). In contrast, in mating-stimulated rats, many cFos-ir neurons were present in the rostral to caudal parts of the PAG, particularly in the lateral area (**Figure 1B**). The number of cFos-ir neurons in the lateral PAG in these rats was fourfold greater than that in control rats ($P < 0.05$, **Figure 1C**).

PROJECTION OF MATING-STIMULATED cFos-EXPRESSING NEURONS IN THE LATERAL PAG

To investigate whether cFos-expressing lateral PAG neurons induced by a mating stimulus project to the MRF, FG was injected into the MRF of female rats prior to mating stimulus. The injection of FG extended through the reticular formation (RF), including the MRF, and caudal pontine RF (PRF), with a longitudinal distance from 11.28 to 12.48 mm posterior to the bregma in the brain atlas (Paxinos and Watson, 2006) (**Figure 2A**). This area included the gigantocellular reticular nucleus (Gi), the gigantocellular reticular nucleus ventral (GiV) and alpha (GiA) regions, and the lateral paragigantocellular nucleus, in which neurons found neuroanatomically (Daniels et al., 1999) and electrophysiologically (Sakuma and Pfaff, 1980) have been suggested to be involved in lordosis. Many FG-ir neurons were distributed bilaterally with an ipsilateral dominance through the rostral to caudal regions of the lateral PAG (**Figure 2B**). In non-stimulated rats, there were a few cFos-ir and FG and cFos double-ir neurons in the lateral PAG (**Figure 2C**). In contrast, many FG and cFos double-ir neurons were found in the lateral PAG in mating-stimulated rats (**Figure 2D**). The numbers of FG and cFos-ir, cFos-ir, and FG-ir neurons in the ROI (0.5×0.5 mm) in the lateral PAG were 114.3 ± 7.9, 229.3 ± 19.7, and 644.5 ± 22.2, respectively. The percentage of FG-ir neurons among total cFos-ir neurons was $50.4 \pm 1.7\%$ and that of cFos-ir neurons among total FG-ir neurons was $17.9 \pm 1.5\%$ (**Table 1**). These numbers and percentages were significantly higher ($P < 0.05$) in mating-stimulated rats than in non-stimulated rats, except for FG-ir neurons (**Table 1**).

NEUROCHEMICAL IDENTITY OF MATING-STIMULATED cFos-EXPRESSING NEURONS IN THE LATERAL PAG

We performed double staining for *vGLUT2* mRNA ISH and cFos IHC to examine whether the mating stimulus-induced cFos-expressing neurons in the lateral PAG are glutamatergic. Many *vGLUT2* mRNA-positive neurons were located in the lateral PAG (**Figures 3A,B**). The distribution pattern of *vGLUT2* mRNA-positive neurons was similar to that in a previous study using another type of *vGLUT2* cRNA probe (Oka et al., 2008). Several *vGLUT2* mRNA-positive neurons showed cFos-ir in

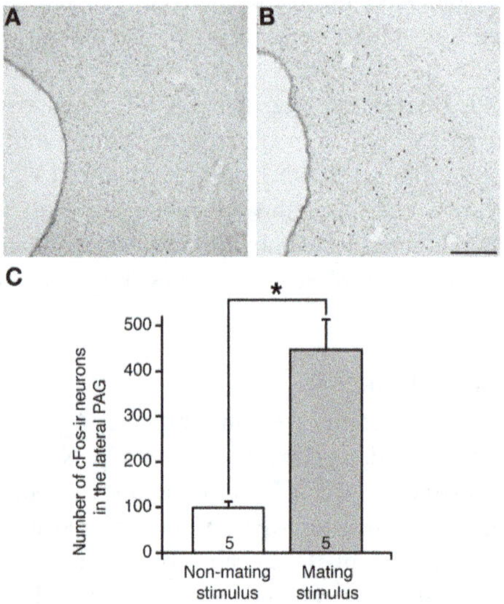

FIGURE 1 | cFos expression in the lateral PAG in representative female rats following (A) non-mating stimulus and (B) mating stimulus. cFos-ir neurons are shown by black dots. **(C)** The mean number of cFos-ir neurons in the lateral PAG in OVX+E2 rats after mating stimulus (solid bar) was significantly higher than that in non-stimulated control rats (open bar) (*$P < 0.05$; Student *t*-test). Values are shown as means ± SEM. The numbers in each column indicate the numbers of animals used. Scale bar, 100 μm.

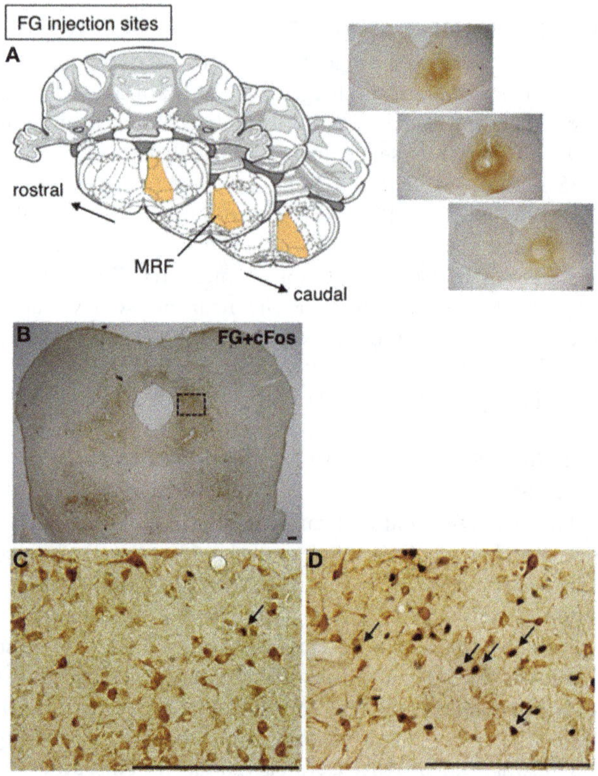

FIGURE 2 | (A) Coronal sections from the rat brain atlas of Paxinos and Watson (2006), showing the position of the MRF and representative photomicrographs showing the site of FG injection in the RF. **(B)** Representative photomicrographs of the caudal part of the lateral PAG in rat after injection of FG into the RF. High magnification of FG-ir (brown) and cFos-ir (black) neurons in the caudal part of the lateral PAG in a non-stimulated control rat **(C)** and a mating-stimulated rat **(D)**. Arrows show FG-ir neurons with cFos-ir in nuclei. Scale bar: 200 μm.

Table 1 | Numbers and percentages of FG and cFos immunoreactive neurons in the lateral PAG in female rats after FG injection into the RF with or without mating stimulus.

	Number of neurons			Percentages (%)	
	FG and cFos	cFos	FG	FG/cFos	cFos/FG
Non-stimulus	31.0 ± 3.0	71.7 ± 8.3	709.7 ± 41.0	43.5 ± 1.5	4.4 ± 1.5
Mating-stimulus	114.3 ± 7.9*	229.3 ± 19.7*	644.5 ± 22.2	50.4 ± 1.7*	17.9 ± 1.5*

$P < 0.05$ compared with the non-stimulated rats.

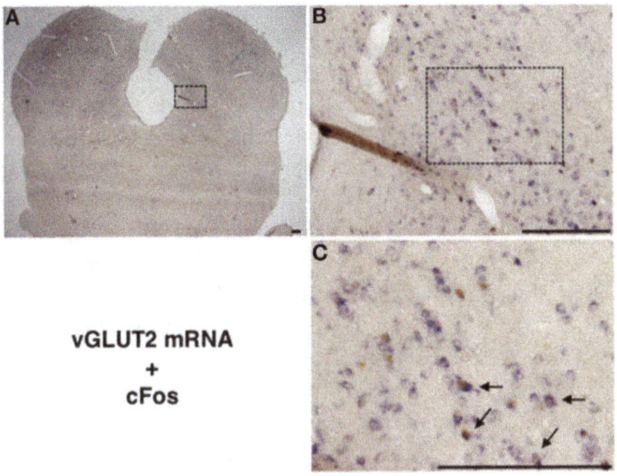

FIGURE 3 | (A) Representative photomicrographs showing vGLUT2 mRNA (purple) *in situ* hybridization and cFos (brown) immunohistochemistry in the caudal part of the lateral PAG. **(B)** High magnification of the square in **(A)**. **(C)** Enlarged view of several neurons in the square in **(B)**. Arrows show vGLUT2 mRNA and Fos-ir neurons. Scale bar: 200 μm.

nuclei (**Figure 3C**). The number of *vGLUT2* mRNA-positive and cFos-ir neurons, cFos-ir neurons, and *vGLUT2* mRNA-positive neurons in the ROI (0.5 × 0.5 mm) in the lateral PAG were 74.8 ± 11.1, 131.0 ± 11.5, and 421.2 ± 31.0, respectively. The percentage of *vGLUT2* mRNA-positive neurons among total cFos-ir neurons was 55.6 ± 3.9% and that of cFos-ir neurons among total *vGLUT2* mRNA-positive neurons was 17.4 ± 1.6% (**Table 2**). There were no hybridization signals in brain sections incubated with sense probes for *vGLUT2* (data not shown).

PROJECTION OF *vGLUT2*-POSITIVE NEURONS IN THE LATERAL PAG TO THE MRF

We investigated whether MRF-projecting lateral PAG neurons were positive for *vGLUT2* mRNA using double fluorescence staining for *vGLUT2* mRNA ISH and FG IHC with enhancement of ISH signals by biotin-tyramide. Two out of 3 rats received a successful FG injection into the RF. Among FG-ir neurons, 75% were positive for *vGLUT2* mRNA in the lateral PAG ipsilateral to the injection site (**Figure 4**).

Table 2 | Numbers and percentages of vGLUT2 mRNA-positive and cFos immunoreactive neurons in the lateral PAG in female rats after mating stimulus.

Number of neurons			Percentages (%)	
vGLUT2 and cFos	cFos	vGLUT2	vGLUT2/ cFos	cFos/ vGLUT2
74.8 ± 11.1	131.0 ± 11.5	421.2 ± 31.0	55.6 ± 3.9	17.4 ± 1.6

N = 6; 8 sections in each rats.

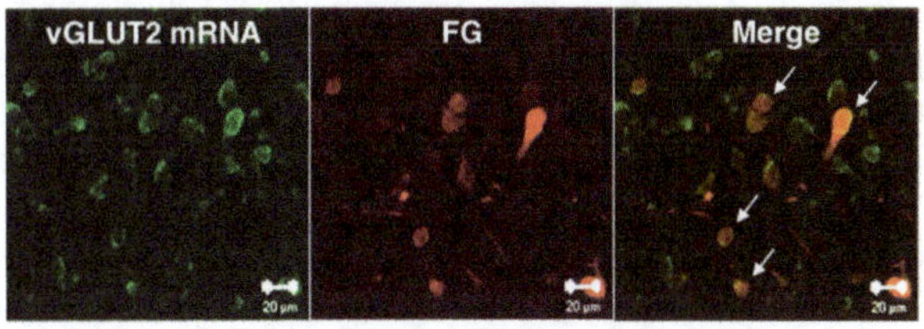

FIGURE 4 | Confocal microscope images showing vGLUT2 mRNA-positive (green) and FG-ir (red) neurons in the caudal part of lateral PAG. Arrows indicate vGLUT2 mRNA-positive and FG-ir double-stained neurons. Scale bars: 20 μm.

DISCUSSION

The results of the study show that (1) a mating stimulus activates neurons in the lateral PAG, (2) 50% of lateral PAG neurons activated by the mating stimulus project to the RF, (3) 56% of these neurons are glutamatergic, and (4) there are glutamatergic neurons projecting to the RF. The PAG and MRF are essential sites for lordosis behavior in female rats (Pfaff, 1980) and there is a clear relationship between glutamate and induction of lordosis (Gargiulo et al., 1992; Gargiulo and Donoso, 1995; Landa et al., 2009). Our findings provide further evidence that glutamatergic neurons in the lateral PAG project to the MRF and are involved in lordosis in female rats.

The PAG receives input from many brain areas, including the forebrain, hypothalamus, and brainstem, and has reciprocal efferent neurons linked with these brain areas (Paxinos, 2004). Functionally, the PAG is associated with modulation of pain and defensive behavior, in addition to lordosis (Paxinos, 2004). Thus, although we and others have shown increased cFos expression by VCS of mating or manual probing in the PAG (Tetel et al., 1993; Pfaus et al., 1996), the function of the activated PAG neurons is still not understood. In the current study, half of the mating-induced cFos-expressing neurons in the lateral PAG were found to project to the RF (MRF and PRF) using a retrograde tracer, and the MRF has also been implicated in induction of lordosis. For example, lesions in the MRF disrupt lordosis (Zemlan et al., 1983) and electrical stimulation of the MRF causes an EMG response in lordosis-inducing muscles (Femano et al., 1984). Moreover, PAG neurons are antidromically activated by electrical stimulation of the MRF in female rats (Sakuma and Pfaff, 1980). These results suggest that sensory information induced by a mount stimulus has afferent inputs in the lateral PAG and activates neurons projecting to the MRF, after which MRF neurons cause lordosis behavior in female rats.

Contradictory effects of glutamate on lordosis have been found. Icv injection of NMDA accelerated lordosis in low estrogen-primed OVX rats that rarely showed lordosis (Gargiulo and Donoso, 1995; Landa et al., 2009); whereas local injection of NMDA into the VMH inhibited lordosis in estrogen- and progesterone-treated OVX rats that showed frequent lordosis behavior (Georgescu and Pfaus, 2006). In similar rats, subcutaneous injection of MK-801, a NMDA antagonist, inhibited lordosis (Fleischmann et al., 1991), but injection into the ventral tegmental area increased lordosis (Petralia et al., 2007). In another study, an increase in lordosis induced by progesterone and luteinizing hormone-releasing hormone (LHRH) was inhibited by icv administration of a NMDA antagonist (Gargiulo et al., 1992). These results suggest condition- or region-specific effects of glutamate on lordosis behavior.

In the current study, using *vGLUT2 in situ* hybridization, we first showed activation of lateral PAG glutamatergic neurons by mating stimulus in OVX + E2 rats, indicating involvement of PAG glutamatergic neurons in lordosis. Double fluorescence for *vGLUT2* mRNA ISH and FG IHC showed the presence of lateral PAG glutamatergic neurons projecting to the RF. mRNAs for the NMDA receptor and its subunit are abundant in the MRF (Keifer and Carr, 2000; Matsuda et al., 2002). It is also likely that the NMDA receptor in the MRF is involved in lordosis because activation of lordosis-relevant muscles by electrical stimulation of the MRF was more effective in rats with additional NMDA in the MRF, compared with controls (Robbins et al., 1992). Triple-labeled histological analysis for cFos, FG IHC, and *vGLUT2* mRNA ISH was not performed, but we suggest that lateral PAG glutamatergic neurons with axonal connections to the MRF are an important neural pathway for induction of lordosis.

Several lines of evidence suggest that many neurotransmitters are related to regulation of lordosis. Thus, microinfusion of LHRH (Sakuma and Pfaff, 1983), prolactin (Harlan et al., 1983), and substance P (Dornan et al., 1987) into the PAG induces lordosis. Findings for immunoreactive nerve terminals in the PAG (Ljungdahl et al., 1978; Liposits and Setalo, 1980; Harlan et al., 1983) suggest that these peptides may be neurotransmitters or neuromodulaters that convey a mount stimulus from the spinal cord or estrogen information from the VMH to PAG glutamatergic neurons to induce lordosis.

In this study, half of mating-induced cFos-expressing neurons were not FG-ir in the lateral PAG. Some hypothalamic nuclei have an increased number of cFos-expressing neurons after mating stimulus, but not following a manual sensory stimulus of the flank and rump (Pfaus et al., 1993). Sensory stimulation of the flank and rump by a male forefoot during mount behavior is important for lordosis in female rats because denervation of the perineum, tail base, posterior rump and ventral flanks suppresses lordosis (Kow, 1976). The mating stimulus from male rats in the current study included sensory stimuli of the flank and rump and VCS in females, which suggests that the stimulus also induces activation of lateral PAG neurons that are not associated with lordosis. There are afferent projections from the PAG to the thalamus and parabrachial nucleus, which are related to cognition and pain (Sim and Joseph, 1992; Krout et al., 1998). Thus, FG-negative cFos-expressing neurons in the lateral PAG may have a role in modulating the nociceptive mechanism during lordosis. In addition, half of mating-induced cFos-expressing neurons were not glutamatergic in the lateral PAG. GABA- or neurotensin-expressing neural cell bodies are present in the PAG (Paxinos, 2004) and GABA is involved in lordosis behavior (Wada et al., 2008). This indicates that GABA neurons are a candidate for the neurons activated by mating stimulus in the lateral PAG.

We previously showed cFos IHC following ISH using a *Kiss1* DIG-labeling probe (Adachi et al., 2007). In the current study, cFos IHC following *vGLUT2* mRNA ISH was performed using the same technique, except for the difference in the DIG-labeling probe. However, cFos expression in the combination of cFos IHC with *vGLUT2* ISH was lower than that in cFos and FG double-IHC. This may have occurred because incubation with the *vGLUT2* DIG-labeling probe at 55°C might have masked an antigenic determinant of cFos for our antibody.

The precise activated area of the MRF in lordosis is not completely clear. We investigated mating stimulus-induced cFos expression in the MRF, but did not detect a cFos signal in this procedure (data not shown). Immediate early genes, including cFos, are sometimes not induced in brain regions containing neurons with spontaneous and high baseline firing rates prior to stimulation of areas such as the MRF (Pfaus and Heeb, 1997). In the current study, the widespread distribution of FG in the RF indicates the presence of mating stimulus-activated glutamatergic neurons in the lateral PAG projecting to the MRF. Our data raise the possibility that MRF neurons distributed around glutamatergic terminals from the lateral PAG can influence lordosis. Further studies are needed to address the glutamatergic influences on these neurons in regulation of lordosis.

ACKNOWLEDGMENTS

We thank Atsuko Yashiro and Nobunari Tomura for providing experimental support. This work was supported by Grants-in-Aid for Scientific Research from the Ministry of Education, Science, Sports, Culture and Technology, Japan (KAKENHI 24300128 to Mitsuhiro Kawata and 25870621 to Shunji Yamada).

REFERENCES

Adachi, S., Yamada, S., Takatsu, Y., Matsui, H., Kinoshita, M., Takase, K., et al. (2007). Involvement of anteroventral periventricular metastin/kisspeptin neurons in estrogen positive feedback action on luteinizing hormone release in female rats. *J. Reprod. Dev.* 53, 367–378. doi: 10.1262/jrd.18146

Calizo, L. H., and Flanagan-Cato, L. M. (2003). Hormonal-neural integration in the female rat ventromedial hypothalamus: triple labeling for estrogen receptor-alpha, retrograde tract tracing from the periaqueductal gray, and mating-induced Fos expression. *Endocrinology* 144, 5430–5440. doi: 10.1210/en.2003-0331en.2003-0331

Daniels, D., Miselis, R. R., and Flanagan-Cato, L. M. (1999). Central neuronal circuit innervating the lordosis-producing muscles defined by transneuronal transport of pseudorabies virus. *J. Neurosci.* 19, 2823–2833.

Dornan, W. A., Malsbury, C. W., and Penney, R. B. (1987). Facilitation of lordosis by injection of substance P into the midbrain central gray. *Neuroendocrinology* 45, 498–506. doi: 10.1159/000124781

Femano, P. A., Schwartz-Giblin, S., and Pfaff, D. W. (1984). Brain stem reticular influences on lumbar axial muscle activity. I. effective sites. *Am. J. Physiol.* 246, R389–R395.

Fleischmann, A., Vincent, P. A., and Etgen, A. M. (1991). Effects of non-competitive NMDA receptor antagonists on reproductive and motor behaviors in female rats. *Brain Res.* 568, 138–146. doi: 10.1016/0006-8993(91)91389-I

Gargiulo, P. A., and Donoso, A. O. (1995). Interaction between glutamate and luteinizing hormone-releasing hormone (LHRH) in lordosis behavior and luteinizing hormone release (LH): further studies on NMDA receptor mediation. *Physiol. Behav.* 58, 169–173. doi: 10.1016/0031-9384(95)00040-P

Gargiulo, P. A., Munoz, V., and Donoso, A. O. (1992). Inhibition by N-methyl-D-aspartic acid (NMDA) receptor antagonist of lordosis behavior induced by estrogen followed by progesterone or luteinizing hormone-releasing hormone (LHRH) in the rat. *Physiol. Behav.* 52, 737–739. doi: 10.1016/0031-9384(92)90407-S

Georgescu, M., and Pfaus, J. G. (2006). Role of glutamate receptors in the ventromedial hypothalamus in the regulation of female rat sexual behaviors I. Behavioral effects of glutamate and its selective receptor agonists AMPA, NMDA and kainate. *Pharmacol. Biochem. Behav.* 83, 322–332. doi: 10.1016/j.pbb.2006.02.016

Harlan, R. E., Shivers, B. D., and Pfaff, D. W. (1983). Midbrain microinfusions of prolactin increase the estrogen-dependent behavior, lordosis. *Science* 219, 1451–1453. doi: 10.1126/science.6828874

Keifer, J., and Carr, M. T. (2000). Immunocytochemical localization of glutamate receptor subunits in the brain stem and cerebellum of the turtle Chrysemys picta. *J. Comp. Neurol.* 427, 455–468. doi: 10.1002/1096-9861(20001120)427:3<455::AID-CNE11>3.0.CO;2-X

Kow, L. M. (1976). Sensory requirements for the lordosis reflex in female rats. *Brain Res.* 101, 47–66. doi: 10.1016/0006-8993(76)90987-2

Krout, K. E., Jansen, A. S., and Loewy, A. D. (1998). Periaqueductal gray matter projection to the parabrachial nucleus in rat. *J. Comp. Neurol.* 401, 437–454.

Landa, A. I., Gargiulo, A. J., Gargiulo, M. M., Cabrera, R. J., Bregonzio, C., Lafuente Sanchez, J. V., et al. (2009). Alpha and beta noradrenergic mediation of NMDA glutamatergic effects on lordosis behaviour and plasmatic LH concentrations in the primed female rat. *J. Neural Transm.* 116, 551–557. doi: 10.1007/s00702-009-0217-x

Liposits, Z., and Setalo, G. (1980). Descending luteinizing hormone-releasing hormone (LH-RH) nerve fibers to the midbrain of the rat. *Neurosci. Lett.* 20, 1–4. doi: 10.1016/0304-3940(80)90223-2

Ljungdahl, A., Hokfelt, T., and Nilsson, G. (1978). Distribution of substance P-like immunoreactivity in the central nervous system of the rat–I. Cell bodies and nerve terminals. *Neuroscience* 3, 861–943. doi: 10.1016/0306-4522(78)90116-1

Lonstein, J. S., and Stern, J. M. (1998). Site and behavioral specificity of periaqueductal gray lesions on postpartum sexual, maternal, and aggressive behaviors in rats. *Brain Res.* 804, 21–35. doi: 10.1016/S0006-8993(98)00642-8

Matsuda, K., Kamiya, Y., Matsuda, S., and Yuzaki, M. (2002). Cloning and characterization of a novel NMDA receptor subunit NR3B: a dominant subunit that reduces calcium permeability. *Brain Res. Mol. Brain Res.* 100, 43–52. doi: 10.1016/S0169-328X(02)00173-0

Oka, T., Tsumori, T., Yokota, S., and Yasui, Y. (2008). Neuroanatomical and neurochemical organization of projections from the central amygdaloid nucleus to the nucleus retroambiguus via the periaqueductal gray in the rat. *Neurosci. Res.* 62, 286–298. doi: 10.1016/j.neures.2008.10.004

Paxinos, G. (2004). *The Rat Nervous System.* San Diego, CA: Gulf Professional Publishing.

Paxinos, G., and Watson, C. (2006). *The Rat Brain in Stereotaxic Coordinates.* San Diego, CA: Hard Cover Edn. Access Online via Elsevier.

Petralia, S. M., Debold, J. F., and Frye, C. A. (2007). MK-801 infusions to the ventral tegmental area and ventromedial hypothalamus produce opposite effects on lordosis of hormone-primed rats. *Pharmacol. Biochem. Behav.* 86, 377–385. doi: 10.1016/j.pbb.2007.01.005

Pfaff, D. W. (1980). *Estrogens and Brain Function: Neural Analysis of a Hormone-Controlled Mammalian Reproductive Behavior.* New York, NY: Springer-Verlag.

Pfaus, J. G., and Heeb, M. M. (1997). Implications of immediate-early gene induction in the brain following sexual stimulation of female and male rodents. *Brain Res. Bull.* 44, 397–407. doi: 10.1016/S0361-9230(97)00219-0

Pfaus, J. G., Kleopoulos, S. P., Mobbs, C. V., Gibbs, R. B., and Pfaff, D. W. (1993). Sexual stimulation activates c-fos within estrogen-concentrating regions of the female rat forebrain. *Brain Res.* 624, 253–267. doi: 10.1016/0006-8993(93)90085-2

Pfaus, J. G., Marcangione, C., Smith, W. J., Manitt, C., and Abillamaa, H. (1996). Differential induction of Fos in the female rat brain following different amounts of vaginocervical stimulation: modulation by steroid hormones. *Brain Res.* 741, 314–330. doi: 10.1016/S0006-8993(96)00985-7

Robbins, A., Pfaff, D. W., and Schwartz-Giblin, S. (1992). Reticulospinal and reticuloreticular pathways for activating the lumbar back muscles in the rat. *Exp. Brain Res.* 92, 46–58. doi: 10.1007/BF00230382

Robbins, A., Schwartz-Giblin, S., and Pfaff, D. W. (1990). Ascending and descending projections to medullary reticular formation sites which activate deep lumbar back muscles in the rat. *Exp. Brain Res.* 80, 463–474. doi: 10.1007/BF00227988

Rubin, B. S., and Barfield, R. J. (1983). Induction of estrous behavior in ovariectomized rats by sequential replacement of estrogen and progesterone to the ventromedial hypothalamus. *Neuroendocrinology* 37, 218–224. doi: 10.1159/000123546

Sakuma, Y., and Pfaff, D. W. (1979a). Facilitation of female reproductive behavior from mesensephalic central gray in the rat. *Am. J. Physiol.* 237, R278–R284.

Sakuma, Y., and Pfaff, D. W. (1979b). Mesencephalic mechanisms for integration of female reproductive behavior in the rat. *Am. J. Physiol.* 237, R285–R290.

Sakuma, Y., and Pfaff, D. W. (1980). Covergent effects of lordosis-relevant somatosensory and hypothalamic influences on central gray cells in the rat mesencephalon. *Exp. Neurol.* 70, 269–281. doi: 10.1016/0014-4886(80)90026-6

Sakuma, Y., and Pfaff, D. W. (1983). Modulation of the lordosis reflex of female rats by LHRH, its antiserum and analogs in the mesencephalic central gray. *Neuroendocrinology* 36, 218–224. doi: 10.1159/000123459

Sim, L. J., and Joseph, S. A. (1992). Serotonin and substance P afferents to parafascicular and central medial nuclei. *Peptides* 13, 171–176. doi: 10.1016/0196-9781(92)90159-Z

Takanami, K., Sakamoto, H., Matsuda, K., Hosokawa, K., Nishi, M., Prossnitz, E. R., et al. (2010). Expression of G protein-coupled receptor 30 in the spinal somatosensory system. *Brain Res.* 1310, 17–28. doi: 10.1016/j.brainres.2009.11.004

Tetel, M. J., Getzinger, M. J., and Blaustein, J. D. (1993). Fos expression in the rat brain following vaginal-cervical stimulation by mating and manual probing. *J. Neuroendocrinol.* 5, 397–404. doi: 10.1111/j.1365-2826.1993.tb00500.x

Wada, S., Yamada, S., and Yamanouchi, K. (2008). Additive inhibition of lordosis by simultaneous treatments with GABA(A) and GABA(B) receptor agonists, muscimol and baclofen, in female rats. *Pharmacol. Biochem. Behav.* 90, 590–593. doi: 10.1016/j.pbb.2008.04.020

Yamada, S., Uenoyama, Y., Deura, C., Minabe, S., Naniwa, Y., Iwata, K., et al. (2012). Oestrogen-dependent suppression of pulsatile luteinising hormone secretion and kiss1 mRNA expression in the arcuate nucleus during late lactation in rats. *J. Neuroendocrinol.* 24, 1234–1242. doi: 10.1111/j.1365-2826.2012.02330.x

Yamada, S., Uenoyama, Y., Kinoshita, M., Iwata, K., Takase, K., Matsui, H., et al. (2007). Inhibition of metastin (kisspeptin-54)-GPR54 signaling in the arcuate nucleus-median eminence region during lactation in rats. *Endocrinology* 148, 2226–2232. doi: 10.1210/en.2006-1529

Zemlan, F. P., Kow, L. M., and Pfaff, D. W. (1983). Effect of interruption of bulbospinal pathways on lordosis, posture, and locomotion. *Exp. Neurol.* 81, 177–194. doi: 10.1016/0014-4886(83)90167-X

Ziegler, D. R., Cullinan, W. E., and Herman, J. P. (2002). Distribution of vesicular glutamate transporter mRNA in rat hypothalamus. *J. Comp. Neurol.* 448, 217–229. doi: 10.1002/cne.10257

Ziegler, D. R., Edwards, M. R., Ulrich-Lai, Y. M., Herman, J. P., and Cullinan, W. E. (2012). Brainstem origins of glutamatergic innervation of the rat hypothalamic paraventricular nucleus. *J. Comp. Neurol.* 520, 2369–2394. doi: 10.1002/cne.23043

20

The mechanisms underlying sexual differentiation of behavior and physiology in mammals and birds: relative contributions of sex steroids and sex chromosomes

Fumihiko Maekawa[1]*, Shinji Tsukahara[2], Takaharu Kawashima[3], Keiko Nohara[1] and Hiroko Ohki-Hamazaki[4]*

[1] *Molecular Toxicology Section, Center for Environmental Health Sciences, National Institute for Environmental Studies, Tsukuba, Japan*
[2] *Division of Life Science, Graduate School of Science and Engineering, Saitama University, Saitama, Japan*
[3] *Ecological Genetics Research Section, Center for Environmental Biology and Ecosystem Studies, National Institute for Environmental Studies, Tsukuba, Japan*
[4] *College of Liberal Arts and Sciences, Kitasato University, Sagamihara, Japan*

Correspondence:
Fumihiko Maekawa, Molecular Toxicology Section, Center for Environmental Health Sciences, National Institute for Environmental Studies, 16-2 Onogawa, Tsukuba, 305-8506, Japan
e-mail: fmaekawa@nies.go.jp;
Hiroko Ohki-Hamazaki, College of Liberal Arts and Sciences, Kitasato University, 1-15-1 Kitasato, Minami-ku, Sagamihara, Kanagawa 252-0373, Japan
e-mail: hamazaki@kitasato-u.ac.jp

From a classical viewpoint, sex-specific behavior and physiological functions as well as the brain structures of mammals such as rats and mice, have been thought to be influenced by perinatal sex steroids secreted by the gonads. Sex steroids have also been thought to affect the differentiation of the sex-typical behavior of a few members of the avian order Galliformes, including the Japanese quail and chickens, during their development *in ovo*. However, recent mammalian studies that focused on the artificial shuffling or knockout of the sex-determining gene, *Sry*, have revealed that sex chromosomal effects may be associated with particular types of sex-linked differences such as aggression levels, social interaction, and autoimmune diseases, independently of sex steroid-mediated effects. In addition, studies on naturally occurring, rare phenomena such as gynandromorphic birds and experimentally constructed chimeras in which the composition of sex chromosomes in the brain differs from that in the other parts of the body, indicated that sex chromosomes play certain direct roles in the sex-specific differentiation of the gonads and the brain. In this article, we review the relative contributions of sex steroids and sex chromosomes in the determination of brain functions related to sexual behavior and reproductive physiology in mammals and birds.

Keywords: sexual differentiation of the brain, neurosteroids, birds, rodents, chimera

INTRODUCTION

In most eukaryotic species, sex differences exist within aspects of behavior as well as physiology. Since typical sexual behaviors and reproductive physiology are crucial to produce offspring, it is important to understand the mechanism of sexual differentiation in the brain in conjunction with sex-specific behaviors and physiology. From the standpoint of environmental science, several external factors from the industrialized world can impair reproduction. Studies have shown that the specific chemicals called endocrine disruptors can influence sexual differentiation in many species (Colborn et al., 1993). It has been reported that bisphenol-A and organotin compounds are examples of such endocrine disruptors that mimic and/or antagonize the functions of sex steroids and impair sexual differentiation in wildlife (Flint et al., 2012; Lewis and Ford, 2012). Therefore, research has been conducted on how such chemicals affect sex steroid-dependent organization of various organs, including the brain, during development, in order to protect wildlife and humans from potential endocrine disruptors (Frye et al., 2012). On the other hand, the knowledge regarding sexual differentiation has increased with progress in basic research (Arnold, 2004; Arnold and Chen, 2009) and the endpoints for investigating how environmental chemicals impair normal sexual differentiation might be updated subsequently. In this article, we review the relative contribution of gonadal steroids and sex chromosomes to the differentiation of brain functions related to the sexual behavior and reproductive physiology in mammals and birds by focusing on the recent findings.

CHROMOSOMAL COMPOSITIONS AND GONADAL SEX DETERMINATION IN MAMMALS AND BIRDS

The molecular mechanism of gonadal development in mammals and birds has been studied extensively. In most mammals, the males have one X chromosome and one Y chromosome whereas females have two X chromosomes. The gene *Sry/SRY*, located on the Y chromosome has been shown to be critical for testis development in most mammals (Gubbay et al., 1990; Sinclair et al., 1990; Koopman et al., 1991). The mechanism of testis determination in mammals is similar to that of the gonadal sex determination system of some teleost fish whose sex is determined by the specific gene *DMY* located on the Y chromosome (Matsuda et al., 2002). The sex chromosomes of birds are designated Z and W, where male birds have two Z chromosomes, while female birds have one Z chromosome and one W chromosome. The *DMRT1* gene on the Z chromosome, which encodes the doublesex and mab-3-related transcription factor 1 (DMRT1), is required for testis determination in birds of the order *Galliformes* (Smith et al., 2009). Birds lack a global mechanism of dosage compensation to equalize the expression of genes between sexes on the Z chromosome(s). Moreover, male-biased gene expression in gonads has been reported for most genes located on the Z chromosome, with variable levels of expression depending on the locus (Mank and Ellegren, 2009). *DMRT1* in the order *Galliformes* is an example of such a gene and the amount of DMRT1 produced from expression of the single *DMRT1* gene on the single Z chromosome in females is insufficient to induce the formation of a testis. It has also been reported that knockdown of DMRT1 by RNA interference in the male chicken gonadal primordium results in feminization of the gonads (Smith et al., 2009). Therefore, the lower level of *DMRT1* expression presumably induces the gonadal primordium to develop into ovary. Dosage compensation seems to occur on the Z chromosome at a gene-by-gene level in avian organs besides the gonads, such as the brain (Mank and Ellegren, 2009). This fact is the basis for the argument that sex chromosomes autonomously regulate sexual physiology and function in somatic tissues.

GONADAL HORMONE-DEPENDENT SEXUAL DIFFERENTIATION IN THE MAMMALIAN BEHAVIOR

In contrast to gonadal development, evidence suggests that sexual behavior is masculinized and defeminized during the perinatal or postnatal period by androgen secreted by the testes, irrespective of *Sry* expression in the brain. The action of testicular androgens in the developing brain is critical to the expression of the male-typical pattern of behaviors in mammals (Phoenix et al., 1959; Arnold and Gorski, 1984). In rodents, testosterone secreted by the testes is locally converted to 17β-estradiol (E2) by the cytochrome P450 enzyme, aromatase, in the brain, and E2 in turn, masculinizes/defeminizes the brain (MacLusky and Naftolin, 1981).

In rat, which is one of the most popular mammalian models for studying sexual differentiation in the brain, testosterone is first detected in the testes on embryonic day 15.5 and testosterone synthesis in the testes peaks at approximately, embryonic day 18.5 (Warren et al., 1973). Testicular testosterone synthesis as well as plasma testosterone concentrations decrease sharply after birth. Since the plasma testosterone level in rats from day 18 of gestation to day 5 postpartum is higher in male than in female rats (Weisz and Ward, 1980), the male brain is exposed to higher levels of testosterone than female brain. Therefore, this perinatal period is considered to be a critical period for sexual differentiation in the rat brain (MacLusky and Naftolin, 1981) and this hypothesis was then supported by the experiments described below.

Injection of female rats with either testosterone propionate (TP) or E2 during the perinatal period resulted in decreased ability to display female sexual behaviors in adulthood (Phoenix et al., 1959). In female mice, knockout of α-fetoprotein that binds to estrogen, thus protecting the developing female brain from exposure to estrogen, has been reported to cause reduction in lordosis, a manifestation of female sexual behavior, and an increase in expression of the male-typical sexual behavior, that is, mounting (Bakker et al., 2006). In addition, it has been reported that estrogen receptor (ER)- α–knockout males exhibited decreased frequency of intromission, another male-typical sexual behavior (Ogawa et al., 1997). Based on these results, the differentiation of stereotypic pattern of sexual behavior in rodents is thought to be, at least in part, due to the effects of sex steroids. Sex-specific copulatory behavior is assumed to be accompanied by structural changes in the brain. Various studies demonstrating morphological sex differences in the brains of rats and mice discussed below.

GONADAL HORMONE-DEPENDENT SEXUAL DIMORPHIC NUCLEI IN THE MAMMALIAN BRAIN

Certain brain nuclei exhibit sex differences, in terms of volume and number of neurons and/or synapses and are generally referred to as sexually dimorphic nuclei. Difference in volume of the nuclei is attributable to the differences in number of neurons. Gorski et al. discovered a nucleus in the preoptic region that shows morphological sex differences in rats (Gorski et al., 1978, 1980); this nucleus is now known as the sexually dimorphic nucleus of the preoptic area (SDN-POA), though its physiological functions are still unknown. The SDN-POA is significantly larger and contains more neurons in male than in female rats. Similarly, the volume of the calbindin-D28K-immunoreactive area in the SDN-POA is 2–4 times larger in male than in female rats (Simerly et al., 1997; Sickel and McCarthy, 2000; Orikasa et al., 2007). Moreover, following neonatal castration, the SDN-POA volume in adult male rat decreased (Gorski et al., 1978), whereas injection of TP in females during the early developmental period resulted in an increase in the SDN-POA volume in adult female rats to match that of adult male rats (Gorski et al., 1978; Dohler et al., 1984). On the other hand, injection of TP in adult rats has no effect on the volume of the SDN-POA. These findings suggest that testosterone synthesized in the rat testes affects the brain during development and not during adulthood, to increase the volume of the SDN-POA. Injection of E2 instead of TP in postnatal female rats also increased the size of their SDN-POA during adulthood. Injection of an ER-α agonist, and not an ER-β agonist, mimicked the effect of E2 (Patchev et al., 2004). The effects of estrogen, which is converted from androgen by aromatization and then binds to ER-α during the perinatal period, may be essential to establish the sexual dimorphism in the SDN-POA in rats.

During development, gonadal steroids also influence the sexually dimorphic formation of the principal nucleus of the bed nuclei of the stria terminalis (BNSTp). The BNSTp of the adult male rats is larger and contains more neurons than that of adult females (del Abril et al., 1987; Hines et al., 1992). Perinatal orchidectomy of males and perinatal androgenization of females by injection of TP prevent the occurrence of sexual dimorphism in BNSTp (Guillamon et al., 1988; Chung et al., 2000). Inactivation of androgen receptor results in feminization of the testes, which then show an ovary-like phenotype, and also reduction in the volume of the BNSTp in male rats (Durazzo et al., 2007). Sex differences in the volume and number of neurons in BNSTp do not occur in mice deficient in either aromatase or the ER-α gene, because of feminization of BNSTp in males (Tsukahara et al., 2011). On the other hand, mice deficient in the ER-β gene show sex differences in BNSTp (Tsukahara et al., 2011). These results suggest that estrogen is synthesized from androgen and that its effects, exerted through binding to ER-α during the perinatal and/or adult stage, appear to be involved in the male-typical formation of the BNSTp in mice. It has recently been reported that, in the BNST, gene expression of *Brs3*, *Cckar* and *Sytl4*, was sexually dimorphic, and regulated female and male sexual behaviors (Xu et al., 2012). However, since expression of these genes was altered by gonadectomy, sexual dimorphism was suspected to be attributable to the effect of sex steroids at the adult stage. More recently, it has been reported that the number of CRH neurons in the BNST (Fukushima et al., 2013) can be altered by TP injection in the perinatal period.

In contrast to the effects of sex steroids on the SDN-POA and BNSTp, the size of the anteroventral periventricular nucleus of POA (AVPV) in rats was reduced by androgens or estrogens during the perinatal period (Ito et al., 1986; Patchev et al., 2004). Injection of an ER-α agonist or an ER-β agonist in the perinatal period has been shown to decrease the neuronal cell density in the AVPV in female rats (Patchev et al., 2004), indicating that this reduction in neuronal cell density in the AVPV is an effect of estrogen mediated through binding to either ER-α or ER-β. The AVPV in female rats contains a greater numbers of tyrosine-hydroxylase (TH) mRNA-positive, dopaminergic neurons (Simerly et al., 1985) and Kiss1 mRNA-positive neurons (Kauffman et al., 2007) than the AVPV in male rats. Perinatal orchidectomy in males and perinatal treatment with testosterone in females resulted in an increase and decrease, respectively, in the number of TH mRNA-positive neurons in the AVPV (Simerly, 1989). In addition, perinatal treatment with TP in females decreased the number of Kiss1 mRNA-positive neurons (Kauffman et al., 2007).

INVESTIGATION OF SEXUAL DIFFERENTIATION IN THE BRAIN, BY GONADAL HORMONES AND SEX CHROMOSOMES USING TRANSGENIC APPROACHES IN MICE

There is accumulating evidence that a certain type of sexual differentiation in the brain is attributable to mechanisms that are independent of steroid hormones. The mouse model specific to this phenomenon called "four core genotypes" (FCG) was made possible by bioengineering techniques that created a mismatch between gonadal sex and chromosomal sex (XX vs. XY). This FCG model provides a breakthrough in the understanding of how sex chromosomes affect sexual differentiation in the brain. Based on observations in the FCG mouse model, the investigators reported that the latency and frequency of copulatory behavior are somewhat influenced by sex chromosomes (Park et al., 2008). However, sexual orientation seems to be mainly determined by differences in gonadal sex and subsequent secretion of sex steroids. This finding is generally consistent with the results of studies in which the sexual differentiation in the brain was examined after hormonal manipulation during the critical period. Indeed, the FCG model revealed that expression of progesterone receptor, which is inducible under the control of estrogen, is also dependent on gonadal sex (Wagner et al., 2004). On the other hand, aggression manifested in the form of attacks against intruders and parenting studied in pup-retrieval tests, have been reported to be regulated by chromosomal sex as well as by gonadal sex steroids (Gatewood et al., 2006). The aggression score, based on the proportion of mice that attacked intruders and the latency of attacking on first trial, was reported to increase in the presence of either testes or Y chromosome. By contrast, parental behavior, scored by latency to retrieve pups and number of pups retrieved, was low in the presence of either testes or Y chromosome. The sexual orientation of social behavior, including sniffing and play behavior in juvenile mice has been reported to be organized, at least in part, by the interaction between gonadal sex and chromosomal sex (Cox and Rissman, 2011). Therefore, neural circuits in the brain, responsible for social communications such as aggression, sniffing, and play behavior, may be differentiated not only by gonadal hormones, but also by the sex chromosome complement. In addition, the differentiation of neural circuits related to nociception, drug abuse, and autoimmune disease is related to the chromosomal sex, although the precise mechanisms by which chromosomal sex affects the neuronal circuits are not yet known. Taken together, the differentiation of core sexual behavior might be predominantly under the control of gonadal hormones, whereas the sex differentiation of various other aspects of physiology and behavior, including social communications might be determined, at least in part, by the interaction of gonadal hormones and sex chromosomes in mice.

EFFECTS OF CHROMOSOMAL SEX ON THE STRUCTURE AND GENE EXPRESSION IN THE BRAIN

The sexual dimorphism of midbrain dopaminergic neurons in rodents is reported to be controlled directly by chromosomal sex. Mice that have a Y chromosome, irrespective of their gonadal sex, have more dopaminergic neurons in their midbrain than mice that have only X chromosomes (Carruth et al., 2002). Expression of *Sry*, located on the Y chromosome in the male brain, has been reported to directly affect TH expression in the dopaminergic neurons of the substantia nigra (Dewing et al., 2006). In the lateral septum, on the other hand, both testosterone and the presence of a Y chromosome in male mice have been reported to increase the number of vasopressin neural fibers (De Vries et al., 2002). De Vries et al. revealed that XY males whose *Sry* gene was lost from the Y chromosome but had the heterotopic *Sry* transgene show a higher density of vasopressin fibers in the lateral septum than XX "males" with a heterotopic *Sry* transgene, whereas XY "females" whose *Sry* gene was lost from Y chromosome showed a higher density of vasopressin fibers in the area compared to the XX females (De Vries et al., 2002). These reports suggest that certain genes that are located on the Y chromosome, other than *Sry* affect the sexually dimorphic structure of the brain in mice. In association with such structural differences caused by sex chromosomes, expression of the genes located on X and Y chromosomes is also sexually dimorphic in the mouse brain (Xu et al., 2002; Dewing et al., 2003).

In addition, substantial differences in expression between sex-specific parental alleles on the X chromosome have been reported in the mouse brain (Gregg et al., 2010a). One study demonstrated that sex-specific imprinted genes whose expression differs between paternal and maternal alleles are mostly found in the hypothalamic area in the female brain (Gregg et al., 2010a), although early studies showed that maternal and paternal influence occurs in the cortex and in the hypothalamus, respectively (Allen et al., 1995; Keverne et al., 1996). On the other hand, paternal bias of autosomal genes in the brain was also reported (Gregg et al., 2010b). Understanding the epigenetic process that underlies the mechanism of parental bias would open up a new avenue of research on sex chromosomal effects in the brain.

GONADAL HORMONE-DEPENDENT SEXUAL DIFFERENTIATION IN THE AVIAN BRAIN

The Japanese quail is an animal model that has been used to examine how sex steroids determine the sexual differentiation in the brains of birds (Balthazart et al., 1983). The mating behavior of Japanese quail is sexually dimorphic: males strut and crow in front of the females and mount them (Adkins and Pniewski, 1978), whereas females never exhibit mounting behavior, even when injected with testosterone at adulthood (Adkins, 1975; Balthazart et al., 1983). It has been reported that in the adult male quail, estradiol produced by aromatization of testosterone in the brain induces male mounting behavior and that the testosterone metabolite 5-hydrotestosterone in the adult male induces strutting and crowing (Adkins and Pniewski, 1978; Balthazart et al., 1985). In contrast, exposure of male Japanese quail embryos to either testosterone or estrogen prior to day 12 of incubation resulted in significant reduction of mounting behavior at adult stage, indicating that actions of testosterone and estrogen at embryonic stage demasculinize male-type copulatory behavior at adulthood (Adkins-Regan, 1987). On the other hand, administration of an anti-estrogen agent to females prior to day 9 of incubation masculinizes their copulatory behavior (Adkins-Regan and Garcia, 1986). These results suggest that the order *Galliformes* and mammals are different in terms of the developmental effects of steroids. More specifically, the neuronal circuit related to copulatory behavior is masculinized in mammals by estrogen produced from testosterone in the brain, whereas it is feminized and de-masculinized in *Galliformes* by estrogen secreted from the ovary. As for plasma steroids in Japanese quail, it has been reported that from day 10 of incubation to hatching, estrogen concentrations are higher in females than in males, and conversely, testosterone concentrations are higher in males than in females (Ottinger et al., 2001). Therefore, the mechanism protecting the male quail brain from testosterone exposure has been postulated but is still under debate. Since a high activity of 5β-reductase has been reported in the embryonic male brain (Balthazart and Ottinger, 1984), this enzyme possibly metabolizes testosterone into 5β-dihydrotestosterone instead of E2 and protects the male brain from being de-masculinized by testosterone exposure (Balthazart and Ottinger, 1984). Taken together, these results suggest that endogenous estrogen secreted by the ovary is sufficient to differentiate the neuronal circuits related to copulatory behavior into the female-type in quail, but the precise mechanism by which the male brain escapes from feminization remains unclear.

SEXUAL DIFFERENTIATION IN THE SONG CONTROL SYSTEM IN THE AVIAN BRAIN

Song performance of the zebra finch is observed only in males and song-related nuclei including the nucleus hyperstriatum ventrale, pars caudale (HVc), and the nucleus robustus archistriatalis (RA) have been reported to be sexually dimorphic. The song performance is affected by developmental exposure of steroids. Double treatment, consisting of either estrogen or testosterone during hatching and testosterone at the adult stage, enables females to sing (Gurney and Konishi, 1980), indicating that the presence of estrogen in the brain during development can masculinize the song-related nuclei. Thus, there may be a difference between the actions of steroids on sexual behavior in *Galliformes* and on song performance of *Passeriformes* during development. Although the source of estradiol in the song control system during development of the zebra finch was long unknown, male brain slices containing the HVc and the RA regions have been found to produce more estrogen than corresponding female brain slices (Holloway and Clayton, 2001). This suggests that estrogen produced locally in the HVc and/or the RA contributes to masculinization of song-related nuclei. Indeed, various steroid-synthesizing enzymes are expressed in the zebra finch brain (Schlinger and Remage-Healey, 2012) and the same is true for the Japanese quail brain (Tsutsui, 2011). Studies performed by Remage-Healey et al. (2010, 2013) suggested that neurosteroids rapidly produced in the brain are important for social interaction via modulation of song production and perception of acoustic signals.

GONADAL HORMONE-INDEPENDENT SEXUAL DIFFERENTIATION OF THE AVIAN BRAIN

It has been suspected that genes located on the sex chromosome act in a cell-autonomous manner in brain cells to differentiate song-related circuits. Findings from a naturally-occurring gynandromorphic finch whose right and left sides show different sex genetics, demonstrated that the sexually dimorphic neural circuit for the song system is differentiated in part due to chromosomal sex. Most interestingly, the expression level of androgen receptor in the one half showed a masculine phenotype as compared to the other half, despite the identical influence of steroid hormones on both sides (Agate et al., 2003). Similar chromosomal sex influences on the sex difference of somatic tissues may also apply to *Galliformes*. The coloration, wattle, and leg spur of gynandromorphic chicken were observed to be different on the right and left, indicating that cell-autonomous sex determination in somatic cells occurs in *Galliformes* as well as in *Passeriformes* (Zhao et al., 2010).

INVESTIGATION OF AVIAN SEXUAL DIFFERENTIATION USING A CHIMERA IN WHICH THE SEX CHROMOSOMAL SET IN THE BRAIN DIFFERS FROM THAT FOR OTHER SOMATIC TISSUES

To determine whether the sex of the brain affects brain function and behavior, chimeras were constructed, in which the brains of two embryos were switched. The pioneering work by Nicole Le Douarin showed that developmental fate of cells can be monitored by creating quail-chick chimeras (Le Douarin and Jotereau, 1975). By a surgical method using a microscalpel, the brain primordium of a chick embryo at 1.5 days after incubation of the egg could be replaced by that of a quail embryo (Balaban et al., 1988; Teillet et al., 1991). By applying a similar method, the male (female) brain could be replaced by the female (male) brain of conspecies in *Galliformes.*

The first study with chimeras that have a brain with different chromosomal sex was conducted in Japanese quail (Gahr, 2003). In this study, the forebrain primordia were switched between two embryos before gonadal differentiation. The results showed that the chimeras with female karyotype in the forebrain but a male karyotype in other tissues did not exhibit mounting and exhibited only rudimentary crowing behavior. Since the adult chimeras showed low plasma level of testosterone which is required for male-type copulatory behavior, their impaired reproductive behaviors were attributable to their lower testosterone level. The volume of the preoptic area (POA) which is known to be dependent on plasma testosterone level (Panzica et al., 1987) was also reported to be feminized in the chimeras (Gahr, 2003). Therefore, it is speculated that male-typical chromosomal set complement is required in the forebrain of the quail, so that gonadotropin regulation can maintain testicular function in males.

On the other hand, we recently analyzed chicken chimeras with a brain of different chromosomal sex (Maekawa et al., 2013). However, in contrast to the previously observed results in Japanese quail chimeras, we did not observe any abnormalities in male-typical copulatory behavior and spermatogenesis in the chicken chimeras that had a male karyotype in gonads and a female karyotype in their brain. Rather, sexual maturation was delayed and an irregular ovulatory cycle was exhibited in the chimeras that had a female karyotype in their gonads and male karyotype in their brains. This abnormality in sexual maturation and ovulatory cycle was not reported in the previous study conducted with Japanese quail. Since the baseline gonadotropin level in chicken chimeras that had a female karyotype in their gonads and male karyotype in their brains was comparable to that in female chickens, we hypothesized that irregular oviposition in the chimeras is caused by a timing mismatch of the gonadotropin surge due to the male-type chromosomal sex in the brain.

Meanwhile, we also found that overall sexually dimorphic behavior, judged based on the results of the open field test and tests of sexual behavior, was not influenced by brain chromosomal sex. This suggests that gonadal steroids may determine brain function related to overall sexual dimorphic behavior. In addition, the blood steroid level of the chicken chimeras was not affected by the sex of the brain, which was different from the sex of the remaining tissues; the sexual dimorphism of the BNSTp, a nucleus that is thought to be related to sexual identity in humans, was dependent on gonadal hormones.

Only two studies of brain chimeras, one in Japanese quail and another in chicken, have ever been conducted. Both studies showed that brain chromosomal sex directly affects reproductive physiology, albeit with substantial discrepancies when compared in the details. We speculated the following three possible explanations for these discrepancies of pathology, resulting from transplantation:

1) *Species difference*: A comparison between the genome of quail and chicken revealed that chromosome rearrangements may have occurred between these two *Galliformes* species over 35 million years ago (Kayang et al., 2006). A draft Japanese quail genome sequence was assembled by means of next-generation sequencing technology (Kawahara-Miki et al., 2013). The results suggested that the genomes of Japanese quail and chicken were closely related while being more distantly related to the genome of the zebra finch (Kawahara-Miki et al., 2013). However, genomic variation (Kawahara-Miki et al., 2013) and differences in reproductive physiology (Yoshimura, 2013) between Japanese quail and chicken have been found and such differences may affect pathology.
2) *Differences between the methods of transplantation*: In the study conducted on Japanese quail chimera, only the forebrain was transplanted, whereas the total brain primordium was transplanted in our study of chicken chimera. Indeed, our preliminary results in quail-chick transplantation revealed that the midbrain in which the dopaminergic neurons are known to show sexual dimorphism under sex chromosomal control in mammals was not exchanged by forebrain transplantation.
3) *Rejection*: In our study of chicken chimera, the female tissue transplanted into male bodies was rejected at the time of sexual maturation (Maekawa et al., 2013). Since the rejection was strictly sex combination-dependent, we speculated that the rejection was attributable to the expression of a female-specific antigen coded by gene(s) on the W chromosome. Daily injection of an immunosuppressant was necessary to evaluate behavior and physiology of chicken chimeras that had a female karyotype in the brain and male karyotype in the rest of their body. On the other hand, no rejection was reported in the study on Japanese quail. It is possible that a mild rejection occurred in Japanese quail chimeras that had a female karyotype in the forebrain and male karyotype in the rest of their body. In fact, we experienced that the partial transplantation of the brain primordium led to a mild rejection, which did not cause the death of the chicken chimera.

Additional studies of Japanese quail and chicken chimeras that are created by the same experimental protocol would be necessary to fully understand whether the fundamental rule of brain sexual differentiation exists in *Galliformes.*

POSSIBLE SIMILARITIES IN SEXUAL DIFFERENTIATION OF BEHAVIOR AND PHYSIOLOGY IN MAMMALS AND BIRDS

Finally, we describe possible similarities in sexual differentiation of behavior and physiology in mammals and birds (**Table 1**).

SEX DIFFERENCES IN SEXUAL BEHAVIOR AND BRAIN STRUCTURES

The sexual orientation of murine copulatory behavior is mainly determined by exposure of mice to sex steroids during development. Similarly, the sexual orientation of chicken copulatory behavior, including mounting in males and adopting a receptive posture in females, has been found in our study to be determined by gonadal sex. Taken together, the above results suggest that overall sexual orientation of the copulatory behavior of both mammals and birds may be regulated by gonadal hormones. The brain nuclei related to sexual functions, namely the SDN-POA and BNST in mammals and the BNST in the chicken, are reported to be differentiated in a sexual dimorphic manner mainly by

Table 1 | Possible similarities of sex differences in brain, physiology and behavior in mammals and birds.

	Similarities	Typical literatures
1	Sex differentiation of core sexual behavior is mainly induced by the exposure of gonadal hormones during development	Arnold and Chen, 2009; Maekawa et al., 2013 (also, 2–5)
2	The structure of BNST (M > F) is sexually differentiated mainly by the exposure of gonadal hormones during development	Tsukahara et al., 2011
3	Sex chromosomes in brain affects sexual dimorphism observed in communication such as song production in bird and social behavior in mouse	Agate et al., 2003; Cox and Rissman, 2011
4	Sex-biased local synthesis of neuroestrogen (M > F)	Hojo et al., 2009, 2014
5	Sexual differentiation of neuronal structures related to circadian timing could be affected by sex chromosomes in the brain	Kuljis et al., 2013

gonadal hormones. On the other hand, song performance in male zebra finches and sexual dimorphism observed in mice social behavior were reported to be affected by the sex chromosomes in the brain. Studies on a variety of species of mammals and birds may lead to a clear understanding of the precise interaction between such behaviors and the effect of sex chromosome in the brain or gonadal hormones.

NEUROSTEROID PRODUCTION

There is direct and indirect evidence that estrogen is locally produced in the songbird brain and that its concentration is higher in the specific brain nuclei in males. The estradiol level in whole brain, at embryonic day 21 and at 13 months of age has been found to be significantly higher in males than in females, even though the plasma estradiol level in females was higher (Maekawa et al., 2013). Moreover, chicken chimeras that had a female karyotype in their gonads and male karyotype in their brains had higher estradiol level in the brain relevant to male phenotype. Conversely, chimeras that had a female karyotype in their brains and male karyotype in their gonads had lower estradiol level relevant to female phenotype. These findings provide the first clear evidence that local estradiol production in the chicken brain is regulated by the chromosomal sex in the brain (**Figure 1**). Neuroestrogen has been reported to regulate the socio-sexual behavior in Japanese quail (Ubuka et al., 2014), although it remains uncertain whether sex difference of neuroestrogen is related to certain behavioral and physiological functions. In rat, the hippocampus has been shown to synthesize steroid hormones, which show sexual dimorphic concentrations (Hojo et al., 2004, 2014). The estradiol level of the female hippocampus at all stages of the estrous cycle was much lower than in the male (Hojo et al., 2009), and this finding is consistent with the results showing higher estradiol level in the brain of male zebra finch and chickens. The common mechanism underlying the sex-biased local synthesis of neuroestrogen in mammals and birds could be further elucidated by focused research on the expression of steroid-synthesizing enzymes.

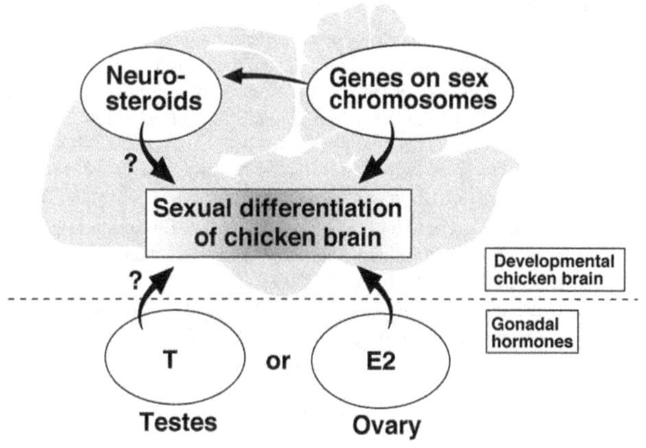

FIGURE 1 | Schematic diagram of the factors related to sexual differentiation of chicken brain.

CIRCADIAN TIMING

Chicken chimeras that have a male karyotype in the brain and female karyotype in their gonads have an irregular ovulatory cycle (Maekawa et al., 2013). The circadian timing of ovulation was delayed in the chimera, indicating that the neural circuit responsible for the timing of ovulation may be differentiated under the influence of chromosomal sex of the brain. It has been reported that mice having the XX chromosomal complement have longer activity duration than mice having the XY chromosomal complement irrespective of their gonadal sex (Kuljis et al., 2013), suggesting that sex chromosomal effect in mouse brain affects the circadian biological clock. Thus, the sex differences of neuronal structures related to determination of or mediating circadian timing may provide an alternative target to elucidate sex-related brain function. Elucidation of the defect in circadian timing of ovulation found in chicken chimeras may provide new insights into the relationship between the biological clock and sex differences.

CONCLUDING REMARKS

In this review, we summarized the mechanisms underlying sexual differentiation of the behavior and physiology in mammals and birds. From a classical viewpoint, perinatal sex steroids secreted by the gonads differentiate the sex-specific behavioral and physiological functions as well as brain structures both in mammals and birds. However, recent studies suggest that brain sex chromosomes directly affect the sexual differentiation of certain types of behavior and physiology. Especially, our study using chicken chimeras revealed that brain sex chromosomes directly influence neurosteroid synthesis.

In the context of environmental sciences examining harmful effects of endocrine disruptors, several studies have been conducted to investigate how endocrine disruptors affect the production and secretion of steroid hormones, how they impair ligand-binding of steroid hormones to their receptors, and their effects on tissues. Based on the findings described in this review, the effects of endocrine disruptors on local steroid production in the brain should be considered as the focus for further investigation of the harmful effects of endocrine disruptors.

ACKNOWLEDGMENTS

This work was supported by Grant-in-Aid for Scientific Research (B) (23310043), (C) (24590307) from Japan Society for the Promotion of Science (JSPS) and by the National Institute for Environmental Studies [14309][14013] to Fumihiko Maekawa.

REFERENCES

Adkins, E. K. (1975). Hormonal basis of sexual differentiation in the Japanese quail. *J. Comp. Physiol. Psychol.* 89, 61–71. doi: 10.1037/h0076406

Adkins, E. K., and Pniewski, E. E. (1978). Control of reproductive behavior by sex steroids in male quail. *J. Comp. Physiol. Psychol.* 92, 1169–1178. doi: 10.1037/h0077523

Adkins-Regan, E. (1987). Sexual differentiation in birds. *Trends Neurosci.* 10, 517–522. doi: 10.1016/0166-2236(87)90133-0

Adkins-Regan, E., and Garcia, M. (1986). Effect of flutamide (an antiandrogen) and diethylstilbestrol on the reproductive behavior of Japanese quail. *Physiol. Behav.* 36, 419–425. doi: 10.1016/0031-9384(86)90308-2

Agate, R. J., Grisham, W., Wade, J., Mann, S., Wingfield, J., Schanen, C., et al. (2003). Neural, not gonadal, origin of brain sex differences in a gynandromorphic finch. *Proc. Natl. Acad. Sci. U.S.A.* 100, 4873–4878. doi: 10.1073/pnas.0636925100

Allen, N. D., Logan, K., Lally, G., Drage, D. J., Norris, M. L., and Keverne, E. B. (1995). Distribution of parthenogenetic cells in the mouse brain and their influence on brain development and behavior. *Proc. Natl. Acad. Sci. U.S.A.* 92, 10782–10786. doi: 10.1073/pnas.92.23.10782

Arnold, A. P. (2004). Sex chromosomes and brain gender. *Nat. Rev. Neurosci.* 5, 701–708. doi: 10.1038/nrn1494

Arnold, A. P., and Chen, X. (2009). What does the "four core genotypes" mouse model tell us about sex differences in the brain and other tissues? *Front. Neuroendocrinol.* 30:1–9. doi: 10.1016/j.yfrne.2008.11.001

Arnold, A. P., and Gorski, R. A. (1984). Gonadal steroid induction of structural sex differences in the central nervous system. *Annu. Rev. Neurosci.* 7, 413–442. doi: 10.1146/annurev.ne.07.030184.002213

Bakker, J., De Mees, C., Douhard, Q., Balthazart, J., Gabant, P., Szpirer, J., et al. (2006). Alpha-fetoprotein protects the developing female mouse brain from masculinization and defeminization by estrogens. *Nat. Neurosci.* 9, 220–226. doi: 10.1038/nn1624

Balaban, E., Teillet, M. A., and Le Douarin, N. (1988). Application of the quail-chick chimera system to the study of brain development and behavior. *Science* 241, 1339–1342. doi: 10.1126/science.3413496

Balthazart, J., and Ottinger, M. A. (1984). 5β-reductase activity in the brain and cloacal gland of male and female embryos in the Japanese quail (Coturnix coturnix Japonica). *J. Endocrinol.* 102, 77–81. doi: 10.1677/joe.0.1020077

Balthazart, J., Schumacher, M., and Malacarne, G. (1985). Interaction of androgens and estrogens in the control of sexual behavior in male Japanese quail. *Physiol. Behav.* 35, 157–166. doi: 10.1016/0031-9384(85)90330-0

Balthazart, J., Schumacher, M., and Ottinger, M. A. (1983). Sexual differences in the Japanese quail: behavior, morphology, and intracellular metabolism of testosterone. *Gen. Comp. Endocrinol.* 51, 191–207. doi: 10.1016/0016-6480(83)90072-2

Carruth, L. L., Reisert, I., and Arnold, A. P. (2002). Sex chromosome genes directly affect brain sexual differentiation. *Nat. Neurosci.* 5, 933–934. doi: 10.1038/nn922

Chung, W. C., Swaab, D. F., and De Vries, G. J. (2000). Apoptosis during sexual differentiation of the bed nucleus of the stria terminalis in the rat brain. *J. Neurobiol.* 43, 234–243. doi: 10.1002/(SICI)1097-4695(20000605)43:3%3C234::AID-NEU2%3E3.3.CO;2-V

Colborn, T., vom Saal, F. S., and Soto, A. M. (1993). Developmental effects of endocrine-disrupting chemicals in wildlife and humans. *Environ. Health Perspect.* 101, 378–384. doi: 10.1289/ehp.93101378

Cox, K. H., and Rissman, E. F. (2011). Sex differences in juvenile mouse social behavior are influenced by sex chromosomes and social context. *Genes Brain Behav.* 10, 465–472. doi: 10.1111/j.1601-183X.2011.00688.x

del Abril, A., Segovia, S., and Guillamon, A. (1987). The bed nucleus of the stria terminalis in the rat: regional sex differences controlled by gonadal steroids early after birth. *Brain Res.* 429, 295–300. doi: 10.1016/0165-3806(87)90110-6

De Vries, G. J., Rissman, E. F., Simerly, R. B., Yang, L. Y., Scordalakes, E. M., Auger, C. J., et al. (2002). A model system for study of sex chromosome effects on sexually dimorphic neural and behavioral traits. *J. Neurosci.* 22, 9005–9014.

Dewing, P., Chiang, C. W., Sinchak, K., Sim, H., Fernagut, P. O., Kelly, S., et al. (2006). Direct regulation of adult brain function by the male-specific factor SRY. *Curr. Biol.* 16, 415–420. doi: 10.1016/j.cub.2006.01.017

Dewing, P., Shi, T., Horvath, S., and Vilain, E. (2003). Sexually dimorphic gene expression in mouse brain precedes gonadal differentiation. *Brain Res. Mol. Brain Res.* 118, 82–90. doi: 10.1016/S0169-328X(03)00339-5

Dohler, K. D., Coquelin, A., Davis, F., Hines, M., Shryne, J. E., and Gorski, R. A. (1984). Pre- and postnatal influence of testosterone propionate and diethylstilbestrol on differentiation of the sexually dimorphic nucleus of the preoptic area in male and female rats. *Brain Res.* 302, 291–295. doi: 10.1016/0006-8993(84)90242-7

Durazzo, A., Morris, J. A., Breedlove, S. M., and Jordan, C. L. (2007). Effects of the testicular feminization mutation (tfm) of the androgen receptor gene on BSTMPM volume and morphology in rats. *Neurosci. Lett.* 419, 168–171. doi: 10.1016/j.neulet.2007.04.033

Flint, S., Markle, T., Thompson, S., and Wallace, E. (2012). Bisphenol A exposure, effects, and policy: a wildlife perspective. *J. Environ. Manage.* 104, 19–34. doi: 10.1016/j.jenvman.2012.03.021

Frye, C. A., Bo, E., Calamandrei, G., Calzà, L., Dessì-Fulgheri, F., Fernández, M., et al. (2012). Endocrine disrupters: a review of some sources, effects, and mechanisms of actions on behaviour and neuroendocrine systems. *J. Neuroendocrinol.* 24, 144–159. doi: 10.1111/j.1365-2826.2011.02229.x

Fukushima, A., Furuta, M., Kimura, F., Akema, T., and Funabashi, T. (2013). Testosterone exposure during the critical period decreases corticotropin-releasing hormone-immunoreactive neurons in the bed nucleus of the stria terminalis of female rats. *Neurosci. Lett.* 534, 64–68. doi: 10.1016/j.neulet.2012.11.065

Gahr, M. (2003). Male Japanese quails with female brains do not show male sexual behaviors. *Proc. Natl. Acad. Sci. U. S. A.* 100, 7959–7964. doi: 10.1073/pnas.1335934100

Gatewood, J. D., Wills, A., Shetty, S., Xu, J., Arnold, A. P., Burgoyne, P. S., et al. (2006). Sex chromosome complement and gonadal sex influence aggressive and parental behaviors in mice. *J. Neurosci.* 26, 2335–2342. doi: 10.1523/JNEUROSCI.3743-05.2006

Gorski, R. A., Gordon, J. H., Shryne, J. E., and Southam, A. M. (1978). Evidence for a morphological sex difference within the medial preoptic area of the rat brain. *Brain Res.* 148, 333–346. doi: 10.1016/0006-8993(78)90723-0

Gorski, R. A., Harlan, R. E., Jacobson, C. D., Shryne, J. E., and Southam, A. M. (1980). Evidence for the existence of a sexually dimorphic nucleus in the preoptic area of the rat. *J. Comp. Neurol.* 193, 529–539. doi: 10.1002/cne.901930214

Gregg, C., Zhang, J., Butler, J. E., Haig, D., and Dulac, C. (2010a). Sex-specific parent-of-origin allelic expression in the mouse brain. *Science* 329, 682–685. doi: 10.1126/science.1190831

Gregg, C., Zhang, J., Weissbourd, B., Luo, S., Schroth, G. P., Haig, D., et al. (2010b). High-resolution analysis of parent-of-origin allelic expression in the mouse brain. *Science* 329, 643–648. doi: 10.1126/science.1190830

Gubbay, J., Collignon, J., Koopman, P., Capel, B., Economou, A., Münsterberg, A., et al. (1990). A gene mapping to the sex-determining region of the mouse Y chromosome is a member of a novel family of embryonically expressed genes. *Nature* 346, 245–250. doi: 10.1038/346245a0

Guillamon, A., Segovia, S., and del Abril, A. (1988). Early effects of gonadal steroids on the neuron number in the medial posterior region and the lateral division of the bed nucleus of the stria terminalis in the rat. *Dev Brain Res.* 44, 281–290. doi: 10.1016/0165-3806(88)90226-X

Gurney, M. E., and Konishi, M. (1980). Hormone-induced sexual differentiation of brain and behavior in zebra finches. *Science* 208, 1380–1383. doi: 10.1126/science.208.4450.1380

Hines, M., Allen, L. S., and Gorski, R. A. (1992). Sex differences in subregions of the medial nucleus of the amygdala and the bed nucleus of the stria terminalis of the rat. *Brain Res.* 579, 321–326. doi: 10.1016/0006-8993(92)90068-K

Hojo, Y., Hattori, T. A., Enami, T., Furukawa, A., Suzuki, K., Ishii, H. T., et al. (2004). Adult male rat hippocampus synthesizes estradiol from pregnenolone by cytochromes P450 17alpha and P450 aromatase localized in neurons. *Proc. Natl. Acad. Sci. U.S.A.* 101, 865–870. doi: 10.1073/pnas.2630225100

Hojo, Y., Higo, S., Ishii, H., Ooishi, Y., Mukai, H., Murakami, G., et al. (2009). Comparison between hippocampus-synthesized and circulation-derived sex steroids in the hippocampus. *Endocrinology* 150, 5106–5112. doi: 10.1210/en.2009-0305

Hojo, Y., Okamoto, M., Kato, A., Higo, S., Sakai, F., Soya, H., et al. (2014). Neurosteroid synthesis in adult female rat hippocampus, including androgens and allopregnanolone. *J. Steroids Hormone Sci.* S4, 002. doi: 10.4172/2157-7536.S4-002

Holloway, C. C., and Clayton, D. F. (2001). Estrogen synthesis in the male brain triggers development of the avian song control pathway *in vitro*. *Nat. Neurosci.* 4, 170–175. doi: 10.1038/84001

Ito, S., Murakami, S., Yamanouchi, K., and Arai, Y. (1986). Perinatal androgen decreases the size of the sexually dimorphic medial preoptic nucleus in the rat. *Proc. Jpn. Acad. Ser. B.* 62, 408–411. doi: 10.2183/pjab.62.408

Kauffman, A. S., Gottsch, M. L., Roa, J., Byquist, A. C., Crown, A., Clifton, D. K., et al. (2007). Sexual differentiation of Kiss1 gene expression in the brain of the rat. *Endocrinology* 148, 1774–1783. doi: 10.1210/en.2006-1540

Kawahara-Miki, R., Sano, S., Nunome, M., Shimmura, T., Kuwayama, T., Takahashi, S., et al. (2013). Next-generation sequencing reveals genomic features in the Japanese quail. *Genomics* 101, 345–353. doi: 10.1016/j.ygeno.2013.03.006

Kayang, B. B., Fillon, V., Inoue-Murayama, M., Miwa, M., Leroux, S., Fève, K., et al. (2006). Integrated maps in quail (*Coturnix japonica*) confirm the high degree of synteny conservation with chicken (*Gallus gallus*) despite 35 million years of divergence. *BMC Genomics* 7:101. doi: 10.1186/1471-2164-7-101

Keverne, E. B., Fundele, R., Narasimha, M., Barton, S. C., and Surani, M. A. (1996). Genomic imprinting and the differential roles of parental genomes in brain development. *Brain Res. Dev. Brain Res.* 92, 91–100. doi: 10.1016/0165-3806(95)00209-X

Koopman, P., Gubbay, J., Vivian, N., Goodfellow, P., and Lovell-Badge, R. (1991). Male development of chromosomally female mice transgenic for Sry. *Nature* 351, 117–121. doi: 10.1038/351117a0

Kuljis, D. A., Loh, D. H., Truong, D., Vosko, A. M., Ong, M. L., McClusky, R., et al. (2013). Gonadal- and sex-chromosome-dependent sex differences in the circadian system. *Endocrinology* 154, 1501–1512. doi: 10.1210/en.2012-1921

Le Douarin, N. M., and Jotereau, F. V. (1975). Tracing of cells of the avian thymus through embryonic life in interspecific chimeras. *J. Exp. Med.* 142, 17–40. doi: 10.1084/jem.142.1.17

Lewis, C., and Ford, A. T. (2012). Infertility in male aquatic invertebrates: a review. *Aquat. Toxicol.* 120–121, 79–89. doi: 10.1016/j.aquatox.2012.05.002

MacLusky, N. J., and Naftolin, F. (1981). Sexual differentiation of the central nervous system. *Science* 211, 1294–1302. doi: 10.1126/science.6163211

Maekawa, F., Sakurai, M., Yamashita, Y., Tanaka, K., Haraguchi, S., Yamamoto, K., et al. (2013). A genetically female brain is required for a regular reproductive cycle in chicken brain chimeras. *Nat. Commun.* 4, 1372. doi: 10.1038/ncomms2372

Mank, J. E., and Ellegren, H. (2009). All dosage compensation is local: gene-by-gene regulation of sex-biased expression on the chicken Z chromosome. *Heredity (Edinb).* 102, 312–320. doi: 10.1038/hdy.2008.116

Matsuda, M., Nagahama, Y., Shinomiya, A., Sato, T., Matsuda, C., Kobayashi, T., et al. (2002). DMY is a Y-specific DM-domain gene required for male development in the medaka fish. *Nature* 417, 559–563. doi: 10.1038/nature751

Ogawa, S., Lubahn, D. B., Korach, K. S., and Pfaff, D. W. (1997). Behavioral effects of estrogen receptor gene disruption in male mice. *Proc. Natl. Acad. Sci. U.S.A.* 94, 1476–1481. doi: 10.1073/pnas.94.4.1476

Orikasa, C., Kondo, Y., and Sakuma, Y. (2007). Transient transcription of the somatostatin gene at the time of estrogen-dependent organization of the sexually dimorphic nucleus of the rat preoptic area. *Endocrinology* 148, 1144–1149. doi: 10.1210/en.2006-1214

Ottinger, M. A., Pitts, S., and Abdelnabi, M. A. (2001). Steroid hormones during embryonic development in Japanese Quail: plasma, gonadal, and adrenal levels. *Poult. Sci.* 80:795–799. doi: 10.1093/ps/80.6.795

Panzica, G. C., Viglietti-Panzica, C., Calacagni, M., Anselmetti, G. C., Schumacher, M., and Balthazart, J. (1987). Sexual differentiation and hormonal control of the sexually dimorphic medial preoptic nucleus in the quail. *Brain Res.* 416, 59–68. doi: 10.1016/0006-8993(87)91496-X

Park, J. H., Burns-Cusato, M., Dominguez-Salazar, E., Riggan, A., Shetty, S., Arnold, A. P., et al. (2008). Effects of sex chromosome aneuploidy on male sexual behavior. *Genes Brain Behav.* 7, 609–617. doi: 10.1111/j.1601-183X.2008.00397.x

Patchev, A. V., Gotz, F., and Rohde, W. (2004). Differential role of estrogen receptor isoforms in sex-specific brain organization. *FASEB J.* 18, 1568–1570. doi: 10.1096/fj.04-1959fje

Phoenix, C. H., Goy, R. W., Gerall, A. A., and Young, W. C. (1959). Organizing action of prenatally administered testosterone propionate on the tissues mediating mating behavior in the female guinea pig. *Endocrinology* 65, 369–382. doi: 10.1210/endo-65-3-369

Remage-Healey, L., Coleman, M. E., Oyama, R. K., and Schlinger, B. A. (2010). Brain estrogens rapidly strengthen auditory encoding and guide song preference in a songbird. *Proc. Natl. Acad. Sci. U.S.A.* 107, 3852–3857. doi: 10.1073/pnas.0906572107

Remage-Healey, L., Jeon, S. D., and Joshi, N. R. (2013). Recent evidence for rapid synthesis and action of oestrogens during auditory processing in a songbird. *J. Neuroendocrinol.* 25, 1024–1031. doi: 10.1111/jne.12055

Schlinger, B. A., and Remage-Healey, L. (2012). Neurosteroidogenesis: insights from studies of songbirds. *J. Neuroendocrinol.* 24, 16–21. doi: 10.1111/j.1365-2826.2011.02150.x

Sickel, M. J., and McCarthy, M. M. (2000). Calbindin-D28k immunoreactivity is a marker for a subdivision of the sexually dimorphic nucleus of the preoptic area of the rat: developmental profile and gonadal steroid modulation. *J. Neuroendocrinol.* 12, 397–402. doi: 10.1046/j.1365-2826.2000.00474.x

Simerly, R. B. (1989). Hormonal control of the development and regulation of tyrosine hydroxylase expression within a sexually dimorphic population of dopaminergic cells in the hypothalamus. *Mol. Brain Res.* 6, 297–310. doi: 10.1016/0169-328X(89)90075-2

Simerly, R. B., Swanson, L. W., and Gorski, R. A. (1985). The distribution of monoaminergic cells and fibers in a periventricular preoptic nucleus involved in the control of gonadotropin release: immunohistochemical evidence for a dopaminergic sexual dimorphism. *Brain Res.* 330, 55–64. doi: 10.1016/0006-8993(85)90007-1

Simerly, R. B., Zee, M. C., Pendleton, J. W., Lubahn, D. B., and Korach, K. S. (1997). Estrogen receptor-dependent sexual differentiation of dopaminergic neurons in the preoptic region of the mouse. *Proc. Natl. Acad. Sci. U.S.A.* 94, 14077–14082. doi: 10.1073/pnas.94.25.14077

Sinclair, A. H., Berta, P., Palmer, M. S., Hawkins, J. R., Griffiths, B. L., Smith, M. J., et al. (1990). A gene from the human sex-determining region encodes a protein with homology to a conserved DNA-binding motif. *Nature* 346, 240–244. doi: 10.1038/346240a0

Smith, C. A., Roeszler, K. N., Ohnesorg, T., Cummins, D. M., Farlie, P. G., Doran, T. J., et al. (2009). The avian Z-linked gene DMRT1 is required for male sex determination in the chicken. *Nature* 461, 267–271. doi: 10.1038/nature08298

Teillet, M. A., Naquet, R., Le Gal La Salle, G., Merat, P., Schuler, B., and Le Douarin, N. M. (1991). Transfer of genetic epilepsy by embryonic brain grafts in the chicken. *Proc. Natl. Acad. Sci. U.S.A.* 88, 6966–6970. doi: 10.1073/pnas.88.16.6966

Tsukahara, S., Tsuda, M. C., Kurihara, R., Kato, Y., Kuroda, Y., Nakata, M., et al. (2011). Effects of aromatase or estrogen receptor gene deletion on masculinization of the principal nucleus of the bed nucleus of the stria terminalis of mice. *Neuroendocrinology* 94, 137–147. doi: 10.1159/000327541

Tsutsui, K. (2011). Neurosteroid biosynthesis and function in the brain of domestic birds. *Front. Endocrinol. (Lausanne).* 2:37. doi: 10.3389/fendo.2011.00037

Ubuka, T., Haraguchi, S., Tobari, Y., Narihiro, M., Ishikawa, K., Hayashi, T., et al. (2014). Hypothalamic inhibition of socio-sexual behaviour by increasing neuroestrogen synthesis. *Nat. Commun.* 5, 3061. doi: 10.1038/ncomms4061

Wagner, C. K., Xu, J., Pfau, J. L., Quadros, P. S., De Vries, G. J., and Arnold, A. P. (2004). Neonatal mice possessing an Sry transgene show a masculinized pattern of progesterone receptor expression in the brain independent of sex chromosome status. *Endocrinology* 145, 1046–1049. doi: 10.1210/en.2003-1219

Warren, D. W., Haltmeyer, G. C., and Eik-Nes, K. B. (1973). Testosterone in the fetal rat testis. *Biol. Reprod.* 8, 560–565.

Weisz, J., and Ward, I. L. (1980). Plasma testosterone and progesterone titers of pregnant rats, their male and female fetuses, and neonatal offspring. *Endocrinology* 106, 306–316. doi: 10.1210/endo-106-1-306

Xu, J., Burgoyne, P. S., and Arnold, A. P. (2002). Sex differences in sex chromosome gene expression in mouse brain. *Hum. Mol. Genet.* 11, 1409–1419. doi: 10.1093/hmg/11.12.1409

Xu, X., Coats, J. K., Yang, C. F., Wang, A., Ahmed, O. M., Alvarado, M., et al. (2012). Modular genetic control of sexually dimorphic behaviors. *Cell* 148, 596–607. doi: 10.1016/j.cell.2011.12.018

Yoshimura, T. (2013). Thyroid hormone and seasonal regulation of reproduction. *Front. Neuroendocrinol.* 34:157–166. doi: 10.1016/j.yfrne.2013.04.002

Zhao, D., McBride, D., Nandi, S., McQueen, H. A., McGrew, M. J., Hocking, P. M., et al. (2010). Somatic sex identity is cell autonomous in the chicken. *Nature* 464, 237–242. doi: 10.1038/nature08852

21

Electrophysiological characterization of male goldfish (*Carassius auratus*) ventral preoptic area neurons receiving olfactory inputs

Wudu E. Lado[1,2], David C. Spanswick[3,4], John E. Lewis[1] and Vance L. Trudeau[1]*

[1] Department of Biology, University of Ottawa, Ottawa, ON, Canada
[2] Department of Cell and Systems Biology, University of Toronto, Toronto, ON, Canada
[3] Warwick Medical School, University of Warwick, Coventry, UK
[4] Department of Physiology, Monash University, Clayton, VIC, Australia

***Correspondence:**
Vance L. Trudeau, University Research Chair in Neuroendocrinology, Department of Biology, Centre for Advanced Research in Environmental Genomics, University of Ottawa, 20 Marie Curie, Ottawa, ON K1N 6N5, Canada
e-mail: trudeauv@uottawa.ca

Chemical communication via sex pheromones is critical for successful reproduction but the underlying neural mechanisms are not well-understood. The goldfish is a tractable model because sex pheromones have been well-characterized in this species. We used male goldfish forebrain explants *in vitro* and performed whole-cell current clamp recordings from single neurons in the ventral preoptic area (vPOA) to characterize their membrane properties and synaptic inputs from the olfactory bulbs (OB). Principle component and cluster analyses based on intrinsic membrane properties of vPOA neurons ($N = 107$) revealed five (I–V) distinct cell groups. These cells displayed differences in their input resistance (R_{input}: I < II < IV < III = V), time constant (TC: I = II < IV < III = V), and threshold current ($I_{threshold}$: I > II = IV > III = V). Evidence from electrical stimulation of the OB and application of receptor antagonists suggests that vPOA neurons receive monosynaptic glutamatergic inputs via the medial olfactory tract, with connectivity varying among neuronal groups [I (24%), II (40%), III (0%), IV (34%), and V (2%)].

Keywords: ventral preoptic area, male goldfish, monosynaptic glutamatergic projections

INTRODUCTION

Chemical communication plays a vital role in vertebrate reproduction. Biologically-active sex pheromones have evolved across the animal kingdom to convey reproductive information to conspecifics (Dulac and Torello, 2003). However, in most cases, the neural circuitry associated with the processing of sex pheromones is poorly understood. Chemical communication is especially important in animals like goldfish because they rely on external fertilization and often live in turbid waters. These fish have evolved sex pheromones to synchronize spawning between the sexes and thus ensure reproductive success. Further, the goldfish is an attractive model to study the neural substrates of chemical communication because it is one of the few vertebrates whose sex pheromones have been fully characterized (Stacey et al., 1989; Sorensen et al., 1991; Dulka, 1993).

Studies of male goldfish indicate that sex pheromones from females regulate male sexual behavior and milt production by inducing the release of luteinizing hormone (LH) from the male pituitary gland through stimulation of gonadotropin-releasing hormone (GnRH) in the POA (Stacey, 1983; Kobayashi et al., 1986, 2002; Trudeau, 1997). The POA controls the release of LH (Peter et al., 1990; Chang et al., 2000; Trudeau et al., 2000a,b) via a signaling pathway involving dopamine (DA), which tonically inhibits both GnRH and LH release (Peter and Paulencu, 1980; Kah et al., 1987; Sloley et al., 1992; Popesku et al., 2011). Coupled to the GABAergic inputs this area receives from the ventral telencephali pars ventralis (Vv) (Martinoli et al., 1990; Trudeau et al., 2000b), the vPOA may be the site where DA suppression of GnRH is removed to allow increased GnRH levels to elicit LH release and subsequent spawning.

To characterize the neural pathways underlying the OB and POA networks, we have developed a novel *in vitro* explant preparation of the goldfish forebrain (Trudeau et al., 2000b). The adult goldfish brain is small and relatively unmyelinated making it attractive for patch clamp electrophysiology. In addition, the explant preserves the underlying neural circuitry yet allows for easy access to neurons on the ventral surface of the brain.

Here, we first describe the intrinsic membrane properties of neurons in the vPOA. Based on these properties, we suggest that vPOA neurons comprise five different subgroups. We then characterized the synaptic projections from the OB to the vPOA. In the goldfish and the closely related Crucian carp, the lateral olfactory tract (LOT) transmits food-related odors (Dulka, 1993; Hamdani et al., 2001a,b) while the medial olfactory tract (MOT) conveys exclusively pheromonal and social signals (Demski and Dulka, 1984; Sorensen et al., 1991; Hamdani et al., 2000). Here, we demonstrate that there are functional glutamatergic projections from the OB to the POA through the MOT.

MATERIALS AND METHODS

EXPERIMENTAL ANIMALS

This study was approved by the animal care committee of the University of Ottawa and carried out in accordance with the guidelines of Canadian Council on Animal Care. Common goldfish *(Carassius auratus)* weighing 15–40 g were purchased from a commercial supplier (Aleong's International Inc., Mississauga, ON, Canada). Fish were acclimated to 18°C, fed and maintained on a simulated photoperiod as previously reported (Trudeau et al., 1991). Only male goldfish were used throughout the study. During spawning season, sexually mature males were easily discernable by their distinctive tubercles and some readily expressed milt when their anogenital area was gently pressed. After the spawning season and during recrudescence, when tubercles are not always evident, sex was confirmed post-mortem by visual inspection of the testes.

Fish were anesthetized by immersion in 0.05% tricaine methanesulphonate (TMS) prior to dissection of the brain explant. Briefly, after severing the spinal cord, the skull was carefully opened with surgical scissors to expose the brain. The brain was dissected out from the skull cavity by cutting the optic nerves, and then removing the whole brain with olfactory bulbs still attached. The explant was attached to a Petri-dish ventral side up at the level of the spinal cord and cerebellum with cyanoacrylate glue, and placed in a bath with ice-cold artificial cerebrospinal fluid (ACSF) of the following composition [mM]: 127 NaCl, 1.9 KCl, 1.2 KH_2PO_4, 2.4 $CaCl_2$, 1.3 $MgCl_2$, 26 $NaHCO_3$, 10 D-glucose; gassed with carbogen (95 O_2, 5% CO_2); pH adjusted to 7.4 with NaOH. The ACSF was modified from rats' ACSF (Spanswick et al., 1998) and it was similar to others (ACSF) in other fish such as *Apteronotus leptorhynchus* (Kotecha et al., 1997) and *C. auratus* (Wilkie et al., 2008). When magnesium-free solution was used, $MgCl_2$ was omitted from the ACSF.

The meninges were removed with fine forceps to expose the ventral telencephalon and access the vPOA; then a transverse cut using a razor blade was made posterior to the hypothalamus to free the brain from the dish. The brain was then transferred carefully to a custom-built recording chamber perfused at room temperature with ACSF at a rate of 2–4 ml/min. The brain explant was mounted with the ventral side up and then held between two custom-made nylon grids where it was allowed to recover for 1 h prior to recordings; all recordings were made in the 7 h following dissection. Neuroanatomical nomenclature in this study follows that of Anglade et al. (1993). Our vPOA corresponded to *nucleus preopticus periventricularis* as depicted in Plate 43 of the goldfish brain atlas (Peter and Gill, 1975).

ELECTROPHYSIOLOGICAL RECORDINGS

Electrophysiological recordings were made based on previous methods for rat spinal cord and hypothalamus (Spanswick et al., 1998). Whole-cell patch clamp recordings using a Multiclamp 700B amplifier (Molecular Devices) in current clamp mode, were obtained from vPOA neurons ($N = 107$) in the *in vitro* forebrain explants at room temperature (~18–20°C) from 120 fish. Patch pipettes (5–8 MΩ) were fabricated from borosilicate filament glass (Sutter Instrument Co., Novata, CA, USA) using a horizontal pipette puller (P2000; Sutter Instrument Co., Novata, CA, USA) and filled with intracellular solution of the following composition [mM]: 140 K-gluconate, 10 KCl, 1 sucrose, 2 Na_2ATP, 1 EGTA-Na_4 plus 10 HEPES and pH adjusted to 7.4 with KOH modified from Spanswick et al. (1998).

Using the anterior commissure and optic chiasm as landmarks, patch electrodes were guided to the vPOA under visual control of a dissecting microscope. Seal formation was monitored on an oscilloscope. Once a gigaohm seal (typically $> 5\,G\Omega$) was achieved, whole-cell access was made by gentle suction. Series resistance was $< 25\,M\Omega$.

To measure synaptic connectivity, a bipolar stimulating electrode was inserted into one of the olfactory bulbs (OBs). Postsynaptic potentials (PSPs) in the vPOA were elicited by single pulse electrical stimulation (5–30 V, 0.2 ms pulse duration) of the ipsilateral OB via a stimulus isolation unit (Digitimer Ltd., model DS2). Data acquisition and experimental control was performed using pCLAMP 9.2 software (Molecular Devices). Data were low-pass filtered at 2 kHz and acquired at 10 kHz and later analyzed offline using CLAMPFIT 9.2 software (Molecular Devices).

PHARMACOLOGICAL AGENTS

To characterize the pharmacological properties of the connectivity from the OB to the vPOA neurons, we used 6-cyano-7-nitroquinoxaline-2, 3-dione (CNQX; Tocris), an α-amino-3-hydroxy-5-methyl-4-isoxazolepropionic acid (AMPA/kainate) receptor antagonist; and D-2-amino-5-phosphonopentanoic acid (D-APV; Tocris), an N-Methyl-D-aspartic acid or N-Methyl-D-aspartate (NMDA) receptor antagonist. Drugs were made up as stock solutions, CNQX in DMSO (Sigma-Aldrich) and D-APV in distilled water, then, diluted in Mg^{2+} free ACSF. The final concentration of DMSO was always < 0.1%. Typically, Mg^{2+} free ACSF and the drugs were applied sequentially for 10 min each to the recording chamber before any attempts at recordings to allow sufficient equilibration time.

DATA ANALYSIS

Intrinsic membrane properties of vPOA neurons were characterized by patch clamp electrophysiology to determine whether they constituted distinct populations. After achieving whole cell access, the resting membrane potential (RMP) which is the baseline potential in the absence of any current stimulus was measured in current clamp mode ($I = 0$ nA). In addition, properties related to spontaneous action potential production was measured (**Figure 1A**): Spike amplitude (SA) was measured from the shoulder of the rising phase (~threshold) to the peak; spike width (S_{width}) was measured at the width of half-maximal from the peak to the afterhyperpolarization (AHP); AHP was determined from the threshold to the peak of the hyperpolarization following the action potential (note that only the fast component of the AHP was considered in this study); after-depolarization potential (ADP) was measured from the hyperpolarization peak to the ADP peak. For neurons that showed spontaneous activity, the coefficient of variation of the interspike interval (the interval between successive spikes) was calculated over a 90 s time window (CV_{spikes} = SD/mean). Neurons were then stimulated with 1 s hyperpolarizing and depolarizing current steps (2–30 pA) from a holding potential of −60 mV to measure a number of other

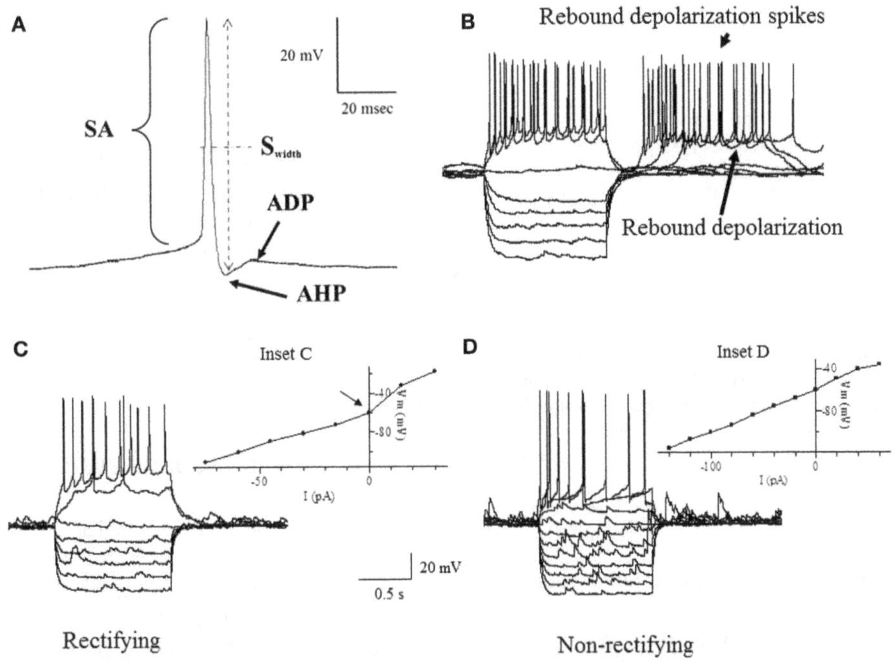

FIGURE 1 | Traces of some of the intrinsic membrane properties used in our statistical analyses. **(A)** Depicts the AHP (after hyperpolarization potential), APA (action potential amplitude), APD (action potential duration) and ADP (after depolarization potential). **(B)** Shows the RD (rebound depolarization) and RDS (rebound depolarization spikes). **(C,D)** demonstrate the current to voltage relationship (IV) where **(C)** is rectifying as shown by the arrow at the inflection point (Inset C) and **(D)** is non-rectifying (Inset D). APA was measured from the shoulder at threshold shown by the arrowhead. APD was the width of the AP measured from the shoulder at threshold shown by the arrowhead. See definitions in Materials and Methods section.

intrinsic membrane properties (**Figures 1B–D**): current threshold ($I_{threshold}$) is the minimum current required to elicit an action potential; spike threshold ($S_{threshold}$) is the number of spikes elicited by the minimum current i.e., at $I_{threshold}$; the presence or absence of a rebound depolarization (RD) after a hyperpolarizing current step; the presence or absence of rebound depolarization spikes (RDS), rebound spike frequency (RS) is the action potential frequency during the RD; the presence or absence of H current (I_H) which is associated with non-selective cation channels; rectification (Rec) refers to a non-linearity in the current-voltage (IV) relationship (Siegelbaum and Koester, 2000) (compare insets in **Figures 1C,D**); the input resistance (R_{input}), which is the slope of the IV curve; membrane time constant (TC) is the time for the hyperpolarization response to reach two-thirds of its plateau value; soma membrane capacitance (C_{soma}) is calculated as TC/R_{input} (Abbud and Smith, 1995).

A principle component analysis (PCA; SPSS Inc.; 2006, v.15) was used to reduce the set of intrinsic membrane properties to a number of independent uncorrelated variables. For this analysis, all properties that were characterized by their presence or absence, i.e., RD, RDS, I_H and Rec were assigned binary values (0, 1). The PCA variables were then used to cluster (SPSS Inc.; 2006, v.15) the neurons into groups. An unsupervised cluster analysis was performed to classify neurons, similar to previous studies (Ward, 1963; Krimer et al., 2005; Sosulina et al., 2006; Andjelic et al., 2009). This method consisted of grouping individual neurons based on the Euclidean distance between their respective PCA loadings.

Postsynaptic potentials (PSP) data were characterized by the peak amplitude (the height of the evoked PSP measured from baseline to peak), the latency (the time between the OB stimulus and beginning of PSP rise), 10–90% rise time (measured from the shoulder of the rise to the peak) and 90%–10% decay time (determined from 90% of the peak of the PSP to 10% above baseline) (**Figure 2**). To measure variability in the latency and rise time, the mean, standard deviation (SD) and coefficient of variation (CV); (SD/mean) was calculated over 4 stimulus trials in each cell.

All data generated by the PCA were tested for normality and homogeneity of variance, and either an analysis of variance (ANOVA) or a Kruskal-Wallis (KW) analysis was used for between group comparisons where appropriate (SPSS Inc.; 2006, v.15). *Post-hoc* analyses consisted of paired *t*-tests and Tukey's (SPSS Inc.; 2006, v.15). Unless otherwise stated, data are reported as mean ± s.e.m.

RESULTS

HETEROGENEITY OF INTRINSIC MEMBRANE PROPERTIES

To characterize the population of vPOA neurons, a number of intrinsic membrane properties were quantified (see Materials and Methods). We used a Principle Component Analysis (PCA) to determine the set of properties that could best distinguish neuronal subgroups. The PCA revealed seven significant properties (loading factor) [RD (0.92), R_{input} (0.87), SA (0.77), $S_{threshold}$ (0.80), RS (0.82), I_H (0.78), and Rec (0.83)] (**Table 1**). A subsequent cluster analysis of these variables revealed five distinct neuronal subgroups (denoted I, II, III, IV, and V). In the following, we

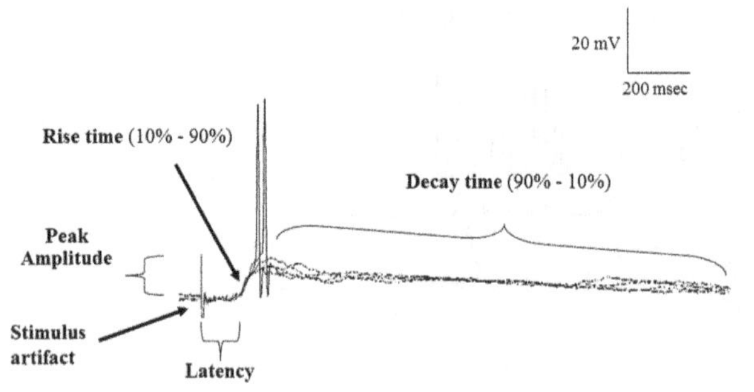

FIGURE 2 | Samples of a continuous recording showing superimposed EPSPs evoked in POA neurons following stimulation of the olfactory bulb under normal (ACSF) conditions and highlighting the properties of EPSPs measured. Note that evoked EPSPs could give rise to action potential firing and showed constant latency and rise time, consistent with a monosynaptic origin.

compare the membrane properties across the different subgroups (**Table 2**).

Since the data from our PCA failed the normality test ($P > 0.05$), it was transformed to its square root equivalent; and statistical analyses performed. Neuronal subgroups were found to differ in their R_{input} [$F_{(4, 106)} = 325.93$, $P = 0.001$], TC [$F_{(4, 106)} = 13.63$, $P = 0.001$] and $I_{threshold}$ [$F_{(4, 106)} = 3.86$, $P = 0.006$] but not ADP [$F_{(4, 106)} = 1.35$, $P = 0.25$]. *Tukey's post-hoc* analyses showed that R_{input} was different in each neuronal cluster with V = III > IV > II > I (**Figure 3A**). Similarly, the TC of neurons in clusters III and V were higher than IV which in turn was higher than those in clusters I and II (**Figure 3B**). In addition, $I_{threshold}$ for neurons in cluster I was greater than II which in turn was greater than for IV greater than III and V neurons (**Figure 3C**). Since the rectification (Rec) and RS were categorical variables, *post-hoc* comparisons were performed using KW analyses: rectification was not significant [$\chi^2_{(4)} = 1.55$; $P = 0.818$] nor was RS [$\chi^2_{(4)} = 10.28$; $P = 0.036$, Bonferroni correction, $P > 0.005$].

Overall, our analyses showed that only R_{input}, TC and $I_{threshold}$ were significantly different between groups ($P < 0.05$), while rectification and RS were not ($P > 0.05$). Together, the R_{input}, TC and C_{soma} constitute the passive membrane properties of the cell. Note that the TC is directly proportional to the product of the R_{input} and C_{soma} [TC = $R_{input} \cdot C_{soma}$] (Molleman, 2003). The calculated C_{soma} (after its transformation to the reciprocal of its square root to normalize the data) was also statistically different between neuronal groups [$F_{(4, 106)} = 25.89$, $P = 0.001$], with *Tukey's post-hoc* indicating that I > II > IV > III = V (**Figure 3D**). Since capacitance is proportional to membrane area (Hille, 2001), the differences we observe between neuronal groups can be at least partially explained by neuronal size.

PROPERTIES OF POSTSYNAPTIC POTENTIALS: INPUTS FROM THE OLFACTORY BULB

Given these putative subgroups of vPOA neurons, we next set out to determine their inputs from the olfactory bulb (OB). Of the 107 vPOA cells tested, 50 received synaptic inputs from the OB. The ratio of connected to unconnected neurons in each cluster was: I: 59% (12/23); II: 60% (20/38); III: 0% (0/4); IV: 53% (17/36); and V: 19% (1/6).

The PSPs were reliably evoked with latencies of approximately 90 ms. The small coefficients of variation (CV) of the latency (1.5%) and rise-time (2.2%) within cells are not consistent with a multi-synaptic pathway (for which latency is expected to be more variable). Given the consistency of the synaptic response, we suggest that these connections are monosynaptic (Spanswick et al., 1998). Since the distance from the OB to the POA is about 9 mm, a latency of 100 ms suggests an estimated conduction velocity similar to the slowest conduction velocity (~0.1 m/s) reported in olfactory nerves of the tench at similar temperatures (Dubois-Dauphin et al., 1980).

BIOCHEMICAL PROPERTIES OF THE POSTSYNAPTIC POTENTIALS OF vPOA

To characterize the pharmacological properties of the PSP in vPOA ($N = 13$) neurons, goldfish brain explants were perfused sequentially with normal ACSF, Mg^{++}-free ACSF (MFACSF), 20 μM D-APV and 10 μM CNQX before washing off both drugs with normal saline. The latency, peak amplitude rise and decay times of the evoked PSPs were then measured and compared under the different recording conditions. **Figure 4** shows representative data from a vPOA neuron. The Mg^{2+}free ACSF increased the PSP compared to normal saline. The glutamate antagonist APV partially blocked the evoked response. The residual response was subsequently blocked completely by CNQX, indicating that the PSPs had a dual component and were mediated by glutamate acting on both NMDARs and AMPARs (**Figure 4**). Indeed, when AMPARs alone were blocked with CNQX (data not shown; $N = 10$), no EPSPs were evoked suggesting that activation of NMDARs requires preceding depolarization via AMPARs to overcome voltage-dependent Mg^{2+} block.

A statistical analysis on data obtained from POA neurons ($N = 13$) did not find significant differences ($P > 0.05$) in their PSP latencies and rise times between the different perfusion media, but their decay times differed significantly between MFACSF vs. ACSF [$F_{(1, 12)} = 16.11$, $P = 0.002$] and MFACSF vs. APV [$F_{(1, 12)} = 16.59$, $P = 0.002$]. *Post-hoc* analysis indicated that POA neurons in MFACSF had a longer decay time than in either ACSF [$t_{(13)} = 3.76$, $p = 0.002$] or APV [$t_{(13)} = 4.07$, $p = 0.002$] (**Figure 5**). These data show that the evoked PSPs had a biphasic response, with APV partially blocking the slower and longer lasting NMDAR component, revealing a faster and shorter lasting AMPAR component that was completely blocked by CNQX.

SECTIONING THE LATERAL OLFACTORY TRACT WHILE RECORDING FROM THE vPOA

To determine if the OB to vPOA projection is mediated through the MOT, we sectioned the LOT ($N = 3$) while leaving the medial tract intact. We found that PSPs evoked in vPOA neurons by OB stimulation did not differ from those evoked under control conditions for latency, rise time, peak amplitude and decay times (KW analysis; $P > 0.05$). Cutting the MOT ($N = 10$) while leaving the LOT intact did not elicit any response consistent with studies which have shown that the MOT innervates targets in area

Table 1 | The rotated component matrix of variables used in our principle component analysis.

Property/Loaded factors	1	2	3	4	5	6	7
RMP (mV)	−0.247	0.151	−0.075	−0.014	−0.217	0.692	−0.314
TC (msec)	0.224	0.769	0.210	−0.065	0.120	−0.160	0.228
R_{input} (GΩ)	−0.113	**0.870**	0.030	0.026	−0.151	0.041	−0.035
AHP (mV)	−0.320	0.152	0.664	−0.081	0.000	−0.085	−0.240
SA (mV)	0.209	0.003	**0.770**	−0.104	0.033	−0.261	0.159
$I_{threshold}$ (pA)	−0.056	−0.368	0.057	0.794	−0.001	−0.238	0.120
$S_{threshold}$ (Hz)	0.228	0.299	0.037	**0.797**	−0.057	0.122	−0.073
S_{width} (ms)	−0.061	−0.043	−0.784	−0.340	0.043	−0.189	−0.092
CV	−0.038	0.285	−0.172	0.218	−0.720	−0.086	−0.225
RS	0.171	0.086	−0.079	0.056	**0.782**	−0.018	−0.126
ADP (mV)	0.397	−0.397	0.223	−0.173	−0.409	−0.051	−0.148
I_H	0.041	−0.184	−0.058	−0.053	−0.094	**0.783**	0.305
Rec	−0.134	0.135	0.031	0.031	0.039	0.044	**0.819**
RD	**0.916**	−0.066	−0.002	0.040	0.076	−0.093	0.032
RDS	0.877	0.136	0.007	0.136	0.135	−0.035	−0.179

*Loaded factors in bold show measurements that were subsequently used for our cluster analysis. See definitions in Materials and Methods section and **Figure 1**. Extraction Method: Principal Component Analysis. Rotation Method: Varimax with Kaiser Normalization. Rotation converged in 8 iterations.*

Table 2 | Intrinsic membrane properties of POA neurons measured in ACSF.

Property/Clusters	I ($N = 23$)	II ($N = 38$)	III ($N = 4$)	IV ($N = 36$)	V ($N = 6$)
RMP (mV)	−56.5 ± 2.2	−58.2 ± 1.4	−57.1 ± 4.5	−56 ± 1.4	−54.3 ± 2.1
TC (ms)	47.6 ± 5.2	47.0 ± 2.7	92.9 ± 15.3	66.2 ± 3.9	110.3 ± 10.8
R_{input} (GΩ)	0.42 ± 0.04	1.0 ± 0.03	3.7 ± 0.15	2.0 ± 0.07	5.9 ± 0.04
C_{soma} (pF)	144.3 ± 24	45.8 ± 2.8	24.9 ± 3.7	34.3 ± 3.4	19.2 ± 2.8
AHP (mV)	12.2 ± 1.3	10.2 ± 0.8	13.7 ± 5.8	11.0 ± 1.0	15.4 ± 3.7
SA (mV)	56.1 ± 2.7	52.6 ± 2.3	60.7 ± 5.7	53.1 ± 1.9	54.3 ± 4.5
$I_{threshold}$ (pA)	13.0 ± 2.0	8.2 ± 1.2	3.9 ± 0.8	6.0 ± 0.7	3.3 ± 0.8
$S_{threshold}$ (Hz)	3.3 ± 0.6	2.4 ± 0.3	2 ± 0.4	3.5 ± 0.4	5.3 ± 1.0
CV	1.1 ± 0.1	1.1 ± 0.1	1.0 ± 0.1	1.1 ± 0.1	2.3 ± 0.6
ADP (mV)	1.4 ± 0.4	1.6 ± 0.4	–	0.6 ± 0.2	0.12 ± 0.0

*RMP (resting membrane potential); TC (membrane time constant); R_{input} (input resistance); C_m (membrane capacitance); AHP (after hyperpolarization potential); APA (action potential amplitude); TI (action potential threshold current); ST (number of spikes at threshold current); APD (action potential duration); CV (coefficient of variation); ADP (after depolarization potential). Not shown are variables for rectifying and RS. See definitions in Materials and Methods section and **Figure 1**.*

dorsalis and area ventralis while the LOT projects only to area dorsalis (Levine and Dethier, 1985). Furthermore, pharmacological manipulations influenced the recorded EPSPs in similar ways for both cut and intact LOTs for latency, rise time, peak amplitude and decay times (KW analysis; $P > 0.05$). Sectioning both the medial and LOTs abolished the PSPs completely. This confirms that the pathway we describe from OB to POA is via the MOT.

DISCUSSION

Female sex pheromones regulate reproduction in male goldfish through the olfactory system (Partridge et al., 1976; Sorensen et al., 1991; Dulka, 1993; Stacey et al., 2003; Chung-Davidson et al., 2008). Previous anatomical studies have shown direct neuronal pathways from the OB to POA in the teleost brain (Forlano and Bass, 2011). With whole-cell patch clamp recordings, we show for the first time that these connections are functional and glutamatergic. In addition, we show that these synapses involve both N-methyl-D-aspartate (NMDAR) and α-amino-3-hydroxy-5-methyl-4-isoxazolepropionic acid receptors (AMPAR). We also provide evidence, with a thorough characterization of electrophysiological properties, that neurons of the vPOA comprise several subgroups.

The POA is an important hypophysiotropic center that regulates reproduction in vertebrates. Electrical stimulation of this area has been shown to elicit sperm release (Demski, 1983; Dulka and Demski, 1986; Dulka, 1993; Dominguez, 2009); sexual calling (Schmidt, 1968); nest-building and courtship (Demski and Knigge, 1971) in several vertebrate models. Conversely, lesioning the POA impairs reproduction in male goldfish thereby underscoring the importance of this neural system (Hart et al.,

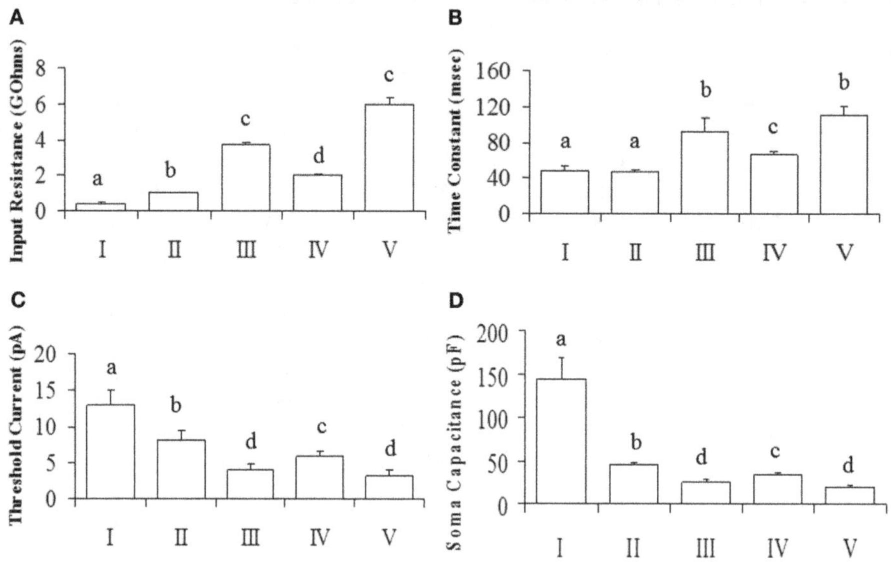

FIGURE 3 | Intrinsic membrane properties of POA neurons. Neurons were made up of connected ($N = 50$) and unconnected ($N = 57$) neurons to the OB. **(A)** The input resistance showing group differences. **(B)** The time constant, indicating differences between groups. **(C)** The threshold current differences between groups. Results are presented as mean ± s.e.m. for convenience. Letters represent groups that differed significantly ($P < 0.005$) from each other with Bonferroni corrections. **(D)** Soma capacitances of the different neuronal groups.

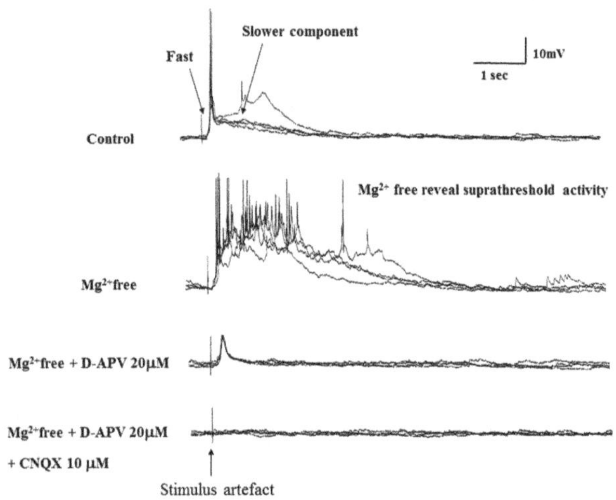

FIGURE 4 | Evoked EPSPs in a POA neuron under different recording conditions. After achieving whole cell access, recordings were made in current-clamp mode. Typically, neurons were perfused sequentially with normal ACSF, Mg^{2+}free ACSF, 20 μM AP-5 (in Mg^{2+}free ACSF) and 10 μM CNQX (in Mg^{2+}free ACSF) for 10 min each before recordings.

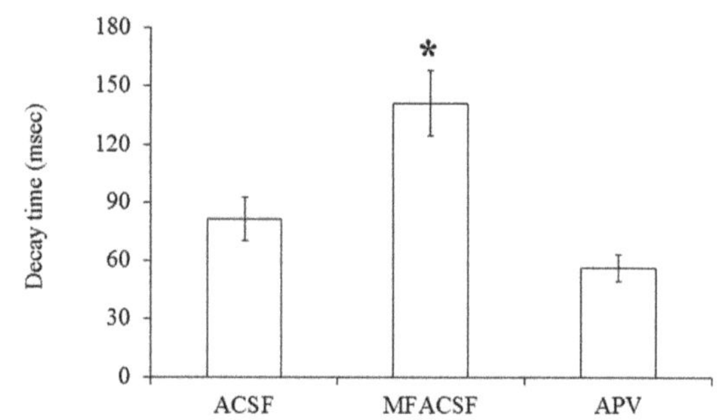

FIGURE 5 | The PSP decay time of POA neurons connected to the OB under the different perfusions (normal ACSF, Mg^{2+} free ACSF (MFACSF) and APV). Error bars denote s.e.m. Asterisks (*) statistical significance ($P < 0.05$) between perfusions.

1973; Kyle and Peter, 1982; Kyle et al., 1982; Koyama et al., 1984; Sorensen et al., 1991; Dulka, 1993).

HETEROGENEITY OF NEURONAL ELECTRICAL PROPERTIES

We recorded from neurons in the vPOA while stimulating the OB. Our analysis revealed five subgroups of vPOA neurons, each with distinct intrinsic membrane properties and variable connectivity to the OB. Indeed, the POA has been shown to contain a plethora of cells immunoreactive to substance P (Sharma et al., 1989), GnRH (Peter et al., 1990, 2003; Parhar et al., 2001), γ-aminobutyric acid (GABA) (Martinoli et al., 1990), glutamate (Anglade et al., 1993), somatostatin (Canosa et al., 2004), CRF (Olivereau et al., 1984), secretoneurin (Canosa et al., 2011) vasotocin (Parhar et al., 2001) and tyrosine hydroxylase (Hornby et al., 1987). Thus, this heterogeneity in electrophysiological profiles may reflect functionally diverse classes of vPOA neurons. Further work is required to determine if these electrophysiological "signatures" correspond to chemical phenotypes, exhibiting differential projections and functional roles.

PROPERTIES OF POSTSYNAPTIC POTENTIALS: INPUTS FROM OLFACTORY BULB

Electrical stimulation of the OB evoked PSPs in vPOA neurons. These PSPs gave rise to action potentials at the peak of their responses in some cases. The evoked excitatory PSPs (EPSPs) had consistent and constant latencies and rise times with small coefficient of variation suggesting they arise through monosynaptic inputs from the OB (Spanswick et al., 1998). The conduction velocities of the inputs from the OB to the POA were similar to those found previously in other systems (Gasser, 1956; Potapov and Gusel'nikova, 1976b). The relatively slow conduction is consistent with propagation through unmyelinated olfactory fibers (Westerman and Wilson, 1968; Potapov and Gusel'nikova, 1976a; Farbman, 1992). The conduction velocity of the inputs from the OB to the vPOA was estimated to be 0.1 m/s, which was similar to the pike (Gasser, 1956) and slower, by four times, than that reported by Kandel (1964) in the goldfish for the larger POA magnocellular neurons projecting to the neural lobe of the pituitary gland when stimulated antidromically.

BIOCHEMICAL PROPERTIES OF THE SYNAPTIC CONNECTIONS

Anatomical connections between the OB and vPOA have been established previously through tract-tracings (Levine and Dethier, 1985; Anglade et al., 1993), but their functional nature remains unclear. To investigate the possible role of glutamate in chemical communication, we perfused the goldfish brain explant sequentially with ACSF, APV, and CNQX in Mg^{2+}free ACSF while stimulating the OB to measure the latency, amplitude, rise time, decay time and duration of the evoked potentials in the vPOA (**Figure 4**). Mg^{2+}free ACSF enhanced the evoked EPSPs compared to normal ACSF. The NMDAR antagonist APV partially blocked the EPSPs leaving a fast acting and short lasting component that was subsequently completely blocked by CNQX, suggesting that the evoked PSP was mediated by glutamate acting on NMDARs and AMPARs, respectively. Receptors for AMPA may therefore be required to depolarize the cells (from their resting state) sufficiently to relieve the Mg^{2+} blockage of NMDARs (Gotz et al., 1997; Spanswick et al., 1998). Bath application of drugs allows for the possibility that the observed effects are indirect and involve peripheral pathways. However, given that the latency and rising phase of the evoked response is very consistent and remains so during drug application, the effects are likely direct.

The complete blockage of the evoked PSPs by the glutamatergic antagonists suggests that glutamate plays an important role in mediating chemical communication between the OB and vPOA. Since the POA is important for the regulation of reproductive behaviors, it may receive pheromonal cues from the OB to integrate milt release and spawning in male goldfish (Kyle and Peter, 1982; Kyle et al., 1982). The use of glutamate signaling through NMDA receptors may therefore be a mechanism to induce the sustained neuronal firing required to trigger an LH surge when sex pheromones are detected. To our knowledge, this is the first pharmacological characterization of second order neurons in the teleost olfactory system linked to reproduction.

A monosynaptic glutamatergic connection from the OB to the vPOA complements and extends our understanding of the neural circuitry involved in the control of goldfish reproduction. Previously, Trudeau et al. (2000b) demonstrated the existence of monosynaptic GABAergic projections from the Vv to the vPOA. Indeed, GABA plays a central role in male goldfish reproduction by suppressing the DAergic inhibition of LH release (Trudeau et al., 1993). This suggests that there are interactions between diverse sets of neurotransmitters and neurohormones that regulate reproduction in male goldfish. The Vv may therefore modulate the glutamatergic inputs from the OB to the vPOA to regulate some aspects of reproductive behavior or hormone release.

ROLE OF GLUTAMATE IN GOLDFISH REPRODUCTION

Previous studies have shown that intraperitoneal injections of male goldfish with either monosodium glutamate (MSG) (Sloley et al., 1992) or NMDA (Trudeau et al., 2000b) or AMPA (Trudeau et al., 2000b; Popesku et al., 2011) rapidly induces LH release. Furthermore, in rainbow trout it has been shown that the LH response to NMDA is blocked by APV or a GnRH receptor antagonist, indicating that glutamate modulates LH release through stimulation of GnRH (Flett et al., 1994), similar to the situation in mammalian models (Kocsis et al., 2003). Moreover, Peter et al. (1980) has shown that MSG injections in goldfish causes cellular degeneration in the POA, demonstrating excitotoxic actions of glutamate on POA neurons. Additionally, in rats it has been shown that glutamate injections in the POA or electrical stimulation of the POA decreases the latency between intromissions thereby increasing ejaculation frequency (Dominguez, 2009). Glutamate in the POA therefore plays an important role in vertebrate reproduction.

SECTIONING THE LATERAL OLFACTORY TRACT

We employed olfactory tract sectioning to determine if the glutamatergic projection to the vPOA was via the MOT or the LOT. The EPSPs recorded in vPOA cells in explants with a transected LOT had the same amplitude and duration as those with the LOT intact. These EPSPs were modulated by APV and CNQX in the same way as in intact preparations. In other experiments, sectioning the MOT while leaving the LOT intact did not elicit PSPs in vPOA neurons indicating that the OB to vPOA projection we have studied is via the MOT and not the LOT. This supports previous studies indicating unequivocally that sex pheromones signals in goldfish are mediated exclusively by the MOT indeed tract tracing studies have shown that while the MOT projects to area dorsalis and area ventralis of the telencephalon the LOT only innervates targets in the area dorsalis (Levine and Dethier, 1985; Sorensen et al., 1991).

CONCLUSION

We describe an electrophysiological basis for classifying neurons of the vPOA. Further, we provide evidence that the synaptic connections from the OB to the vPOA are monosynaptic and glutamatergic. These connections from the OB to vPOA may play a role in facilitating spermiation and steroidogenesis (Peter and Paulencu, 1980; Peter et al., 1980; Kyle and Peter, 1982). While speculative at this point, the olfactory glutamatergic projections we identified may represent pathways that integrate pheromonal signals from females that stimulate reproductive hormone release and male sexual behavior in the spawning period.

AUTHOR CONTRIBUTIONS

Wudu E. Lado, Vance L. Trudeau and David C. Spanswick designed the experiment. Wudu E. Lado and David C. Spanswick performed the experiment. Wudu E. Lado, John E. Lewis and Vance L. Trudeau analyzed the results and wrote the paper.

ACKNOWLEDGMENTS

We thank Dr. Andrew Whyment for invaluable advice and Bill Fletcher for technical assistance during the preparation of this manuscript. We acknowledge with appreciation Dr. Leo Renaud for his early support and encouragement to pursue this study. Funding from the University of Ottawa, NSERC to John E. Lewis and Vance L. Trudeau and OGS to Wudu E. Lado is gratefully acknowledged.

REFERENCES

Abbud, R., and Smith, M. S. (1995). Do GnRH neurons express the gene for the NMDA receptor? *Brain Res.* 690, 117–120. doi: 10.1016/0006-8993(95)00610-3

Andjelic, S., Gallopin, T., Cauli, B., Hill, E. L., Roux, L., Badr, S., et al. (2009). Glutamatergic nonpyramidal neurons from neocortical layer VI and their comparison with pyramidal and spiny stellate neurons. *J. Neurophysiol.* 101, 641–654. doi: 10.1152/jn.91094.2008

Anglade, I., Zandbergen, T., and Kah, O. (1993). Origins of the pituitary innervation in the goldfish. *Cell Tissue Res.* 273, 345–355. doi: 10.1007/BF00312837

Canosa, L. F., Cerda-Reverter, J. M., and Peter, R. E. (2004). Brain mapping of three somatostatin encoding genes in the goldfish. *J. Comp. Neurol.* 474, 43–57. doi: 10.1002/cne.20097

Canosa, L. F., Lopez, G. C., Scharrig, E., Lesaux-Farmer, K., Somoza, G. M., Kah, O., et al. (2011). Forebrain mapping of secretoneurinâ€ like immunoreactivity and its colocalization with isotocin in the preoptic nucleus and pituitary gland of goldfish. *J. Comp. Neurol.* 519, 3748–3765. doi: 10.1002/cne.22688

Chang, J. P., Johnson, J. D., Van Goor, F., Wong, C. J., Yunker, W. K., Uretsky, A. D., et al. (2000). Signal transduction mechanisms mediating secretion in goldfish gonadotropes and somatotropes. *Biochem. Cell Biol.* 78, 139–153. doi: 10.1139/o00-011

Chung-Davidson, Y. W., Rees, C. B., Bryan, M. B., and Li, W. (2008). Neurogenic and neuroendocrine effects of goldfish pheromones. *J. Neurosci.* 28, 14492–14499. doi: 10.1523/JNEUROSCI.3589-08.2008

Demski, L. S. (1983). *Behavioural Effects of Electrical Stimulation of the Brain.* Ann Arbor, MI: University of Michigan Press.

Demski, L. S., and Dulka, J. G. (1984). Functional-anatomical studies on sperm release evoked by electrical stimulation of the olfactory tract in goldfish. *Brain Res.* 291, 241–247. doi: 10.1016/0006-8993(84)91256-3

Demski, L. S., and Knigge, K. M. (1971). The telencephalon and hypothalamus of the bluegill (*Lepomis macrochirus*): evoked feeding, aggressive and reproductive behavior with representative frontal sections. *J. Comp. Neurol.* 143, 1–16. doi: 10.1002/cne.901430102

Dominguez, J. M. (2009). A role for preoptic glutamate in the regulation of male reproductive behavior. *Neuroscientist* 15, 11. doi: 10.1177/1073858408322679

Dubois-Dauphin, M., Dã Ving, K. B., and Holley, A. (1980). Topographical relation between the olfactory bulb and the olfactory tract in tench (*Tinca tinca* L). *Chem. Senses* 5, 159–169. doi: 10.1093/chemse/5.2.159

Dulac, C., and Torello, A. T. (2003). Molecular detection of pheromone signals in mammals: from genes to behaviour. *Nat. Rev. Neurosci.* 4, 551–562. doi: 10.1038/nrn1140

Dulka, J. G. (1993). Sex pheromone systems in goldfish: comparisons to vomeronasal systems in tetrapods. *Brain Behav. Evol.* 42, 265–280. doi: 10.1159/000114166

Dulka, J. G., and Demski, L. S. (1986). Sperm duct contractions mediate centrally evoked sperm release in goldfish. *J. Exp. Zool.* 237, 271–279. doi: 10.1002/jez.1402370213

Farbman, A. I. (1992). *Cell Biology of Olfaction.* New York, NY: Cambridge University Press.

Flett, P. A., Van Der Kraak, G., and Leatherland, J. F. (1994). Effects of excitatory amino acids on *in vivo* and *in vitro* gonadotropin and growth hormone secretion in testosterone-primed immature rainbow trout, *Oncorhynchus mykiss*. *J. Exp. Zool.* 268, 390–399. doi: 10.1002/jez.1402680508

Forlano, P. M., and Bass, A. H. (2011). Neural and hormonal mechanisms of reproductive-related arousal in fishes. *Horm. Behav.* 59, 616–629. doi: 10.1016/j.yhbeh.2010.10.006

Gasser, H. S. (1956). Olfactory nerve fibers. *J. Gen. Physiol.* 39, 473–496. doi: 10.1085/jgp.39.4.473

Gotz, T., Kraushaar, U., Geiger, J., Lubke, J., Berger, T., and Jonas, P. (1997). Functional properties of AMPA and NMDA receptors expressed in identified types of basal ganglia neurons. *J. Neurosci.* 17, 204–215.

Hamdani, E. H., Alexander, G., and Doving, K. B. (2001a). Projection of sensory neurons with microvilli to the lateral olfactory tract indicates their participation in feeding behaviour in crucian carp. *Chem. Senses* 26, 1139–1144. doi: 10.1093/chemse/26.9.1139

Hamdani, E. H., Kasumyan, A., and Doving, K. B. (2001b). Is feeding behaviour in crucian carp mediated by the lateral olfactory tract? *Chem. Senses* 26, 1133–1138. doi: 10.1093/chemse/26.9.1133

Hamdani, E. H., Stabell, O. B., Alexander, G., and Doving, K. B. (2000). Alarm reaction in the crucian carp is mediated by the medial bundle of the medial olfactory tract. *Chem. Senses* 25, 103–109. doi: 10.1093/chemse/25.1.103

Hart, B. L., Haugen, C. M., and Peterson, D. M. (1973). Effects of medial preoptic-anterior hypothalamic lesions on mating behavior of male cats. *Brain Res.* 54, 177–191. doi: 10.1016/0006-8993(73)90043-7

Hille, B. (2001). *Ion Channels of Excitable Membranes.* Sunderland, MA: Sinauer.

Hornby, P. J., Piekut, D. T., and Demski, L. S. (1987). Localization of immunoreactive tyrosine hydroxylase in the goldfish brain. *J. Comp. Neurol.* 261, 1–14. doi: 10.1002/cne.902610102

Kah, O., Dulka, J. G., Dubourg, P., Thibault, J., and Peter, R. E. (1987). Neuroanatomical substrate for the inhibition of gonadotrophin secretion in goldfish: existence of a dopaminergic preoptico-hypophyseal pathway. *Neuroendocrinology* 45, 451–458. doi: 10.1159/000124774

Kandel, E. R. (1964). Electrical properties of hypothalamic neuroendocrine cells. *J. Gen. Physiol.* 47, 691–717. doi: 10.1085/jgp.47.4.691

Kobayashi, M., Aida, K., and Hanyu, I. (1986). Pheromone from ovulatory female goldfish induces gonadotropin surge in males. *Gen. Comp. Endocrinol.* 63, 451–455. doi: 10.1016/0016-6480(86)90145-0

Kobayashi, M., Sorensen, P. W., and Stacey, N. E. (2002). Hormonal and pheromonal control of spawning behavior in the goldfish. *Fish Physiol. Biochem.* 26, 71–84. doi: 10.1023/A:1023375931734

Kocsis, K., Kiss, J., Csaki, A., and Halasz, B. (2003). Location of putative glutamatergic neurons projecting to the medial preoptic area of the rat hypothalamus. *Brain Res. Bull.* 61, 459–468. doi: 10.1016/S0361-9230(03)00180-1

Kotecha, S., Eley, D., and Turner, R. (1997). Tissue printed cells from teleost electrosensory and cerebellar structures. *J. Comp. Neurol.* 386, 277–292.

Koyama, Y., Satou, M., Oka, Y., and Ueda, K. (1984). Involvement of the telencephalic hemispheres and the preoptic area in sexual behavior of the male goldfish, *Carassius auratus*: a brain-lesion study. *Behav. Neural Biol.* 40, 70–86. doi: 10.1016/S0163-1047(84)90182-1

Krimer, L. S., Zaitsev, A. V., Czanner, G., Kröner, S., González-Burgos, G., Povysheva, N. V., et al. (2005). Cluster analysis–based physiological classification and morphological properties of inhibitory neurons in layers 2–3 of monkey dorsolateral prefrontal cortex. *J. Neurophysiol.* 94, 3009. doi: 10.1152/jn.00156.2005

Kyle, A. L., and Peter, R. E. (1982). Effects of forebrain lesions on spawning behaviour in the male goldfish. *Physiol. Behav.* 28, 1103–1109. doi: 10.1016/0031-9384(82)90183-4

Kyle, A. L., Stacey, N. E., and Peter, R. E. (1982). Ventral telencephalic lesions: effects on bisexual behavior, activity, and olfaction in the male goldfish. *Behav. Neural Biol.* 36, 229–241. doi: 10.1016/S0163-1047(82)90855-X

Levine, R. L., and Dethier, S. (1985). The connections between the olfactory bulb and the brain in the goldfish. *J. Comp. Neurol.* 237, 427–444. doi: 10.1002/cne.902370402

Martinoli, M. G., Dubourg, P., Geffard, M., Calas, A., and Kah, O. (1990). Distribution of GABA-immunoreactive neurons in the forebrain of the goldfish, *Carassius auratus*. *Cell Tissue Res.* 260, 77–84. doi: 10.1007/BF00297492

Molleman, A. (2003). *Patch Clamping: An Introductory Guide to Patch Clamp Electrophysiology*. Chichester: Wiley Online Library.

Olivereau, M., Ollevier, F., Vandesande, F., and Verdonck, W. (1984). Immunocytochemical identification of CRF-like and SRIF-like peptides in the brain and the pituitary of cyprinid fish. *Cell Tissue Res.* 237, 379–382. doi: 10.1007/BF00217162

Parhar, I. S., Tosaki, H., Sakuma, Y., and Kobayashi, M. (2001). Sex differences in the brain of goldfish: gonadotropin-releasing hormone and vasotocinergic neurons. *Neuroscience* 104, 1099–1110. doi: 10.1016/S0306-4522(01)00153-1

Partridge, B. L., Liley, N. R., and Stacey, N. E. (1976). The role of pheromones in the sexual behaviour of the goldfish. *Anim. Behav.* 24, 291–299. doi: 10.1016/S0003-3472(76)80037-1

Peter, R. E., and Gill, V. E. (1975). A stereotaxic atlas and technique for forebrain nuclei of the goldfish, *Carassius auratus*. *J. Comp. Neurol.* 159, 69–101. doi: 10.1002/cne.901590106

Peter, R. E., Kah, O., Paulencu, C. R., Cook, H., and Kyle, A. L. (1980). Brain lesions and short-term endocrine effects of monosodium L-glutamate in goldfish, *Carassius auratus*. *Cell Tissue Res.* 212, 429–442. doi: 10.1007/BF00236508

Peter, R. E., and Paulencu, C. R. (1980). Involvement of the preoptic region in gonadotropin release-inhibition in goldfish, *Carassius auratus*. *Neuroendocrinology* 31, 133–141. doi: 10.1159/000123064

Peter, R. E., Prasada Rao, P. D., Baby, S. M., Illing, N., and Millar, R. P. (2003). Differential brain distribution of gonadotropin-releasing hormone receptors in the goldfish. *Gen. Comp. Endocrinol.* 132, 399–408. doi: 10.1016/S0016-6480(03)00084-4

Peter, R. E., Yu, K. L., Marchant, T. A., and Rosenblum, P. M. (1990). Direct neural regulation of the teleost adenohypophysis. *J. Exp. Zool.* S4, 84–89. doi: 10.1002/jez.1402560415

Popesku, J. T., Mennigen, J. A., Chang, J. P., and Trudeau, V. L. (2011). Dopamine D1 receptor blockage potentiates AMPA-stimulated luteinising hormone release in the goldfish. *J. Neuroendocrinol.* 23, 302–309. doi: 10.1111/j.1365-2826.2011.02114.x

Potapov, A. A., and Gusel'nikova, A. A. (1976a). [Electrotonic interaction of secondary neurons of the carp olfactory bulb]. *Neirofiziologiia* 8, 490–496.

Potapov, A. A., and Gusel'nikova, K. G. (1976b). Electrotonic interaction between secondary neurons of the carp olfactory bulb. *Neurophysiology* 8, 375–380. doi: 10.1007/BF01063598

Schmidt, R. S. (1968). Preoptic activation of frog mating behavior. *Behaviour* 30, 239–257.

Sharma, S. C., Berthoud, V. M., and Breckwoldt, R. (1989). Distribution of substance P-like immunoreactivity in the goldfish brain. *J. Comp. Neurol.* 279, 104–116. doi: 10.1002/cne.902790109

Siegelbaum, S. A., and Koester, J. (2000). "Ion channels," in *Principles of Neural Science*, eds E. R. Kandel, J. H. Schwartz, and M. T. Jessel (New York, NY: McGraw Hill), 105–124.

Sloley, B. D., Kah, O., Trudeau, V. L., Dulka, J. G., and Peter, R. E. (1992). Amino acid neurotransmitters and dopamine in brain and pituitary of the goldfish: involvement in the regulation of gonadotropin secretion. *J. Neurochem.* 58, 2254–2262. doi: 10.1111/j.1471-4159.1992.tb10971.x

Sorensen, P. W., Hara, T. J., and Stacey, N. E. (1991). Sex pheromones selectively stimulate the medial olfactory tracts of male goldfish. *Brain Res.* 558, 343–347. doi: 10.1016/0006-8993(91)90790-3

Sosulina, L., Meis, S., Seifert, G., Steinhäuser, C., and Pape, H. C. (2006). Classification of projection neurons and interneurons in the rat lateral amygdala based upon cluster analysis. *Mol. Cell. Neurosci.* 33, 57–67. doi: 10.1016/j.mcn.2006.06.005

Spanswick, D., Renaud, L. P., and Logan, S. D. (1998). Bilaterally evoked monosynaptic EPSPs, NMDA receptors and potentiation in rat sympathetic preganglionic neurones *in vitro*. *J. Physiol.* 509(pt 1), 195–209. doi: 10.1111/j.1469-7793.1998.195bo.x

Stacey, N. (1983). Hormones and pheromones in fish sexual behavior. *Bioscience* 33, 552–556. doi: 10.2307/1309204

Stacey, N., Chojnacki, A., Narayanan, A., Cole, T., and Murphy, C. (2003). Hormonally derived sex pheromones in fish: exogenous cues and signals from gonad to brain. *Can. J. Physiol. Pharmacol.* 81, 329–341. doi: 10.1139/y03-024

Stacey, N. E., Sorensen, P. W., Van Der Kraak, G. J., and Dulka, J. G. (1989). Direct evidence that 17a,20b-dihydroxy-4-pregnen-3-one functions as a goldfish primer pheromone: preovulatory release is closely associated with male endocrine responses. *Gen. Comp. Endocrinol.* 75, 62–70. doi: 10.1016/0016-6480(89)90008-7

Trudeau, V. L. (1997). Neuroendocrine regulation of gonadotrophin II release and gonadal growth in the goldfish, *Carassius auratus*. *Rev. Reprod.* 2, 55–68. doi: 10.1530/ror.0.0020055

Trudeau, V. L., Kah, O., Chang, J. P., Sloley, B. D., Dubourg, P., Fraser, E. J., et al. (2000a). The inhibitory effects of g-aminobutyric acid (GABA) on growth hormone secretion in the goldfish are modulated by sex steroids. *J. Exp. Biol.* 203, 1477–1485.

Trudeau, V. L., Peter, R. E., and Sloley, B. D. (1991). Testosterone and estradiol potentiate the serum gonadotropin response to gonadotropin-releasing hormone in goldfish. *Biol. Reprod.* 44, 951–960. doi: 10.1095/biolreprod44.6.951

Trudeau, V. L., Sloley, B. D., and Peter, R. E. (1993). Testosterone enhances GABA and taurine but not N-methyl-D,L-aspartate stimulation of gonadotropin secretion in the goldfish: possible sex steroid feedback mechanisms. *J. Neuroendocrinol.* 5, 129–136. doi: 10.1111/j.1365-2826.1993.tb00372.x

Trudeau, V. L., Spanswick, D., Fraser, E. J., Lariviere, K., Crump, D., Chiu, S., et al. (2000b). The role of amino acid neurotransmitters in the regulation of pituitary gonadotropin release in fish. *Biochem. Cell Biol.* 78, 241–259. doi: 10.1139/o99-075

Ward, J. H. (1963). Hierarchical grouping to optimize an objective function. *J. Am. Stat. Assoc.* 58, 236–244. doi: 10.1080/01621459.1963.10500845

Westerman, R., and Wilson, J. A. (1968). The fine structure of the olfactory tract in the teleost *Carassius carassius* L. *Zeitschrift für Zellforschung und Mikroskopische Anatomie* 91, 186–199. doi: 10.1007/BF00364310

Wilkie, M. P., Pamenter, M. E., Alkabie, S., Carapic, D., Shin, D. S., and Buck, L. T. (2008). Evidence of anoxia-induced channel arrest in the brain of the goldfish (*Carassius auratus*). *Comp. Biochem. Physiol. C Toxicol. Pharmacol.* 148, 355–362. doi: 10.1016/j.cbpc.2008.06.004

22

Universality and diversity in the signal transduction pathway that regulates seasonal reproduction in vertebrates

Yusuke Nakane[1] and Takashi Yoshimura[1,2,3,4]*

[1] Laboratory of Animal Physiology, Department of Applied Molecular Biosciences, Graduate School of Bioagricultural Sciences, Nagoya University, Nagoya, Japan
[2] Institute of Transformative Bio-Molecules (WPI-ITbM), Nagoya University, Nagoya, Japan
[3] Avian Bioscience Research Center, Graduate School of Bioagricultural Sciences, Nagoya University, Nagoya, Japan
[4] Division of Seasonal Biology, Department of Environmental Biology, National Institute for Basic Biology, Okazaki, Japan

***Correspondence:**
Takashi Yoshimura, Institute of Transformative Bio-Molecules (WPI-ITbM), Nagoya University, Furo-cho, Chikusa-ku, Nagoya 464-8601, Japan
e-mail: takashiy@agr.nagoya-u.ac.jp

Most vertebrates living outside the tropical zone show robust physiological responses in response to seasonal changes in photoperiod, such as seasonal reproduction, molt, and migration. The highly sophisticated photoperiodic mechanism in Japanese quail has been used to uncover the mechanism of seasonal reproduction. Molecular analysis of quail mediobasal hypothalamus (MBH) revealed that local thyroid hormone activation within the MBH plays a critical role in the photoperiodic response of gonads. This activation is accomplished by two gene switches: thyroid hormone-activating (DIO2) and thyroid hormone-inactivating enzymes (DIO3). Functional genomics studies have shown that long-day induced thyroid-stimulating hormone (TSH) in the pars tuberalis (PT) of the pituitary gland regulates DIO2/3 switching. In birds, light information received directly by deep brain photoreceptors regulates PT TSH. Recent studies demonstrated that Opsin 5-positive cerebrospinal fluid (CSF)-contacting neurons are deep brain photoreceptors that regulate avian seasonal reproduction. Although the involvement of TSH and DIO2/3 in seasonal reproduction has been confirmed in various mammals, the light input pathway that regulates PT TSH in mammals differs from that of birds. In mammals, the eye is the only photoreceptor organ and light information received by the eye is transmitted to the pineal gland through the circadian pacemaker, the suprachiasmatic nucleus. Nocturnal melatonin secretion from the pineal gland indicates the length of night and regulates the PT TSH. In fish, the regulatory machinery for seasonal reproduction, from light input to neuroendocrine output, has been recently demonstrated in the coronet cells of the saccus vasculosus (SV). The SV is unique to fish and coronet cells are CSF-contacting neurons. Here, we discuss the universality and diversity of signal transduction pathways that regulate vertebrate seasonal reproduction.

Keywords: circadian rhythm, pars tuberalis, saccus vasculosus, deep brain photoreceptor, thyroid-stimulating hormone, thyroid hormone, cerebrospinal fluid-contacting neuron, coronet cell

INTRODUCTION

Animals that reproduce year-round (e.g., human beings and mice) are so-called non-seasonal breeders. However, in most animals living outside of tropical zones, gametogenesis occurs during a particular period of the year. This allows the animals to produce offspring in a favorable season. Such animals are called seasonal breeders. The timing of the breeding period is related to the length of the gestation or incubation period. Animals that mate in spring-summer (e.g., hamsters, quail, and medaka) are called long-day breeders, whereas those that mate in fall-winter (e.g., sheep, emu, and salmon) are called short-day breeders.

INVOLVEMENT OF THE MEDIOBASAL HYPOTHALAMUS IN THE REGULATION OF SEASONAL REPRODUCTION IN BIRDS

The photoperiodic responses of seasonally breeding birds are so robust and rapid that they provide excellent models for the study of seasonal reproduction. Avian gonads change size seasonally, increasing or decreasing more than one hundred-fold within a few weeks. For example, when Japanese quail (*Coturnix japonica*) kept under short-day conditions are transferred to long-day conditions, an increase in plasma gonadotropin (luteinizing hormone: LH) concentration is observed by the end of the first long day and spermatogenesis is accomplished within 2 weeks (Nicholls et al., 1983). Because quail can be readily obtained from quail farms, it has been frequently used for the study of photoperiodism. Quail has been used as a model to explore the center that regulates seasonal reproduction. Lesions of the mediobasal hypothalamus (MBH), including the median eminence (ME) and infundibular nucleus (IN), or the dorsal MBH result in low plasma LH concentration and attenuate testicular growth under long-day conditions (Sharp and Follett, 1969; Davies and Follett, 1975). Electrical stimulation of the MBH increases plasma LH concentration (Konishi et al., 1987) and testicular growth (Ohta et al., 1984). Birds are receiving light information within the brain and local illumination of the MBH induces testicular development, suggesting the presence of deep brain photoreceptors within the MBH (Homma et al., 1979). In addition, expression of the neuronal activation marker, c-*Fos*, was observed within the ME and IN in response to a single long-day stimulus (Meddle and Follett, 1995, 1997). Therefore, the MBH is considered to be the center for seasonal reproduction in birds.

LOCAL THYROID HORMONE ACTIVATION DRIVEN BY PARS TUBERALIS THYROTROPIN IS THE KEY FOR ELICITING PHOTOPERIODIC RESPONSE IN BIRDS

Lack of genome information had been a barrier to avian research for long time. However, differential subtractive hybridization analysis has revealed that long-day stimuli induce mRNA that encode type 2 deiodinase (DIO2) in the ependymal cells (ECs) (also known as tanycytes) lining the ventro-lateral walls of the third ventricle within the MBH (Yoshimura et al., 2003) (**Figure 1**). DIO2 is a thyroid hormone-activating enzyme that converts prohormone thyroxine (T_4) to bioactive 3,5,3′-triiodothyronine (T_3). Subsequently, long day suppression of type 3 deiodinase (DIO3) was reported. DIO3 is a thyroid hormone-inactivating enzyme that converts T_4 and T_3 to inactive metabolites rT_3 and T_2. These reciprocal gene switches, *DIO2/3*, appear to be the key for regulation of seasonal reproduction in quail (Yasuo et al., 2005). Indeed, T_3 was up-regulated by these gene switches in the MBH under long-day conditions. In addition, ICV administration of T_3 mimicked long day-induced testicular growth under short-day conditions and infusion of DIO2 inhibitor blocked testicular growth under long-day conditions (Yoshimura et al., 2003). It is well established that thyroid hormone is essential for brain development and is also critical for adult brain plasticity (Bernal, 2005). Indeed, T_3 is reported to cause morphological changes in gonadotropin-releasing hormone (GnRH) nerve terminals and glial cells in the ME (Yamamura et al., 2006). Most GnRH nerve terminals are covered with glial cells and do not touch the basal lamina of the perivascular space of portal capillaries under short-day conditions. Under long-day conditions, however, many GnRH nerve terminals are in direct contact with the basal lamina. T_3 implantation under short-day conditions mimics these morphological changes and results in testicular development (Yamamura et al., 2006). These findings suggest that local activation of thyroid hormone within the MBH is a critical event for the seasonal regulation of GnRH secretion.

The availability of genome sequences in avian species has provided an opportunity to employ a functional genomics approach to photoperiodism research. Using a functional genomics approach, long-day induction of *TSHB* mRNA, which encodes the β subunit of thyroid-stimulating hormone (TSH), was observed in the par tuberalis (PT) of the pituitary gland. This *TSHB* induction preceded *DIO2/3* switching by about 4 h. Localization of TSH receptor (TSHR) was observed in the ECs where *DIO2/3* are expressed, suggesting that PT TSH may act on the TSHR expressed in the ECs to regulate *DIO2/3* switching. Indeed, ICV infusion of TSH drives *DIO2/3* switching and testicular growth, even under short-day conditions (Nakao et al., 2008) (**Figure 1**). However, the transport system of PT TSH to the ECs remains unclear.

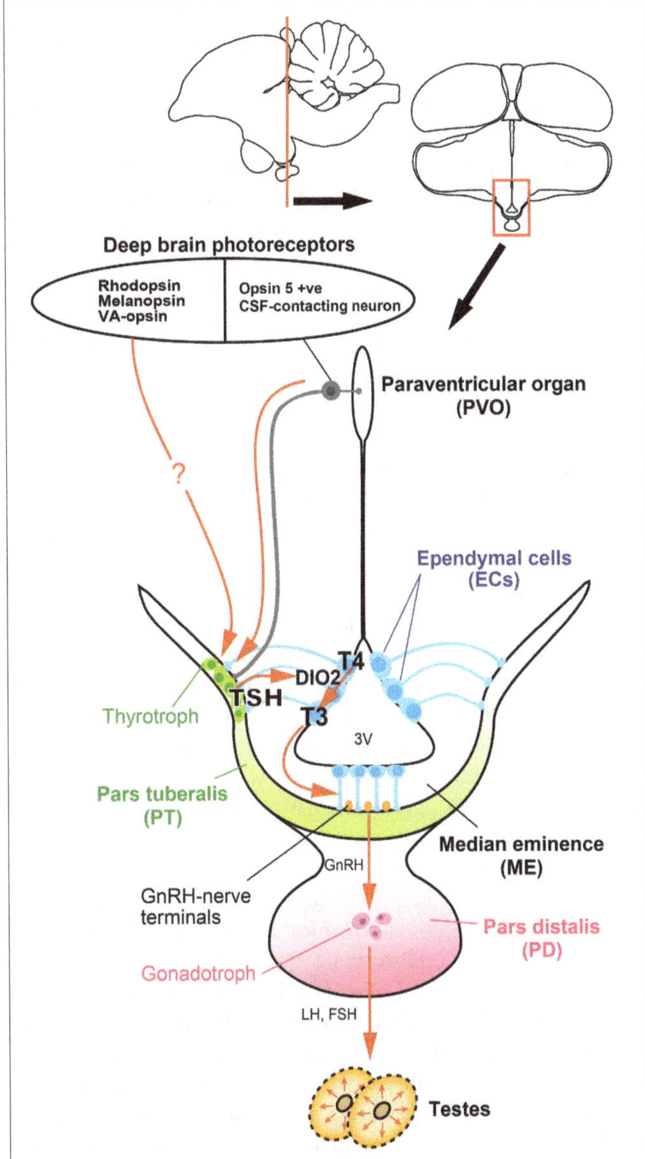

FIGURE 1 | Signal transduction pathway regulating seasonal reproduction in birds. Light information received by deep brain photoreceptors is transmitted to the pars tuberalis (PT) of the pituitary gland, a regulatory hub for seasonal reproduction. Long day-induced thyrotropin (TSH) in the PT acts on ependymal cells to induce a thyroid hormone-activating enzyme, DIO2. The bioactive thyroid hormone, T_3 is converted by DIO2 from the prohormone, T_4. T_3 regulates seasonal morphological changes in GnRH nerve terminals and glial processes, thereby regulating or modulating GnRH secretion.

INVOLVEMENT OF DEEP BRAIN PHOTORECEPTORS IN AVIAN SEASONAL REPRODUCTION

Although the eye is the only photoreceptor organ in mammals, photoreceptive organs in non-mammalian vertebrates include eyes, pineal organs, and deep brain photoreceptors. Photocapability in the deep brain was first demonstrated in European minnows, in which it controls changes in skin color (von Frisch, 1911). Subsequently, evidence of a deep brain photoreceptor that regulates seasonal reproduction in ducks was reported. Blind ducks continue to show photoperiodic responses, whereas enveloping the heads of ducks with black caps blocks testicular responses (Benoit, 1935). Moreover, injection of India ink under the scalp in pinealectomized sparrows abolishes the photoperiodic response (Menaker et al., 1970). Both pinealectomized and blinded quail are reported to undergo gonadal development in response to light cues (Siopes and Wilson, 1974). In addition, photo-stimulation of the hypothalamus using light fiber and light-emitting beads prompts testicular development in sparrows (Yokoyama et al., 1978) and Japanese quail (Homma et al., 1979). It has been confirmed that a broad spectrum of light penetrates into the brains of various vertebrate species (Hartwig and van Veen, 1979; Foster and Follett, 1985; Oishi and Ohashi, 1993).

Many groups have tried to identify deep brain photoreceptors. Several rhodopsin family proteins (e.g., rhodopsin (RH), melanopsin (OPN4), and vertebrate ancient (VA)-opsin) were reported to be localized in the avian deep brain region (Silver et al., 1988; Wada et al., 1998; Chaurasia et al., 2005; Halford et al., 2009). In addition, a novel opsin called Opsin 5 (OPN5: also known as neuropsin) was recently reported to be localized in the paraventricular organ (PVO) within the MBH (Nakane et al., 2010; Yamashita et al., 2010). This is intriguing because lesions around the PVO block the photoperiodic responses of gonads in Japanese quail (Sharp and Follett, 1969). Immunohistochemical analysis of OPN5 revealed its presence in the cerebrospinal fluid (CSF)-contacting neurons (**Figure 2A**). The CSF-contacting neurons in the PVO have long been a candidate deep brain photoreceptor because the retina and pineal organ evaginate from the diencephalon (around the third ventricle where the PVO is located) and the CSF-contacting neurons resemble photoreceptor cells in the developing retina (Vigh-Teichmann et al., 1980). Functional analysis demonstrated that OPN5 is a short-wavelength sensitive photopigment (Nakane et al., 2010; Yamashita et al., 2010) and long-day stimulation with short-wavelength light triggered testicular growth in eye-patched and pinealectomized quail (Nakane et al., 2010). Therefore, OPN5-expressing, CSF-contacting neurons in the PVO may be deep brain photoreceptors that are important for seasonal reproduction in birds (**Figures 1, 2A**).

In summary, a series of quail studies have uncovered the signal transduction cascade that regulates seasonal reproduction, from photoreceptors to neuroendocrine output, in birds (**Figure 1**). That is, light information received by deep brain photoreceptors (e.g., OPN5, RH, OPN4, VA-opsin, etc.) is transmitted to the PT and long-day induced TSH secreted from the PT acts on TSHR to regulate DIO2/3 switching in the ECs. Bioactive T_3 converted from T_4 by DIO2 causes morphological changes in GnRH nerve terminals and glial processes in the ME, thereby regulating seasonal changes in GnRH secretion.

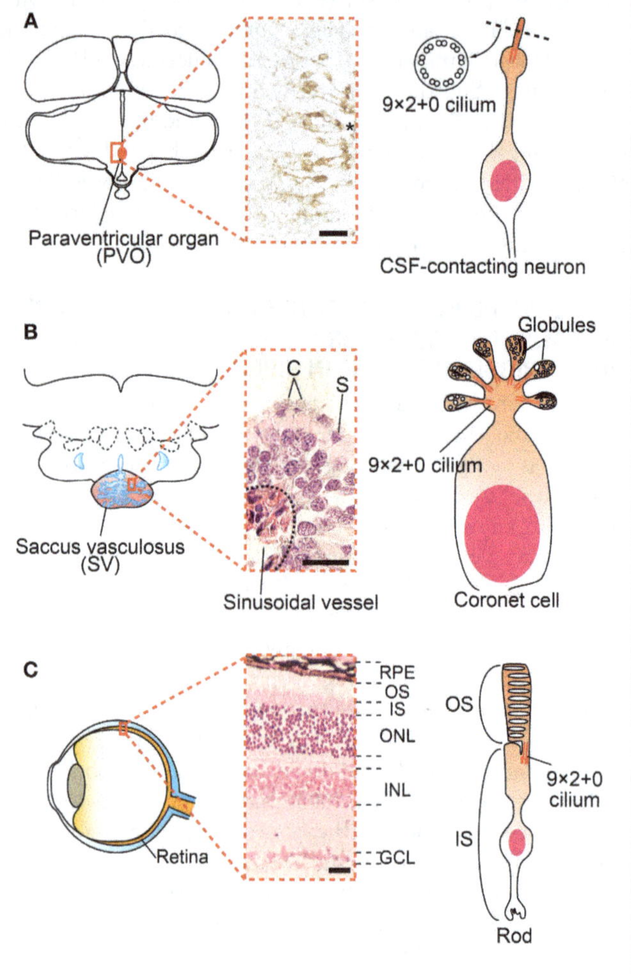

FIGURE 2 | Family of cerebrospinal fluid (CSF)-contacting neurons. (A) Schematic drawings and picture of OPN5 positive CSF-contacting neurons in the paraventricular organ (PVO) of quail. **(B)** Schematic drawing and picture of coronet cells in the salmon saccus vasculosus (SV). The SV consists of coronet cells (C) and supporting cells (S). Globules of coronet cells are based on $9 \times 2 + 0$ cilia. **(C)** Schematic drawing and picture of a mammalian retina and photoreceptor. The outer segments of rod and cone cells are also based on $9 \times 2 + 0$ cilia. *third ventrile. RPE, retinal pigment epithelium, OS, outer segment, IS, inner segment, ONL, outer nuclear layer, INL inner nuclear layer, GCL, ganglion cell layer. Scale bars indicate 20 μm.

SIGNAL TRANSDUCTION CASCADE FOR SEASONAL REPRODUCTION IN MAMMALS

Thyroidectomy blocks the transition of seasonal reproductive state in sheep (Moenter et al., 1991), and it has been known for several decades that thyroid hormone is involved in the regulation of mammalian seasonality (Nicholls et al., 1988). However, its precise mode of action was unknown. After the discovery of photoperiodic *DIO2/3* switching in birds, photoperiodic regulation of *DIO2* and/or *DIO3* within the MBH was reported in a number of mammalian species, such as hamsters (Watanabe et al., 2004, 2007; Revel et al., 2006; Barrett et al., 2007; Freeman et al., 2007; Yasuo et al., 2007a), rats (Yasuo et al., 2007b), mice (Ono et al., 2008) and even in short-day breeding sheep (Hanon et al., 2008) and goats (Yasuo et al., 2006). Therefore, local thyroid hormone activation within the MBH is considered to be central in the regulation of seasonal reproduction in mammals (**Figure 3**). However, in marked contrast with birds, the eye is the only photoreceptor organ. Light information is transmitted to the pineal gland through the circadian pacemaker, the suprachiasmatic nucleus (SCN). In mammals, photoperiodic information is decoded based on the duration of melatonin secretion by the pineal gland (Reiter, 1980; Yamazaki et al., 1999). Therefore, pinealectomy abolishes seasonal responses and melatonin administration mimics the effect of short photoperiod in mammals. Thus, melatonin is considered to play a deterministic role in mammalian seasonal reproduction (Reiter, 1980). Although melatonin controls *DIO2/3* switching, melatonin receptors are absent in the ECs where *DIO2/3* are expressed (Schuster et al., 2000; Song and Bartness, 2001). In contrast, melatonin receptors are densely expressed in the PT (Williams and Morgan, 1988; Wittkowski et al., 1988; Reppert et al., 1994; Klosen et al., 2002; Dardente et al., 2003). Therefore, it was predicted that TSH secreted from the PT may mediate the melatonin action to regulation of *DIO2/3* switching in mammals. This hypothesis was tested using TSHR and melatonin receptor knockout mice (Ono et al., 2008; Yasuo et al., 2009). Melatonin administration had no effect on *DIO2/3* switching in the TSHR and MT1 melatonin receptor null mice, whereas melatonin affected *DIO2/3* switching in MT2 null mice. This suggests that melatonin acts on the MT1 melatonin receptor to regulate *DIO2/3* switching through the TSH-TSHR signaling pathway in mammals (**Figure 3**).

The RF-amides such as kisspeptin, a ligand for the G protein coupled receptor, GPR54, and RFamide-related peptide 3 (RFRP-3) are involved in the regulation of GnRH secretion (Clements et al., 2001; Kotani et al., 2001; Muir et al., 2001; Ohtaki et al., 2001; Clarke et al., 2008). Seasonal regulation of kisspeptin and RFRP-3 has been reported in hamsters (Revel et al., 2006, 2008). Administration of TSH to Djungarian and Syrian hamsters induces the expression of kisspeptin and RFRP-3 as well as gonadal development under short-day conditions (Klosen et al., 2013). T_3 also provoked significant testicular growth and kisspeptin expression in Siberian hamsters (*Phodopus sungorus*) under short-day conditions (Henson et al., 2013). This suggests that long-day induces TSH and, following the activation of thyroid hormone by DIO2, regulates kisspeptin, RFRP-3 and the hypothalamic-pituitary-gonadal (HPG)-axis in mammalian species.

SIGNAL TRANSDUCTION CASCADE FOR SEASONAL REPRODUCTION IN FISH

Fish also show marked seasonal changes in physiology and behavior. Medaka (*Oryzias latipes*), are long-day seasonal breeders, and their gonads develop in response to elongated day-length (Koger et al., 1999). Salmonids, short-day seasonal breeders, show distinct photoperiodic responses, such as migration and parr-smolt transformation. Smoltification is closely linked to thyroid hormone (Robertson, 1949; Nishikawa et al., 1979). Although all fishes examined have had higher circulating levels of melatonin during the night than during the day, there are few reliable data consistent with a major physiological role for melatonin in the seasonal reproduction of fish (Urasaki, 1976; Garg, 1989; Masuda et al., 2005; Borg, 2010). This is in marked contrast to mammals, but is similar to birds. Fish do not have anatomically distinct PTs, a regulatory hub of seasonal reproduction in birds and mammals. Thus, the signal transduction pathway for fish seasonal reproduction remains unknown.

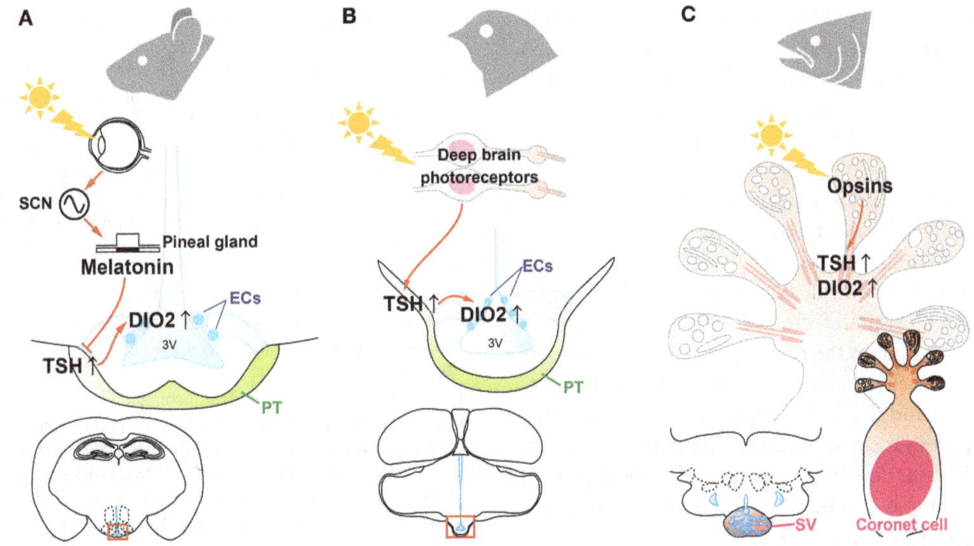

FIGURE 3 | Universality and diversity of signal transduction pathways that regulate seasonal reproduction in vertebrates. (A) Eyes are the only photoreceptor organ in mammals. Light information is transmitted through the suprachiasmatic nucleus (SCN) to the pineal gland. Photoperiodic information is encoded by the pattern of melatonin secretion from the pineal gland. Melatonin regulates the "springtime hormone," TSH, in the pars tuberalis (PT) of the pituitary gland. **(B)** In contrast to mammals, light information is directly received by deep brain photoreceptors in birds and is then transmitted to the PT to induce TSH. **(C)** In fish, all of the machinery required for seasonal reproduction (from photoreceptors to neuroendocrine output) is located in the saccus vasculosus (SV).

A recent study of masu salmon (*Oncorhynchus masou masou*) revealed that key elements for vertebrate seasonal reproduction, such as photopigments, TSH, TSHR, and DIO2, are expressed in the saccus vasculosus (SV). The SV is an organ only observed in fish and is located at the floor of the hypothalamus, posterior to the pituitary gland. Although its existence was first described in the 17th century (Collins, 1685), its physiological function remained a mystery for several centuries. In the SV, a folded EC layer makes a chamber that is directly connected to the third ventricle. Abundant sinusoidal vessels cover the whole external surface of the SV. The EC layer of the SV mainly consists of coronet cells and supporting cells (Sueiro et al., 2007). The coronet cells have morphologically specialized features; globules occupy the apical cellular structures of these cells (**Figure 2B**). Each globule has $9 \times 2 + 0$ cilia, as do photoreceptors in the retina (**Figure 2C**) and CSF-contacting neurons in the PVO (**Figure 2A**). The coronet cells also possess manifold primary vesicles (Jansen et al., 1982; Vigh and Vigh-Teichmann, 1998). Therefore, the coronet cells are considered to be CSF-contacting neurons.

Immunohistochemical analysis has revealed localization of photopigments (OPN4 and SWS1), TSH, and DIO2 in coronet cells (Nakane et al., 2013). The expression of these photoperiodic regulatory mechanisms within the SV implies that the SV plays a pivotal role as a seasonal sensor in fish. Indeed, isolated SVs respond to photoperiodic changes in *in vitro* and ablation of the SV prevents photoperiodically-induced gonadal development (Nakane et al., 2013). This suggests that coronet cells have multiple functions, including photoreception and neuroendocrine output (**Figure 3**).

CONCLUSION REMARKS

The mechanisms of seasonal time measurement were a mystery for long time. However, recent studies have uncovered the signal transduction pathway that regulates seasonal reproduction in birds, mammals, and fish. These studies revealed the universality (i.e., signal transduction machineries) and diversity (responsible cells or organs) of these mechanisms among vertebrate species (**Figure 3**). This is similar to the structural and functional evolution of the pineal organ (Korf, 1994; Falcón et al., 2009). In non-mammalian vertebrates, the pinealocyte contains photoreceptors, the circadian clock, and neuroendocrine output in the form of melatonin. In marked contrast with non-mammalian vertebrates, the mammalian pinealocyte is specialized as a neuroendocrine organ for melatonin secretion. This is why the pineal organ is generally referred to as the pineal gland in mammals. As expressed by Ernst Haeckel's phrase "ontogeny recapitulates phylogeny," the rat pineal gland responds to light during the postnatal period (Zweig et al., 1966; Tosini et al., 2000; Fukuhara and Tosini, 2003). Because multi-functionality is considered to be a general feature of ancient cell types (Arendt, 2008), coronet cells appear to be the ancestral vertebrate seasonal sensors.

ACKNOWLEDGMENTS

This work is supported by the Funding Program for Next Generation World Leading Researchers (NEXT Program) initiated by the Council for Science and Technology Policy (CSTP) (LS055) and JSPS KAKENHI grant number 26000013. WPI-ITbM is supported by World Premier International Research Center Initiative (WPI), MEXT, Japan.

REFERENCES

Arendt, D. (2008). The evolution of cell types in animals: emerging principles from molecular studies. *Nat. Rev. Genet.* 9, 868–882. doi: 10.1038/nrg2416

Barrett, P., Ebling, F. J., Schuhler, S., Wilson, D., Ross, A. W., Warner, A., et al. (2007). Hypothalamic thyroid hormone catabolism acts as a gatekeeper for the seasonal control of body weight and reproduction. *Endocrinology* 148, 3608–3617. doi: 10.1210/en.2007-0316

Benoit, J. (1935). Le role des yeux dans l'action stimulante de la lumiere sure le developpement testiulaire chez le canard. *CR. Soc. Bio. (Paris.)* 118, 669–671.

Bernal, J. (2005). Thyroid hormones and brain development. *Vitam. Horm.* 71, 95–122. doi: 10.1016/S0083-6729(05)71004-9

Borg, B. (2010). "Photoperiodism in fishes," in *Photoperiodism: The Biological Calendar*, eds R. J. Nelson, D. L. Denlinger, and D. E. Somers (New York, NY: Oxford University Press), 371–398.

Chaurasia, S. S., Rollag, M. D., Jiang, G., Hayes, W. P., Haque, R., Natesan, A., et al. (2005). Molecular cloning, localization and circadian expression of chicken melanopsin (Opn4): differential regulation of expression in pineal and retinal cell types. *J. Neurochem.* 92, 158–170. doi: 10.1111/j.1471-4159.2004.02874.x

Clarke, I. J., Sari, I. P. Qi, Y., Smith, J. T., Parkington, H. C., Ubuka, T., Iqbal, J., et al. (2008). Potent action of RFamide-related peptide-3 on pituitary gonadotropes indicative of a hypophysiotropic role in the negative regulation of gonadotropin secretion. *Endocrinology* 149, 5811–5821. doi: 10.1210/en.2008-0575

Clements, M. K., McDonald, T. P., Wang, R., Xie, G., O'Dowd, B. F., George, S. R., et al. (2001). FMRFamide-related neuropeptides are agonists of the orphan G-protein-coupled receptor GPR54. *Biochem. Biophys. Res. Commun.* 284, 1189–1193. doi: 10.1006/bbrc.2001.5098

Collins, S. (1685). *A Systeme of Anatomy*. London: Thomas Newcomb.

Dardente, H., Klosen, P., Pévet, P., and Masson-Pévet, M. (2003). MT1 melatonin receptor mRNA expressing cells in the pars tuberalis of the European hamster: effect of photoperiod. *J. Neuroendocrinol.* 15, 778–786. doi: 10.1046/j.1365-2826.2003.01060.x

Davies, D. T., and Follett, B. K. (1975). Electrical stimulation of the hypothalamus and luteinizing hormone secretion in Japanese quail. *J. Endocrinol.* 67, 431–443. doi: 10.1677/joe.0.0670431

Falcón, J., Besseau, L., Fuentès, M., Sauzet, S., Magnanou, E., and Boeuf, G. (2009). Structural and functional evolution of the pineal melatonin system in vertebrates. *Ann. N. Y. Acad. Sci.* 1163, 101–111. doi: 10.1111/j.1749-6632.2009.04435.x

Foster, R. G., and Follett, B. K. (1985). The involvement of a rhodopsin-like photopigment in the photoperiodic response of the Japanese quail. *J. Comp. Physiol. A* 157, 519–528. doi: 10.1007/BF00615153

Freeman, D. A., Teubner, B. J., Smith, C. D., and Prendergast, B. J. (2007). Exogenous T_3 mimics long day lengths in Siberian hamsters. *Am. J. Physiol. Regul. Integr. Comp. Physiol.* 292, 2368–2372. doi: 10.1152/ajpregu.00713.2006

Fukuhara, C., and Tosini, G. (2003). Induction of photosensitivity in cultured rat pineal affects Aa-nat regulation. *Brain Res. Dev. Brain Res.* 142, 219–221. doi: 10.1016/S0165-3806(03)00067-1

Garg, S. K. (1989). Effect of pinealectomy, eye enucleation, and melatonin treatment on ovarian activity and vitellogenin levels in the catfish exposed to short photoperiod or long photoperiod. *J. Pineal. Res.* 7, 91–104. doi: 10.1111/j.1600-079X.1989.tb00658.x

Halford, S., Pires, S. S., Turton, M., Zheng, L., González-Menéndez, I., Davies, W. L., et al. (2009). VA opsin-based photoreceptors in the hypothalamus of birds. *Curr. Biol.* 19, 1396–1402. doi: 10.1016/j.cub.2009.06.066

Hanon, E. A., Lincoln, G. A., Fustin, J. M., Dardente, H., Masson-Pévet, M., Morgan, P. J., et al. (2008). Ancestral TSH mechanism signals summer in a photoperiodic mammal. *Curr. Biol.* 18, 1147–1152. doi: 10.1016/j.cub.2008.06.076

Hartwig, H. G., and van Veen, T. (1979). Spectral characteristics of visible radiation penetrating into the brain and stimulating extraretinal photoreceptors. *J. Comp. Physiol.* 130, 277–282. doi: 10.1007/BF00614615

Henson, J. R., Carter, S. N., and Freeman, D. A. (2013). Exogenous T_3 elicits long day-like alterations in testis size and the RFamides Kisspeptin and gonadotropin-inhibitory hormone in short-day Siberian hamsters. *J. Biol. Rhythms* 28, 193–200. doi: 10.1177/0748730413487974

Homma, K., Ohta, M., and Sakakibara, Y. (1979). "Photoinducible phase of the Japanese quail detected by direct stimulation of the brain," in *Biological Rhythms and their Central Mechanism,* eds M. Suda, O. Hayaishi, and H. Nakagawa (Amsterdam: Elsevier, North-Holland Biomedical Press), 85–94.

Jansen, W. F., Burger, E. H., and Zandbergen, M. A. (1982). Subcellular localization of calcium in the coronet cells and tanycytes of the saccus vasculosus of the rainbow trout, Salmo gairdneri. *Ann. N. Y. Acad. Sci.* 117, 217–227.

Klosen, P., Bienvenu, C., Demarteau, O., Dardente, H., Guerrero, H., Pévet, P., et al. (2002). The mt1 melatonin receptor and RORb receptor are co-localized in specific TSH-immunoreactive cells in the pars tuberalis of the rat pituitary. *J. Histochem. Cytochem.* 50, 1647–1657. doi: 10.1177/002215540205001209

Klosen, P., Sébert, M. E., Rasri, K., Laran-Chich, M. P., and Simonneaux, V. (2013). TSH restores a summer phenotype in photoinhibited mammals via the RF-amides RFRP3 and kisspeptin. *FASEB J.* 27, 2677–2686. doi: 10.1096/fj.13-229559

Koger, C. S., Teh, S. J., and Hinton, D. E. (1999).Variations of light and temperature regimes and resulting effects on reproductive parameters in medaka (*Oryzias latipes*). *Biol. Reprod.* 61, 1287–1293. doi: 10.1095/biolreprod61.5.1287

Konishi, H., Foster, R. G., and Follett, B. K. (1987). Evidence for a daily rhythmicity in the acute release of LH in response to electrical stimulation in the Japanese quail. *J. Comp. Physiol. A* 161, 315–319. doi: 10.1007/BF00615251

Korf, H. W. (1994). The pineal organ as a component of the biological clock. Phylogenetic and ontogenetic considerations. *Ann. N. Y. Acad. Sci.* 31, 13–42. doi: 10.1111/j.1749-6632.1994.tb56818.x

Kotani, M., Detheux, M., Vandenbogaerde, A., Communi, D., Vanderwinden, J. M., Le Poul, E., et al. (2001). The metastasis suppressor gene KiSS-1 encodes kisspeptins, the natural ligands of the orphan G protein-coupled receptor GPR54. *J. Biol. Chem.* 276, 34631–34636. doi: 10.1074/jbc.M104847200

Masuda, T., Iigo, M., and Aida, K. (2005). Existence of an extra-retinal and extra-pineal photoreceptive organ that regulates photoperiodism in gonadal development of an Osmerid teleost, ayu (*Plecoglossus altivelis*). *Comp. Biochem. Physiol. A. Mol. Integr. Physiol.* 140, 414–422. doi: 10.1016/j.cbpb.2005.01.004

Meddle, S. L., and Follett, B. K. (1995). Photoperiodic activation of fos-like immunoreactive protein in neurones within the tuberal hypothalamus of Japanese quail. *J. Comp. Physiol. A.* 176, 79–89. doi: 10.1007/BF00197754

Meddle, S. L., and Follett, B. K. (1997). Photoperiodically driven changes in Fos expression within the basal tuberal hypothalamus and median eminence of Japanese quail. *J. Neurosci.* 17, 8909–8918.

Menaker, M., Roberts, R., Elliott, J., and Underwood, H. (1970). Extraretinal light perception in the sparrow. III. The eyes do not participate in photoperiodic photoreception. *Proc. Natl. Acad. Sci. U.S.A.* 67, 320–325. doi: 10.1073/pnas.67.1.320

Moenter, S. M., Woodfill, C. J., and Karsch, F. J. (1991). Role of the thyroid gland in seasonal reproduction: thyroidectomy blocks seasonal suppression of reproductive neuroendocrine activity in ewes. *Endocrinology* 128, 1337–1344. doi: 10.1210/endo-128-3-1337

Muir, A. I., Chamberlain, L., Elshourbagy, N. A., Michalovich, D., Moore, D. J., Calamari, A., et al. (2001). AXOR12, a novel human G protein-coupled receptor, activated by the peptide KiSS-1. *J. Biol. Chem.* 276, 28969–28975. doi: 10.1074/jbc.M102743200

Nakane, Y., Ikegami, K., Iigo, M., Ono, H., Takeda, K., Takahashi, D., et al. (2013). The saccus vasculosus of fish is a sensor of seasonal changes in day length. *Nat. Commun.* 4, 2108. doi: 10.1038/ncomms3108

Nakane, Y., Ikegami, K., Ono, H., Yamamoto, N., Yoshida, S., Hirunagi, K., et al. (2010). A novel mammalian neural tissue opsin (Opsin5) is a deep brain photoreceptor in birds. *Proc. Natl. Acad. Sci. U.S.A.* 107, 15264–15268. doi: 10.1073/pnas.1006393107

Nakao, N., Ono, H., Yamamura, T., Anraku, T., Takagi, T., Higashi, K., et al. (2008). Thyrotrophin in the pars tuberalis triggers photoperiodic response. *Nature* 452, 317–311. doi: 10.1038/nature06738

Nicholls, T. J., Follett, B. K., Goldsmith, A. R., and Pearson, H. (1988). Possible homologies between photorefractoriness in sheep and birds: the effect of thyroidectomy on the length of the ewe's breeding season. *Reprod. Nutr. Dev.* 28, 375–385. doi: 10.1051/rnd:19880304

Nicholls, T. J., Follett, B. K., and Robinson, J. E. (1983). A photoperiodic response in gonadectomized Japanese quail exposed to a single long day. *J. Endocrinol.* 97, 121–126. doi: 10.1677/joe.0.0970121

Nishikawa, K., Hirashima, T., Suzuki, S., and Suzuki, M. (1979). Changes in circulating L-thyroxine and L-triiodothyronine of the masu salmon, *Oncorhynchus masou* accompaning the smoltification, measured by radioimmunoassay. *Endocrinol. Jpn.* 26, 731–735. doi: 10.1507/endocrj1954.26.731

Ohta, M., Wada, M., and Homma, K. (1984). Induction of rapid testicular growth in quail by phasic electrical stimulation of the hypothalamic photosensitive area. *J. Comp. Physiol. A* 154, 583–589. doi: 10.1007/BF00610171

Ohtaki, T., Shintani, Y., Honda, S., Matsumoto, H., Hori, A., Kanehashi, K., et al. (2001). Metastasis suppressor gene KiSS-1 encodes peptide ligand of a G-protein-coupled receptor. *Nature* 411, 613–617. doi: 10.1038/35079135

Oishi, T., and Ohashi, K. (1993). Effects of wavelengths of light on the photoperiodic gonadal response of blinded-pinealectomized Japanese quail. *Zoolog. Sci.* 10, 757–762.

Ono, H., Hoshino, Y., Yasuo, S., Watanabe, M., Nakane, Y., Murai, A., et al. (2008). Involvement of thyrotropin in photoperiodic signal transduction in mice. *Proc. Natl. Acad. Sci. U.S.A.* 105, 18238–18242. doi: 10.1073/pnas.0808952105

Reiter, R. J. (1980). The pineal and its hormones in the control of reproduction in mammals. *Endocr. Rev.* 1, 109–131. doi: 10.1210/edrv-1-2-109

Reppert, S. M., Weaver, D. R., and Ebisawa, T. (1994). Cloning and characterization of a mammalian melatonin receptor that mediates reproductive and circadian responses. *Neuron* 13, 1177–1185. doi: 10.1016/0896-6273(94)90055-8

Revel, F. G., Saboureau, M., Pévet, P., Mikkelsen, J. D., and Simonneaux, V. (2006). Melatonin regulates type 2 deiodinase gene expression in the Syrian hamster. *Endocrinology* 147, 4680–4687. doi: 10.1210/en.2006-0606

Revel, R. G., Saboureau, M., Pévet, P., Simonneaux, V., and Mikkelsen, J. D. (2008). RFamide-related peptide gene is a melatonin-driven photoperiodic gene. *Endocrinology* 149, 902–912. doi: 10.1210/en.2007-0848

Robertson, O. H. (1949). Production of the silvery smolt stage in rainbow trout by intramuscular injection of mammalian thyroid extract and thyrotropic hormone. *J. Exp. Zool.* 110, 337–355 doi: 10.1002/jez.1401100303

Schuster, C., Gauer, F., Guerrero, H., Lakhdar-Ghazal, N., Pévet, P., and Masson-Pévet, M. (2000). Photic regulation of mt1 melatonin receptors in the Siberian hamster pars tuberalis and suprachiasmatic nuclei: involvement of the circadian clock and intergeniculate leaflet. *J. Neuroendocrinol.* 12, 207–216. doi: 10.1046/j.1365-2826.2000.00039.x

Sharp, P. J., and Follett, B. K. (1969). The effect of hypothalamic lesions on gonadotrophin release in Japanese quail (*Coturnix coturnix japonica*). *Neuroendocrinology* 5, 205–218. doi: 10.1159/000121861

Silver, R., Witkovsky, P., Horvath, P., Alones, V., Barnstable, C. J., and Lehman, M. N. (1988). Coexpression of opsin- and VIP-like-immunoreactivity in CSF-contacting neurons of the avian brain. *Cell Tissue Res.* 253, 189–198. doi: 10.1007/BF00221754

Siopes, T. D., and Wilson, W. O. (1974). Extraocular modification of photoreception in intact and pinealectomized coturnix. *Poult. Sci.* 53, 2035–2041. doi: 10.3382/ps.0532035

Song, C. K., and Bartness, T. J. (2001). CNS sympathetic outflow neurons to white fat that express MEL receptors may mediate seasonal adiposity. *Am. J. Physiol. Regul. Integr. Comp. Physiol.* 281, R666–R672.

Sueiro, C., Carrera, I., Ferreiro, S., Molist, P., Adrio, F., Anadón, R., et al. (2007). New insights on saccus vasculosus evolution: a developmental and immunohistochemical study in Elasmobranchs. *Brain Behav. Evol.* 70, 187–204. doi: 10.1159/000104309

Tosini, G., Doyle, S., Geusz, M., and Menaker, M. (2000). Induction of photosensitivity in neonatal rat pineal gland. *Proc. Natl. Acad. Sci. U.S.A.* 97, 11540–11544. doi: 10.1073/pnas.210248297

Urasaki, H. (1976). The role of pineal and eyes in the photoperiodic effect on the gonad of the medaka, *Oryzias latipes. Chronobiologia* 3, 228–234.

Vigh, B., and Vigh-Teichmann, I. (1998). Actual problems of the cerebrospinal fluid-contacting neurons. *Microsc. Res. Tech.* 41, 57–83.

Vigh-Teichmann, I., Röhlich, P., Vigh, B., and Aros, B. (1980). Comparison of the pineal complex,retina and cerebrospinal fluid contacting neurons by immunocytochemical antirhodopsin reaction. *Z. Mikrosk. Anat. Forsch.* 94, 623–640.

von Frisch, K. (1911). Beitrage zur physiologie der pigmentzellen in der fischhaut. *Pflü. Arch. Gesammte. Physiol. Menschen. Tiere.* 138, 319–387. doi: 10.1007/BF01680752

Wada, Y., Okano, T., Adachi, A., Ebihara, S., and Fukada, Y. (1998). Identification of rhodopsin in the pigeon deep brain. *FEBS Lett.* 424, 53–56. doi: 10.1016/S0014-5793(98)00138-0

Watanabe, M., Yasuo, S., Watanabe, T., Yamamura, T., Nakao, N., Ebihara, S., et al. (2004). Photoperiodic regulation of type 2 deiodinase gene in Djungarian hamster: Possible homologies between avian and mammalian photoperiodic regulation of reproduction. *Endocrinology* 145, 1546–1549. doi: 10.1210/en.2003-1593

Watanabe, T., Yamamura, T., Watanabe, M., Yasuo, S., Nakao, N., Dawson, A., et al. (2007). Hypothalamic expression of thyroid hormone-activating and -inactivating enzyme genes in relation to photorefractoriness in birds and mammals. *Am. J. Physiol. Regul. Integr. Comp. Physiol.* 292, 568–572. doi: 10.1152/ajpregu.00521.2006

Williams, L. M., and Morgan, P. J. (1988). Demonstration of melatonin-binding sites on the pars tuberalis of the rat. *J. Endocrinol.* 119, 1–3. doi: 10.1677/joe.0.119R001

Wittkowski, W., Bergmann, M., Hoffmann, K., and Pera, F. (1988). Photoperiod-dependent changes in TSH-like immunoreactivity of cells in the hypophysial pars tuberalis of the Djungarian hamster, *Phodopus sungorus*. *Cell Tissue Res.* 251, 183–187. doi: 10.1007/BF00215463

Yamamura, T., Yasuo, S., Hirunagi, K., Ebihara, S., and Yoshimura, T. (2006). T_3 implantation mimics photoperiodically reduced encasement of nerve terminals by glial processes in the median eminence of Japanese quail. *Cell Tissue Res.* 324, 175–179. doi: 10.1007/s00441-005-0126-8

Yamashita, T., Ohuchi, H., Tomonari, S., Ikeda, K., Sakai, K., and Shichida, Y. (2010). Opn5 is a UV-sensitive bistable pigment that couples with Gi subtype of G protein. *Proc. Natl. Acad. Sci. U.S.A.* 107, 22084–22089. doi: 10.1073/pnas.1012498107

Yamazaki, S., Goto, M., and Menaker, M. (1999). No evidence for extraocular photoreceptors in the circadian system of the Syrian hamster. *J. Biol. Rhythms* 14, 197–201. doi: 10.1177/074873099129000605

Yasuo, S., Nakao, N., Ohkura, S., Iigo, M., Hagiwara, S., Goto, A., et al. (2006). Long-day suppressed expression of type 2 deiodinase gene in the mediobasal hypothalamus of the Saanen goat, a short-day breeder: Implication for seasonal window of thyroid hormone action on reproductive neuroendocrine axis. *Endocrinology* 147, 432–440. doi: 10.1210/en.2005-0507

Yasuo, S., Watanabe, M., Iigo, M., Nakamura, T. J., Watanabe, T., Takagi, T., et al. (2007b). Differential response of type 2 deiodinase gene expression tophotoperiod between photoperiodic Fischer 344 and nonphotoperiodic Wistar rats. *Am. J. Physiol. Regul. Integr. Comp. Physiol.* 292, 1315–1319. doi: 10.1152/ajpregu.00396.2006

Yasuo, S., Watanabe, M., Nakao, N., Takagi, T., Follett, B. K., Ebihara, S., et al. (2005). The reciprocal switching of two thyroid hormone-activating and -inactivating enzyme genes is involved in the photoperiodic gonadal response of Japanese quail. *Endocrinology* 146, 2551–2554. doi: 10.1210/en.2005-0057

Yasuo, S., Yoshimura, T., Ebihara, S., and Kolf, H. W. (2009). Melatonin transmits photoperiodic signals through the MT1 melatonin receptor. *J. Neurosci.* 29, 2885–2889. doi: 10.1523/JNEUROSCI.0145-09.2009

Yasuo, S., Yoshimura, T., Ebihara, S., and Korf, H. W. (2007a). Temporal dynamics of type 2 deiodinase expression after melatonin injections in Syrian hamsters. *Endocrinology* 148, 3608–3617. doi: 10.1210/en.2007-0497

Yokoyama, K., Oksche, A., Darden, T. R., and Farner, D. S. (1978). The sites of encephalic photoreception in phosoperiodic induction of the growth of the testes in the white-crowned sparrow. *Zonotrichia leucophrys gambelii*. *Cell Tissue Res.* 189, 441–467. doi: 10.1007/BF00209132

Yoshimura, T., Yasuo, S., Watanabe, M., Iigo, M., Yamamura, T., Hirunagi, K. et al. (2003). Light-induced hormone conversion of T_4 to T_3 regulates photoperiodic response of gonads in birds. *Nature* 426, 178–181. doi: 10.1038/nature02117

Zweig, M., Snyder, S. H., and Axelrod, J. (1966). Evidence for a nonretinal pathway of light to the pineal gland of newborn rats. *Proc. Natl. Acad. Sci. U.S.A.* 56, 515–520. doi: 10.1073/pnas.56.2.515

23

Ultradian oscillation in expression of four melatonin receptor subtype genes in the pineal gland of the grass puffer, a semilunar-synchronized spawner, under constant darkness

Taro Ikegami[1], Yusuke Maruyama[2], Hiroyuki Doi[3], Atsuhiko Hattori[2] and Hironori Ando[4]*

[1] Department of Chemistry, Biology, and Marine Science, Faculty of Science, University of the Ryukyus, Okinawa, Japan
[2] Department of Biology, College of Liberal Arts and Sciences, Tokyo Medical and Dental University, Ichikawa, Japan
[3] Shimonoseki Marine Science Museum "Kaikyokan," Shimonoseki Academy of Marine Science, Yamaguchi, Japan
[4] Sado Marine Biological Station, Faculty of Science, Niigata University, Sado, Japan

***Correspondence:**
Hironori Ando, Sado Marine Biological Station, Faculty of Science, Niigata University, 87 Tassha, Sado 952-2135, Japan
e-mail: hando311@cc.niigata-u.ac.jp

Melatonin receptor gene expression as well as melatonin synthesis and secretion activities were examined in the pineal gland of the grass puffer, which exhibits unique lunar/tidal cycle-synchronized mass spawing: spawning occurs before high tide on the day of spring tide during spawing season. Melatonin synthesizing activity was assessed by the abundance of arylalkylamine *N*-acetyltransferase 2 (AANAT2) mRNA. The amount of *aanat2* mRNA was low during light phase and initiated to increase after the light was turned off. The secretion of melatonin from primary pineal organ culture was stimulated after the light was turned off and ceased immediately after the light was turned on. The expression levels of four melatonin receptor subtype genes (*mel*$_{1a}$*1.4*, *mel*$_{1a}$*1.7*, *mel1b*, and *mel1c*) showed synchronous variations, and the levels tended to be high during the dark phase under light/dark conditions. These results suggest that the action of melatonin on the pineal gland is highly dependent on light and photoperiod, possibly with stronger action during night time. Under constant darkness, the expression of four melatonin receptor subtype genes showed unique ultradian oscillations with the period of 14.0–15.4 h, suggesting the presence of a circatidal oscillator in the pineal gland. The present results indicate that melatonin may serve local chronobiological functions in the pineal gland. These cyclic expressions of melatonin receptor genes in the pineal gland may be important in the control of the lunar/tidal cycle-synchronized mass spawning in the grass puffer.

Keywords: arylalkylamine *N*-acetyltransferase, circadian rhythm, circatidal rhythm, melatonin receptor, pineal gland, puffer, reproduction, ultradian rhythm

INTRODUCTION

Melatonin is produced mainly in the pineal gland and retina in fish, and its plasma concentration is higher during night-time than daytime. This daily rhythm of circulating melatonin informs the organism about the time within a day, whereas the duration of the nocturnal elevation of melatonin that corresponds to photoperiod informs the organism about the season within a year (Reiter, 1993). Melatonin has been implicated in a wide variety of physiological and behavioral functions, such as circadian and seasonal rhythms, reproduction, growth, antioxidant action, immune response, sleep, feeding, locomotor activity, and depression (Pandi-Perumal et al., 2006; Falcón et al., 2010).

The actions of melatonin are mediated via melatonin receptors that belong to the G protein-coupled receptor superfamily (Reppert et al., 1996). In vertebrates, there are three types of melatonin receptors, Mel$_{1a}$ (MT1), Mel$_{1b}$ (MT2), and Mel$_{1c}$. Mel$_{1a}$ and Mel$_{1b}$ have been identified in all vertebrate species investigated, whereas Mel$_{1c}$ has been found only in non-mammalian species (Ebisawa et al., 1994; Reppert et al., 1995). Furthermore, two different subtypes of Mel$_{1a}$ (Mel$_{1a}$1.4 and Mel$_{1a}$1.7) have been identified in zebrafish (Reppert et al., 1995), rainbow trout (Mazurais et al., 1999), goldfish (Ikegami et al., 2009a), grass puffer (Ikegami et al., 2009b), and mudskipper (Hong et al., 2014). Accordingly, phylogenetic analyses have shown that there are four subtypes of melatonin receptor genes in fish (Reppert et al., 1995).

Synchronous reproduction is crucial to reproductive success in most vertebrate species. The daily and seasonal control of reproduction involves cyclic and photoperiod-dependent changes in the activity of neurons secreting hypothalamic neuropeptides such as kisspeptin, gonadotropin-inhibitory hormone (GnIH) and gonadotropin-releasing hormone (GnRH) (Khan and Kauffman, 2012; Williams and Kriegsfeld, 2012; Simonneaux et al., 2013). These changes are brought in part by melatonin signals that transmit daily and photoperiodic information via melatonin receptors (Ubuka et al., 2005; Revel et al., 2008; Simonneaux et al., 2009; Yasuo et al., 2009). However, the mode of melatonin action on the reproductive neuroendocrine system remains to be determined.

The grass puffer (*Takifugu niphobles*) exhibits unique reproductive physiology and behavior that are synchronized with seasonal, lunar, and daily cycles. During the spawning season from spring to early summer, spawning occurs only during spring tide every 2 weeks (Yamahira, 2004; Motohashi et al., 2010; Ando et al., 2013). The fish aggregate at a certain seashore location for spawning that takes place in groups of 10–60 individuals, of which one is female. The fish usually aggregate at the spawning ground 2.5–3 h before high tide at night. Then, spawning starts 1.5–2 h before high tide and continues for 1 h during the rising tidal phase (Motohashi et al., 2010). Therefore, the timing of spawning is tightly connected with lunar and tidal rhythms as well as daily rhythm. Since we are aware of the time and place of the spawning, we can obtain spawning fish easily by dip net at the spawning bed. Thus, the grass puffer provides a unique animal model for studying the neuroendocrine mechanisms underlying the seasonal, lunar, and circadian control of reproduction.

Lunar-synchronized reproduction has been reported in a wide variety of organisms, particularly those living in shallow waters and reef areas. In these organisms, changes in moonlight and tide are considered to act as an environmental cue that entrains an internal clock for the synchronization of reproduction. However, the molecular mechanisms for lunar-synchronized spawning are poorly understood (Leatherland et al., 1992; Takemura et al., 2004a). In the golden rabbitfish, which spawns around the first quarter moon, the plasma levels of melatonin at midnight are higher on the day of new moon than full moon. This lunar phase-dependent variation in the plasma melatonin concentrations is critical for the occurrence of the lunar-synchronized spawning in the golden rabbitfish (Takemura et al., 2004b). The levels of melatonin receptor gene expression for *mt1* and mel_{1c} showed variations depending on moonlight brightness in the pineal gland (Park et al., 2014). In addition, the levels of mudskipper $mel_{1a}1.4$ expression in the diencephalon show a lunar cycle-dependent variation with two peaks at the first and last lunar quarters when the fish spawns (Hong et al., 2014). These facts suggest that melatonin signals may play a key role in transmitting the photoperiodic information of moonlight to the reproductive neuroendocrine system in the hypothalamus.

Our previous studies on the grass puffer spawning rhythm also showed possible involvement of melatonin signals in the control of the semilunar-synchronized spawning. In the diencephalon, all four melatonin receptor subtype genes are synchronously expressed with daily and circadian variations under light/dark (LD) and constant darkness (DD) conditions, respectively (Ikegami et al., 2009b). In addition, not only kisspeptin (*kiss2*) and its receptor (*kiss2r*) genes but also LPXRFamide peptide gene (*lpxrfa*), fish ortholog of GnIH gene, and its receptor (*lpxrfa-r*) gene clearly showed daily and circadian oscillations in expression, and their expression patterns are almost synchronized with each other (Shahjahan et al., 2011; Ando et al., 2014). These results indicate that melatonin signals are highly dependent on light/dark cycle in the diencephalon, and melatonin may have an important role in the cyclic expressions of *kiss2*/*kiss2r* and *lpxrfa*/*lpxrfa-r* in the grass puffer.

In the present study, to further elucidate the role of melatonin signals in the control of the semilunar-synchronized spawning, daily and circadian oscillations in expression of the four melatonin receptor subtype genes were examined in the pineal gland of grass puffer. The pineal gland is one of the master clocks in fish (Falcón et al., 2009), and melatonin may have a local action on the pineal gland via melatonin receptor that leads to the production of the semilunar-synchronized spawning rhythm. In addition, daily and circadian changes in melatonin synthesis and secretion from the pineal gland was examined by cloning and expression analyses of gene encoding arylalkylamine-*N*-acetyltransferase (AANAT) 2, a rate-limiting enzyme in melatonin synthesis, and by measurement of melatonin secreted from primary pineal organ culture.

MATERIALS AND METHODS

ANIMALS

Mature grass puffer of both sexes were caught by dip net at a spawning ground in Tomioka Bay, Kumamoto, Japan during spawning period in July and August 2009 and July 2010. They were transferred to the Fishery Research Laboratory Station, Kyushu University, Fukutsu, Japan and were kept in indoor tanks (500 l) with flow of seawater and under natural photoperiod (14L:10D, exact time of dawn and dusk were as follows: 5:20 and 19:30 in July 2009; 5:35 and 19:15 in August 2009; 5:25, and 19:25 in July 2010). The fish were fed commercial pellets equivalent to 1% of body weight (BW) at 9 a.m. daily. The experimental procedures followed the guidance approved by the Animal Care and Use Committees of Kyushu University, Fukuoka, Japan and Niigata University, Niigata, Japan.

SAMPLE COLLECTION

Daily variations of melatonin receptor and AANAT2 genes were examined by real-time PCR using the fish obtained in July 2009 ($n = 56$, 49 males, 50.0 ± 1.6 g in BW and 7 females, 49.9 ± 1.9 g in BW, July 18–19, age of the moon 26.0/middle tide, time of high tide 20:17, time of low tide 13:35) and July 2010 ($n = 108$, all males, 44.9 ± 0.7 g in BW, July 23–25, age of the moon 12.0/middle tide, time of high tide 21:33, time of low tide 15:17). The fish were transferred into indoor tanks (60 l) and acclimatized at 22°C for 6 days under natural photoperiod (14L:10D). After 3 days of fasting, the fish were anesthetized in 0.03% MS222, and killed by decapitation at 3 h intervals for 1 day at Zeitgeber time (ZT) 3, ZT6, ZT9, ZT12, ZT15, ZT18, ZT21, and ZT24 in 2009 ($n = 7$ for each time point) and for 2 days in 2010 ($n = 6$ for each time point). The whole brain including the pineal gland was removed and soaked in RNA*later* (Ambion, TX, USA) and was kept at 4°C for 1 day. The pineal gland was removed from the brain under a stereoscopic microscope and immediately frozen in liquid nitrogen and stored at −80°C.

For circadian variation, the fish obtained in August 2009 ($n = 62$, 48 males, 44.7 ± 1.4 g in BW and 14 females, 60.6 ± 3.3 g in BW, August 3–4, age of the moon 13.0/spring tide, time of high tide 21:37, time of low tide 15:22) and July 2010 ($n = 136$, 132 males, 45.2 ± 0.7 g in BW and 4 females, 47.9 ± 4.5 g in BW, July 7–9, age of the moon 25.0/middle tide, time of high tide 19:47, time of low tide 13:05) were acclimatized in the indoor tanks (60 l) for 6 days as described above. Then, the fish were left under DD condition without feeding for 3 days. The fish were anesthetized in 0.03% MS222 and killed by decapitation at 3 h intervals for 1 day at circadian time (CT) 3, CT6, CT9, CT12, CT15, CT18, CT21, and CT24 in 2009 ($n = 6$–7 for each time point) and for 2 days in 2010 ($n = 8$ for each time point). The whole brain including the pineal gland was removed under red dim light, and soaked in RNA*later* (Ambion, TX, USA). The pineal gland was collected as described above.

REAL–TIME PCR ASSAY OF MELATONIN RECEPTOR mRNAs

Real–time PCR assay was carried out as described previously (Ikegami et al., 2009b). Briefly, total RNA was extracted from the pineal gland and 200 ng of total RNA was used for synthesis of first strand cDNA by reverse transcription reaction using Multiscribe Reverse Transcriptase (Applied Biosystems, USA) according to the manufacturer's instruction. PCR reaction mixture (10 μl) contained 2 μl of sample cDNA, 0.2 μM of forward and reverse primers (**Table 1**) and 5 μl of SYBR Premix DimerEraser (Takara, Ohtsu, Japan). Amplification was carried out at 95°C for 30 s, followed by 40 cycles at 95°C for 5 s, 55°C for 30 s, and 72°C for 30 s. Specific amplification of each subtype cDNA was verified by melting curve analysis, gel electrophoresis of the product. The cross-reactivity with other subtype mRNAs in each assay was less than 0.29%. The slope and correlation coefficient (r) of the standard curve and the intra- and inter-assay coefficients of variation (CVs) in each assay are shown in Supplementary Table 1.

PARTIAL CLONING OF *aanat2* AND REAL–TIME PCR ASSAY

Genomic DNA of grass puffer was prepared from blood using a Puregene DNA Purification Kit (Gentra, MN, USA). In order to design primers for cloning the grass puffer *aanat2*, the genome database of tiger puffer (http://uswest.ensembl.org/Takifugu_rubripes/Info/Index) were BLAST searched. There are three *aanats* (*aanat1a*, *aanat1b*, and *aanat2*) in the tiger puffer genome, and all of them consist of 3 exons. PCR primers for the grass puffer *aanat2* were designed in the region from intron 1 to exon 3 (**Table 1**). PCR amplification using the grass puffer genomic DNA as template DNA was performed using a HotStar Taq Master Mix (Qiagen, Japan). Amplification was carried out at 95°C for 15 min, followed by 35 cycles of 94°C for 30 s, 53°C for 30 s and 72°C for 1 min, and finally by additional 10 min at 72°C. The PCR fragment of expected size was purified by a StrataPrep PCR Purification Kit (Stratagene, CA, USA) and cloned into a pGEM-T easy cloning vector (Promega, USA). The purified plasmid DNA was sequenced by a CEQ8800 DNA Analysis System (Beckman, Coulter).

Real–time PCR assay of *aanat2* mRNA was carried out as described above. PCR reaction mixture (10 μl) contained 2 μl of sample, 0.2 μM of forward and reverse primers (**Table 1**) and 5 μl of SYBR Premix DimerEraser (Takara, Ohtsu, Japan). Amplification was carried out at 95°C for 30 s, followed by 40 cycles at 95°C for 5 s, 55°C for 30 s, and 72°C for 30 s. Specific amplification of *aanat2* cDNA was verified by melting curve analysis and gel electrophoresis of the product. The slope, r, intra-assay CV, and inter-assay CV are shown in Supplementary Table 1.

Table 1 | Primers used in the present study.

	Forward primer	Reverse primer
REAL-TIME PCR FOR MELATONIN RECEPTOR mRNAs		
Mel1a1.4	GGCTCTTCACAGCCAGCTA	CGGAACTTGAAGACGATCAG
Mel1a1.7	TGGACTCGGTCTGAGCCAG	TCACGAAGCACCATGGTACAG
Mel1b	CCATAGATCCGTCCCACGTA	TGTTGAGCAGGCCATAGATG
Mel1c	ACGGAGACGTCGCGTTG	TCATGACGTTGGTCAACACG
PARTIAL CLONING OF *aanat2 cDNA*		
AANAT2	TCCTCACCTCGACTCTGTC	TGGAAGTGCATGTTGGATATG
REAL-TIME PCR FOR *aanat2 mRNA*		
AANAT2	ATCCACGTGTTGTCAGTACACC	AAGTCCTCGCAGATGAGCAG

PRIMARY ORGAN CULTURE OF THE PINEAL GLAND

The pineal gland was dissected out from adult grass puffer at ZT10, and were transferred to RPMI medium containing 20 mM HEPES, 9 mM sodium bicarbonate, penicillin (100 U/ml), streptomycin (100 U/ml) and fungizone (0.25 mg/ml), and pre-incubated at 20°C for 4 h. Two pineal glands were placed on sterile glass wool in a superfusion chamber (5 mm in diameter, 20 mm in height). The medium was superfused to keep the volume in the chamber 0.2 ml. The entire apparatus including the culture medium stock and the culture chamber was placed in an incubator at 20°C. A white fluorescent light was set in the incubator, and light intensity at the surface of the incubation chamber was approximately 1400 lux. The pineal glands were maintained for 1 day under LD condition (14L:10D) and then the light was turned off to keep them under DD condition for 31 h. The culture medium was continuously pumped at a rate of 1 ml/h and the perfusate was collected hourly by a fraction collector (FRAC-200, Amersham Biosciences). This primary culture experiment using two pineal glands was repeated four times.

MELATONIN MEASUREMENT

The melatonin concentrations in the culture medium were measured as described previously (Itoh et al., 1997). Melatonin was extracted from 0.3 ml of perfusate by mixing with chloroform (4 ml) and distilled water (1 ml). After centrifugation at 3000 rpm for 1 min, the aqueous phase was discarded and the organic phase was evaporated with a vacuum evaporator. The extracts were redissolved in 300 μl of HPLC mobile phase solution consisting of 50 mM ammonium acetate and 30% methanol (vol/vol), adjusted to pH 4.8 with acetic acid. After centrifugation at 500 × g for 1 min at room temperature, the supernatant was filtrated through a Millex LH 0.45 μm filter unit (Millipore, Bedford, MA, USA) and subjected to chromatography using a CAPCELL PAC C18 MGII 5 μm column (4.6 × 250 mm) (Shiseido, Tokyo, Japan) and RF-10AXL fluorometric detector (Shimadzu, Kyoto, Japan). The detector was operated at an excitation wavelength of 280 nm and an emission wavelength of 340 nm. All separations were performed isocratically at mobile phase flow rate of 0.8 ml/min and 40°C. The fraction corresponding to the authentic melatonin peak was collected. Peaks were identified by retention time and melatonin was quantified by peak area. The limit of sensitivity of the assay was as low as 1 pg for a 2:1 signal-to-noise ratio. Intra- and inter-assay CVs were 0.52% ($n = 3$) and 1.15% ($n = 5$), respectively. Melatonin was obtained from Sigma (St. Louis, MO, USA).

STATISTICAL ANALYSIS

The amounts of melatonin receptor and *aanat2* mRNAs are expressed as means ± SEM. Data were analyzed by one-way analysis of variance (ANOVA) followed by Tukey's test or Games–Howell's multiple comparisons test to assess statistically significant differences among the different time points in the daily and circadian variation experiments. The periodicity of daily and circadian variations was calculated with COSINOR (http://www.circadian.org/softwar.html).

RESULTS

DAILY AND CIRCADIAN VARIATIONS IN MELATONIN SECRETION FROM THE PINEAL GLAND

The secretion pattern of melatonin from the pineal gland was examined using the primary organ culture system. Under LD conditions, the medium melatonin concentrations significantly increased during dark phase and quickly dropped after exposure to light (**Figure 1**). During the light phase, the medium melatonin levels remained at almost zero. This daily change was repeated at least for 3 days under the LD conditions in this culture system (data not shown). Under DD conditions, the medium melatonin levels showed a circadian variation with lowest levels at CT9 (middle of subjective light phase), but the levels were significantly higher than that at ZT9 (0.07 ± 0.01 ng/ml at ZT9 vs. 0.68 ± 0.05 ng/ml at CT9, $n = 4$, $p < 0.001$ by t-test). The levels were initiated to increase at the end of subjective light phase. The COSINOR analysis revealed a significant circadian rhythm with 23.7 h period ($p < 0.001$).

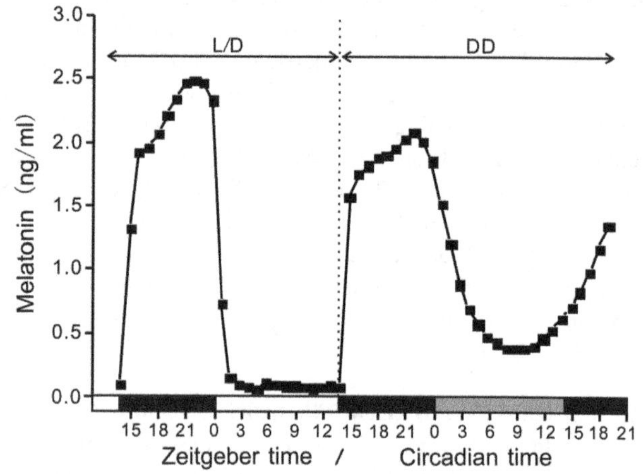

FIGURE 1 | Daily and circadian changes in melatonin secretion from the pineal gland *in vitro*. Two pineal glands were placed in a superfusion chamber and maintained for 1 day under LD condition (14L:10D, 1400 lux at the surface of the incubation chamber) and then the light was turned off to keep them under DD condition for 31 h. The culture medium was collected hourly by a fraction collector, and the concentrations of melatonin in the perfusate were determined by high performance liquid chromatography. This primary culture experiment using two pineal glands was repeated four times and a representative profile is shown.

DAILY AND CIRCADIAN OSCILLATIONS IN EXPRESSION OF *aanat2* IN THE PINEAL GLAND

Partial DNA sequence determined for the grass puffer *aanat2* was 454 bp including exons 2–3 (Accession No. LC010911). The coding region of 383 bp encodes a predicted AANAT2 protein that contains conserved regions including C/c-1, D/c-1, D/c-2, and motifs A and B (Supplementary Figure 1). The nucleotide sequence similarity of *aanat2* between grass puffer and tiger puffer is 98.2%.

Under LD conditions, the absolute amounts of *aanat2* mRNA were low during the light phase and significantly increased at the end of the light phase or during the dark phase, although the peak levels and positions were different (3×10^6 copies/μg RNA at ZT21 in 2009 and approximately 11×10^6 copies/μg RNA at ZT12-15 in 2010 (**Figure 2**). The COSINOR analyses for the variations in 2009 and 2010 revealed significant daily rhythms with 19.3 h period ($p < 0.05$) and 21.0 h period ($p < 0.001$), respectively.

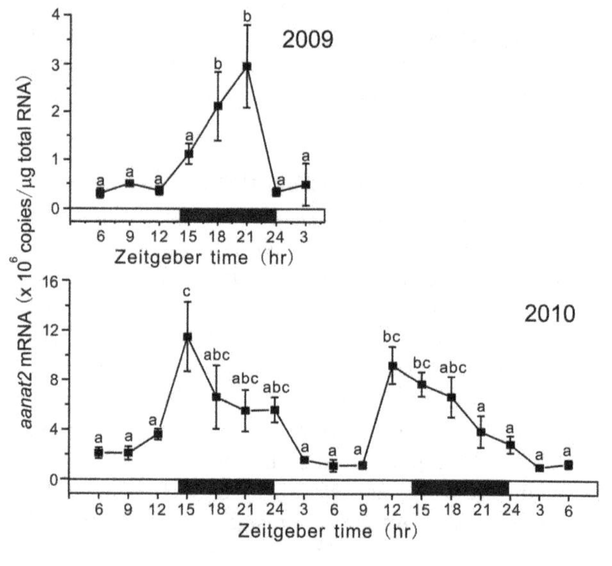

FIGURE 2 | Daily variations in the amounts of *aanat2* mRNA in the pineal gland. The fish were kept under natural photoperiod (14L:10D), and the brain samples were taken at 3 h intervals for 1 day at ZT3, ZT6, ZT9, ZT12, ZT15, ZT18, ZT21, and ZT24 in 2009 ($n = 7$ for each time point) and for 2 days in 2010 ($n = 6$ for each time point). Values accompanied by different letters are statistically significantly different ($p < 0.05$).

Under DD conditions, *aanat2* showed circadian oscillation, but the profiles were different between 2009 and 2010 (**Figure 3**). In 2009, the mRNA levels showed a peak at CT9 and the lowest level at CT18 with a significant circadian rhythm with 18.3 h period ($p < 0.01$). In 2010, *aanat2* showed a somewhat different circadian oscillation to that in 2009: the low levels of mRNA continued for longer period from CT21 to CT6 with a significant circadian rhythm with 24.0 h period ($p < 0.001$).

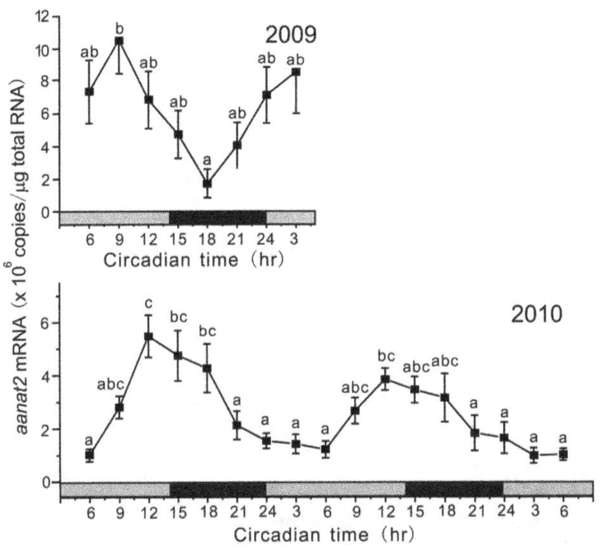

FIGURE 3 | Circadian variations in the amounts of *aanat2* mRNA in the pineal gland. The fish were kept under constant darkness condition for 3 days, and then the brain samples were taken under red dim light at 3 h intervals for 1 day at CT3, CT6, CT9, CT12, CT15, CT18, CT21, and CT24 in 2009 ($n = 6$–7 for each time point) and for 2 days in 2010 ($n = 8$ for each time point). Values accompanied by different letters are statistically significantly different ($p < 0.05$).

DAILY AND ULTRADIAN OSCILLATIONS IN EXPRESSION OF FOUR MELATONIN RECEPTOR SUBTYPE GENES IN THE PINEAL GLAND

In the pineal gland, the absolute amounts of melatonin receptor subtype mRNAs were comparable for $mel_{1a}1.4$, $mel_{1a}1.7$, and mel_{1b} with highest levels of mel_{1b} mRNA (**Figure 4**). The amounts of mel_{1c} mRNA were as low as approximately one thirtieth those of mel_{1b} mRNA. In 2009 under LD conditions, the mRNA amounts of $mel_{1a}1.4$, $mel_{1a}1.7$, and mel_{1c} showed a synchronous daily variation with a sharp peak at ZT18, whereas mel_{1b} showed a somewhat arrhythmic expression pattern. In 2010, the expression levels of four melatonin receptor subtype genes showed a synchronous variation for 2 days. The levels tended to be high during the dark phase, although these changes were less cyclic.

Under DD conditions, all subtype genes showed a synchronous ultradian oscillation in expression (**Figure 5**). In 2009, all four subtype genes showed synchronous variations with two peaks at CT9 (middle of subjective light phase) and CT24 (start of subjective light phase). The COSINOR analyses revealed significant circadian rhythms with 14.6 h period for $mel_{1a}1.4$ ($p < 0.05$), 15.4 h period for $mel_{1a}1.7$ ($p < 0.05$), and 14.5 h period for mel_{1b} ($p < 0.05$). In 2010, the four subtype genes also exhibited ultradian oscillation in expression continuously for 2 days. The COSINOR analyses revealed significant circadian rhythms with 15.4 h period for $mel_{1a}1.4$ ($p < 0.01$), 14.5 h period for $mel_{1a}1.7$ ($p < 0.001$), 14.9 h period for mel_{1b} ($p < 0.01$), and 14.0 h period for mel_{1c} ($p < 0.001$).

DISCUSSION

In the present study, melatonin receptor gene expression as well as melatonin synthesis and secretion activites were examined in the pineal gland of grass puffer, a semilunar-synchronized spawner. Melatonin synthesizing activity was assessed by the abundance of *aanat2* mRNA, which encodes a rate-limiting enzyme in the conversion of serotonin to melatonin. The amount of *aanat2* mRNA were low during light phase and was initiated to increase after the light was turned off. The secretion of melatonin from the pineal organ culture was drastically stimulated after the light was turned off and ceased immediately after the light turned on. Accordingly, the melatonin synthesis and secretion is certainly dependent on light, and melatonin is secreted only during dark phase. On the other hand, four melatonin receptor subtype genes mostly showed synchronous expression with a peak during dark phase. These results suggest that the action of melatonin on the pineal gland is highly dependent on light and photoperiod, possibly with stronger action during night time. Interestingly, the four melatonin receptor genes showed unique ultradian oscillations with the period of 14.0–15.4 h under DD conditions. To our knowledge, this is the first description of ultradian oscillation in melatonin receptor gene expression under DD conditions. This unique ultradian expression of melatonin receptor genes may be involved in the control of the semilunar-synchronized spawning rhythm in the grass puffer.

In this study, we identified three *aanats* in the tiger puffer genome, and a partial nucleotide sequence of the grass puffer *aanat2* was determined. Two *aanat* genes, *aanat1* and *aanat2*, have been identified in teleosts (Coon et al., 1999; Benyassi et al., 2000; Shi et al., 2004; Zilberman-Peled et al., 2004; Vuilleumier et al., 2007). In addition, two subtypes of *aanat1* genes, *aanat1a* and *aanat1b*, have been predicted in the genomes of tiger puffer and medaka (Falcón et al., 2009), and their cDNAs were isolated from the Senegalese sole retina (Isorna et al., 2011). *aanat1* is mainly expressed in the retina, whereas *aanat2* is expressed exclusively in the pineal gland. The deduced grass puffer AANAT2 contains plausible arylalkylamine binding domains (C/c-1, D/c-1, and D/c-2) (Klein et al., 1997), and highly conserved regions of *N*-acetyltransferase superfamily (motifs A and B). Site directed mutagenesis in yeast MAK3 and human spermidine/spermine *N*-acetyltransferases revealed that motifs A and B are important to maintain enzyme activities (Tercero et al., 1992; Coleman et al., 1996). The nocturnal expression of the grass puffer *aanat2* was apparent in both 2009 and 2010 (**Figure 2**), and this is well-consistent with the nocturnal secretion of melatonin *in vitro* (**Figure 1**). Under DD conditions, the grass puffer *aanat2* exhibited cyclic expression patterns with a peak at CT9 in 2009 and at CT12 or CT15 in 2010. The profiles of *aanat2* expression were somewhat different between 2009 and 2010 possibly due to variation in natural light conditions in the 2 years. It is assumed that the grass puffer *aanat2* expression shows daily and circadian oscillation through regulation by the internal circadian clock, as reported in other species (Foulkes et al., 1997; Coon et al., 1999; Kashiwagi et al., 2013).

Melatonin secreted from the pineal gland has been shown to be involved in the control of daily and seasonal rhythms in many physiological and behavioral functions through melatonin receptors. The present study demonstrated cyclic changes in expression of all four melatonin receptor genes in the pineal

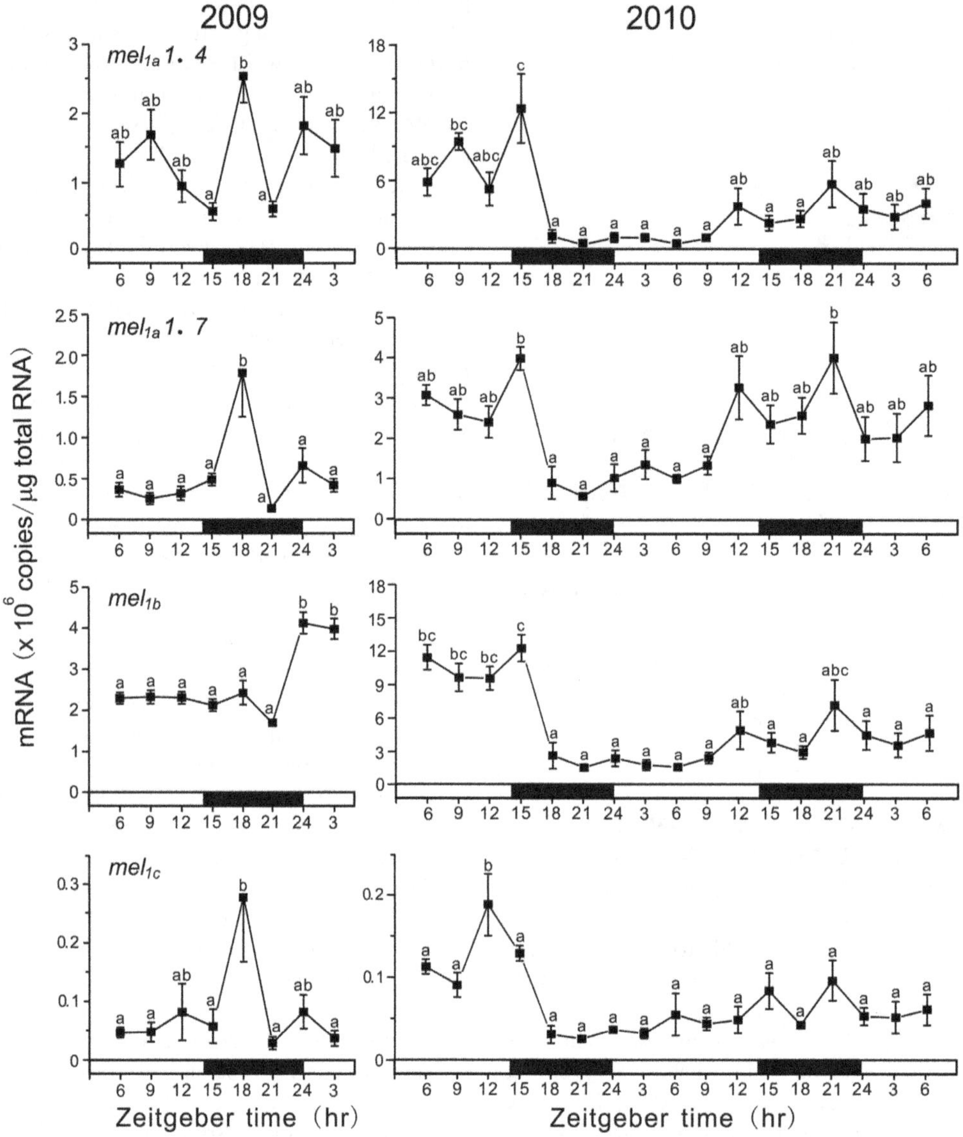

FIGURE 4 | Daily variations in the amounts of four melatonin receptor subtype mRNAs in the pineal gland. The fish were kept under natural photoperiod (14L:10D), and the brain samples were taken at 3 h intervals for 1 day at ZT3, ZT6, ZT9, ZT12, ZT15, ZT18, ZT21, and ZT24 in 2009 ($n = 7$ for each time point) and for 2 days in 2010 ($n = 6$ for each time point). Values accompanied by different letters are statistically significantly different ($p < 0.05$).

gland, and their expression patterns are mostly synchronized. It is thus conceivable that melatonin may serve local functions in the pineal gland that are most probably connected to rhythmic processes. In mammals, melatonin has been shown to play a role in resetting the circadian pacemaker activity in the suprachiasmatic nucleus (SCN) via MT2 (Liu et al., 1997). Melatonin directly influences on the electrical and metabolic activities of the SCN, resulting in the phase-shifting effect and also a significant increase in amplitude of the oscillations (Pévet et al., 2002). Since in fish the master circadian clock is considered to be located in the pineal organ in addition to eyes and probably hypothalamus (Falcón et al., 2009), the pineal melatonin may exhibit a local action on the activity of circadian clock. The expression of the four melatonin receptor genes tended to increase during the dark phase (**Figure 4**), indicating that melatonin's chronobiotic effect is certainly dependent on light and time. Taken together with the nocturnal melatonin secretion, the effect may be more drastic during the dark phase.

The daily oscillation in expression of melatonin receptor genes has been reported in the brain of various fish species (Park et al., 2006, 2007a,b; Ikegami et al., 2009a,b; Confente et al., 2010; Chai et al., 2013). In the diencephalon of grass puffer, all four subtype genes showed a peak at ZT15 under LD conditions like in the pineal gland (Ikegami et al., 2009b). Similarly, ZT-dependent fluctuations in expression of the four melatonin receptor genes were observed in the grass puffer retina and optic tectum, although in some cases including the pineal glands in 2010, the mRNA amounts showed arrhythmic variations. This

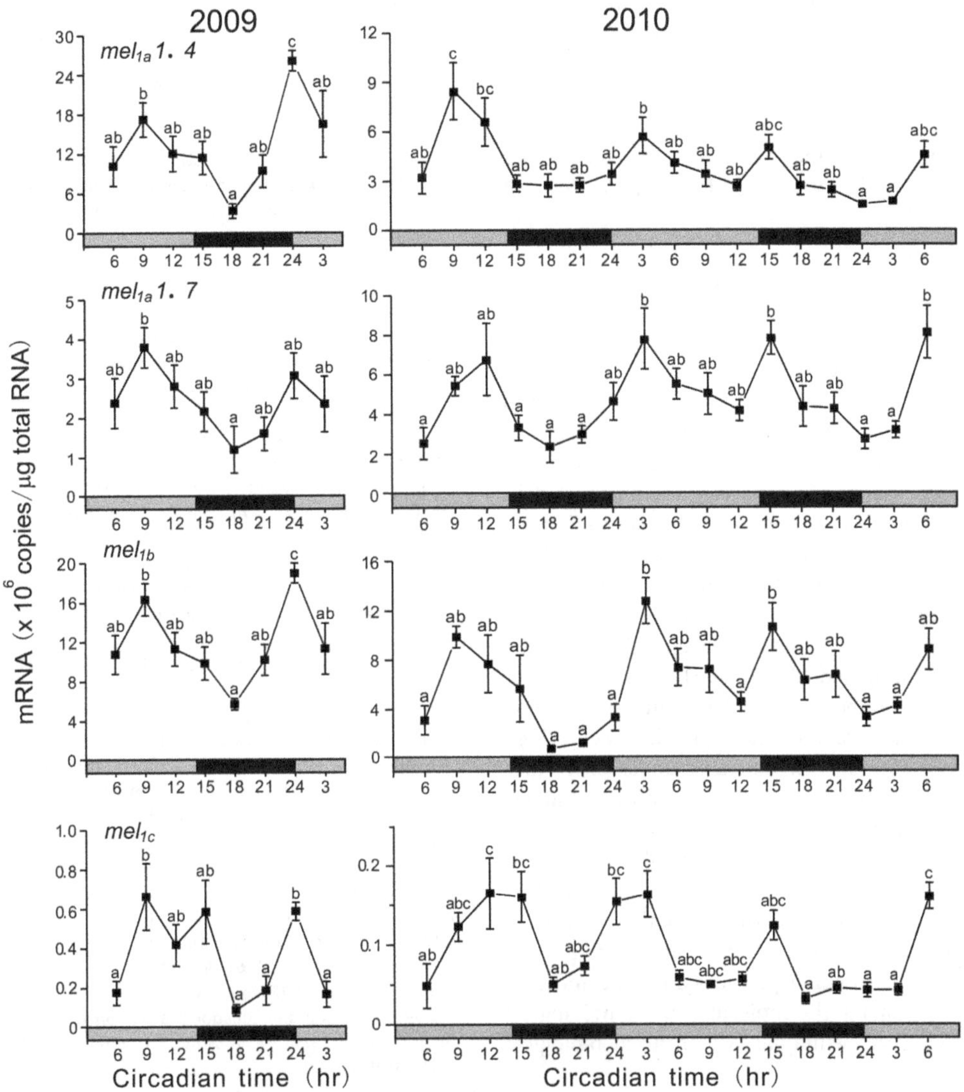

FIGURE 5 | Ultradian variations in the amounts of four melatonin receptor subtype mRNAs in the pineal gland. The fish were kept under constant darkness condition for 3 days, and then the brain samples were taken under red dim light at 3 h intervals for 1 day at CT3, CT6, CT9, CT12, CT15, CT18, CT21, and CT24 in 2009 ($n = 6$–7 for each time point) and for 2 days in 2010 ($n = 8$ for each time point). Values accompanied by different letters are statistically significantly different ($p < 0.05$).

might be due to effects on melatonin receptor gene expression of some other environmental and internal conditions, such as water temperature, nutrition, sexual maturation, and infection (immune response) (Pandi-Perumal et al., 2006; Falcón et al., 2010). Nevertheless, it is of considerable interest to note that in the grass puffer diencephalon, *kiss2*/*kiss2r* and *lpxrfa*/*lpxrfa-r* also showed daily and mostly synchronized oscillations (Shahjahan et al., 2011; Ando et al., 2014). These results suggest that the reproductive neuroendocrine activity may be cyclic within a day under the control of melatonin signals directly or indirectly via circadian clock in the pineal gland (Ando et al., 2013, 2014). The involvement of MT1 in the control of *gnrh1* expression through *kiss2* was reported in the orange-spotted grouper (Chai et al., 2013).

Recently, studies on melatonin receptor gene expression in lunar-dependent spawner indicated that their expressions are dependent on the lunar phase, e.g., *mt1* and mel_{1c} in the pineal gland of golden rabbitfish (Park et al., 2014) and $mel_{1a}1.4$ in the diencephalon of mudskipper (Hong et al., 2014). Thus, the melatonin signals may play a key role in transmitting the photoperiodic information of moonlight to the reproductive neuroendocrine system. Taking together with the clear daily and circadian expressions of kisspeptin and LPXRFa genes in the grass puffer (Shahjahan et al., 2011; Ando et al., 2014), it is possible that the lunar cycle-dependent changes in the melatonin/melatonin receptor levels may produce lunar-related oscillations of kisspeptin and LPXRFa gene expressions in addition to the daily oscillations. So far, the plasma melatonin levels could not be determined in the grass puffer due to the presence of interfering material in the assay, and monthly variations of the plasma melatonin levels and melatonin receptor gene expression are currently under investigation.

Under DD conditions, all four melatonin receptor genes showed ultradian oscillations with the period of 14.0–15.4 h in both 2009 and 2010 (**Figure 5**). This unique ultradian rhythm in melatonin receptor gene expression leads us to speculate that this rhythm might be related to circatidal rhythm, the period of which is 12.4 h, and there must be a circasemidian clock in the pineal gland of the grass puffer in addition to the circadian clock. Circatidal rhythms have been reported in behavioral and physiological activities of various marine aminals, for example in crab (Saigusa, 2002; Chabot et al., 2004), cumacean (Akiyama, 2004), cricket (Satoh et al., 2008) and ragworm (Last et al., 2009). On the other hand, circasemidian rhythms have been reported in humans (Wan et al., 1992; Hayashi et al., 2002; Tarquini et al., 2005). Interestingly, the combination of a circatidal oscillator with a circadian oscillator can produce circasemilunar oscillations which enable an animal to synchronize its rhythms with the environmental situation that reoccurs every 15 days at the same time of day (Bünning and Müller, 1961). It should be of considerable interest and importance to determine if this ultradian rhythm of melatonin receptor gene expression is entrained with the tidal changes when the fish are reared under such situation. If so, the pineal gland would be able to produce semilunar oscillations of melatonin signals without changes in moonlight. Alternatively, there may be a circasemilunar oscillator that can be entrained with moonlight (Neumann, 1989). Although further studies will be needed to examine which hypothesis is correct for the semilunar spawning rhythm of grass puffer, the present results indicate that the grass puffer provides a unique and useful animal model for studying the molecular and physiological mechanisms underlying the semilunar-synchronized biological rhythm.

In conclusion, in the grass puffer pineal gland, the activity of melatonin synthesis and secretion was solely dependent on light and time, and melatonin is secreted only during dark phase. Four melatonin receptor subtype genes mostly showed synchronous expression with a peak during dark phase, suggesting that melatonin may serve local chronobiotic functions in the pineal gland that might be influenced by moonlight. Moreover, the four melatonin receptor genes showed unique ultradian oscillations under DD conditions with the period of 14.0–15.4 h, suggesting the presence of a circasemidian oscillator. Taken together, the cyclic expressions of melatonin receptor genes may be important in the control of the semilunar-synchronized spawning rhythm in the grass puffer.

ACKNOWLEDGMENTS

We are grateful to Dr. Eiji Motohashi, Dr. M. Shahjahan, Mr. Atsushi Suda, Mr. Takeshi Yoshihara, and laboratory members of the Fishery Research Laboratory Station, Kyushu University, for their help in keeping and sampling fish. This study was supported by Grants-in-Aid from the Ministry of Education, Science, Sports, Science, and Technology, Japan.

REFERENCES

Akiyama, T. (2004). Entrainment of the circatidal swimming activity rhythm in the cumacean *Dimorphostylis asiatica* (Crustacea) to 12.5-hour hydrostatic pressure cycles. *Zool. Sci.* 21, 29–38. doi: 10.2108/0289-0003(2004)21[29:EOTCSA]2.0.CO;2

Ando, H., Ogawa, S., Shahjahan, M., Ikegami, T., Doi, H., Hattori, A., et al. (2014). Diurnal and circadian oscillations in expression of kisspeptin, kisspeptin receptor and gonadotrophin-releasing hormone 2 genes in the grass puffer, a semilunar-synchronised spawner. *J. Neuroendocrinol.* 26, 459–467. doi: 10.1111/jne.12165

Ando, H., Shahjahan, M., and Hattori, A. (2013). Molecular neuroendocrine basis of lunar-related spawning in grass puffer. *Gen. Comp. Endocrinol.* 181, 211–214. doi: 10.1016/j.ygcen.2012.07.027

Benyassi, A., Schwartz, C., Coon, S. L., Klein, D. C., and Falcón, J. (2000). Melatonin synthesis: arylalkylamine *N*-acetyltransferases in trout retina and pineal organ are different. *Neuroreport* 11, 255–258. doi: 10.1097/00001756-200002070-00006

Bünning, E., and Müller, D. (1961). Wie messen organismen lunare zyklen? *Z. Naturforsch.* 16b, 391–395.

Chabot, C. C., Kent, J., and Watson, W. H. III. (2004). Circatidal and circadian rhythms of locomotion in *Limulus polyphemus*. *Biol. Bull.* 207, 72–75. doi: 10.2307/1543630

Chai, K. E., Liu, X., Zhang, Y., and Lin, H. (2013). Day-night and reproductive cycle profiles of *melatonin receptor*, *kiss*, and *gnrh* expression in orange-spotted grouper (*Epinephelus coioides*). *Mol. Reprod. Dev.* 80, 535–548. doi: 10.1002/mrd.22191

Coleman, C. S., Huang, H., and Pegg, A. E. (1996). Structure and critical residues at the active site of spermidine/spermine-N^1-acetyltransferase. *Biochem. J.* 316, 697–701.

Confente, F., Rendón, M., Besseau, L., Falcón, J., and Muñoz-Cueto, J. A. (2010). Melatonin receptors in a pleuronectiform species, *Solea senegalensis*: cloning, tissue expression, day-night and seasonal variations. *Gen. Comp. Endocrinol.* 167, 202–214. doi: 10.1016/j.ygcen.2010.03.006

Coon, S. L., Bégay, V., Deurloo, D., Fálcon, J., and Klein, D. C. (1999). Two arylalkylamine *N*-acetyltransferase genes mediate melatonin synthesis in fish. *J. Biol. Chem.* 274, 9076–9082. doi: 10.1074/jbc.274.13.9076

Ebisawa, T., Karne, S., Lerner, M. R., and Reppert, S. M. (1994). Expression cloning of a high-affinity melatonin receptor from *Xenopus* dermal melanophores. *Proc. Natl. Acad. Sci. U.S.A.* 91, 6133–6137. doi: 10.1073/pnas.91.13.6133

Falcón, J., Besseau, L., Fuentès, M., Sauzet, S., Magnanou, E., and Boeuf, G. (2009). Structural and functional evolution of the pineal melatonin system in vertebrates. *Ann. N. Y. Acad. Sci.* 1163, 101–111. doi: 10.1111/j.1749-6632.2009.04435.x

Falcón, J., Migaud, H., Muñoz-Cueto, J. A., and Carrillo, M. (2010). Current knowledge on the melatonin system in teleost fish. *Gen. Comp. Endocrinol.* 165, 469–482. doi: 10.1016/j.ygcen.2009.04.026

Foulkes, N. S., Whitmore, D., and Sassone-Corsi, P. (1997). Rhythmic transcription: the molecular basis of circadian melatonin synthesis. *Biol. Cell.* 89, 487–494. doi: 10.1016/S0248-4900(98)80004-X

Hayashi, M., Morikawa, T., and Hori, T. (2002). Circasemidian 12 h cycle of slow wave sleep under constant darkness. *Clin. Neurophysiol.* 113, 1505–1516. doi: 10.1016/S1388-2457(02)00168-2

Hong, L. Y., Hong, W. S., Zhu, W. B., Shi, Q., You, X. X., and Chen, S. X. (2014). Cloning and expression of melatonin receptors in the mudskipper *Boleophthalmus pectinirostris*: their role in synchronizing its semilunar spawning rhythm. *Gen. Comp. Endocrinol.* 195, 138–150. doi: 10.1016/j.ygcen.2013.11.004

Ikegami, T., Azuma, K., Nakamura, M., Suzuki, N., Hattori, A., and Ando, H. (2009a). Diurnal expressions of four subtypes of melatonin receptor genes in the optic tectum and retina of goldfish. *Comp. Biochem. Physiol. Part A* 152, 219–224. doi: 10.1016/j.cbpa.2008.09.030

Ikegami, T., Motohashi, E., Doi, H., Hattori, A., and Ando, H. (2009b). Synchronized diurnal and circadian expressions of four subtypes of melatonin receptor genes in the diencephalon of a puffer fish with lunar-related spawning cycles. *Neurosci. Lett.* 462, 58–63. doi: 10.1016/j.neulet.2009.06.076

Isorna, E., Aliaga-Guerrero, M., M'Rabet, A. E., Servili, A., Falcón, J., and Muñoz-Cueto, J. A. (2011). Identification of two arylalkylamine *N*-acetyltranferase 1 genes with different developmental expression profiles in the flatfish

Solea senegalensis. *J. Pineal Res.* 51, 434–444. doi: 10.1111/j.1600-079X.2011.00907.x

Itoh, M. T., Hattori, A., and Sumi, Y. (1997). Hydroxyindole-O-methyltransferase activity assay using high-performance liquid chromatography with fluorometric detection: determination of melatonin enzymatically formed from N-acetylserotonin and S-adenosyl-L-methionine. *J. Chromatogr. B Biomed. Sci. Appl.* 692, 217–221. doi: 10.1016/S0378-4347(96)00503-8

Kashiwagi, T., Park, Y. J., Park, J. G., Imamura, S., Takeuchi, Y., Hur, S. P., et al. (2013). Moonlight affects mRNA abundance of arylalkylamine *N*-acetyltransferase in the retina of a lunar-synchronized spawner, the gold-lined spinefoot. *J. Exp. Zool. A Ecol. Genet. Physiol.* 319, 505–516. doi: 10.1002/jez.1814

Khan, A. R., and Kauffman, A. S. (2012). The role of kisspeptin and RFamide-related peptide-3 neurones in the circadian-timed preovulatory luteinising hormone surge. *J. Neuroendocrinol.* 24, 131–143. doi: 10.1111/j.1365-2826.2011.02162.x

Klein, D. C., Coon, S. L., Roseboom, P. H., Weller, J. L., Bernard, M., Gastel, J. A., et al. (1997). The melatonin rhythm-generating enzyme: molecular regulation of serotonin *N*-acetyltransferase in the pineal gland. *Recent. Prog. Horm. Res.* 52, 307–357.

Last, K. S., Bailhache, T., Kramer, C., Kyriacou, C. P., Rosato, E., and Olive, P. J. (2009). Tidal, daily, and lunar-day activity cycles in the marine polychaete *Nereis virens*. *Chronobiol. Int.* 26, 167–183. doi: 10.1080/07420520902774524

Leatherland, J. F., Farbridge, K. J., and Boujard, T. (1992). "Lunar and semi-lunar rhythms in fishes," in *Rhythms in Fishes*, ed M. A. Ali (New York, NY: Plenum Press), 83–107.

Liu, C., Weaver, D. R., Jin, X., Shearman, L. P., Pieschl, R. L., Gribkoff, V. K., et al. (1997). Molecular dissection of two distinct actions of melatonin on the suprachiasmatic circadian clock. *Neuron* 19, 91–102. doi: 10.1016/S0896-6273(00)80350-5

Mazurais, D., Brierley, I., Anglade, I., Drew, J., Randall, C., Bromage, N., et al. (1999). Central melatonin receptors in the rainbow trout: comparative distribution of ligand binding and gene expression. *J. Comp. Neurol.* 409, 313–324. doi: 10.1002/(SICI)1096-9861(19990628)409:2<313::AID-CNE11>3.0.CO;2-1

Motohashi, E., Yoshihara, T., Doi, H., and Ando, H. (2010). Aggregating behavior of grass puffer, *Takifugu niphobles*, observed in aquarium during the spawning period. *Zool. Sci.* 27, 559–564. doi: 10.2108/zsj.27.559

Neumann, D. (1989). Circadian components of semilunar and lunar timing mechanisms. *J. Biol. Rhythms.* 4, 285–294. doi: 10.1177/074873048900400213

Pandi-Perumal, S. R., Srinivasan, V., Maestroni, G. J., Cardinali, D. P., Poeggeler, B., and Hardeland, R. (2006). Melatonin: nature's most versatile biological signal? *FEBS J.* 273, 2813–2838. doi: 10.1111/j.1742-4658.2006.05322.x

Park, Y. J., Park, J. G., Hiyakawa, N., Lee, Y. D., Kim, S. J., and Takemura, A. (2007a). Diurnal and circadian regulation of a melatonin receptor, MT1, in the golden rabbitfish, *Siganus guttatus*, *Gen. Comp. Endocrinol.* 150, 253–262. doi: 10.1016/j.ygcen.2006.08.011

Park, Y. J., Park, J. G., Jeong, H. B., Takeuchi, Y., Kim, S. J., Lee, Y. D., et al. (2007b). Expression of the melatonin receptor Mel1c in neural tissues of the reef fish *Siganus guttatus*. *Comp. Biochem. Physiol. A Mol. Integr. Physiol.* 147, 103–111. doi: 10.1016/j.cbpa.2006.11.027

Park, Y. J., Park, J. G., Kim, S. J., Lee, Y. D., Rahman, M. S., and Takemura, A. (2006). Melatonin receptor of a reef fish with lunar-related rhythmicity: cloning and daily variations. *J. Pineal Res.* 41, 166–174. doi: 10.1111/j.1600-079X.2006.00350.x

Park, Y. J., Park, J. G., Takeuchi, Y., Hur, S. P., Lee, Y. D., Kim, S. J., et al. (2014). Influence of moonlight on mRNA expression patterns of melatonin receptor subtypes in the pineal organ of a tropical fish. *Mar. Genomics.* 14, 67–70. doi: 10.1016/j.margen.2013.10.006

Pévet, P., Bothorel, B., Slotten, H., and Saboureau, M. (2002). The chronobiotic properties of melatonin. *Cell Tissue Res.* 309, 183–191. doi: 10.1007/s00441-002-0584-1

Reiter, R. J. (1993). The melatonin rhythm: both a clock and a calendar. *Experientia* 49, 654–664. doi: 10.1007/BF01923947

Reppert, S. M., Weaver, D. R., Cassone, V. M., Godson, C., and Kolakowski, L. F. Jr. (1995). Melatonin receptors are for the birds: molecular analysis of two receptor subtypes differentially expressed in chick brain. *Neuron* 15, 1003–1015. doi: 10.1016/0896-6273(95)90090-X

Reppert, S. M., Weaver, D. R., and Godson, C. (1996). Melatonin receptors step into the light: cloning and classification of subtypes. *Trends Pharmacol. Sci.* 17, 100–102. doi: 10.1016/0165-6147(96)10005-5

Revel, F. G., Saboureau, M., Pévet, P., Simonneaux, V., and Mikkelsen, J. D. (2008). RFamide-related peptide gene is a melatonin-driven photoperiodic gene. *Endocrinology* 149, 902–912. doi: 10.1210/en.2007-0848

Saigusa, M. (2002). Hatching controlled by the circatidal clock, and the role of the medulla terminalis in the optic peduncle of the eyestalk, in an estuarine crab *Sesarma haematocheir*. *J. Exp. Biol.* 205, 3487–3504.

Satoh, A., Yoshioka, E., and Numata, H. (2008). Circatidal activity rhythm in the mangrove cricket *Apteronemobius asahinai*. *Biol. Lett.* 4, 233–236. doi: 10.1098/rsbl.2008.0036

Shahjahan, M., Ikegami, T., Osugi, T., Ukena, K., Doi, H., Hattori, A., et al. (2011). Synchronised expressions of LPXRFamide peptide and its receptor genes: seasonal, diurnal and circadian changes during spawning period in grass puffer. *J. Neuroendocrinol.* 23, 39–51. doi: 10.1111/j.1365-2826.2010.02081.x

Shi, Q., Ando, H., Coon, S. L., Sato, S., Ban, M., and Urano, A. (2004). Embryonic and post-embryonic expression of arylalkylamine *N*-acetyltransferase and melatonin receptor genes in the eye and brain of chum salmon (*Oncorhynchus keta*). *Gen. Comp. Endocrinol.* 136, 311–321. doi: 10.1016/j.ygcen.2004.01.004

Simonneaux, V., Ancel, C., Poirel, V. J., and Gauer, F. (2013). Kisspeptins and RFRP-3 act in concert to synchronize rodent reproduction with seasons. *Front. Neurosci.* 7:22. doi: 10.3389/fnins.2013.00022

Simonneaux, V., Ansel, L., Revel, F. G., Klosen, P., Pévet, P., and Mikkelsen, J. D. (2009). Kisspeptin and the seasonal control of reproduction in hamsters. *Peptides* 30, 146–153. doi: 10.1016/j.peptides.2008.06.006

Takemura, A., Rahman, M. S., Nakamura, S., Park, Y. J., and Takano, K. (2004a). Lunar cycles and reproductive activity in reef fishes with particular attention to rabbitfishes. *Fish Fisheries* 5, 317–328. doi: 10.1111/j.1467-2679.2004.00164.x

Takemura, A., Susilo, E. S., Rahman, M. D., and Morita, M. (2004b). Perception and possible utilization of moonlight intensity for reproductive activities in a lunar-synchronized spawner, the golden rabbitfish. *J. Exp. Zool.* 301A, 844–851. doi: 10.1002/jez.a.105

Tarquini, R., Mazzoccoli, G., Dolenti, S., Gaudiano, P., Comuni, C., Laffi, G., et al. (2005). Circasemidian rather than circadian variation of circulating osteoprotegerin in clinical health. *Biomed. Pharmacother.* 59, S225–S228. doi: 10.1016/S0753-3322(05)80036-8

Tercero, J. C., Riles, L. E., and Wickner, R. B. (1992). Localized mutagenesis and evidence for post-transcriptional regulation of MAK3. A putative N-acetyltransferase required for double-stranded RNA virus propagation in *Saccharomyces cerevisiae*. *J. Biol. Chem.* 267, 20270–20276.

Ubuka, T., Bentley, G. E., Ukena, K., Wingfield, J. C., and Tsutsui, K. (2005). Melatonin induces the expression of gonadotropin-inhibitory hormone in the avian brain. *Proc. Natl. Acad. Sci. U.S.A.* 102, 3052–3057. doi: 10.1073/pnas.0403840102

Vuilleumier, R., Boeuf, G., Fuentes, M., Gehring, W. J., and Falcón, J. (2007). Cloning and early expression pattern of two melatonin biosynthesis enzymes in the turbot (*Scophthalmus maximus*). *Eur. J. Neurosci.* 25, 3047–3057. doi: 10.1111/j.1460-9568.2007.05578.x

Wan, C., Wang, Z., Cornélissen, G., and Halberg, F. (1992). Age, gender and circadian or circasemidian blood pressure and heart rate variation of children. *Chronobiologia.* 19, 121–129.

Williams, W. P. I. I., and Kriegsfeld, L. J. (2012). Circadian control of neuroendocrine circuits regulating female reproductive function. *Front. Endocrinol.* 3:60. doi: 10.3389/fendo.2012.00060

Yamahira, K. (2004). How do multiple environmental cycles in combination determine reproductive timing in marine organisms? A model and test. *Funct. Ecol.* 18, 4–15. doi: 10.1046/j.0269-8463.2004.00795.x

Yasuo, S., Yoshimura, T., Ebihara, S., and Korf, H. W. (2009). Melatonin transmits photoperiodic signals through the MT1 melatonin receptor. *J. Neurosci.* 29, 2885–2889. doi: 10.1523/JNEUROSCI.0145-09.2009

Zilberman-Peled, B., Benhar, I., Coon, S. L., Ron, B., and Gothilf, Y. (2004). Duality of serotonin-*N*-acetyltransferase in the gilthead seabream (*Sparus aurata*): molecular cloning and characterization of recombinant enzymes. *Gen. Comp. Endocrinol.* 138, 139–147. doi: 10.1016/j.ygcen.2004.05.007

24

Restoration of tryptophan hydroxylase functions and serotonin content in the Atlantic croaker hypothalamus by antioxidant treatment during hypoxic stress

Md. Saydur Rahman* and Peter Thomas

Marine Science Institute, University of Texas at Austin, Port Aransas, TX, USA

***Correspondence:**
Md. Saydur Rahman, Marine Science Institute, University of Texas at Austin, 750 Channel View Drive, Port Aransas, TX 78373, USA
e-mail: rahman@utexas.edu

Antioxidants are prototypical scavengers of oxygen-free radicals and have been shown to prevent neuroendocrine dysfunction in vertebrates during oxidative stress. In the present study, we investigated whether antioxidant treatment can reverse hypoxia-induced down-regulation of hypothalamic tryptophan hydroxylase (TPH) and serotonergic functions in Atlantic croaker. Hypothalamic neuronal contents of TPH-1 and TPH-2 proteins, serotonin (5-hydroxytryptamine, 5-HT) and its precursor, 5-hydroxytryptophan (5-HTP) as well as hypothalamic TPH-1 and TPH-2 mRNA expression and TPH activity were measured in croaker after exposure to hypoxia and treatment with pharmacological agents. Multiple injections of *N*-ethylmaleimide, a sulfhydryl alkylating agent, caused comparable decreases in hypothalamic TPHs functions and 5-HT contents to that induced by hypoxia exposure (dissolved oxygen: 1.7 mg/L for 4 weeks) which were partially restored by repeated injections with a nitric oxide synthase (NOS)-inhibitor and/or vitamin E. Double-labeled immunohistochemical results showed that TPHs and 5-HT neurons were co-expressed with neuronal NOS (nNOS, a neuroenzyme) that catalyzes the production of nitric oxide, a free radical, in hypothalamic neurons. These results suggest that hypoxia-induced impairment of TPH and serotonergic functions are mediated by nNOS and involve the generation of free radicals and a decrease in the antioxidant status. This study provides, to our knowledge, the first evidence of a protective role for an antioxidant in maintaining neural TPHs functions and 5-HT regulation in an aquatic vertebrate during hypoxic stress.

Keywords: neuroenzyme, neurotransmitter, antioxidant, fish, brain, hypoxia

INTRODUCTION

The brains of vertebrates are particularly susceptible to decreases in oxygen levels (Lahiri et al., 2006). A deficiency of oxygen and/or antioxidant status often results in neural dysfunction in vertebrates (Zingg and Azzi, 2004; Lahiri et al., 2006; Traber and Stevens, 2011). Impairment of neural functions often occurs when aquatic vertebrates, particularly fish, are frequently exposed to low oxygen conditions in their environment (Thomas and Rahman, 2009; Wu, 2009). The neurons that synthesize the neurotransmitter serotonin (5-HT) appear to be especially sensitive to low oxygen levels. Tryptophan hydroxylase (TPH) is the rate-limiting enzyme in 5-HT synthesis and minor changes in TPH activity can cause drastic changes in 5-HT content and serotonergic functions. TPH is an oxygen-liable neuroenzyme, and maintenance of adequate oxygen levels is essential for maintaining its enzymatic activity (Kuhn et al., 1980). Therefore, the extreme sensitivity of serotonergic functions to alterations in neuronal levels of oxygen are largely due to this requirement of TPH (Roberts and Fitzpatrick, 2013). The serotonergic system in teleosts differs from that in mammals because the 5-HT neurons controlling reproductive neuroendocrine functions are mainly localized in the hypothalamic region, separate from those controlling other neuronal functions of 5-HT in the CNS (Jacobs and Azmitia, 1992; Khan and Thomas, 1993; Mohammad-Zadeh and Gwaltney-Brant, 2008). Thus, the teleost hypothalamus is an excellent vertebrate model for examining the effects of hypoxia on serotonergic functions specifically controlling reproductive neuroendocrine functions and the molecular mechanisms involved.

Hypoxia (dissolved oxygen concentration <2.0 mg/L defined as hypoxia, Diaz and Rosenberg, 2008) is a severe environmental stress that has pronounced effects on reproduction by impairing gonadal development and gonadotropin secretion from the pituitary (Thomas et al., 2007; Wu, 2009; Thomas and Rahman, 2012). Hypoxia also disrupts brain functions by decreasing neuropeptide and neurotransmitter levels and neuroenzyme activities (Hedner and Lundborg, 1979; Thomas et al., 2007; Wu, 2009; Gilany and Vafakhah, 2010; Kumar, 2011). In recent *in vivo* studies, we have shown that hypoxia markedly decreases TPHs (TPH isoforms: TPH-1 and TPH-2) immunoreactive (IR) neuronal expression, mRNA and protein levels, and TPH activity

Abbreviations: TPH, tryptophan hydroxylase; 5-HT, 5-hydroxytryptamine; 5-HTP, 5-hydroxytryptophan; NOS, nitric oxide synthase; NO, nitric oxide; ROS, reactive oxygen species; RNS, reactive nitrogen species; DO, dissolved oxygen; IR, immunoreactive; REA, radioenzymatic assay; HPLC, high-performance liquid chromatography; NEM, *N*-ethylmaleimide, NAME, *Nω*-nitro-L-arginine methyl ester; Vit E, vitamin E; AOX, antioxidant.

in the hypothalamus of Atlantic croaker, a relatively hypoxia-tolerant marine fish (Rahman and Thomas, 2009). We have also shown that these declines in TPH expression are accompanied by decreases in hypothalamic 5-hydroxytryptophan (5-HTP, an immediate precursor of 5-HT) and 5-HT contents, and gonadotropin-releasing hormone-I (GnRH-I) mRNA levels in croaker hypothalamus (Thomas et al., 2007; Rahman et al., 2011). These hypoxia-induced neuroendocrine dysfunctions also lead to decreased pituitary luteinizing hormone secretion and plasma sex steroid hormone levels, resulting in impairment of gonadal development and reproductive success in croaker and other teleost fishes (Thomas et al., 2007; Wu, 2009). Experimental *in vivo* studies in tetrapods have also shown that hypoxia decreases TPH activity and 5-HT contents in neonatal and adult rat brains (Davis et al., 1973; Hedner and Lundborg, 1979; Poncet et al., 1997). Collectively, these studies indicate that serotonergic transmission in vertebrates is extremely susceptible to disturbance by hypoxia.

Antioxidants such as vitamin A, C, and E, are essential nutrients necessary for optimal growth, development, and reproduction in animals (Evans and Bishop, 1922; Traber and Stevens, 2011). Among them, vitamin E (Vit E) is a potent antioxidant which regulates neuronal function(s) and maintains cellular integrity (Muller, 2010). Vit E also plays an important role in cell signaling (Azzi, 2007). Mounting evidence has also accumulated that Vit E exerts protective effects against oxidative stress and prevents the propagation of reactive oxygen species (ROS, such as superoxide anion, O_2^-; hydroxyl radical, OH·) and reactive nitrogen species (RNS, such as nitric oxide, NO; peroxynitrate, $ONOO^-$) (Chow, 1991; Chow et al., 1999; Traber and Stevens, 2011). Numerous studies have reported that hypoxia increases cellular O_2^- and NO levels which induce oxidative stress, leading to increased neuronal apoptosis and necrosis (Cazevieille et al., 1993; Tagami et al., 1998; Yamagata et al., 2010). Subsequently, overproduced of O_2^- and NO rapidly react with each other to generate $ONOO^-$, a highly reactive molecule, which attacks neurons, cells, and tissues as well as depleting antioxidant enzymes activities (Freidovich, 1999; Kelm, 1999; Lièvre et al., 2000). Several lines of evidence indicate that NO and $ONOO^-$ directly inactivate the enzymatic activity of TPH and exposure of this enzyme to oxidizing conditions rapidly destroys its catalytic function (Kuhn and Arthur, 1996, 1997a,b; Kuhn and Geddes, 1999, 2000). Therefore, we hypothesize that under hypoxic conditions when large amounts and varieties of radicals are produced, administration of Vit E may restore TPH activity as well as serotonergic functions in the vertebrate brain.

The aims of the present study were to investigate whether treatment with Vit E reverses the inhibitory effects of hypoxia on TPH levels and TPH activity and 5-HT content in the hypothalamic tissues of Atlantic croaker. We investigated the role of nitric oxide synthase (NOS, an enzyme) in the hypoxia-induced effects on hypothalamic serotonergic function by investigating whether TPH and 5-HT expression could be restored by systemic administration of a NOS-inhibitor. Finally, to evaluate the potential role of alterations sulfhydryl (SH) groups on TPH in hypoxia impairment of serotonergic functions, we tested whether the hypoxia effects are mimicked by treatment with a SH alkylating agent.

MATERIALS AND METHODS

CHEMICALS

L-[5-^{3}H]-tryptophan citation (27 Ci/mmol) and 5-hydroxy tryptamine (5-HT, serotonin) were purchased from Amersham Biosciences (Piscataway, NJ) and Sigma-Aldrich (St. Louis, MO), respectively. Rabbit polyclonal anti-TPH-1 and -TPH-2 antibodies and TPHs peptides were generous gifts from Dr. Donald M. Kuhn, Wayne State University School of Medicine, Detroit, MI and the specificity of both antibodies has been demonstrated previously (Sakowski et al., 2006). Commercially available antibodies, rabbit anti-5-HT, goat polyclonal to rabbit IgG (HRP), and rabbit anti-actin were purchased from ImmunoStar (Hudson, WI), SouthernBiotech (Birmingham, AL), and Novus Biologicals (Littleton, CO), respectively. Materials for molecular biology were obtained from Agilent Technologies (La Jolla, CA), Promega (Madison, WI), and Invitrogen (Carlsbad, CA). All other chemicals were purchased from Sigma-Aldrich and Fisher Scientific (Pittsburgh, PA).

EXPERIMENTAL FISH

Juvenile (year 1) Atlantic croaker, *Micropogonias undulatus* (10–11 cm length; 25–35 g body weight, BW), were purchased from local bait shops during the summer and transported to fish holding facilities at the University of Texas Marine Science Institute, Port Aransas, Texas. Fish were treated with Paracide-F (Argent Chemical, Redmond, WA) at 170 ppm in seawater to minimize parasite infections and transferred to large indoor recirculating seawater tanks (5000 L) and maintained under ambient temperature (22–23°C) and photoperiod (13D:11L) for 3 months by which time they had become sexually mature. Chopped shrimp were fed to the fish once a day (3% BW/day).

EXPERIMENT: EFFECTS OF HYPOXIA AND PHARMACOLOGICAL AGENTS ON TPH AND 5-HT REGULATION

Sexually mature croakers were stocked into 12 tanks (30 mixed-sex fish/tank) with a recirculating seawater system (capacity 2025 l, including biological filter) under constant temperature/photoperiod conditions (22 ± 1°C, 13D:11L) for 1 month prior to experimentation. The hypoxia experimental setup used in this study has been described previously (Rahman and Thomas, 2009). Briefly, six tanks were maintained under normoxic conditions (dissolved oxygen, DO: 6.5 mg/L) and the other six tanks were assigned hypoxia treatments (1.7 mg DO/L). The DO levels in the hypoxia exposure tanks were lowered by reducing the aeration gradually with air regulators and adjusted until the DO level reached 1.7 mg/L which was achieved within 2 days. DO, pH, and temperature levels were measured with a YSI multiprobe meter (YSI 556 Multiprobe System, YSI Incorporated, Yellow Springs, OH) three times a day in the morning, afternoon and night. Ammonia and nitrite levels were monitored using Hach kits (HACH, Loveland, CO) three times a week. There were no major changes of the physio-chemical parameters (pH 7.7–7.9, ammonia 0.1–0.2 mg/L, and nitrite 0.01–0.02 mg/L) during the experimental periods.

Fish were anesthetized with quinaldine sulfate (20 mg/L), rapidly weighed and received intraperitoneal (i.p.) injections with vehicle, *N*-ethylmaleimide (NEM, a chemical which covalently modifies sulfhydryl groups in the reactive center of enzymes), $N\omega$-nitro-L-arginine methyl ester (NAME, an inhibitor of nitric oxide synthase), or vitamin E (α-tocopherol, an antioxidant) every 4 days for 4 weeks (6 i.p. injections of 1 μg NEM, 1 μg NAME, or 1 μg Vit E/g BW). At the end of the experiments, the fish were sacrificed under deep anesthesia using quinaldine sulfate (20 mg/L), following guidelines and ethical rules approved by the University of Texas at Austin Animal Care and Use Committee (IACUC, protocol# 09022701). Brain tissues were quickly excised, frozen in liquid nitrogen and stored at −80°C. Hypothalamic tissues were excised from frozen brain samples with the aid of a croaker brain atlas (Khan and Thomas, 1993) for RNA extraction, protein determination, and neurotransmitter measurement. For radioenzymatic assay, hypothalamic tissue samples were separated from fresh brain samples. For immunohistochemical detection, whole brains were fixed in ice cold paraformaldehyde solution.

SINGLE- AND DOUBLE-IMMUNOFLUORESCENCE STAINING OF TPHs AND 5-HT NEURONS

Details the single-immufluorescence staining methods were used in this study have been described previously (Rahman and Thomas, 2009, 2013). Briefly, whole brains were stored in paraformaldehyde solution (4% paraformaldehyde in 0.01 M phosphate-buffered saline, PBS, pH 7.4) overnight at 4°C. The following day, brains were dehydrated in a series of ethanol solutions, embedded in paraffin (Paraplast, Sigma-Aldrich), and sectioned at 10 μm on a rotary microtome in transverse and sagittal planes. Sections were mounted on superfrost plus slides (Fisher Scientific), deparaffinized in xylene, dehydrated in a series of ethanol solutions, and rinsed with PBS. Endogenous peroxidase activity was blocked with 5% H_2O_2 for 10 min at room temperature. Sections were treated in retrieval solution (1 mM Tris, pH 9.0, with 0.5 mM EGTA) for 10 min to facilitate the immunoreactions. Nonspecific binding was prevented by blocking in PBS containing 1% BSA. The immunofluorescent signals of TPHs and 5-HT neurons in croaker hypothalamus were amplified by tyramide signal amplification solution (Molecular Probes, Eugene, OR) using a signal-labeling technique. Sections were incubated with TPH-1, TPH-2, or 5-HT antibodies at a dilution of 1:100 overnight at 4°C. For peptide block controls, each antigenic TPHs peptide was diluted in blocking buffer (400 ng/ml) containing it's respective antibody (dilution: 1:100) and preabsorbed overnight at 4°C. The fluorescence signal was amplified by adding Alexa Fluor 594 or Alexa Fluor 488 goat anti-rabbit secondary antibodies (dilution 1:500, Invitrogen) and incubating for 1 h in the dark. The sections were rinsed three times in PBS and mounted with Prolong Gold antifade reagent (Invitrogen). The presence of the fluorescent-labeled TPH-1, TPH-2 and 5-HT neurons was examined using a Nikon Eclipse E600 microscope (Nikon, Japan) with fluorescein red and green filters. The image was captured by CoolSNAP camera (Photometrics, Tucson, AZ), and the intensity of each neuron was quantified by NIH ImageJ analysis software (http://rsb.info.nih.gov/ij/), a computer-assisted scientific image processing program (Schneider et al., 2012), according to Collins (2007).

A double-immunofluorescence method described by Kroeber et al. (1998) which employs two primary antibodies raised in the same species was used with minor modifications to detect neuronal NOS (nNOS) and TPHs or 5-HT in the same neurons. Briefly, rabbit polyclonal anti-nNOS antibody (SC-1025, Santa Cruz, CA) was purified by Melon Gel IgG purification column (catalog# 45206, Thermo Fisher Scientific, Rockford, IL). The IgG purified antibody was then directly labeled with DyLight-488 antibody (catalog# 53024, Thermo Scientific) according to the manufacturer's protocol. Sections were incubated with unlabeled rabbit TPH-1, TPH-2, or 5-HT primary antibodies (1:100) overnight at 4°C, rinsed three times with PBS and incubated with fluorescent Rhodamine Red-X conjugated goat anti-rabbit secondary antibody (1:500; Jackson Immunoresearch, West Grove, PA) for 1 h in the dark. Sections were rinsed with PBS, and incubated with 5% normal rabbit serum in PBS-T (PBS with 0.3% TritonX-100) to occupy any free binding site for rabbit antibody remaining on the secondary antibody. Sections were then blocked with blocking solution (3% normal goat serum and 0.3% TritonX-100 in PBS) for 1 h at room temperature, rinsed three times with PBS, and incubated with anti-nNOS-DyLight 488 labeled-antibody (1:500) at 4°C overnight in a humidified chamber the dark. Sections were then rinsed three times in PBS and mounted in Fluoromount-G solution (a non-fluorescing solution, SouthernBiotech). The presence of the double-labeled immunofluorescence signal was visualized using a confocal microscope (Nikon Eclipse C2, Nikon, Japan).

WESTERN BLOT ANALYSIS OF TPHs PROTEINS

TPH-1 and -2 protein levels in hypothalamic tissues were determined by Western blot analysis as described previously (Rahman and Thomas, 2009). Briefly, a protease inhibitor cocktail was added to the homogenization buffer (HEPES buffer containing 25 mM HEPES, 10 mM NaCl, 1 mM EDTA, 1 mM dithioerythritol, pH 7.6) to prevent degradation of TPH proteins during homogenization. The tissue homogenate were centrifuged at 10,000 ×g for 15 min at 4°C and the supernatant was used for Western blot analysis. The proteins were solubilized by boiling in SDS loading buffer (0.5 M Tris-HCl, 0.5% Bromophenol Blue, 10% glycerol) and cooled on ice for 5 min. The solubilized protein was resolved on a 10% SDS-PAGE gel, transferred onto a immuno-blot polyvinyl difluoride membrane (PVDF membrane, Bio-Rad, Hercules, CA) and blocked with 5% nonfat milk in TBS-T buffer (50 mM Tris, 100 mM NaCl, 0.1% Tween 20, pH 7.4) for 1 h. Membranes were rinsed with TBS-T buffer and probed with primary rabbit anti-TPHs (dilution: 1:1000) or anti-actin (1:10,000; Novus Biologicals) antibodies overnight at 4°C. Membranes were then washed with TBS-T, and incubated for 2 h with a goat polyclonal to rabbit IgG (HRP) secondary antibody (1: 4000; SouthernBiotech). The protein was visualized by the addition of chemiluminescent substrate (Pierce, Rockford, IL) and photographed on Hyperfilm (Amersham Biosciences). The intensities of TPHs and actin protein bands were estimated by ImageJ software to quantify the relative TPHs protein expression.

QUANTITATIVE REAL-TIME PCR (qRT-PCR) ANALYSIS OF TPH mRNAs

To determine the expression of TPH-1 and TPH-2 mRNAs in croaker hypothalamic, qRT-PCR analyses were performed on total RNA using a one step SYBR Green qRT-PCR method

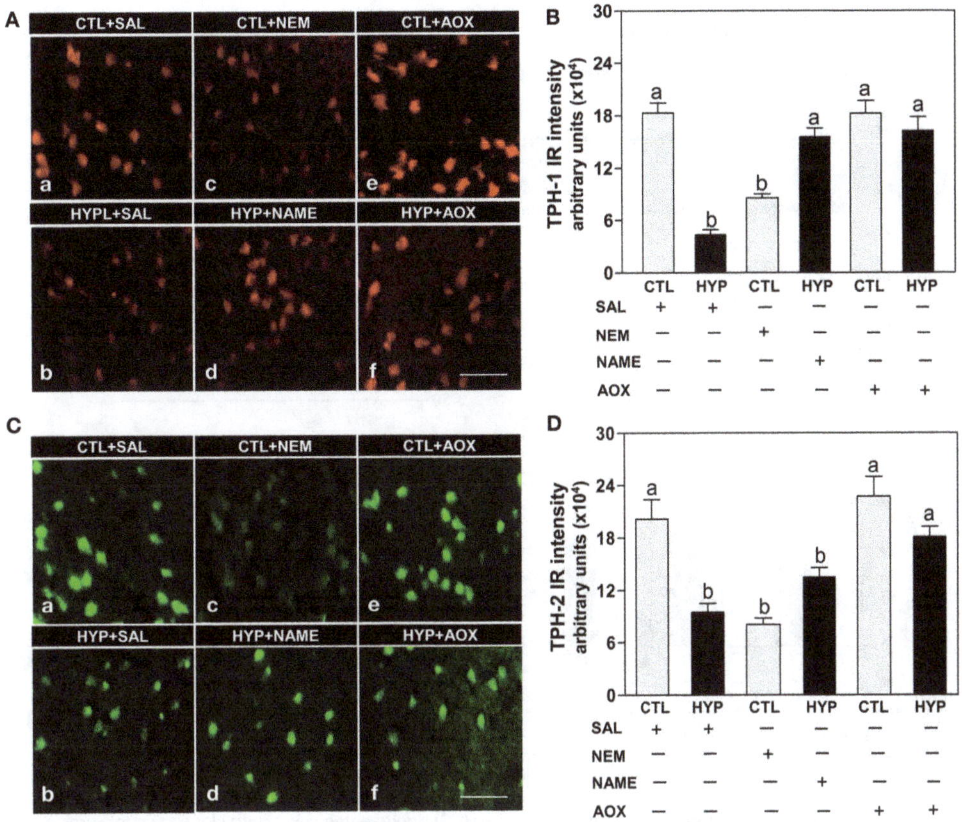

FIGURE 1 | Interactive effects of hypoxia and pharmacological agents that modulate generation of reactive oxygen and nitrogen species (ROS and RNS) on expression of TPHs proteins in croaker hypothalamic neurons assessed by immunohistochemistry. Effects of hypoxia (dissolved oxygen, DO: 1.7 mg/L for 4 weeks; note: here and in subsequent figures exposure duration only refers to period fish were exposed to target DO; fish were previously exposed to declining DO for additional 2-day adjustment period) exposure and pharmacological treatments with *N*-ethylmaleimide (NEM, a chemical which covalently modifies sulfhydryl groups in the reactive center of enzymes), *N*ω-nitro-L-arginine methyl ester (NAME, an inhibitor of nitric oxide synthase) and vitamin E (an antioxidant, AOX) on immunohistochemical (IHC) expression and immunoreactive (IR) intensity of TPH-1 **(A,B)** and TPH-2 **(C,D)** neurons in croaker hypothalamus. **(A,C)** Representative IHC micrographs of TPHs neurons in hypothalamic sections from fish after the various treatments. Scale bar = 20 μm. **(B,D)** IR staining intensity of the fluorescent-labeled TPHs neurons assayed by fluorescein filter with Nikon Eclipse microscope, and the IR staining intensity of each neuron estimated by ImageJ software (http://rsb.info.nih.gov/ij/) according to Collins (2007). Each value represents the mean ±s.e.m. ($N = 25$–33 neurons). Significant differences as compared to control (CTL) identified with a multiple range test, Fisher's PLSD, are indicated with different letters ($P < 0.05$). SAL, saline; CTL, control; HYP, hypoxia.

as described previously (Rahman and Thomas, 2012, 2013). Briefly, RNA was extracted from hypothalamic tissues using TRI reagent (Sigma-Aldrich) and treated with DNase (Promega) to prevent genomic DNA contamination. Afterwards the RNA was quantified with a NanoDrop 2000C (Thermo Fisher Scientific) and stored at −80°C until use. qRT-PCR analyses were performed using a Brilliant II SYBR Green QRT-PCR master mix kit (Agilent Technologies, La Jolla, CA) in a 25 μl reaction mixture containing 12.5 μl of 2× SYBR-QRT-PCR master mix, 1 μl of RT/RNase block enzyme mixture, 125 nM of each primer, and 2.5 ng of total RNA. The gene-specific primers used for amplification of croaker TPHs mRNA were as follows: TPH-1 (forward: 5′-GAAGACGTGGGGAGTT GTGT-3′ and reverse: 5′-ACAGTGGAAAACACGGAAGG-3′; GenBank accession number EU730759) and TPH-2 (forward: 5′-ATGTTTGACCCGAAGACGAC-3′ and reverse: 5′-GTGTTCATC TTCCCCAGAGC-3′ primers; EU730760). The thermocycler conditions for amplification were 50°C for 30 min, 95°C for 10 min, and 40 cycles of 95°C for 30 s, 55°C for 1 min and 72°C for 30 s. Dissociation curve analyses were performed immediately after the amplification cycles at 95°C for 15 min, 50°C for 15 s. Each transcript level was normalized on the basis of the amplification of croaker 18S rRNA (primers: forward 5′-AGAAACGGCTACCACATCCA-3′ and reverse 5′-TCCCGAGATCCAACTACGAG-3′; AY866435). The mean of threshold cycle (C*t*) was used for the analysis and the relative expression levels of croaker TPHs mRNA against 18S rRNA were calculated using the $2^{-\Delta\Delta Ct}$ method (Livak and Schmittgen, 2001).

RADIOENZYMATIC ASSAY (REA) OF TPH ACTIVITY

TPH activity was measured by REA (Vrana et al., 1993) using [^{3}H]-tryptophan tracer and validated for croaker brain as described previously (Khan and Thomas, 2001; Rahman and Thomas, 2009, 2013). Briefly, hypothalamic tissues were sonicated in HEPES buffer (pH 7.6). Twenty five μl of tissue

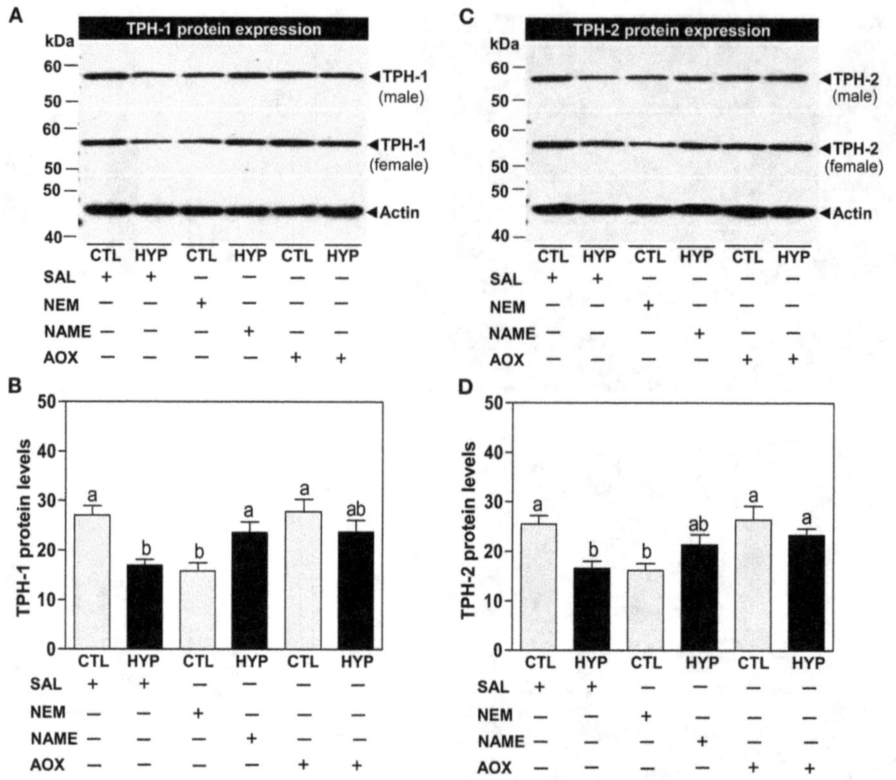

FIGURE 2 | Interactive effects of hypoxia and pharmacological agents that modulate generation of ROS and RNS on TPHs protein expression determined by Western blot analysis in croaker hypothalamus. Effects of hypoxia (DO: 1.7 mg/L for 4 weeks) exposure and pharmacological treatments with NEM, NAME, and AOX on immunoreactive (IR) expression and IR intensity of TPH-1 **(A,B)** and TPH-2 **(C,D)** protein in croaker hypothalamus. **(A,C)** Representative Western blot shown for samples from individual male and female fish after the various treatments. **(B,D)** IR protein intensity estimated by ImageJ software. Each bar represents mean ±s.e.m. ($N = 8$, results from both sexes were combined because they were not significantly different). Fisher's PLSD, are indicated with different letters ($P < 0.05$). SAL, saline; CTL, control; HYP, hypoxia.

homogenate was added to 25 μl of reaction mixture containing 0.05 mM tryptophan, 50 mM HEPES (pH 7.6), 5 mM DTT, 0.01 mM $Fe(NH_4)_2(SO_4)_2$, 0.5 mM 6-MPH_4, 0.1 mg/ml catalase, and 1 μCi L-[5-^{3}H]-tryptophan. The reaction mixture was incubated at 25°C for 20 min in a water bath and stopped by addition of 500 μl of ice-cold 7.5% charcoal in 1 M HCl. The reaction mixture was centrifuged at 14,000 ×*g* for 2 min and the supernatant (200 μl) was added to 3 ml of CytoScint scintillation cocktail (MP Biomedicals, Irvine, CA). The radioactivity was measured by a liquid scintillation counter (Beckman LS 6000SC, Beckman Instruments, Fullerton, CA). The radioactivity derived from each assay was normalized to total protein present in the homogenate as determined by Bradford protein assay. Each assay was done in duplicate and the mean value was expressed as nmol tryptophan converted/mg protein/h.

HIGH-PERFORMANCE LIQUID CHROMATOGRAPHY (HPLC) WITH ELECTROCHEMICAL DETECTION ANALYSIS OF 5-HT AND 5-HTP CONTENTS

5-HTP and 5-HT concentrations in hypothalamic tissues were determined by reversed-phase HPLC with an electrochemical detection citation(Waters 464 Electrochemical Detector and Breeze Software, Milford, MA) system (Saligaut et al., 1986) according to Khan and Thomas (1997) with minor modifications. Briefly, the frozen hypothalamic tissue samples were sonicated in 0.5 ml of ice-cold perchloric acid (0.2 M) containing 0.1% cysteine, 0.05% sodium bisulfite, and 0.05% EDTA, and centrifuged at 2500 ×*g* for 10 min. The supernatant was filtered through a 0.22 μm Millex-GV filter and immediately injected (50 μl) into the HPLC apparatus. The chromatographic separations were performed by C18 reverse phase column (4.6 × 150 mm, Waters) using a mobile phase buffer (0.3 M acetic acid, 0.08 M ammonium hydroxide, 0.1 mM EDTA, and 75% methanol) at a flow-rate of 1 ml/min at room temperature. The peaks of 5-HTP and 5-HT were identified by comparing the retention times with those of 5-HTP and 5-HT standards, and the concentrations were calculated from the areas under the peaks. 5-HTP and 5-HT contents were normalized to total protein present in the homogenate as determined by Bradford protein assay and expressed as ng/mg protein.

STATISTICAL ANALYSES

All of the experimental results were analyzed by One-Way ANOVA followed by Fisher's protected least-significant difference test for multiple comparisons. A *P*-value of less than 0.05 was considered statistically significant. Analyses were performed using Statview (SAS Instituite Inc., Cary, NC) and GraphPad Prism (GraphPad, San Diego, CA) computer software. Data are expressed as mean ± standard error of the mean (s.e.m).

RESULTS

The specificities of the TPHs antibodies for immunohistochemistry (IHC) detection were confirmed by blocking them with specific TPHs peptide antigens (Supplementary Figure 1). Western blot analyses confirmed the presence of immunoreactive (IR) bands of TPHs proteins of the predicted size around 55–56 kDa as shown previously in croaker hypothalamus (Rahman and Thomas, 2009).

Immunohistochemical results showed strong expression and high intensity of TPH-1 immunoreactive (IR) neurons in hypothalami of fish exposed to normoxic control conditions, whereas weak expression and low intensity of TPH-1 IR neurons were observed in hypoxia-exposed (1.7 mg DO/L for 4 weeks) saline-injected control fish (**Figures 1Aa,b,B**). Administration of the sulfhydryl modifying agent, NEM (1 μg/g BW/4 days for 4 weeks), markedly reduced TPH-1 neuronal expression and intensity compared to normoxic saline controls (**Figures 1Ac,B**), whereas treatments with the NOS-inhibitor, NAME, or the antioxidant, vitamin E (1 μg NAME or 1 μg Vit E/g BW/4 days for 4 weeks), restored the hypoxia down-regulation of TPH-1 neuronal expression and intensity (**Figures 1Ad,f,B**). A similar pattern of treatment effects were observed in TPH-2 neurons in croaker hypothalami (**Figures 1C,D**).

Immunoblot results showed that the expression of TPH-1 IR signal was significantly reduced (~37%) in hypoxia-exposed fish compared with controls following normalization to actin protein (**Figures 2A,B**). Treatment with NEM for 4 weeks caused similar decreases in TPH-1 protein expression and levels to those observed after hypoxia exposure, whereas treatments with NAME or Vit E restored TPH-1 protein levels in hypoxia-exposed fish (**Figures 2A,B**). Similar to the TPH-1 IR signal, hypothalamic TPH-2 protein expression and levels were restored after treatments with NAME or vitamin E in hypoxia-exposed fish (**Figures 2C,D**).

Quantitative real-time PCR (qRT-PCR) showed that exposure to hypoxia and treatment with NEM caused comparable decreases in hypothalamic TPH-1 (**Figure 3A**) and TPH-2 (**Figure 3B**) mRNA levels compared to normoxic saline controls, whereas treatments with NAME or Vit E completely and partially restored TPH-1 (**Figure 3A**) and TPH-2 (**Figure 3B**) mRNA levels, respectively, in hypoxia-exposed fish.

The TPH radioenzymatic assay results showed a dramatic decrease (~56%) in hypothalamic TPH activity in hypoxia-exposed fish compared with normoxic saline controls (**Figure 4**). TPH activity was also significantly decreased by treatment with NEM to a level similar to that observed in the hypoxia-exposed fish, whereas TPH activity was markedly restored (~70% for NAME and ~75% for Vit E treatments) in hypoxia-exposed fish by treatment with NAME or Vit E (**Figure 4**).

Immunohistochemical results showed weak expression and low intensity of 5-HT IR in hypothalamic neurons of fish exposed to hypoxia or treatment with NEM compared to normoxic saline controls (**Figures 5Aa-c,B**), whereas NAME or Vit E treatments partially restored 5-HT IR neuronal expression and intensity in hypoxia-exposed fish (**Figures 5A,d,f,B**).

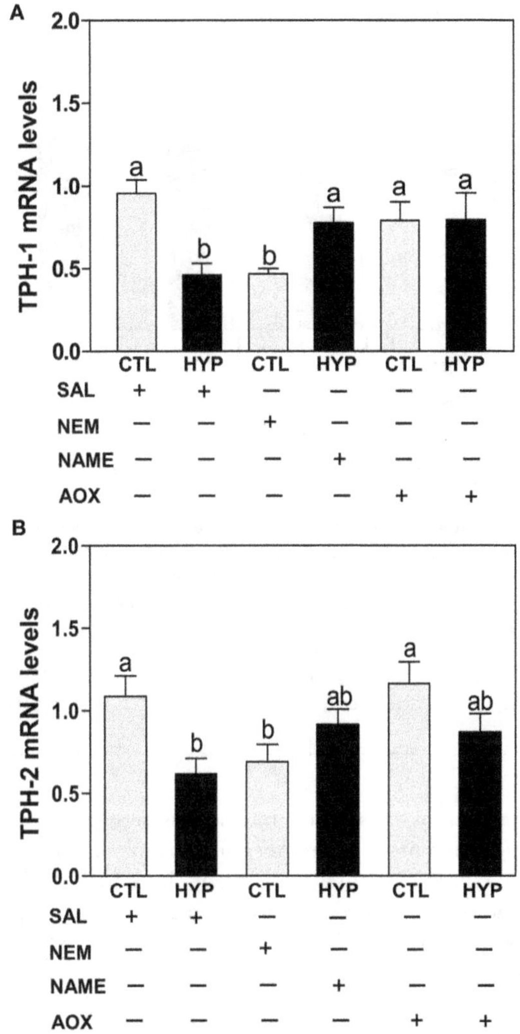

FIGURE 3 | Interactive effects of hypoxia and pharmacological agents that modulate generation of ROS and RNS on TPHs mRNA expression determined by quantitative real-time PCR in croaker hypothalamus. Effects of hypoxia (DO: 1.7 mg/L for 4 weeks) exposure and pharmacological treatments with NEM, NAME, and AOX on expression of TPH-1 **(A)** and TPH-2 **(B)** mRNA levels in croaker hypothalamus. Each bar represents mean ±s.e.m. ($N = 9$–12, results from both sexes were combined because they were not significantly different). Fisher's PLSD, are indicated with different letters ($P < 0.05$). SAL, saline; CTL, control; HYP, hypoxia.

The HPLC results show exposure to hypoxia significantly decreased 5-HTP and 5-HT contents in hypothalamic tissues compared to normoxic saline controls (**Figures 6Aa,b,B,C**). Injection with NEM caused a moderate decrease in 5-HTP content in normoxic fish (**Figures 6Ac,B**), whereas NEM treatment caused a marked decrease 5-HT content similar to that observed in hypoxia-exposed fish (**Figures 6Ac,C**). The hypoxia-induced decreases in 5-HTP and 5-HT contents were restored by treatments with NAME or Vit E in hypoxia-exposed fish (**Figures 6Ad,f,B,C**).

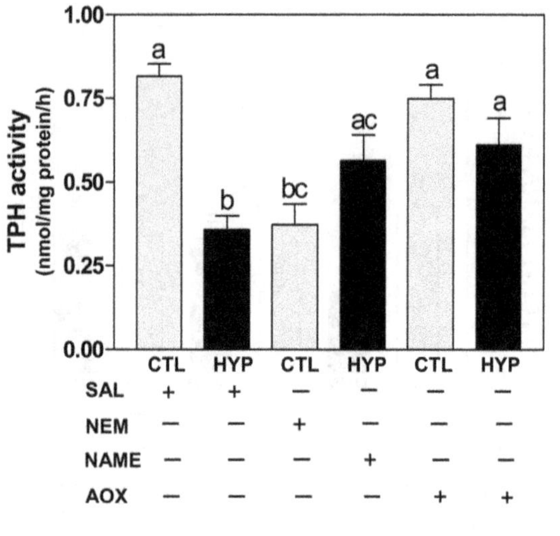

FIGURE 4 | Interactive effects of hypoxia and pharmacological agents that modulate generation of ROS and RNS on TPH activity determined by radioenzymatic assay in croaker hypothalamus. Effects of hypoxia (DO: 1.7 mg/L for 4 weeks) exposure and pharmacological treatments with NEM, NAME, and AOX on TPH activity in croaker hypothalamus. Each bar represents mean ±s.e.m. ($N = 6$–8, results from both sexes were combined because they were not significantly different). Fisher's PLSD, are indicated with different letters ($P < 0.05$). SAL, saline; CTL, control; HYP, hypoxia.

An anatomical basis for the interactions between TPHs or 5-HT neurons and nNOS in croaker hypothalamic was investigated by double-immunofluorescence assay. Immunohistochemical results showed that TPH-1, TPH-2, and 5-HT are co-expressed with nNOS in neurons in croaker hypothalami as seen in the merged images (**Figure 7A**).

DISCUSSION

In this report, several potential components of the mechanism by which hypoxia down-regulates TPHs (TPH-1 and TPH-2) and 5-HT functions in the Atlantic croaker hypothalamus were identified. The observation that repeated injections with vitamin E (Vit E) substantially restored hypothalamic TPHs expression and 5-HT concentrations suggests that increasing the antioxidant status can prevent hypoxia-induced down-regulation of the serotonergic system. In addition, the finding that systemic administration of NOS-inhibitor, NAME, partially reversed the hypoxia down-regulation of TPHs and 5-HT neuronal expression suggests that the hypoxia effects on the serotonergic system are mediated through the enzyme, nNOS. Moreover, the demonstration that TPH and nNOS proteins are co-localized in croaker hypothalamic neurons provides the neuroanotomical basis for close interactions between these two enzymes. Reactive oxygen and nitrogen species (ROS and RNS) are common denominators in all these studies because they are generated during hypoxia and through nNOS and the antioxidant Vit E can block their generation. On the basis of these results we propose that hypoxia causes down-regulation of TPH mRNA expression through the generation of ROS and RNS resulting in reduced TPH protein synthesis and activity and declines in 5-HT levels and neuroendocrine functions (**Figure 7B**). The mechanism(s) by which ROS and RNS alter TPH mRNA expression remains unclear but may involve upregulation of hypoxia-inducible factor-α (HIF-α, an oxygen-sensitive transcription factor) and down-regulation of aromatase (Rahman et al., 2011; Rahman and Thomas, 2013). To our knowledge, this is the first evidence that NOS activity and antioxidant status influence neuronal TPH and 5-HT functions in aquatic vertebrates during hypoxic stress.

The present results showing administration of NAME, an inhibitor of NOS partially restored TPHs (TPH-1 and TPH-2) neuronal, protein and mRNA expressions, TPH activity and 5-HT concentrations in the hypothalamus clearly implicate nNOS activity and nitric oxide (NO) generation as intermediaries in these hypoxia-induced effects. In agreement with these findings, *in vivo* administration of NO inhibitors has been shown to increase neuronal contents of TPH and 5-HT in rat raphe nuclei and 5-HT release from the hippocampus and hypothalamus under normoxic conditions (Kaehler et al., 1999; Wegener et al., 2000; Park et al., 2004). Conversely, administration of *S*-nitroso-*N*-acetypenicillamine (SNAP, a NO-donor) markedly decreases 5-HT contents in the hypothalamus, frontal cortex and raphe nuclei of rat brains under normoxic conditions (Kaehler et al., 1999; Smith and Whitton, 2000), suggesting that expression of both TPH and 5-HT are down-regulated by NO. Several mammalian *in vitro* studies have also been shown that hypoxia increases cellular NO levels, and that excess NO interacts with superoxide radical (O_2^-, a potent ROS) to generate peroxynitrite ($ONOO^-$, a highly diffusible RNS; Beckman and Koppenol, 1996) resulting in oxidative damage in a wide array of cells including neurons (Encinas et al., 2003; Maiti et al., 2010). Consistent with these *in vitro* studies, Maulik et al. (1998) and Mishra et al. (2006) demonstrated that hypoxia increases free radicals and nNOS protein levels in guinea pig and piglets brain tissues *in vivo*. We have recently demonstrated that hypoxia markedly increases plasma NO metabolites (NOx, nitrite, and nitrate), NOS mRNA and protein levels in croaker liver and brain tissues (Rahman and Thomas, 2011; Rahman and Thomas, unpublished observation). These results are consistent with the findings of other teleost studies showing that hypoxia significantly increases plasma NOx concentrations and neural NOS mRNA levels in trout (McNeill and Perry, 2006) and protein carbonyl contents, an indirect measure of ROS (Berlett and Stadtman, 1997), in grouper liver (Yu et al., 2008). Taken together these studies in fish and mammals suggest that hypoxia causes elevated NO-free radical production, such as $ONOO^-$ through an increase in NOS activity that can result in inhibition of TPH expression and activity as well as impairment of serotonergic functions (Kuhn and Geddes, 1999, 2000).

Another significant finding in this study is that Vit E, a potent peroxyl radical scavenger (Traber and Atkinson, 2007), treatment fully restored hypothalamic TPHs neuronal, protein and mRNA expressions, and TPH activity in hypothalamus of hypoxia-exposed fish to those observed in normoxic fish. As predicted, Vit E treatment also restored the immunoreactive 5-HT expression in neurons and the contents of 5-HTP and 5-HT in the hypothalami of hypoxia-exposed fish. The results are consistent with those in an *in vivo* study in rats showing that

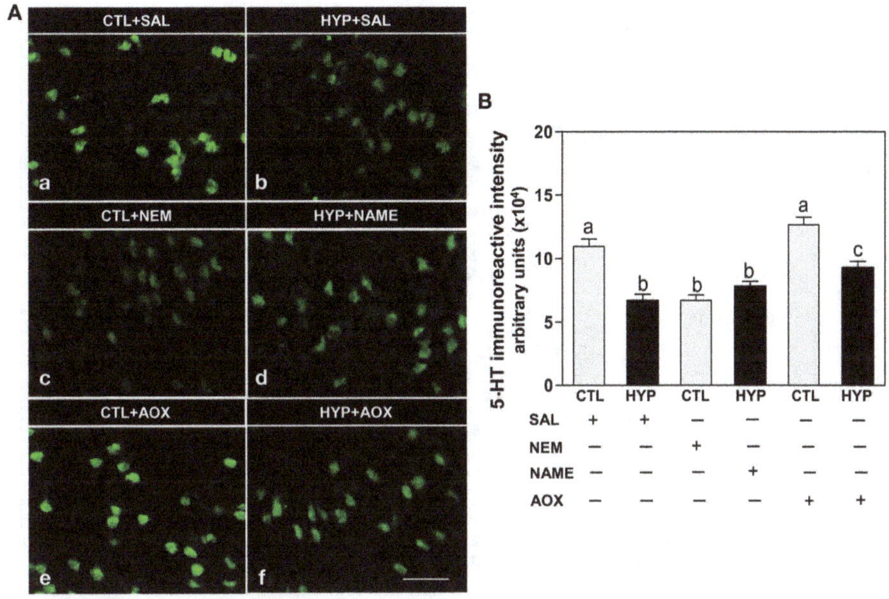

FIGURE 5 | Interactive effects of hypoxia and pharmacological agents that modulate generation of ROS and RNS on 5-HT content in neurons assessed by immunohistochemistry in croaker hypothalamus. Effects of hypoxia (DO: 1.7 mg/L for 4 weeks) exposure and pharmacological treatments with NEM, NAME, and AOX on immunohistochemical (IHC) expression and immunoreactive (IR) intensity of 5-HT neurons in croaker hypothalamus. **(A)** Representative IHC micrographs of 5-HT neurons in hypothalamic sections from fish after the various treatments. Scale bar = 20 μm. **(B)** IR staining intensity of the fluorescent-labeled 5-HT neurons assayed by fluorescein filter with Nikon Eclipse microscope, and the IR staining intensity estimated by ImageJ software. Each value represents the mean ±s.e.m. ($N = 23$–26 neurons). Significant differences as compared to control (CTL) identified with a multiple range test, Fisher's PLSD, are indicated with different letters ($P < 0.05$). SAL, saline; CTL, control; HYP, hypoxia.

hypoxia markedly decreases monoaminergic neurotransmitters such as norepinephrine, dopamine and 5-HT levels in cerebral cortex, hippocampus and striatum, and that the hypoxia-induced decrease in neurotransmitter levels is restored by treatment with Vit E (Yan et al., 2003). Numerous mammalian *in vitro* studies have shown that antioxidants such as Vit C and Vit E decrease cellular oxidative stress and prevent neuronal cell death during hypoxic stress (Chow, 1991; Chow et al., 1999; Yamagata et al., 2010; Traber and Stevens, 2011). Using a primary neuronal culture, Lièvre et al. (2000) showed that Vit E treatment prevents hypoxia-induced apoptosis in rat forebrain neurons. Similarly, Tagami et al. (1998) demonstrated that during exposure to hypoxic conditions, Vit E directly reacts with free radicals to prevent apoptosis in rat cortical neurons. Vit E significantly increases the intracellular antioxidant levels and decreases hydroxyl radical ($OH^{\bullet}$, highly reactive ROS) and lipid peroxidation levels in cultured rat neuronal cells under normoxic conditions (Zhang et al., 2004). Moreover, during hypoxia exposure, Vit E prevents hydrogen peroxide (H_2O_2, a potent ROS) production in cultured human endothelial cells (Martin et al., 1996). We have recently observed that during hypoxia exposure, Vit E attenuates O_2^- production and NOS protein and mRNA levels in croaker liver and brain tissues (Rahman and Thomas, 2011, 2012; Rahman and Thomas, unpublished observation). Importantly, the present results show that the NOS is distinctly co-expressed with TPHs and 5-HT in neurons in croaker hypothalami which is consistent with mammalian studies showing that both TPH and 5-HT neurons are remarkably co-localized with NOS neurons in raphe nuclei (Lopez et al., 2005; Lu et al., 2010). Collectively, our findings together with other tetrapods results suggest that NOS is a mediator of hypoxia-induced down-regulation of TPH and 5-HT function in croaker hypothalamus through it's upregulation of NO production that can be blocked by Vit E.

There are several potential molecular mechanisms of TPH regulation by hypoxia, and by Vit E and ROS or RNS during hypoxia exposure. The available evidence suggests that hypoxia probably down-regulates TPH transcripts through an O_2-dependent mechanism. The O_2-sensitive transcription factor HIF-α, a gene that regulates the expression of numerous genes involved in adaptation to hypoxia (Semenza, 2001; Nikinmaa and Ress, 2005), is likely a key transcriptional regulator of TPH mRNA. Mammalian *in vitro* studies have shown that hypoxia induces cellular ROS levels and that elevated ROS levels leads to increases in HIF-α mRNA and protein levels (Chandel et al., 2000; Pouysségur and Mechta-Grigoriou, 2006). On the contrary, antioxidants prevent hypoxia-induced ROS generation, and HIF-α mRNA and protein accumulation in cultured mammalian cells (Sanjuán-Pla et al., 2005). We have recently shown that hypoxia increases O_2^- generation, HIF-1α mRNA expression, and HIF-2α and endothelial NOS (eNOS) protein levels in croaker liver tissues and treatment with Vit E attenuates all of these hypoxia-induced increases (Rahman and Thomas, 2011, 2012). Vit E is a prototypical scavenger of ROS and RNS, and eliminates the hypoxia-induced activation of HIF-α. Therefore, our results support the idea that the decline of TPHs transcript levels observed during hypoxia exposure could involve the activation of HIF-α that may interact with a

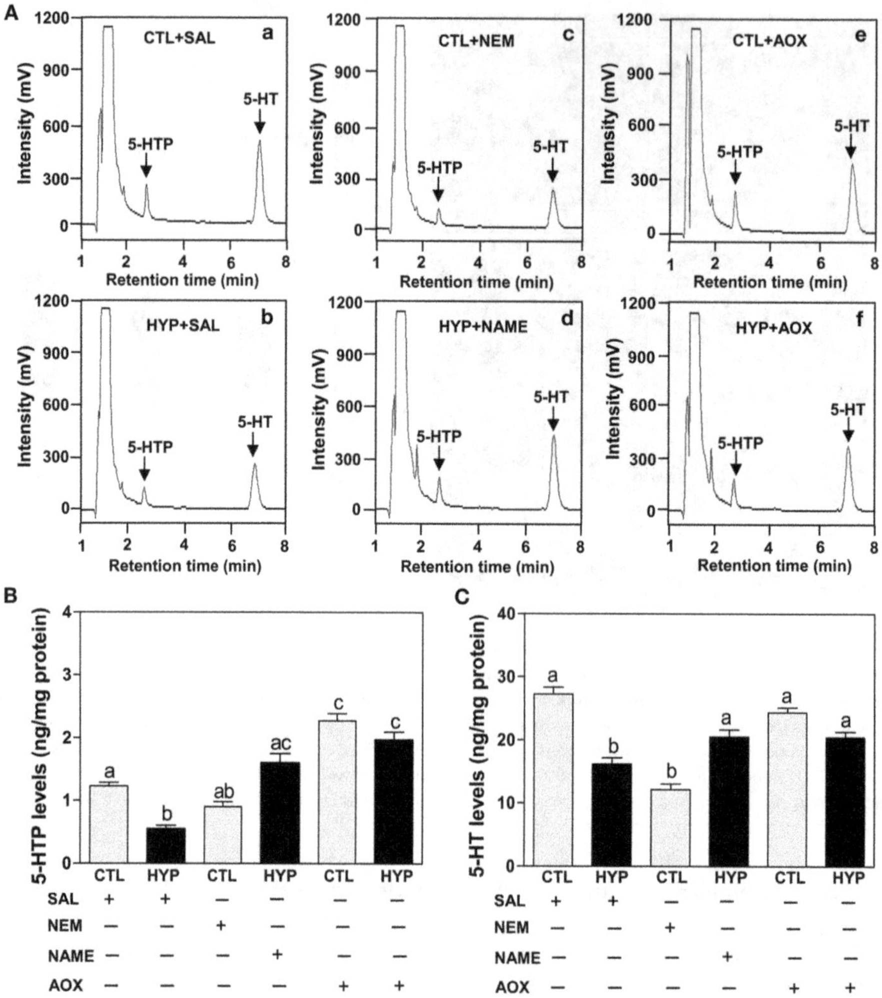

FIGURE 6 | Interactive effects of hypoxia and pharmacological agents that modulate generation of ROS and RNS on 5-HTP and 5-HT levels determined by HPLC in croaker hypothalamus. (A) Reversed-phase HPLC chromatograms of 5-HTP and 5-HT showing that hypothalamic 5-HTP and 5-HT contents from normoxic saline control fish are higher than those in hypoxic (DO: 1.7 mg/L for 4 weeks) and NEM treatment group. **(B,C)** Effects of hypoxia (dissolved oxygen, DO: 1.7 mg/L for 4 weeks) exposure and pharmacological treatments with NEM, NAME, and AOX on 5-HTP **(B)** and 5-HT **(C)** levels in croaker hypothalamus. Each value represents the mean ±s.e.m. ($N = 7$–9, results from both sexes were combined because they were not significantly different). Significant differences identified with a multiple range test, Fisher's PLSD, are indicated with different letters ($P < 0.05$). SAL, saline; CTL, control; HYP, hypoxia.

specific hypoxia-response element in the enhancing region on the TPH promoter causing a decrease in the rate of TPH transcription (Semenza et al., 1996). In addition, the enzymatic activity of TPH may be directly affected by a reduction of O_2concentrations because it uses O_2 as a substrate with the cofactor tetrahydrobiopterin (BH4) required for catalytic conversion of tryptophan to 5-HTP (Cash, 1998). Additional research will be required to determine which of these potential mechanisms have a major influence on serotoneric functions during hypoxia stress.

Hypoxia could also potentially regulate TPH functions through a post-transcriptional mechanism(s). The finding that NEM, a sulfhydryl (SH) blocker that alkylates endogenous SH groups on proteins and peptides, mimics the effects of hypoxia on TPH activity and 5-HT are consistent with such a mechanism. NEM alkylates glutathione (GSH, a major antioxidant present in cells and tissues; Schulz et al., 2000) and cysteine, an amino acid which serves an important role to protect many proteins against oxidative damage (Requejo et al., 2010). The present results are consistent with results of *in vivo* studies showing that NEM treatment drastically suppresses 5-HT content (~43%) in normoxic rat brains (Garzon et al., 1990). *In vitro* studies have also shown that treatment with SH alkalizing agents such as NEM and iodoacetate, suppresses TPH and 5-HT transporter activities in rat brain tissue under normoxic conditions (Kuhn et al., 1980; Wolfel et al., 1989; Wolf and Kuhn, 1992). On the contrary, treatment with various SH agents such as GSH increase TPH activity in rat brain tissues *in vitro* (Kuhn and Arthur, 1997a,b; Hussain and Mitra, 2004), suggesting that the catalytic activity and post-translational modifications of TPH are dependent on endogenous SH residues (Kuhn et al., 1980). We have

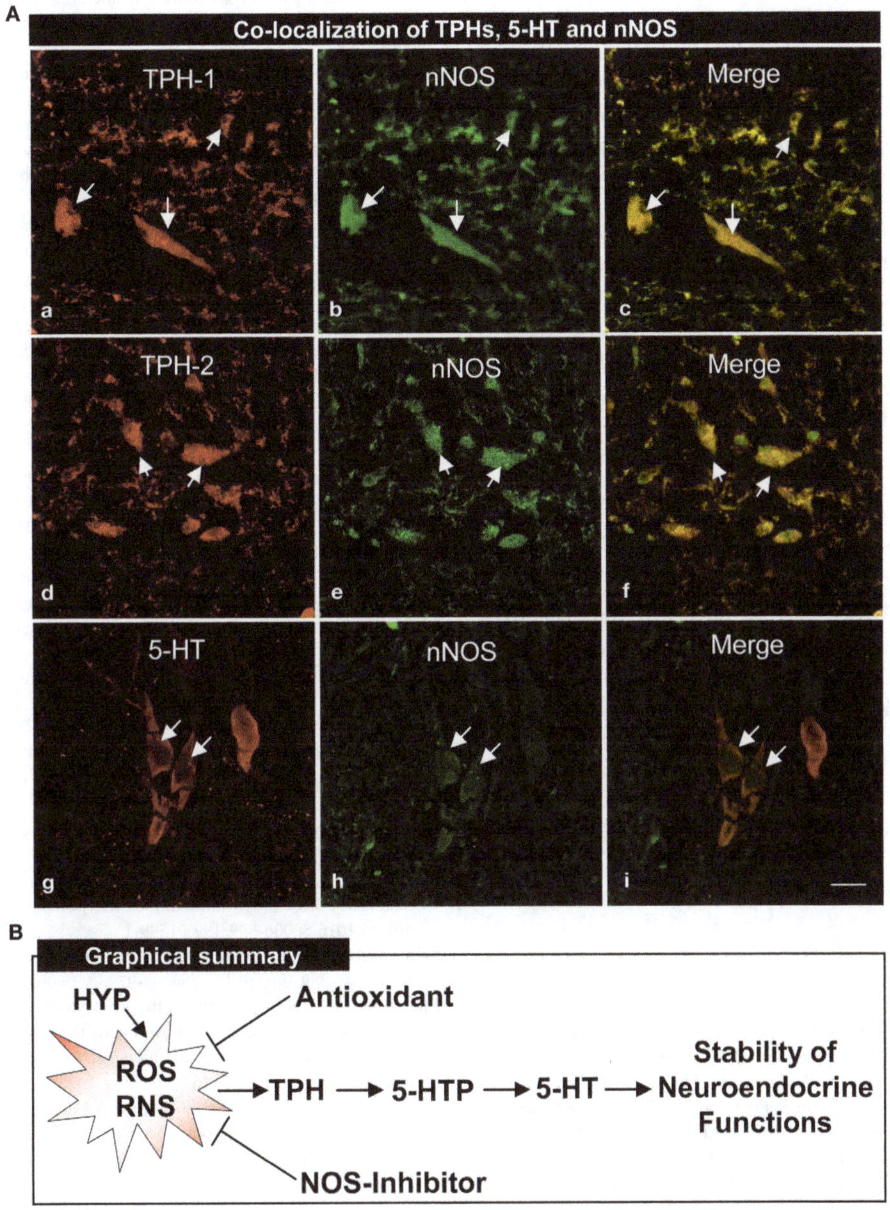

FIGURE 7 | Co-localization of TPHs and 5-HT neurons on neuronal nitric oxide synthase (nNOS) determined by double-immunofluorescence in croaker hypothalamus and proposed model of their interactions (A). Immunohistochemical co-localization of TPH-1 **(a–c)**, TPH-2 **(d–f)** and 5-HT **(g–i)** neurons with nNOS neurons. Scale bar = 5 μm. Arrows indicate neuronal expression of TPH-1, TPH-2, 5-HT, nNOS and their co-expression. **(B)** Proposed model of hypoxia down-regulation of TPH and 5-HT regulation through the generation of reactive oxygen and nitrogen species (ROS and RNS) in croaker hypothalamus. The antioxidant (Vitamin E) and nitric oxide synthase (NOS)-inhibitor block hypoxia-induced down-regulation of TPH activity, 5-HTP, and 5-HT contents and restore the neuroendocrine functions.

no direct evidence in support of this suggestion; however, Kuhn and Arthur (1996, 1997a,b) demonstrated that treatments with various RNS and ROS such as NO and H_2O_2, inactivate TPH activity via SH oxidation in rat brain extracts *in vitro*. Similarly, Hussain and Mitra (2004) have shown that H_2O_2 and exogenous O_2^- suppress TPH activity in rat brain tissues *in vitro*. Interestingly, O_2^- directly reacts with NO to produce $ONOO^-$ which inactivates TPH activity by SH oxidation in rat brain tissues (Kuhn and Geddes, 1999). Together these findings suggest that both ROS and RNS are directly involved in inactivation of TPH (Kuhn and Geddes, 2000), and thus this oxygen-liable enzyme could lose its catalytic activity and post-translational modifications when SH residues are decreased in neural tissues during hypoxic stress. There is considerable evidence that exposure to various stresses such as cold, heat, and hypoxia, lead to increased ROS and RNS levels, resulting in decreases in the total SH residues in blood, brain and hepatic tissues in vertebrates (Beck and Linkenheimer, 1952; Bartlett and Register, 1953; Wideman and Domanska-Janik, 1974; Iyer et al., 1985; Farooqui, 2012).

CONCLUSIONS

The results of the present study indicate that during hypoxic stress, administration of a NOS-inhibitor or Vit E leads to restoration of TPH expression and activity and 5-HT content to normal levels in the croaker hypothalamus. This is the first evidence in an aquatic vertebrate for an involvement of NOS in hypoxia down-regulation of TPH and 5-HT and its reversal by an antioxidant. Essentially, Vit E functions as an antioxidant by scavenging excessive free radicals produced during oxidative stress (Traber and Stevens, 2011). Hypoxia also causes down-regulation of reproductive neuroendocrine function in the croaker hypothalamus (Thomas et al., 2007; Thomas and Rahman, 2012). Current studies are investigating whether Vit E exerts a protective effect on hypothalamic neuronal systems related to reproduction during hypoxia stress.

ACKNOWLEDGMENTS

We gratefully acknowledge the assistance of Susan Lawson, University of Texas Marine Science Institute, for fish care and maintenance of the DO conditions in the experimental tanks. We thank Dr. Richard J. Kline, Department of Biological Sciences, University of Texas at Brownsville, for his expert assistance in confocal microscope. We also thank Stacy Haff, Santa Cruz Biotechnology, Santa Cruz, California, for providing the rabbit anti-nNOS antibody. This study was supported by a grant from the National Science Foundation (grant no. IOS-1119242) to Peter Thomas and Md. Saydur Rahman.

REFERENCES

Azzi, A. (2007). Molecular mechanism of alpha-tocopherol action. *Free Radic. Biol. Med.* 43, 16–21. doi: 10.1016/j.freeradbiomed.2007.03.013

Bartlett, R. G., and Register, U. D. (1953). Effect of cold and restraint on blood and liver nonprotein sulfhydryl compounds. *Proc. Soc. Exp. Biol. Med.* 83, 708–709.

Beck, L. V., and Linkenheimer, W. H. (1952). Effect of shock and clod on mouse liver sulfhydryl. *Proc. Soc. Exp. Biol. Med.* 81, 291–294.

Beckman, J. S., and Koppenol, W. H. (1996). Nitric oxide, superoxide, and peroxynitrite: the good, the bad, and ugly. *Am. J. Physiol.* 271, C1424–C1437.

Berlett, B. S., and Stadtman, E. R. (1997). Protein oxidation in aging, disease, and oxidative stress. *J. Biol. Chem.* 272, 20313–20316. doi: 10.1074/jbc.272.33.20313

Cash, C. D. (1998). Why tryptophan hydroxylase is difficult to purify: a reactive oxygen-derived species-mediated phenomenon that may be implicated in human pathology. *Gen. Pharmacol.* 30, 569–574. doi: 10.1016/S0306-3623(97)00308-X

Cazevieille, C., Muller, A., Meynier, F., and Bonne, C. (1993). Superoxide and nitric oxide cooperation in hypoxia/reoxygenation-induxced neuron injury. *Free Radic. Biol. Med.* 14, 389–395. doi: 10.1016/0891-5849(93)90088-C

Chandel, N. S., McClintock, D. S., Feliciano, C. E., Wood, T. M., Melendez, J. A., Rodriguez, A. M., et al. (2000). Reactive oxygen species generated at mitochondrial complex III stabilize hypoxia-inducible factor-1α during hypoxia. *J. Biol. Chem.* 275, 25130–25138. doi: 10.1074/jbc.M001914200

Chow, C. K. (1991). Vitamin E and oxidative stress. *Free Radic. Biol. Med.* 11, 215–232. doi: 10.1016/0891-5849(91)90174-2

Chow, C. K., Ibrahim, W., Wei, Z., and Chan, A. C. (1999). Vitamin E regulates mitochondrial hydrogen peroxide generation. *Free Radic. Biol. Med.* 27, 580–587. doi: 10.1016/S0891-5849(99)00121-5

Collins, T. J. (2007). ImageJ for microscopy. *Biotechniques* 43, 25–30. doi: 10.2144/000112517

Davis, J. N., Carlsson, A., MacMillan, V., and Siesjö, B. K. (1973). Brain tryptophan hydroxylation: dependence on arterial oxygen tension. *Science* 182, 72–74. doi: 10.1126/science.182.4107.72

Diaz, R. J., and Rosenberg, R. (2008) Spreading dead zones and consequences for marine ecosystems. *Science* 321, 926–929. doi: 10.1126/science.1156401

Encinas, J. M., Serrano, J., Bentura, M. L., Castro-Blanco, S., Fernandez, A. P., and Rodrigo, J. (2003). Nitric oxide system and protein nitration are modified by an acute hypobaric hypoxia in the adult rat hippocampus. *J. Neuropathol. Exp. Neurol.* 62, 863–877.

Evans, H. M., and Bishop, K. S. (1922). On the existence of a hitherto unrecognized dietary factor essential for reproduction. *Science* 56, 650–651. doi: 10.1126/science.56.1458.650

Farooqui, A. A. (2012). "Generation of reactive oxygen species in the brain: signaling for neural cell survival or suicide," in *Oxidative Stress in Vertebrates and Invertebrates: Molecular Aspects of Cell Signaling*, eds T. Farooqui and A. A. Farooqui (Hoboken, NJ: John Wiley & Sons, Inc.), 3–17.

Freidovich, I. (1999). Fundamental aspects of reactive oxygen species, or what's the matter with oxygen? *Ann. N.Y. Acad. Sci.* 893, 13–18. doi: 10.1111/j.1749-6632.1999.tb07814.x

Garzon, J., Lerida, M., Ulibarri, I., and Sanchez-Blazquez, P. (1990). Effect of ICV pertussis toxin and N-ethylmaleimide on the levels of substance P and serotonin in brain spinal cord of the rat. *Life Sci.* 46, 1217–1222. doi: 10.1016/0024-3205(90)90496-E

Gilany, K., and Vafakhah, M. (2010). Hypoxia: a review. *J. Paramed. Sci.* 1, 43–60.

Hedner, T., and Lundborg, P. (1979). Regional changes in monoamine synthesis in the developing rat brain during hypoxia. *Acta Physiol. Scand.* 106, 139–143. doi: 10.1111/j.1748-1716.1979.tb06382.x

Hussain, A. M., and Mitra, A. K. (2004). Effect of reactive oxygen species on the metabolism of tryptophan in rat brain: influence of age. *Mol. Cell. Biochem.* 258, 145–153. doi: 10.1023/B:MCBI.0000012849.16750.00

Iyer, E. M., Dikshit, M. B., and Suryanarayana, S. (1985). Effect of exposure to heart, hypoxia, cold, acceleration, and vibration stress on the total blood sulfhydryl groups in human subjects. *Aviat. Space Environ. Med.* 56, 1097–1101.

Jacobs, B. L., and Azmitia, E. C. (1992). Structure and function of the brain serotonin system. *Physiol. Rev.* 72, 165–229.

Kaehler, S. T., Singewald, N., Sinner, C., and Philippu, A. (1999). Nitric oxide modulates the release of serotonin in the rat hypothalamus. *Brain Res.* 835, 346–349. doi: 10.1016/S0006-8993(99)01599-1

Kelm, M. (1999). Nitric oxide metabolism and breakdown. *Biochim. Biophys. Acta* 1411, 273–289. doi: 10.1016/S0005-2728(99)00020-1

Khan, I. A., and Thomas, P. (1993). Immunocytochemical localization of serotonin and gonadotropin-releasing hormone in the brain and pituitary gland of the Atlantic croaker *Micropogonias undulatus*. *Gen. Comp. Endocrinol.* 91, 167–180. doi: 10.1006/gcen.1993.1116

Khan, I. A., and Thomas, P. (1997). Aroclor 1254-induced alterations in hypothalamic monoamine metabolism in the Atlantic croaker (*Micropogonias undulatus*): correlation with pituitary gonadotropin release. *Neurotoxicology* 18, 553–560.

Khan, I. A., and Thomas, P. (2001). Disruption of neuroendocrine control of luteinizing hormone secretion by Aroclor 1254 involves inhibition of hypothalamic tryptophan hydroxylase activity. *Biol. Reprod.* 64, 955–964. doi: 10.1095/biolreprod64.3.955

Kroeber, S., Schomerus, C., and Korf, H.-W. (1998). A specific and sensitive double-immunofluorescence method for the demonstration of S-antigen and serotonin in trout and rat pinealocytes by means of primary antibodies from the same donor species. *Histochem. Cell Biol.* 109, 309–317. doi: 10.1007/s004180050231

Kuhn, D. M., and Arthur, R. E. Jr. (1996). Inactivation of brain tryptophan hydroxylase by nitric oxide. *J. Neurochem.* 67, 1072–1077. doi: 10.1046/j.1471-4159.1996.67031072.x

Kuhn, D. M., and Arthur, R. E. Jr. (1997a) Inactivation of tryptophan hydroxylase by nitric oxide: enhancement by tetrahydrobiopterin. *J. Neurochem.* 68, 1495–1502. doi: 10.1046/j.1471-4159.1997.68041495.x

Kuhn, D. M., and Arthur, R. Jr. (1997b). Molecular mechanism of the inactivation of tryptophan hydroxylase by nitric oxide: attack on critical sulfhydryls that spare the enzyme iron center. *J. Neurosci.* 17, 7245–7251.

Kuhn, D. M., and Geddes, T. J. (1999). Peroxynitrite inactivates tryptophan hydroxylase via sulfhydryl oxidation. Coincident nitration of enzyme tyrosyl residues has minimal impact on catalytic activity. *J. Biol. Chem.* 274, 29726–29732. doi: 10.1074/jbc.274.42.29726

Kuhn, D. M., and Geddes, T. J. (2000). Molecular footprints of neurotoxic amphetamine action. *Ann. N.Y. Acad. Sci.* 914, 92–103. doi: 10.1111/j.1749-6632.2000.tb05187.x

Kuhn, D. M., Ruskin, B., and Lovenberg, W. (1980). Tryptophan hydroxylase: the role of oxygen, iron, sulfhydryl groups determinants of stability and catalytic activity. *J. Biol. Chem.* 255, 4137–4143.

Kumar, G. K. (2011). Hypoxia. 3. Hypoxia and neurotransmitter synthesis. *Am. J. Physiol. Cell Physiol.* 300, C743–C751. doi: 10.1152/ajpcell.00019.2011

Lahiri, S., Roya, A., Babya, S. M., Hoshia, T., Semenza, G. L., and Prabhakar, N. R. (2006). Oxygen sensing in the body. *Prog. Biophys. Mol. Biol.* 91, 249–286. doi: 10.1016/j.pbiomolbio.2005.07.001

Lièvre, V., Becuwe, P., Bianchi, A., Koziel, V., Franck, P., Schroeder, H., et al. (2000). Free radical production and changes in superoxide dismutases associated with hypoxia/reoxygenation-induced apoptosis of embryonic rat forebrain neurons in culture. *Free Radic. Biol. Med.* 29, 1291–1301. doi: 10.1016/S0891-5849(00)00433-0

Livak, K. J., and Schmittgen, T. D. (2001). Analysis of relative gene expression data using real-time quantitative PCR and the $2^{-\Delta\Delta Ct}$ method. *Methods* 25, 402–408. doi: 10.1006/meth.2001.1262

Lopez, J. M., Moreno, N., Morona, R., Munoz, M., and Gonzalez, A. (2005). Colocalization of nitric oxide synthase and monoamines in neurons of the amphibian brain. *Brain Res. Bull.* 66, 555–559. doi: 10.1016/j.brainresbull.2005.05.008

Lu, Y., Simpson, K. L., Weaver, K. J., and Lin, R. C. S. (2010). Coexpression of serotonin and nitric oxide in the raphe complex: cortical versus subcortical circuit. *Anat. Rec.* 293, 1954–1965. doi: 10.1002/ar.21222

Maiti, P., Singh, S. B., and Ilavazhagan, G. (2010). Nitric oxide system is involved in hypobaric hypoxia-induced oxidative stress in rat brain. *Acta Histochem.*112, 222–232. doi: 10.1016/j.acthis.2008.10.005

Martin, A., Zulueta, J., Hossoun, P., Blumberg, J. B., and Meydani, M. (1996). Effect of vitamin E on hydrogen peroxide production by human vascular endothelial cells after hypoxia/reoxygenation. *Free Radic. Biol. Med.* 20, 99–105. doi: 10.1016/0891-5849(95)02010-1

Maulik, D., Yoshihiro Numagami, Y., Ohnishi, S. T., Mishra, O. P., and Delivoria-Papadopoulos, M. (1998). Direct measurement of oxygen free radicals during *in utero* hypoxia in the fetal guinea pig brain. *Brain Res.* 798, 166–172. doi: 10.1016/S0006-8993(98)00408-9

McNeill, B., and Perry, S. F. (2006). The interactive effects of hypoxia and nitric oxide on catecholamine secretion in rainbow trout (*Oncorhynchus mykiss*). *J. Exp. Biol.* 209, 4214–4223. doi: 10.1242/jeb.02519

Mishra, O. P., Mishra, R., Ashraf, Q. M., and Delivoria-Papadopoulos, M. (2006). Nitric oxide-mediated mechanism of neuronal nitric oxide synthase and inducible nitric oxide synthase expression during hypoxia in the cerebral cortex of newborn piglets. *Neuroscience* 140, 857–863. doi: 10.1016/j.neuroscience.2006.02.060

Mohammad-Zadeh, L. F., and Gwaltney-Brant, S. M. (2008). Serotonin: a review. *J. Vet. Pharmacol. Therap.* 31, 187–199. doi: 10.1111/j.1365-2885.2008.00944.x

Muller, D. P. (2010). Vitamin E and neurological function. *Mol. Nutr. Food Res.* 54, 710–718. doi: 10.1002/mnfr.200900460

Nikinmaa, M., and Ress, B. B. (2005). Oxygen-dependent gene expression in fishes. *Am. J. Physiol. Regul. Integr. Comp. Physiol.* 288, R1079–R1090. doi: 10.1152/ajpregu.00626.2004

Park, C., Cho, K., Ryu, J. H., Shin, K. S., Kim, J., Ahn, H., et al. (2004). 7-Nitroindazole upregulates phosphorylated cAMP response element binding protein, polysialylated-neural cell adhesion molecule and tryptophan hydroxylase expression in the adult rat hippocampus. *Brain Res.* 1008, 120–125. doi: 10.1016/j.brainres.2004.01.055

Poncet, L., Denoroy, L., Dalmaz, Y., and Pequignot, J. M. (1997). Activity of tryptophan hydroxylase and content of indolamines in discrete brain regions after a long-term hypoxic exposure in the rat. *Brain Res.* 765, 122–128. doi: 10.1016/S0006-8993(97)00520-9

Pouysségur, J., and Mechta-Grigoriou, F. (2006). Redox regulation of the hypoxia-inducible factor. *Biol. Chem.* 387, 1337–1346. doi: 10.1515/BC.2006.167

Rahman, M. S., Khan, I. A., and Thomas, P. (2011). Tryptophan hydroxylase: a target for neuroendocrine disruptions. *J. Toxicol. Environ. Health B Crit. Rev.* 14, 473–494. doi: 10.1080/10937404.2011.578563

Rahman, M. S., and Thomas, P. (2009). Molecular cloning, characterization and expression of two tryptophan hydroxylase citation(TPH-1 and TPH-2) genes in the hypothalamus of Atlantic croaker: down-regulation after chronic exposure to hypoxia. *Neuroscience* 158, 751–765. doi: 10.1016/j.neuroscience.2008.10.029

Rahman, M. S., and Thomas, P. (2011). Characterization of three IGFBPs in Atlantic croaker and their regulation during hypoxic stress: potential mechanisms of their upregulation by hypoxia. *Am. J. Physiol. Endocrinol. Metab.* 301, E637–E648. doi: 10.1152/ajpendo.00168.2011

Rahman, M. S., and Thomas, P. (2012). Effects of hypoxia exposure on cytochrome P4501A (CYP1A) expression in Atlantic croaker: molecular mechanisms of CYP1A down-regulation. *PLoS ONE* 7:e40825. doi: 10.1371/journal.pone.0040825

Rahman, M. S., and Thomas, P. (2013). Interactive effects of hypoxia with estradiol-17β on tryptophan hydroxylase activity and serotonin levels in the Atlantic croaker hypothalamus. *Gen. Comp. Endocrinol.* 192, 71–76. doi: 10.1016/j.ygcen.2013.03.001

Requejo, R., Hurd, T. R., Costa, N. J., and Murphy, M. P. (2010). Cysteine residues exposed on protein surfaces are the dominant intramitochondrial thiol and may protect against oxidative damage. *FEBS J.* 277, 1465–1480. doi: 10.1111/j.1742-4658.2010.07576.x

Roberts, K. M., and Fitzpatrick, P. F. (2013). Critical review: mechanisms of tryptophan and tyrosine hydroxylase. *IUMBM Life* 65, 350–357. doi: 10.1002/iub.1144

Sakowski, S. A., Geddes, T. J., Thomas, D. M., Levi, E., Hatfield, J. S., and Kuhn, D. M. (2006). Differential tissue distribution of tryptophan hydroxylase isoforms 1 and 2 as revealed with monospecific antibodies. *Brain Res.* 1085, 11–18. doi: 10.1016/j.brainres.2006.02.047

Saligaut, C., Chretien, P., Daost, M., Moore, N., and Boismare, F. (1986). Dynamic characteristics of dopamine, norepinephrine, and serotonin metabolism in the axonal endings of the rat hypothalamus and striatum during hypoxia: a study using HPLC with electrochemical detection. *Methods Find. Exp. Clin. Pharmacol.* 8, 343–349.

Sanjuán-Pla, A., Cervera, A. M., Apostolova, N., Garcia-Bou, R., Víctor, V. M., Murphy, M. P., et al. (2005). A targeted antioxidant reveals the importance of mitochondrial reactive oxygen species in the hypoxic signaling of HIF-1alpha. *FEBS Lett.* 579, 2669–2674. doi: 10.1016/j.febslet.2005.03.088

Schneider, C. A., Rasband, W. S., and Eliceiri, K. W. (2012). NIH Image to ImageJ: 25 years of image analysis. *Nat. Methods* 9, 671–675. doi: 10.1038/nmeth.2089

Schulz, J. B., Lindenau, J., and Seyfried, J. (2000). Glutathione, oxidative stress and neurodegeneration. *Eur. J. Biochem.* 267, 4904–4911. doi: 10.1016/j.etp.2008.07.005

Semenza, G. L. (2001). HIF-1, O_2, and the 3 PHDs: how animal cells signal hypoxia to the nucleus. *Cell* 107, 1–3. doi: 10.1016/S0092-8674(01)00518-9

Semenza, G. L., Jiang, B. H., Leung, S. W., Passantino, R., Concordet, J. P., Maire, P., et al. (1996). Hypoxia response elements in the aldolase A, enolase 1, and lactate dehydrogenase A gene promoters contain essential binding sites for hypoxia-inducible factor 1. *J. Biol. Chem.* 271, 32529–32537. doi: 10.1074/jbc.271.51.32529

Smith, J. C. E., and Whitton, P. S. (2000). Nitric oxide modulates N-methyl-d-aspartate-evoked serotonin release in the raphe nuclei and frontal cortex of the freely moving rat. *Neurosci. Lett.* 291, 5–8. doi: 10.1016/S0304-3940(00)01378-1

Tagami, M., Yamagata, K., Ikeda, K., Nara, Y., Fujino, H., Kubota, A., et al. (1998). Vitamin E prevents apoptosis in cortical neurons during hypoxia and oxygen reperfusion. *Lab. Invest.* 78, 1415–1429.

Thomas, P., and Rahman, M. S. (2009). Biomarkers of hypoxia exposure and reproductive function in Atlantic croaker: a review with some preliminary findings from the Northern Gulf of Mexico hypoxic zone. *J. Exp. Mar. Biol. Ecol.* 381, S38–S50. doi: 10.1016/j.jembe.2009.07.008

Thomas, P., and Rahman, M. S. (2012). Extensive reproductive disruption, gonadal masculinization, and aromatase suppression in Atlantic croaker collected from an extensive area in the northern Gulf of Mexico hypoxic zone. *Proc. R. Soc. B* 279, 28–38. doi: 10.1098/rspb.2011.0529

Thomas, P., Rahman, M. S., Khan, I. A., and Kummer, J. A. (2007). Widespread endocrine disruption and reproductive impairment in an estuarine fish population exposed to seasonal hypoxia. *Proc. R. Soc. B* 274, 2693–2701. doi: 10.1098/rspb.2007.0921

Traber, M. G., and Atkinson, J. (2007). Vitamin E, antioxidant and nothing more. *Free Radic. Biol. Med.* 43, 4–15. doi: 10.1016/j.freeradbiomed.2007.03.024

Traber, M. G., and Stevens, J. F. (2011). Vitamins C and E: beneficial effects from a mechanistic perspective. *Free Radic. Biol. Med.* 51, 1000–1013. doi: 10.1016/j.freeradbiomed.2011.05.017

Vrana, S. L., Dworkin, S. I., and Vrana, K. E. (1993). Radioenzymatic assay for tryptophan hydroxylase: [^{3}H]H_2O release assessed by charcoal adsorption. *J. Neurosci. Methods* 48, 123–129. doi: 10.1016/S0165-0270(05)80014-7

Wegener, G., Volke, V., and Rosenberg, R. (2000). Endogenous nitric oxide decreases hippocampal levels of serotonin and dopamine *in vivo*. *Br. J. Pharmacol.* 130, 575–580. doi: 10.1038/sj.bjp.0703349

Wideman, J., and Domanska-Janik, K. (1974). Regulation of thiols in the brain. I. Concentrations of thiols and glutathione reductase activity in different parts of the rat brain during hypoxia. *Resuscitation* 3, 27–36. doi: 10.1016/0300-9572(74)90024-0

Wolf, W. A., and Kuhn, D. M. (1992). Role of essential sulfhydryl groups in drug interactions at the neuronal 5-HT transporter: differences between amphetamines and 5-HT uptake inhibitors. *J. Biol. Chem.* 267, 20820–20825.

Wolfel, R., Halbrigge, T., and Graefe, K.-H. (1989). Effects of N-ethylmaleimide on 5-hydroxytryptamine transport and sodium content in rabbit platelets. *Br. J. Pharmacol.* 97, 1308–1314. doi: 10.1111/j.1476-5381.1989.tb12593.x

Wu, R. S. S. (2009). "Effects of hypoxia on fish reproduction and development," in *Hypoxia*, eds J. F. Richards, A. P. Farrell, and C. J. Brauner (San Diego, CA: Academic Press), 80–141.

Yamagata, K., Tagami, M., and Yamori, Y. (2010) Neuronal vulnerability of stroke-prone spontaneously hypertensive rats to ischemia and its prevention with antioxidants such as vitamin E. *Neuroscience* 170, 1–7. doi: 10.1016/j.neuroscience.2010.07.013

Yan, X., Shun-wei, L., Yi, Z., and Jian-jun, Z. (2003). Effect of vitamin E on memory and brain monoaminergic neurotransmitter in chronic episodic hypoxia rat. *Acta Acad. Med. Sinicae* 25, 333–336.

Yu, R. M. K., Ng, P. K. S., Tan, T., Chu, D. L. H., Wu, R. S. S., and Kong. R. Y. C. (2008). Enhancement of hypoxia-induced gene expression in fish liver by the aryl hydrocarbon receptor (AhR) ligand, benzo[*a*]pyrene (B*a*P). *Aqua. Toxicol.* 90, 235–242. doi: 10.1016/j.aquatox.2008.09.004

Zhang, B., Tanaka, J., Yang, L., Yang, L., Sakanaka, M., Hata, R., et al. (2004). Protective effect of vitamin E against focal brain inchemia and neuronal death through induction of target genes of hypoxia-inducible factor-1. *Neuroscience* 126, 433–440. doi: 10.1016/j.neuroscience.2004.03.057

Zingg, J.-M., and Azzi, A. (2004). Non-antioxidant activities of vitamin E. *Curr. Med. Chem.* 11, 1113–1133. doi: 10.2174/0929867043365332

25

Reproduction, smell and neurodevelopmental disorders: genetic defects in different hypogonadotropic hypogonadal syndromes

Hernan Valdes-Socin[1]*, Matilde Rubio Almanza[1], Mariana Tomé Fernández-Ladreda[1], François Guillaume Debray[2], Vincent Bours[2] and Albert Beckers[1]

[1] *Service of Endocrinology, CHU Liège, University of Liège, Liège, Belgium*
[2] *Service of Human Genetics, CHU Liège, University of Liège, Liège, Belgium*

****Correspondence:***
Hernan Valdes-Socin, Service of Endocrinology, Centre Hospitalier Universitaire, Rue de l'Hôpital 1, Liège 4000, Belgium
e-mail: hg.valdessocin@chu.ulg.ac.be

The neuroendocrine control of reproduction in mammals is governed by a neural hypothalamic network of nearly 1500 gonadotropin-releasing hormone (GnRH) secreting neurons that modulate the activity of the reproductive axis across life. Congenital hypogonadotropic hypogonadism (HH) is a clinical syndrome that is characterized by partial or complete pubertal failure. HH may result from inadequate hypothalamic GnRH axis activation, or a failure of pituitary gonadotropin secretion/effects. In man, several genes that participate in olfactory and GnRH neuronal migration are thought to interact during the embryonic life. A growing number of mutations in different genes are responsible for congenital HH. Based on the presence or absence of olfaction dysfunction, HH is divided in two syndromes: HH with olfactory alterations [Kallmann syndrome (KS)] and idiopathic hypogonadotropic hypogonadism (IHH) with normal smell (normosmic IHH). KS is a heterogeneous disorder affecting 1 in 5000 males, with a three to fivefold of males over females. KS is associated with mutations in *KAL1, FGFR1/FGF8, FGF17, IL17RD, PROK2/PROKR2, NELF, CHD7, HS6ST1, FLRT3, SPRY4, DUSP6, SEMA3A, NELF,* and *WDR11* genes that are related to defects in neuronal migration. These reproductive and olfactory deficits include a variable non-reproductive phenotype, including sensorineural deafness, coloboma, bimanual synkinesis, craniofacial abnormalities, and/or renal agenesis. Interestingly, defects in *PROKR2, FGFR1, FGF8, CHD7, DUSP6,* and *WDR11* genes are also associated with normosmic IHH, whereas mutations in *KISS1/KISSR, TAC3/TACR3, GNRH1/GNRHR, LEP/LEPR, HESX1, FSHB,* and *LHB* are only present in patients with normosmic IHH. In this paper, we summarize the reproductive, neurodevelopmental, and genetic aspects of HH in human pathology.

Keywords: reproduction, male, Kallman syndrome, hypogonadotropic hypogonadism, olfaction, kisspeptin, genetics

INTRODUCTION

Reproductive system development and control in mammals is dependent on specific neurons located in the hypothalamus that secrete gonadotropin-releasing hormone-1 (GnRH-1) and control the pituitary–gonadal axis (**Figure 1**). During embryogenesis, these neurons originate in the nasal placode and migrate into the forebrain along the olfactory-vomeronasal nerves (1–3). Alterations in this migratory process lead to defective GnRH-1 secretion, resulting in heterogeneous genetic disorders such as idiopathic hypogonadotropic hypogonadism (IHH), and other reproductive diseases characterized by the reduction in or failure of sexual maturation and competence. Another consequence of these migratory neuronal defects can be olfactory dysfunction. Depending of the affected genes, other neurological developmental disorders can also be encountered (1–4).

Thus, idiopathic hypogonadotropic hypogonadism (IHH) is a genetic disease that can occur with a normal sense of smell (normosmic IHH) or in association with anosmia (Kallmann syndrome; KS). To date, mutations in many genes have been described in relations to KS and/or normosmic IHH (nIHH) (**Tables 1** and **2**). Hypogonadotropic hypogonadism (HH) can also be found in association with other distinctive clinical syndromic conditions, such as Prader Willi syndrome, that are outside the scope of the current review.

In this review, we focus on genetic central hypogonadism, which is more frequently encountered in males than in females. Congenital IHH is a clinically and genetically heterogeneous disorder (3, 4). Although sporadic cases predominate, families with congenital IHH have been reported with X-linked, autosomal dominant (AD) or autosomal recessive (AR) inheritance patterns (1–4). In some families, high variability in reproductive and non-reproductive phenotypic features suggests the presence of complex inheritance. In particular, polygenic (digenic or oligogenic) forms and variable forms of transmission can be found in selected cases (6–11). Indeed, further complexity is added by the remarkable observation

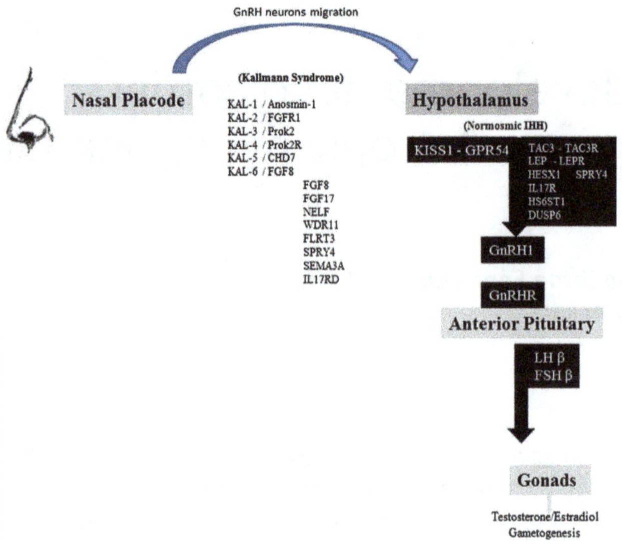

FIGURE 1 | Schematic representation of the reproductive axis and the different genes invalidating mutations participating in Kallman syndrome and nIHH. GnRH neurons migrate from nasal placode to hypothalamus in the first weeks of fetal life. Several genes are represented in the left column: their invalidating mutations are responsible for Kallmann syndrome and olfactory dysfunction. Kiss1 neurons integrate different hormonal, metabolic, circadian inputs from other hypothalamic and brain areas and thus stimulate GnRH neurons firing. Several genes are represented in the right black column, including KISS1-GPR54 system, which invalidating mutations lead to normosmic idiopathic hypogonadotropic hypogonadism. GnRH secretion leads to gonadotropins FSH and LH pituitary release. LH and FSH control sex steroids secretion and gametogenesis [adapted from Valdes-Socin et al. (1), with permission].

of reversibility of the phenotype in some cases of genetically determined hypogonadism (12–16).

THE HUMAN REPRODUCTIVE AXIS

Normal human reproduction and sexual characteristics rely on an intact hypothalamic–pituitary–gonadal axis (HPG; **Figure 1**). Hypogonadism is defined as the insufficient production of sex hormones with or without disturbed gametogenesis. HH results from a dysfunction of the hypothalamic–pituitary axis interfering with control of gonadotropin secretion (1–3, 16).

During life, the activity of the HPG axis has a tri-phasic pattern of "on-off-on." A first phase of activity occurs from the 16th week of intrauterine life as well as in the period between the 4th and 10th weeks of postnatal life (or "mini-puberty"). Mini-puberty is characterized by an increase in gonadotropin and steroid hormone secretion. Gonadotropins and sex hormones levels rise to a lesser extent than in true puberty. After mini-puberty, the HPG axis is repressed ("off") until puberty, when the system is reactivated ("on"). HPG axis activity is maintained throughout adult life in men whereas in women, menopause intervenes, and low sex steroids and compensatory high gonadotropin levels are characteristic (1–3).

The immediate postnatal period can be a window of opportunity for pediatricians and neonatologists to diagnose certain forms of HH. The congenital gonadotropin deficiency phenotype is variable and depends on the gender, the magnitude of the deficit, and the specific genetic abnormalities (**Figure 1**). At the time of puberty, the diagnosis of HH may be suspected due to the absence in the onset of puberty and development of secondary sex characteristics in both sexes. In adulthood, gonadotropin deficiency can be suspected in a woman without breast development or who presents with primary amenorrhea. In adult men, gynecomastia, small testes (<14 mL), penile hypoplasia, and/or oligo-azoospermia raise the clinical suspicion of congenital hypogonadism (1–3).

Table 1 | Genes and phenotype related only with normosmic IHH.

Genes	Locus	Inheritance	Phenotype	Comment
GNRH1 *GNRH-R*	8p21-11.2 4q13.2-3	Autosomal recessive	Normosmic IHH	Cryptorchidism –
KISS1 *KISS1R*	1q32 19p13.3	Autosomal recessive	Normosmic IHH	– –
LEP *LEPR*	7q31.3 1p31	Autosomal recessive	Normosmic IHH	Severe obesity
TAC3 *TACR3*	12q13.3 4q25	Autosomal recessive	Normosmic IHH	– –
DUSP6	12q21.33	Complex trait	Normosmic IHH	–
LHB	19q13.32	Polymorphism and mutations (homozygous and heterozygous)	Normosmic IHH	–
FSHB	11p13	Polymorphism and mutations	Normosmic IHH	–

NORMOSMIC IDIOPATHIC HYPOGONADOTROPIC HYPOGONADISM

The genetic abnormalities described below are infrequent or rare (see **Table 1**). In contrast to KS, patients with nIHH have a normal sense of smell and tend not to have other clinical signs. From a biological point of view, sex steroids secretion and gametogenesis are compromised, but to varying degrees. As it would be expected, reproductive phenotypes are more pronounced in subjects in whom the receptor is inactivated as compared to those harboring hormone inactivating mutations.

GNRH-1 and GNRHR mutations

Gonadotropin-releasing hormone (GnRH) is encoded by the *GNRH1* gene, which is located on chromosome 8p21-11.2. GNRH-1 mutations are rare and have been described in only two families (17, 18). A single homozygous mutation (c.18-19insA) affecting the peptide precursor preproGnRH was described in a Romanian family (17). It encoded a truncated and biologically inactive peptide in a male patient and his sister, both of whom had delayed puberty and normal sense of smell. The phenotype was reversed by pulsatile GnRH administration. Another homozygous *GNRH1* mutation was identified in a prepubertal boy from Armenia, with cryptorchidism and microphallus (18).

Table 2 | Genes, genes product, function, and phenotypes associated to congenital hypogonadism hipogonadotropic with anosmia/hyposmia (KS, Kallmann syndrome).

Genes	Locus	Gene product	Function	Inheritance	Type of hypogonadism	Clinical phenotype
KAL-1 (KS-1)	Xp22.3	Anosmin-1	Migration of GnRH and olfactory neurons	X-linked	Kallmann syndrome or normosmic IHH	Unilateral renal agenesis, synkinesia
FGF8 (KS-6)	10q24	Fibroblast growth factor 8	Migration of GnRH neurons	Autosomal dominant	Kallmann syndrome or normosmic IHH	Cleft lip/relatively common (mid-line defects)
FGFR1 (KS-2)	8p11.22	Fibroblast growth factor receptor	Migration of GnRH neurons	Autosomal dominant	Kallmann syndrome or normosmic IHH	
FGF 17	8p2.3	Fibroblast growth factor 17	Migration of GnRH neurons	Autosomal recessive	Kallmann syndrome or normosmic IHH	
FLRT3	20p12.1	Fibronecting like domain containing leucine enrich transmembrane protein 3	Interaction with FGFR	Complex trait	Kallmann syndrome	FGF network KO mouse is embryonic lethal
DUSP6	12q21.33	Dual specific inhibitor phosphatases	Inhibitor of MAPK pathway	Autosomal recessive	Kallmann syndrome	FGF network
IL17RD	3p14.3	Interleukin-17 receptor	Early stage of GnRH specification	Autosomal recessive	Kallmann syndrome	FGF network
SPRY4	5q31.3	Sprouty homolog interactor with FGFR1	Inhibitor of MAPK pathway	Autosomal recessive	Kallmann syndrome	FGF network
CHD7 (KS-5)	8q12.1-q12.2	Chromatin remodelating factor		Autosomal dominant	Kallmann syndrome or normosmic IHH	CHARGE Syndrome
SEMA3A	7q21.11	Semaphorine 3A	Axonal path finding of GnRH neurons	Autosomal dominant	Kallmann syndrome	–
PROK2 (KS-3)	3p21.1	Prokineticin-2	Migration of GnRH neurons	Autosomal dominant and recessive	Kallmann syndrome or normosmic IHH	Obesity, epilepsy, sleep disorders, fibrous dysplasia, and synkinesia
PROKR2 (KS-4)	20p13	Prok receptor		Kallmann syndrome or normosmic IHH		
NELF	9q34.3	Nasal embrionic LHRH factor	Migration of GnRH neurons	Digenic model (in association wth FGFR1 and HS6ST1)	Kallmann syndrome or normosmic IHH	–
WDR11	10q	WD repeat containing protein family	Development of neurons	Autosomal dominant	Kallmann syndrome or normosmic IHH	–
HS6ST1	2q21	Heparan sulfate 6-O Sulfotransferase	HS modifier Regulates neural branching	Complex trait	Kallmann syndrome or normosmic IHH	–

The *GNRHR* gene (locus on chromosome 4q13.2-3) encodes for the GNRH receptor. There is some variability in clinical expression of *GnRHR* mutations that is due to a partial loss of function. *GNRHR* mutations have been described in about 40–50% of familial AR nIHH cases, and in around 17% of sporadic nIHH (1–3).

KISS1 and GFPR54 mutations

The gene *KISS1* was described originally as a metastasis suppressor gene but it is a key gene in reproduction. It is localized on chromosome 1q32, encoding a protein called kisspeptin, which is, in turn, processed in four peptides Kp10, Kp13, Kp14, and Kp54. Kisspeptins stimulate GnRH neuronal firing and GnRH secretion, which then triggers an increased release of LH and FSH (**Figure 1**). The *KISS1R* gene (locus 19p.13.3), a G-protein-coupled receptor, is also known as the *GPR54* gene, and it is the receptor for kisspeptins. *GPR54* mutations can be compound heterozygous or homozygous (19–22). Loss of function mutations in *KISS1* (20) and *GPR54* cause HH in mice and men (19, 21, 22). Moreover, higher serum kisspeptins levels are found in obese hypogonadal men and in central hypogonadism than in controls (23). In patients with *GPR54* mutations, GnRH deficiency can be partial or complete, permanent, or reversible, and can have a congenital or adult onset. Six homozygous inactivating mutations have been described in 19 individuals with nIHH: their LH and FSH secretion was blunted but normal secretion was restored after exogenous GnRH stimulation (19, 21, 22). Kisspeptins are highly expressed in placenta during pregnancy; different patterns of spatiotemporal expression of *KISS1* and *KISSR* were described in normal and pathological placentas (24).

TAC3R and TAC3 mutations

The *TACR3* gene (chromosome 4q25) encodes the neurokinin 3 receptor (NK3R) and the *TAC3* gene (chromosome 12q13.3) encodes neurokinin B (NKB), its endogenous ligand. nIHH caused by mutations in *TAC3* and *TAC3R* have an AR heritance (25). As well as the *GPR54/Kisspeptin* system, *TACR3/TAC3* pathway stimulates GnRH neurons. In initial studies, defects in either *TAC3* or *TACR3* were found in 11 patients from 5 of 10 families studied, but in none of 50 sporadic cases (25–27). Francou et al. studied the gonadotropin axis dysfunction associated with nCHH due to TAC3/TACR3 mutations: it was related to a low GnRH pulsatile frequency leading to a low frequency of alpha-subunit pulses and to an elevated FSH/LH ratio (27). They suggested that this ratio might be useful for pre-screening nCHH patients for TAC3/TACR3 mutations. In another broad cohort of normosmic IHH patients, 7 of the 16 males and 5 of the 7 females with *TACR3/TAC3* mutations were assessed after discontinuation of therapy: 6 of the 7 males and 4 of the 5 females demonstrated evidence for reversibility of their hypogonadotropism (14).

Leptin (Ob) and leptin receptor mutations

Leptin is an adipocyte secreted protein that ensures a link between body fat and the reproductive axis. HH and severe obesity are seen in humans and ob/ob mice with genetic leptin deficiency. There are at least 12 patients with leptin deficiency and homozygous mutations. In such cases, recombinant leptin administration restores gonadotropin secretion and dramatically reduces body mass index. Defects in the leptin receptor are more common, being identified in 3% of severe early onset obesity patients. Interestingly, the leptin receptor is expressed on kisspeptin neurons whereas leptin administration induces the expression of *Kiss-1* in *ob/ob* mice (3, 28).

LHB mutations

The *LHB* subunit gene is located at chromosome 19q13.32. Five mutations have been published up to now; clinical and molecular data are summarized in **Table 3**. The syndrome of preserved spermatogenesis with androgenic failure (now known to be due to LH deficiency) was described for the first time by Pasqualini and Bur in 1950 (29). The term "fertile eunuch" was then coined to describe these men.

In affected men, sexual differentiation was normal, but the absence of or significantly reduced LH secretion restrained the induction of puberty and altered Leydig cell proliferation and maturation (30–34). These males have impaired spermatogenesis, ranging from azoospermia to oligospermia, which has been linked to the lack of LH stimulation and low intratesticular testosterone action (5, 30–35). In 2004, we described a man with a homozygous missense mutation (G36D) in the *LHB* subunit gene that abrogated subunit dimerization and rendered LH biologically and immunologically inactive (31). Treatment with human chorionic gonadotropin (hCG) induced near normalization of testicular structure (5). The patient and his wife conceived a child by intracytoplasmic sperm injection from ejaculated sperm. The male heterozygous child had normal LH, FSH, and testosterone levels, at the age of 4 weeks (5, 35).

In women, *LHB* mutations lead to a normal pubertal development but they can have primary amenorrhea and micropolycystic ovaries (32–34).

FSHB mutations

The β subunit of FSH (*FSHB*) is located at chromosome 11p13. Three men and four women with inactivating FSH mutations have been reported. Men have normal pubertal development although they have azoospermia, whereas women have abnormal pubertal maturation; in these patients high level of LH are found whereas FSH is low/undetectable. Estrogen and progesterone concentrations are low (1, 2).

Gonadotropins receptor (LHR and FSHR) mutations

Inactivating mutations affecting the gonadotropin receptors contrast with those affecting their ligands in that they are invariably associated with hypergonadotropic hypogonadism; hence, they are not discussed here.

KALLMANN SYNDROME

Kallmann syndrome, involving the characteristic features of HH and anosmia was noted in the historical literature long before being properly characterized as a genetic disorder. A man with delayed puberty and the lack of olfactory bulbs was reported over 150 years ago by the Spanish doctor Aureliano Maestre de San Juan (1828–1890). The German Franz Kallmann (1897–1965) completed in the 1940s a description of hypogonadism and anosmia in two families, establishing the genetic basis of transmission.

Table 3 | Clinical, biological, pathological, and genetic studies in patients with LH deficiency.

	Weiss et al. (30)	Valdes-Socin et al. (31)	Lofrano-Porto et al. (32)	Achard et al. (33)	Basciani et al. (34)
Mutation LH beta	Glut54Arg Homozygous	Glyc36Asp Homozygous	IVS + 1G > C Homozygous	Del10HisProlLeu Homozygous	IVS + 1G > C 12-bp deletion in Exon 2 Heterozygous
Exon localization	Exon 2	Exon 2	Intron 2	Exon 2	Exon 2
LH Functional Studies	Reduced LH bioactivity	Knot cysteine No LH dimerization	Abnormal tertiary structure No LH dimerization	Reduced LH bioactivity	No LH secretion
Plasma LH	LH = 64	LH undetectable	LH undetectable	No detectable LH	LH undetectable
Women	No	No	1, amenorrhea	1, amenorrhea	1, oligomenorrhea
Men	One man, impuberism FSH = 113	One man, impuberism Hypoandrogenism FSH = 23 αSU = 0.8 inhB = N	Two men, high FSH et SUα	One man, impuberism FSH = 20.7 SUα = 1.28 inhB = N High AMH	One man FSH = 8.7 inhB = N
Testis biopsy	Leydig = 0 Arrested SPG	Leydig+ SPG diminished	Leydig = 0 Arrested SPG	Leydig± SPG+	(after hCG) Leydig+ SPG+
Fertility	–	Azoospermia	Azoospermia	Normospermia but abnormal forms.	Oligospermia
Treatment	T2 then hCG	T2 then hCG	T2	T2 then hCG	T2 then hCG

All but one patient (Basciani et al.) are homozygotes for an inactivating βLH mutation.
SU α, alpha subunit; inhB, inhibin B; AMH, antimullerian hormone; SPG, spermatogenesis; T2, testosterone; N, normal; Anorm, abnormal; Dim, dimerization.
Normal values: FSH (2–14 UI/L), LH (2–10 UI/L), alpha subunit (<1.2 mUI/L).

The Swiss scientist, Georges de Morsier (1894–1982) provided the neuropathological description of the syndrome. KS has a prevalence of 1/5000, with a clear male predominance (1–3, 36, 37). Several mechanisms of inheritance and molecular mutations are described here after and summarized in **Table 2**.

Anosmin-1 (KAL-1) mutations

The *KAL-1* gene is located on the X chromosome at Xp22.3. *KAL-1* encodes anosmin-1, a glycoprotein playing an in important role in kidney, respiratory tract, digestive system, and brain embryogenesis (1–3, 37, 38). Anosmin-1 is an adhesion molecule located on cell surface, consistent with the underlying defect of embryonic neuronal migration in KS. Anosmin-1 is mainly involved in growth and migration of GnRH, mitral olfactory cells, and Purkinje cerebellum neurons. Mutations in *KAL-1* gene cause 14% of familial cases of KS and 11% of cases of sporadic cases (1–3, 38). *KAL-1* mutations lead to HH with or without anosmia and may include synkinesis (mirror movements), unilateral renal aplasia, and mid-line abnormalities such as cleft lip/palate (37, 38).

FGF8 (KAL-6), FGF17, and FGFR1 (KAL-2) mutations

The *FGF8* gene (also known as *KAL-6*) is located on chromosome 10q24. Fibroblast growth factors (FGF) interact with FGF tyrosine kinase receptors to mediate growth and development. *FGF8* participates in gastrulation, regionalization of the brain, and organogenesis of the limb and face as an embryonic epithelial factor. *FGF8* and its receptor *FGFR1* are involved in GnRH neuron migration. *FGF8* inactivating mutations can lead to both KS and nIHH with an AD inheritance. Triallelic inheritance has also been described. In addition, cleft lip or palate and other midline defects have been described in patients with *FGF8* and *FGFR1* mutations. Other features such as corpus callosum hypoplasia-agenesis or nose, ear, and finger abnormalities are more specific of *FGFR1* defects (37, 39, 40).

FGF17 is located at chromosome 8p2.3 and *FGF17* has a strong sequence identity with *FGF8*. *FGF17* might be implicated in GnRH neuron biology as an alternative to ligand *FGF8b*. Miraoui et al. have identified FGF17 heterozygous mutations in three patients with congenital HH and anosmia and in another individual. In a sporadic male patient with congenital, HH without anosmia (41).

FGFR1 is located at 8p11.22-p11.23 and *FGFR1* mutations have been identified in 10% of KS. *FGFR1* related KS has an AD inheritance, associated with incomplete penetrance and interfamilial variability. FGFR1 encodes for type 1 FGF receptor, which is expressed in several embryonic tissues. The activation of the FGF–FGFR complex requires two FGF ligands. FLRT3 (Fibronecting like domain containing leucine enrich transmembrane protein 3) also interacts with FGFR (see **Table 2**). In addition, the binding of heparin or HS: heparan sulfate proteoglycan (see HS6ST1 gene later) have been shown to be essential for FGF receptor dimerization and function (38). Mice with Fgfr1$^{-/-}$ mutations and patients with loss-of-function mutations in *FGFR1* have defective GnRH neuron migration (31). Thus, loss of function mutations in *FGFR1* which is involved in the development of the face, lead to the abnormal morphogenesis of the olfactory bulb, while specific gain-of function mutations in *FGFR1* cause craniosynostosis (37, 39–41).

PROK2 and PROKR2 mutations

PROK2 (locus 3p21.1) and *PROKR2* (locus 20p13) genes encode for prokineticin-2 and its receptor (42). Prok2 and prokr2 gene knockout mice both have agenesis or hypoplasia of the olfactory bulbs, in association with HH. In this model, there is also abnormal GnRH neuron migration (43). Its heritance can be AD or AR. Mutations in these genes are described in up to 6% of KS and 3% of nIHH (1–3, 42). In pituitary deficits associated with septo-optical dysplasia, McCabe et al. (44), described a patient with a heterozygous L173R mutation in *PROKR2* gene, while its healthy mother is homozygous for this mutation. As some controversy exists on the pathogenic role of some PROKR2 mutations, the prevalence given should be interpreted cautiously. Indeed, digenic mutations are encountered (i.e., *PROKR2* and *KAL1*), while heterozygous patients (i.e., AD transmission) are present in families with healthy relatives presenting the same genotype. There are no reliable accessory pathognomonic features of *PROK2/PROKR2* function loss: patients have been described with obesity, sleep disorder, fibrous dysplasia, epilepsy, and synkinesia (2, 3, 43, 44).

NELF mutations

The *NELF* gene is located at chromosome 9q34.3. This gene encodes the nasal embryonic LHRH factor. The *NELF* gene is detected in olfactory sensory cells and GnRH cells during embryonic development. It constitutes a guidance molecule for the olfactory axon and GnRH neurons across the nasal region (45). *NELF* mutations have been described in patients with KS, in association with mutations in *FGFR1* or *HS6ST1*, indicating digenic inheritance. More studies are necessary to confirm a relationship between *NELF* and any reproductive and olfactory disorders (2).

WDR11 mutations

The *WDR11* locus is at chromosome 10q26.12 and its heritance is AD. It encodes murine Wdr11 that is expressed in the developing olfactory and GnRH migratory pathway and in the adult hypothalamus. *WDR11* biological function is not well understood: however, Kim et al. identified five different heterozygous mutations in nIHH and KS patients. WDR11 probably also plays an important role in puberty (46).

CHD7 mutations

The *CHD7* gene that encodes a chromatin-remodeling factor is located on chromosome 8q12.1. Mutations (AD inheritance) of this gene can cause CHARGE syndrome (Colobomata, Heart Anomalies, Choanal Atresia, Retardation, Genital, and Ear anomalies). *CHD7* was screened in nearly 200 patients: 7 KS and nIHH patients were found, 3 of them with olfactory abnormalities. CHD7 mutations were identified in 6% of KS and 6% of nIHH, respectively (1, 2, 47, 48). Laittinen et al. described in 2012, a KS patient with a truncating CHD7 mutation that underwent a reversal of central hypogonadism after therapy discontinuation (15).

HS6ST1 mutations

The *HS6ST1* gene (locus 2q.21) encodes a 6-*O*-sulfation enzyme, which is a member of the heparan sulfate enzyme family. The protein is involved in normal neuronal development and may play a role in limb development. In nematodes, HS 6-*O*-sulfate interacts with anosmin-1 and it is involved in function of FGFR1 and FGF8.

HS6ST1 shows complex inheritance patterns, not following autosomal or recessive transmission. *HS6ST1* mutations were found in KS patients in combination with mutations affecting the FGFR1 gene. *HS6ST1* mutations were found in patients who had nIHH or variable degrees of olfactory dysfunction (KS) as well as with either normal or abnormal olfactory structures (49).

IL17RD, DUSP6, and SPRY4 mutations

The *IL17RD* gene (locus 3p14.3) encodes a membrane protein belonging to the interleukin-17 receptor (*IL-17R*) protein family. In a study with eight patients with congenital hypogonadism all had KS, 7/8 had absent puberty, 6/8 showed congenital hearing loss. One *IL17RD* allelic defect is likely to be insufficient, meaning that additional affected alleles in the same and/or other genes must be present to create the phenotype of KS with hearing loss (41).

DUSP6 (locus 12q22-q23) encodes a member of the dual specificity protein phosphatase subfamily. They negatively regulate members of the mitogen-activated protein (MAP) kinase superfamily (25) Three patients were described with DUSP6 and *FGFR1* heterozygous mutation; they were hypogonadic, while one had hearing loss and the two others had abnormal speech. DUSP6$^{-/-}$ mice are however viable and fertile (41).

SPRY4 (locus 5q.31.3) gene encodes a protein (sprouty homolog 4), which is an inhibitor of the receptor-transduced mitogen-activated protein kinase (MAPK) signaling pathway. It is positioned upstream of RAS gene activation and impairs the formation of active GTP-RAS. Diseases associated with SPRY4 include germ cell cancer, and testicular cancer. Miraoui et al. identified four anosmic patients with congenital HH (three females and one male) with heterozygosity for a c.530A-G transition in exon 3 of the SPRY4 gene. Another female patient had a heterozygosity for a c.910G-A transition in exon 3 of the SPRY4 gene. These mutations were not found in 155 controls. One of the patients also had hearing loss and another one had abnormal dentition (41).

HESX1 mutations

The *HESX1* gene (locus 3p14.3) encodes a protein that is a transcriptional repressor in the developing forebrain and pituitary gland (27). *HESX1* plays an important role in the temporal and sequential development of the forebrain, hypothalamus, optic nerve, and posterior pituitary (28). Mutations in *HESX1* have also been described in isolated growth hormone deficiency and combined pituitary deficiency (50, 51). *HESX1* mutations have been described in 1.4% of IHH/KS patients (50, 51), but as in *PROKR2* mutations this prevalence should be interpreted cautiously.

SEMA3A mutations

The *SEMA3A* gene (7q21.11) encodes the semaphorin 3A protein, which regulates axonal path finding and participates in GnRH migration. Deletions and mutations of the *SEMA3A* gene validate a role for *SEMA3A* in KS. Moreover, SEMA3A knockout mice exhibit GnRH dependent hypogonadism and abnormal olfactory bulb innervation (52).

CONCLUSION AND PERSPECTIVES

Kallmann syndrome and nIHH have the potential to unravel the processes behind normal embryonic development and reproductive neuroendocrine maturation (2). The complex biological path from childhood to the onset of human puberty is still incompletely understood (1–3). The molecular mechanism behind IHH remains unknown in a large number of cases. Over the past decade, the same genetic mutations have been described in associated with both KS and nIHH. Moreover, a significant clinical heterogeneity is seen in isolated GnRH deficiency, which might be explained to some extent by oligogenicity (6, 7, 9). In addition, over 60% of central hypogonadic patients have no identifiable mutations, suggesting that yet more disease loci remain to be discovered (1–3). These unidentified genes warrant an integrated research including clinicians, geneticists, and biological investigators to pursue further understanding of these fascinating cases.

ACKNOWLEDGMENTS

We acknowledge the National Fund of Scientific Research (FNRS, Brussels, Belgium), for their financial support and Dr AF Daly for kindly reviewing the manuscript.

REFERENCES

1. Valdes-Socin S, Debray FG, Parent AS, Lebrethon MC, Bourguignon JP, Bours V, et al. How to explore...congenital isolated hypogonadotropic hypogonadism? *Rev Med Liege* (2010) **65**(11):634–41.
2. Semple R, Topaloglu KA. The recent genetics of hypogonadotrophic hypogonadism – novel insights and new questions. *Clin Endocrinol (Oxf)* (2010) **72**(4):427–35. doi:10.1111/j.1365-2265.2009.03687.x
3. Nachtigall LB, Boepple PA, Pralong FP, Crowley WF Jr. Adult-onset idiopathic hypogonadotropic hypogonadism – a treatable form of male infertility. *N Engl J Med* (1997) **336**:410–5. doi:10.1056/NEJM199702063360604
4. Lippincott MF, True C, Seminara SB. Use of genetic models of idiopathic hypogonadotrophic hypogonadism in mice and men to understand the mechanisms of disease. *Exp Physiol* (2013) **98**:1522–7. doi:10.1113/expphysiol.2013.071910
5. Valdes-Socin H, Salvi R, Thiry A, Daly AF, Pralong FP, Gaillard R, et al. Testicular effects of isolated luteinizing hormone deficiency and reversal by long-term human chorionic gonadotropin treatment. *J Clin Endocrinol Metab* (2009) **94**:3–4. doi:10.1210/jc.2008-1584
6. Trarbach EB, Costa EM, Versiani B, de Castro M, Matias Baptista MT, Mendes Garmes H, et al. Novel fibroblast growth factor receptor 1 mutations in patients with congenital hypogonadotropic hypogonadism with and without anosmia. *J Clin Endocrinol Metab* (2006) **91**:4006–12. doi:10.1210/jc.2005-2793
7. Pitteloud N, Acierno JS Jr, Meysing A, Eliseenkova AV, Ma J, Ibrahimi OA, et al. Mutations in fibroblast growth factor receptor 1 cause both Kallmann syndrome and normosmic idiopathic hypogonadotropic hypogonadism. *Proc Natl Acad Sci U S A* (2006) **103**:6281–6. doi:10.1073/pnas.0600962103
8. Pitteloud N, Hayes FJ, Boepple PA, DeCruz S, Seminara SB, MacLaughlin DT, et al. The role of prior pubertal development, biochemical markers of testicular maturation, and genetics in elucidating the phenotypic heterogeneity of idiopathic hypogonadotropic hypogonadism. *J Clin Endocrinol Metab* (2002) **87**:152–60. doi:10.1210/jcem.87.1.8131
9. Sykiotis GP, Plummer L, Hughes VA, Au M, Durrani S, Nayak-Young S, et al. Oligogenic basis of isolated gonadotropin-releasing hormone deficiency. *Proc Natl Acad Sci U S A* (2010) **107**:15140–4. doi:10.1073/pnas.1009622107
10. Fukami M, Maruyama T, Dateki S, Sato N, Yoshimura Y, Ogata T. Hypothalamic dysfunction in a female with isolated hypogonadotropic hypogonadism and compound heterozygous TACR3 mutations and clinical manifestation in her heterozygous mother. *Horm Res Paediatr* (2010) **73**:477–81. doi:10.1159/000313373
11. Lewkowitz-Shpuntoff HM, Hughes VA, Plummer L, Au MG, Doty RL, Seminara SB, et al. Olfactory phenotypic spectrum in idiopathic hypogonadotropic hypogonadism: pathophysiological and genetic implications. *J Clin Endocrinol Metab* (2012) **97**:136–44. doi:10.1210/jc.2011-2041
12. Raivio J, Falardeau A, Dwyer R, Quinton FJ, Hayes VA, Hughes LW, et al. Reversal of idiopathic hypogonadotropic hypogonadism. *N Engl J Med* (2007) **357**:863–73. doi:10.1056/NEJMoa066494
13. Pitteloud N, Acierno JS Jr, Meysing AU, Dwyer AA, Hayes FJ, Crowley WF Jr. Reversible Kallmann syndrome, delayed puberty, and isolated anosmia occurring in a single family with a mutation in the fibroblast growth factor receptor 1 gene. *J Clin Endocrinol Metab* (2005) **90**:1317–22. doi:10.1210/jc.2004-1361
14. Gianetti E, Tusset C, Noel SD, Au MG, Dwyer AA, Hughes VA, et al. TAC3/TACR3 mutations reveal preferential activation of gonadotropin-releasing hormone release by neurokinin B in neonatal life followed by reversal in adulthood. *J Clin Endocrinol Metab* (2010) **95**:2857–67. doi:10.1210/jc.2009-2320
15. Laitinen EM, Tommiska J, Sane T, Vaaralahti K, Toppari J, Raivio T. Reversible congenital hypogonadotropic hypogonadism in patients with CHD7, FGFR1 or GNRHR mutations. *PLoS One* (2012) **7**:e39450. doi:10.1371/journal.pone.0039450
16. Cariboni A, Maggi R. Kallmann's syndrome, a neuronal migration defect. *Cell Mol Life Sci* (2006) **63**(21):2512–26. doi:10.1007/s00018-005-5604-3
17. Bouligand J, Ghervan C, Tello JA, Brailly-Tabard S, Salenave S, Chanson P, et al. Isolated familial hypogonadotropic hypogonadism and a GNRH1 mutation. *N Engl J Med* (2009) **360**:2742–8. doi:10.1056/NEJMoa0900136
18. Chan YM, de Guillebon A, Lang-Muritano M, Plummer L, Cerrato F, Tsiaras S, et al. GNRH1 mutations in patients with idiopathic hypogonadotropic hypogonadism. *Proc Natl Acad Sci U S A* (2009) **106**:11703–8. doi:10.1073/pnas.0903449106
19. de Roux N, Genin E, Carel JC, Matsuda F, Chaussain JL, Milgrom E. Hypogonadotropic hypogonadism due to loss of function of the KiSS1-derived peptide receptor GPR54. *Proc Natl Acad Sci U S A* (2003) **100**:10972–6. doi:10.1073/pnas.1834399100
20. Topaloglu AK, Tello JA, Kotan LD, Ozbek MN, Yilmaz MB, Erdogan S, et al. Inactivating KISS1 mutation and hypogonadotropic hypogonadism. *N Engl J Med* (2012) **366**:629–35. doi:10.1056/NEJMoa1111184
21. Brioude F, Bouligand J, Francou B, Fagart J, Roussel R, Viengchareun S, et al. Two families with normosmic congenital hypogonadotropic hypogonadism and biallelic mutations in KISS1R (KISS1 receptor): clinical evaluation and molecular characterization of a novel mutation. *PLoS One* (2013) **8**(1):e53896. doi:10.1371/journal.pone.0053896
22. Tenenbaum-Rakover Y, Commenges-Ducos M, Iovane A, Aumas C, Admoni O, de Roux N. Neuroendocrine phenotype analysis in five patients with isolated hypogonadotropic hypogonadism due to a L102P inactivating mutation of GPR54. *J Clin Endocrinol Metab* (2007) **92**:1137–44. doi:10.1210/jc.2006-2147
23. Valdes-Socin H, Cavalier E, Beckaert A, Carlisi A, Chavez M, Beckers A. High plasma kisspeptins in obese men with acquired hypogonadism and in men with congenital hypogonadism: pilot study of plasma kisspeptins variations before and after hCG and testosterone administration. *Ann Endocrinol (Paris)* (2011).
24. Valdes-Socin H, Munaut C, Chavez M, Chantrain F, Delbecque K, Delvenne P, et al. Expression and spatio-temporal distribution of KISS1 and its receptor KISSR in human normal and pathological placentae. *Ann Endocrinol (Paris)* (2012) **4**:374. doi:10.1016/j.ando.2012.07.494
25. Topaloglu AK, Reimann F, Guclu M, Yalin AS, Kotan D, Porter KM, et al. TAC3 and TACR3 mutations in familial hypogonadotropic hypogonadism reveal a key role for Neurokinin B in the central control of reproduction. *Nat Genet* (2009) **41**:354–8. doi:10.1038/ng.306
26. Guran T, Tolhurst G, Bereket A, Rocha N, Porter K, Turan S, et al. A novel missense mutation in the first extracellular loop of the neurokinin B receptor causes hypogonadotropic hypogonadism. *J Clin Endocrinol Metab* (2009) **94**:3633–9. doi:10.1210/jc.2009-0551

27. Francou B, Bouligand J, Voican A, Amazit L, Trabado S, Fagart J, et al. Normosmic congenital hypogonadotropic hypogonadism due to TAC3/TACR3 mutations: characterization of neuroendocrine phenotypes and novel mutations. *PLoS One* (2011) **6**:e25614. doi:10.1371/journal.pone.0025614
28. Farooqi IS, Wangensteen T, Collins S, Kimber W, Matarese G, Keogh JM, et al. Clinical and molecular genetic spectrum of congenital deficiency of the leptin receptor. *N Engl J Med* (2007) **356**:237–47. doi:10.1056/NEJMoa063988
29. Pasqualini RQ, Bur GE. Síndrome hipoandrogénico con gametogénesis conservada: clasificación de la insuficiencia testicular. *Rev Asoc Med Argent* (1950) **64**:15–30.
30. Weiss J, Axelrod L, Whitcomb RW, Harris PE, Crowley WF, Jameson JL. Hypogonadism caused by a single amino acid substitution in the subunit of luteinizing hormone. *N Engl J Med* (1992) **326**:179–83. doi:10.1056/NEJM199201163260306
31. Valdes-Socin H, Salvi R, Daly AF, Gaillard RC, Quatresooz P, Tebeu P-M, et al. Hypogonadism in a patient with a mutation in the luteinizing hormone-subunit gene. *N Engl J Med* (2004) **351**:2619–25. doi:10.1056/NEJMoa040326
32. Lofrano-Porto A, Barra GB, Giacomini LA, Nascimento PP, Latronico AC, Casulari LA, et al. Luteinizing hormone mutation and hypogonadism in men and women. *N Engl J Med* (2007) **357**:897–904. doi:10.1056/NEJMoa071999
33. Achard C, Courtillot C, Lahuna O, Me'duri G, Soufir JC, Lie're P, et al. Normal spermatogenesis in a man with mutant luteinizing hormone. *N Engl J Med* (2009) **361**:1856–63. doi:10.1056/NEJMoa0805792
34. Basciani S, Watanabe M, Mariani S, Passeri M, Persichetti A, Fiore D, et al. Hypogonadism in a patient with two novel mutations of the luteinizing hormone –subunit gene expressed in a compound heterozygous form. *J Clin Endocrinol Metab* (2012) **97**:3031–8. doi:10.1210/jc.2012-1986
35. Daly A, Valdes-Socin H, Beckers A. A tall man with hypogonadism. In: Wartofsky L, editor. *Diagnostic Dilemmas: Images in Endocrinology.* Washington DC: The Endocrine Society Press (2011). p. 204–7.
36. Legouis R, Hardelin JP, Levilliers J, Claverie JM, Compain S, Wunderle V, et al. The candidate gene for the X-linked Kallmann syndrome encodes a protein related to adhesion molecules. *Cell* (1991) **67**:423–35. doi:10.1016/0092-8674(91)90193-3
37. Sato N, Katsumata N, Kagami M, Hasegawa T, Hori N, Kawakita S, et al. Clinical assessment and mutation analysis of Kallmann syndrome 1 (KAL1) and fibroblast growth factor receptor 1 (FGR1, or KAL2) in five families and 18 sporadic patients. *J Clin Endocrinol Metab* (2004) **89**:1079–88. doi:10.1210/jc.2003-030476
38. Tsai PS, Gill JC. Mechanisms of disease: insights into X-linked and autosomal-dominant Kallmann syndrome. *Nat Clin Pract Endocrinol Metab* (2006) **2**:160–71. doi:10.1038/ncpendmet0119
39. Dodé C, Levilliers J, Dupont JM, De Paepe A, Le Dû N, Soussi-Yanicostas N, et al. Loss-of-function mutations in FGFR1 cause autosomal dominant Kallmann syndrome. *Nat Genet* (2003) **33**:463–5. doi:10.1038/ng1122
40. Dodé C, Teixeira L, Levilliers J, Fouveaut C, Bouchard P, Kottler ML, et al. Kallmann syndrome: mutations in the genes encoding prokineticin-2 and prokineticin receptor-2. *PLoS Genet* (2006) **2**(10):e175. doi:10.1371/journal.pgen.0020175
41. Miraoui H, Dwyer AA, Sykiotis GP, Plummer L, Chung W, Feng B, et al. Mutations in FGF17, IL17RD, DUPS6, SPRY4, and FLRT3 are identified in individuals with congenital hypogonadotropic hypogonadism. *Am J Hum Genet* (2013) **92**:725–43. doi:10.1016/j.ajhg.2013.04.008
42. Cole LW, Sidis Y, Zhang CK, Quinton R, Plummer L, Pignatelli D, et al. Mutations in prokineticin 2 and prokineticin receptor 2 genes in human gonadotrophin releasing hormone deficiency: molecular genetics and clinical spectrum. *J Clin Endocrinol Metab* (2008) **93**:3551–9. doi:10.1210/jc.2007-2654
43. Matsumoto S, Yamazaki C, Masumoto K, Nagano M, Naito M, Soga T, et al. Abnormal development of the olfactory bulb and reproductive system in mice lacking prokineticin receptor PKR2. *Proc Natl Acad Sci U S A* (2006) **103**:4140–5. doi:10.1073/pnas.0508881103
44. McCabe MJ, Gaston-Massuet C, Gregory LC, Alatzoglou KS, Tziaferi V, Sbai O, et al. Variations in PROKR2, but not PROK2, are associated with hypopituitarism and septo-optic dysplasia. *J Clin Endocrinol Metab* (2013) **98**:547–57. doi:10.1210/jc.2012-3067
45. Kramer PR, Wray S. Novel gene expressed in nasal region influences outgrowth of olfactory axons and migration of luteinizing hormone-releasing hormone (LHRH) neurons. *Genes Dev* (2000) **14**:1824–34.
46. Kim HG, Ahn JW, Kurth I, Ullmann R, Kim HT, Kulharya A, et al. WDR11, a WD protein that interacts with transcription factor EMX1, is mutated in idiopathic hypogonadotropic hypogonadism and Kallmann syndrome. *Am J Hum Genet* (2010) **87**(4):465–79. doi:10.1016/j.ajhg.2010.08.018
47. Kim HG, Kurth I, Lan F, Meliciani I, Wenzel W, Eom SH, et al. Mutations in CHD7, encoding a chromatin-remodeling protein, cause idiopathic hypogonadotropic hypogonadism and Kallmann syndrome. *Am J Hum Genet* (2008) **83**:511–9. doi:10.1016/j.ajhg.2008.09.005
48. Bergman JE, de Ronde W, Jongmans MC, Wolffenbuttel BH, Drop SL, Hermus A, et al. The results of CHD7 analysis in clinically well-characterized patients with Kallmann syndrome. *J Clin Endocrinol Metab* (2012) **97**(5):E858–62. doi:10.1210/jc.2011-2652
49. Tornberg J, Sykiotis GP, Keefe K, Plummer L, Hoang X, Hall JE, et al. Heparan sulfate 6-O-sulfotransferase 1, a gene involved in extracellular sugar modifications, is mutated in patients with idiopathic hypogonadotrophic hypogonadism. *Proc Natl Acad Sci U S A* (2011) **108**:11524–9. doi:10.1073/pnas.1102284108
50. McNay DE, Turton JP, Kelberman D, Woods KS, Brauner R, Papadimitriou A, et al. HESX1 mutations are an uncommon cause of septooptic dysplasia and hypopituitarism. *J Clin Endocrinol Metab* (2007) **92**:691–7. doi:10.1210/jc.2006-1609
51. Newbern K, Natrajan N, Kim H-G, Chorich LP, Halvorson LM, Cameron RS, et al. Identification of HESX1 mutations in Kallmann syndrome. *Fertil Steril* (2013) **99**:1831–7. doi:10.1016/j.fertnstert.2013.01.149
52. Young J, Metay C, Bouligand J, Tou B, Francou B, Maione L, et al. SEMA3A deletion in a family with Kallmann syndrome validates the role of semaphorin 3A in human puberty and olfactory system development. *Hum Reprod* (2012) **27**:1460–5. doi:10.1093/humrep/des022

Permissions

All chapters in this book were first published by Frontiers; hereby published with permission under the Creative Commons Attribution License or equivalent. Every chapter published in this book has been scrutinized by our experts. Their significance has been extensively debated. The topics covered herein carry significant findings which will fuel the growth of the discipline. They may even be implemented as practical applications or may be referred to as a beginning point for another development.

The contributors of this book come from diverse backgrounds, making this book a truly international effort. This book will bring forth new frontiers with its revolutionizing research information and detailed analysis of the nascent developments around the world.

We would like to thank all the contributing authors for lending their expertise to make the book truly unique. They have played a crucial role in the development of this book. Without their invaluable contributions this book wouldn't have been possible. They have made vital efforts to compile up to date information on the varied aspects of this subject to make this book a valuable addition to the collection of many professionals and students.

This book was conceptualized with the vision of imparting up-to-date information and advanced data in this field. To ensure the same, a matchless editorial board was set up. Every individual on the board went through rigorous rounds of assessment to prove their worth. After which they invested a large part of their time researching and compiling the most relevant data for our readers.

The editorial board has been involved in producing this book since its inception. They have spent rigorous hours researching and exploring the diverse topics which have resulted in the successful publishing of this book. They have passed on their knowledge of decades through this book. To expedite this challenging task, the publisher supported the team at every step. A small team of assistant editors was also appointed to further simplify the editing procedure and attain best results for the readers.

Apart from the editorial board, the designing team has also invested a significant amount of their time in understanding the subject and creating the most relevant covers. They scrutinized every image to scout for the most suitable representation of the subject and create an appropriate cover for the book.

The publishing team has been an ardent support to the editorial, designing and production team. Their endless efforts to recruit the best for this project, has resulted in the accomplishment of this book. They are a veteran in the field of academics and their pool of knowledge is as vast as their experience in printing. Their expertise and guidance has proved useful at every step. Their uncompromising quality standards have made this book an exceptional effort. Their encouragement from time to time has been an inspiration for everyone.

The publisher and the editorial board hope that this book will prove to be a valuable piece of knowledge for researchers, students, practitioners and scholars across the globe.

List of Contributors

Gonçalo A. Oliveira
Unidade de Investigação em Eco-Etologia, ISPA - Instituto Universitário, Lisboa, Portugal

Rui F. Oliveira
Unidade de Investigação em Eco-Etologia, ISPA - Instituto Universitário, Lisboa, Portugal
Integrative Behavioural Biology Lab, Instituto Gulbenkian de Ciência, Oeiras, Portugal
Champalimaud Neuroscience Program, Champalimaud Center for the Unknown, Lisboa, Portugal

Yasuo Sakuma
Laboratory of Physiology, University of Tokyo Health Sciences, Tokyo, Japan

Shinji Tsukahara and Moeko Kanaya
Division of Life Science, Graduate School of Science and Engineering, Saitama University, Saitama, Japan

Korehito Yamanouchi
Department of Human Behavior and Environment Sciences, Faculty of Human Sciences, Waseda University, Saitama, Japan

Takashi X. Fujisawa and Akemi Tomoda
Research Center for Child Mental Development, University of Fukui, Fukui, Japan
Department of Child Development, United Graduate School of Child Development, Osaka University, Kanazawa University, Hamamatsu University School of Medicine, Chiba University, University of Fukui, Fukui, Japan

Shiho Tanaka
Research Center for Child Mental Development, University of Fukui, Fukui, Japan

Daisuke N. Saito
Research Center for Child Mental Development, University of Fukui, Fukui, Japan
Department of Child Development, United Graduate School of Child Development, Osaka University, Kanazawa University, Hamamatsu University School of Medicine, Chiba University, University of Fukui, Fukui, Japan
Biomedical Imaging Research Center, University of Fukui, Fukui, Japan

Hirotaka Kosaka
Research Center for Child Mental Development, University of Fukui, Fukui, Japan
Department of Child Development, United Graduate School of Child Development, Osaka University, Kanazawa University, Hamamatsu University School of Medicine, Chiba University, University of Fukui, Fukui, Japan
Department of Neuropsychiatry, Faculty of Medical Sciences, University of Fukui, Fukui, Japan

Ken Ichi Matsuda
Department of Anatomy and Neurobiology, Graduate School of Medical Science, Kyoto Prefectural University of Medicine, Kyoto, Japan

Mumeko C. Tsuda, Mariko Nakata and Sonoko Ogawa
Laboratory of Behavioral Neuroendocrinology, University of Tsukuba, Tsukuba, Japan

Naoko Yamaguchi
Department of Pharmacology, School of Medicine, Aichi Medical University, Nagakute, Japan

Aubrey M. Kelly and James L. Goodson
Department of Biology, Indiana University, Bloomington, IN, USA

Akari Asaba, Tatsuya Hattori, Kazutaka Mogi and Takefumi Kikusui
Department of Animal Science and Biotechnology, Graduate School of Veterinary Medicine, Azabu University, Kanagawa, Japan

Hirotaka Sakamoto
Laboratory of Neuroendocrinology, Ushimado Marine Institute, Graduate School of Natural Science and Technology, Okayama University, Okayama, Japan

Aki Takahashi and Tsuyoshi Koide
Mouse Genomics Resource Laboratory, National Institute of Genetics (NIG), Mishima, Japan
Department of Genetics, SOKENDAI, Mishima, Japan

Toshihiko Shiroishi
Mouse Genomics Resource Laboratory, National Institute of Genetics (NIG), Mishima, Japan
Department of Genetics, SOKENDAI, Mishima, Japan
Mammalian Genetics Laboratory, National Institute of Genetics (NIG), Mishima, Japan

Takayoshi Ubuka and Kazuyoshi Tsutsui
Department of Biology and Center for Medical Life Science, Waseda University, Shinjuku, Tokyo, Japan

Devaleena S. Pradhan
Department of Biology, Georgia State University, Atlanta, GA, USA

Tessa K. Solomon-Lane
Neuroscience Institute, Georgia State University, Atlanta, GA, USA

Matthew S. Grober
Department of Biology, Georgia State University, Atlanta, GA, USA
Neuroscience Institute, Georgia State University, Atlanta, GA, USA

Yutaro Kawaguchi, Akira Nagaoka, Asana Kitami, Tomomi Mitsuhashi, Youichi Hayakawa and Makito Kobayashi
Department of Life Science, International Christian University, Mitaka, Tokyo, Japan

Hirofumi Hashimoto, Takanori Matsuura and Yoichi Ueta
Department of Physiology, School of Medicine, University of Occupational and Environmental Health, Kitakyushu, Japan

Claudia Lieberwirth
Department of Behavioral Science, Utah Valley University, Orem, UT, USA

Zuoxin Wang
Department of Psychology and Program in Neuroscience, Florida State University, Tallahassee, FL, USA

Mayumi Nishi, Noriko Horii-Hayashi and Takayo Sasagawa
Department of Anatomy and Cell Biology, Nara Medical University, Kashihara, Japan

Atsuko Saito and Toshikazu Hasegawa
Department of Cognitive and Behavioral Science, Graduate School of Arts and Sciences, The University of Tokyo, Tokyo, Japan

Hiroki Hamada
Department of General Systems Studies, Graduate School of Arts and Sciences, The University of Tokyo, Tokyo, Japan

Miho Nagasawa and Shohei Mitsui
Department of Animal Science and Biotechnology, Azabu University, Kanagawa, Japan

Takashi Higuchi
Faculty of Medical Sciences, University of Fukui, Fukui, Japan

Kazuo Hiraki
Department of General Systems Studies, Graduate School of Arts and Sciences, The University of Tokyo, Tokyo, Japan
JST, CREST, Tokyo, Japan

Mingkun Liang and Jing Zhong
Department of Basic Research on Social Recognition and Memory, Research Center for Child Mental Development, Kanazawa University, Kanazawa, Japan
Department of Biophysical Genetics, Graduate School of Medical Sciences, Kanazawa University, Kanazawa, Japan

Hong-Xiang Liu, Olga Lopatina and Haruhiro Higashida
Department of Basic Research on Social Recognition and Memory, Research Center for Child Mental Development, Kanazawa University, Kanazawa, Japan

Ryusuke Nakada and Agnes-Mikiko Yamauchi
Department of Biophysical Genetics, Graduate School of Medical Sciences, Kanazawa University, Kanazawa, Japan

Shunji Yamada and Mitsuhiro Kawata
Department of Anatomy and Neurobiology, Kyoto Prefectural University of Medicine, Kyoto, Japan

Fumihiko Maekawa and Keiko Nohara
Molecular Toxicology Section, Center for Environmental Health Sciences, National Institute for Environmental Studies, Tsukuba, Japan

Takaharu Kawashima
Ecological Genetics Research Section, Center for Environmental Biology and Ecosystem Studies, National Institute for Environmental Studies, Tsukuba, Japan

Hiroko Ohki-Hamazaki
College of Liberal Arts and Sciences, Kitasato University, Sagamihara, Japan

Wudu E. Lado
Department of Biology, University of Ottawa, Ottawa, ON, Canada
Department of Cell and Systems Biology, University of Toronto, Toronto, ON, Canada

David C. Spanswick
Warwick Medical School, University of Warwick, Coventry, UK
Department of Physiology, Monash University, Clayton, VIC, Australia

John E. Lewis and Vance L. Trudeau
Department of Biology, University of Ottawa, Ottawa, ON, Canada

Yusuke Nakane
Laboratory of Animal Physiology, Department of Applied Molecular Biosciences, Graduate School of Bioagricultural Sciences, Nagoya University, Nagoya, Japan

Takashi Yoshimura
Laboratory of Animal Physiology, Department of Applied Molecular Biosciences, Graduate School of Bioagricultural Sciences, Nagoya University, Nagoya, Japan
Institute of Transformative Bio-Molecules (WPI-ITbM), Nagoya University, Nagoya, Japan
Avian Bioscience Research Center, Graduate School of Bioagricultural Sciences, Nagoya University, Nagoya, Japan
Division of Seasonal Biology, Department of Environmental Biology, National Institute for Basic Biology, Okazaki, Japan

Taro Ikegami
Department of Chemistry, Biology and Marine Science, Faculty of Science, University of the Ryukyus, Okinawa, Japan

Yusuke Maruyama and Atsuhiko Hattori
Department of Biology, College of Liberal Arts and Sciences, Tokyo Medical and Dental University, Ichikawa, Japan

Hiroyuki Doi
Shimonoseki Marine Science Museum "Kaikyokan," Shimonoseki Academy of Marine Science, Yamaguchi, Japan

Hironori Ando
Sado Marine Biological Station, Faculty of Science, Niigata University, Sado, Japan

Md. Saydur Rahman and Peter Thomas
Marine Science Institute, University of Texas at Austin, Port Aransas, TX, USA

Hernan Valdes-Socin, Matilde Rubio Almanza, Mariana Tomé Fernández-Ladreda and Albert Beckers
Service of Endocrinology, CHU Liège, University of Liège, Liège, Belgium

François Guillaume Debray and Vincent Bours
Service of Human Genetics, CHU Liège, University of Liège, Liège, Belgium

Index

www.ingramcontent.com/pod-product-compliance
Lightning Source LLC
LaVergne TN
LVHW082139200926
848484LV00008B/2076